Thank you r... ,..
history!

Doug Kneed(?)

Hope you find some pleasant memories within —

Rick Nel_

HISTORY IS OUR PRESENT FOR THE FUTURE

DP Rahn

Looking forward to the next chapters

Jeff M[...]

A Specialty Indeed

The History of Emergency Medicine at The Ohio State University

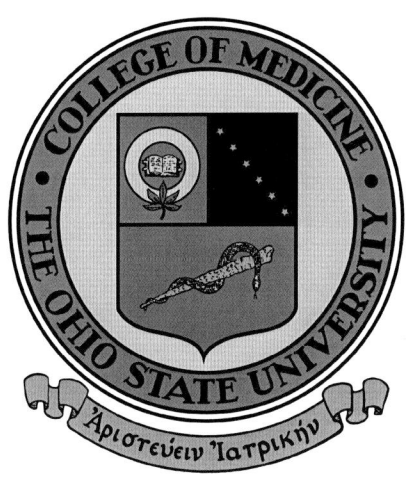

DOUGLAS A. RUND, MD
RICHARD N. NELSON, MD
DAVID P. BAHNER, MD
JEFFREY M. CATERINO, MD, MPH

The Ohio State University
Department of Emergency Medicine
760 Prior Hall
376 W. 10th Avenue
Columbus, OH 43210

Copyright 2023, The Ohio State University
Department of Emergency Medicine

All rights reserved, including the right to reproduce this book
or portions thereof in any form whatsoever.

Cover and page design: Lori Zambito
Front cover: Emergency department, 2022. Insets show emergency care
in 1989 and Division of Emergency Medicine faculty members in 1986.
Back cover: The Ohio State University Medical Center campus

ISBN: 979-8-218-09691-5

Dedication

This history is dedicated to our Emergency Medicine family: faculty, staff, students, residents and fellows who have been part of the journey of The Ohio State University Department of Emergency Medicine, which began in 1978 and continues on—
each year better than the last!

Acknowledgments

This history was made possible with support from The George W. Paulson, MD, Scholar-in Residence Program within the Medical Heritage Center at The Ohio State University Health Sciences Library. The program provides an opportunity for scholars to "publish works on topics of historical medical significance."

The program honors the memory of George W. Paulson, MD, former Professor and Chair of the Department of Neurology, an exceptional medical scholar and dedicated medical historian who wrote so many outstanding learned texts about the history of medicine, particularly at Ohio State. He was a close friend, outstanding neurologist and erudite thinker.

Douglas Rund, MD, who was the first Director of the Division of Emergency Medicine in 1978 and then its first Chair when it became the Department of Emergency Medicine in 1990, was named The George W. Paulson, MD, Scholar-in-Residence for the 2021-2023 period.

The initial application to the scholar-in residence program emphasized that the history of the Department of Emergency Medicine is not a long one: The first faculty members began in 1978. Part of the reasoning for writing the history now is that we have a "window of time" to record the fascinating story of emergency medicine. The founders are "eyewitnesses" to our history and still able to tell the story of our beginning. The Medical Heritage Center (MHC) agreed and has supported us generously. Kristin Rodgers, MHC collections curator, has been enormously helpful. She found historical sources, assisted with research, scanned images, provided guidance to the Ohio State archives, and offered sage and timely advice at all stages of the project.

This work would also not have been possible without Sharon Pfeil, former education coordinator for the Department of Emergency Medicine. She did it all: She transcribed all the interviews, found the photos, arranged chapters, organized and typed text and used her own knowledge of our history to enhance the story. She has a phenomenal work ethic that kept the project going when the efforts of the editors tended to lag. We owe her an enormous debt of gratitude.

Our editor, Lisa Lopez Snyder, a professional writer, editor and project manager with extensive experience in publications and a specialty in academic medicine, has edited the book so carefully. Lori Zambito, our graphic designer, formed each page beautifully and created the cover and design of the book with an artist's experienced eye. Special thanks are also due to Sean Moodie, architectural systems coordinator at Ohio State, for researching and furnishing us with the drawings of previous emergency rooms throughout this history. Mary-Jayne Fortney assisted with providing tireless administrative support and David Way's contacts enabled us to contact all former residents to solicit their contributions. Former residency coordinator Ellen Harr Weatherby provided an outstanding photo collection of residents and faculty over the years.

We are also grateful for all the effort put forth by our current and former faculty and residents, for their contributions and advice and for the recollections of leaders in our specialty who furthered our growth throughout the years.

Finally, we wish to thank our families for their unwavering support and counsel during the long process of creating this book. You provide us with ever present strength and wisdom.

Douglas A. Rund, MD
Richard N. Nelson, MD
David P. Bahner, MD
Jeffrey M. Caterino, MD, MPH

Foreword

It is my distinct pleasure to write the forward for this account of the history of the Department of Emergency Medicine at The Ohio State University. I was hired by Doug Rund right out of my emergency medicine residency at the University of Cincinnati in July 1988. I remember finishing my last shift of residency on a Friday night at 11:00 PM, and starting my first shift at Ohio State the next day at 11 AM. I received the usual orientation at that time, which was a finger pointed in the direction of a large pile of patient charts, with the encouraging words, "You're a smart guy, you'll figure it out." Those were the days!

In all seriousness, the 14 years I spent as a faculty member at Ohio State were some of the most fun and fulfilling years of my career. The Department that the leaders built was a family. The faculty were all family members, related in our mission, and unified in devotion to each other and to the care of our patients. It was a great place for a junior faculty member to have some fun, find a niche and build an academic career. I remember starting in the lab, working alongside Dr. Chuck Brown and Dr. Howie Werman, studying a pig model of cardiac arrest and resuscitation. Chuck had built a nationally recognized program studying the effects of high-dose epinephrine on return of spontaneous circulation after VF arrest. I can remember Chuck coaching and encouraging me as I got ready to present my first paper at the Society for Academic Emergency Medicine on that topic. I was so nervous I was shaking on stage the whole time. The expertise that was shared with me so willingly by senior faculty members defined the culture of the Department.

The Department also had a phenomenal reputation for education. Students and residents loved working with us in the ER. We had great teachers and great clinicians on our faculty from all over the country. The teaching evaluations were stellar and our reputation in the medical school grew year after year. The clinical care we provided spoke for itself. Even though emergency medicine was a fledgling specialty, we earned the respect of our peers by our performance in teaching, research and patient care. I was happy to be a part of the success of the Department for the 14 years I spent at Ohio State.

Good people doing good things can make for an amazing success story. A small number of dedicated, hard-working, mission-driven faculty members turned a small Division of the Department of Preventive Medicine into one of the strongest Departments in the College of Medicine. What follows is the success story of the Department of Emergency Medicine of The Ohio State University. I was honored to be a part of it.

James W. Hoekstra, MD, FACEP

Preface

In some ways, the history of emergency medicine at Ohio State is similar to the history of emergency medicine at universities throughout North America. Following World War II and into the 1950s and 1960s the need for improved emergency care in hospitals became increasingly evident. As the number and complexity of patients needing emergency treatment increased, the quality of care provided in emergency rooms became a concern. Treatment in university hospital emergency rooms was typically provided by house staff: interns and residents. The irony that many of the sickest patients were cared for by the staff with the least education was somehow justified by academic leaders who focused on the *training* mission of academic hospitals.

At Ohio State, in that early era, the Medicine and Surgery departments provided staffing and leadership for the emergency room. In the 1970s leaders in those departments realized that improvements in the emergency room were needed. The most forward looking of them watched national trends to provide answers and ultimately decided that a full-time medical director of the emergency room, a newly-created position, should be recruited. The hospital invited the most highly respected national leaders in emergency medicine of that era to interview. During the interview process they learned about issues that would lead emergency medicine to become the brand-new entrant to the house of academic medicine. The need for a full-time group of faculty physicians to staff the emergency room and supervise residents gradually became apparent. While other academic medical centers around the country were also increasingly realizing this need, questions remained about whether or not emergency medicine actually qualified as a true medical specialty.

In 1977 a director was hired. In 1978 the Division of Emergency Medicine was created in the Department of Preventive Medicine, an established academic department that had served as an "incubator" for new academic departments in the past. The number of emergency medicine faculty grew in the 1980s and leaders began to explore full departmental status. In 1990 the *Division* became the *Department* of Emergency Medicine within the College of Medicine. The department continued to grow with the steady vision of accomplishing all aspects of an academic mission: patient care, education and research.

In many respects, our history at Ohio State is one of struggle. As emergency medicine's specialty recognition grew, faculty and residents were wresting important elements from the grasp of established departments. Emergency procedures were now being performed by emergency physicians and residents—*not* by trainees in medicine or surgery. The sense from outside the Department of Emergency Medicine was that this "newcomer's" educational programs threatened to take financial resources from the common purse and was now controlling the gateway to the hospital. Meanwhile, administrators and other physician leaders had varying degrees of understanding of the department's future vision.

The early leaders of emergency medicine, however, were insistent about the identity of their specialty and took all possible steps to gain acceptance as a specialty in academic medicine: joint authorship of educational materials, joint sponsorship of new educational programs, and excellent teaching for all residents regardless of specialty and joint research endeavors. The unyielding tenacity of the early emergency medicine faculty members eventually prevailed. Emergency Medicine is now an unchallenged specialty, and today, departmental faculty hold key leadership positions across all components of The Ohio State University Wexner Medical Center.

The university archive has only a handful of documents about emergency medicine, so our book attempts to present some of this history drawn from our own reconstruction, relying on our own documents and eyewitness accounts from those who worked to make the department great. Our hope is that ensuing accounts will follow to enrich our historical record.

The current Department of Emergency Medicine includes faculty, residents, fellows, advanced practice practitioners, nurses, a strong research team and an exceptional staff. Philanthropists have been generous. After almost 50 years the department has taken its rightful place among the best in research, clinical care and teaching and, despite the ever-present challenges, the future ahead is bright indeed.

Table of Contents

PART I
Emergency Medicine in the Beginning: 1970 to 1990

Chapter 1	The Prelude: Beginnings of Emergency Medicine *Douglas A. Rund, MD* 1	
Chapter 2	Early Struggles: The Division of Emergency Medicine *Douglas A. Rund, MD, Richard N. Nelson, MD* 25	
Chapter 3	Academic Foundations: The Division of Emergency Medicine in the Department of Preventive Medicine *Douglas A. Rund, MD* 43	
Chapter 4	The Push to Begin: The Residency Program in Emergency Medicine *Richard N. Nelson, MD, Douglas A. Rund, MD* 55	
Chapter 5	A Specialty Indeed: The Road to Department Status – 1981 to 1988 *Douglas A. Rund, MD, Richard N. Nelson, MD* 79	
Chapter 6	Early Research Efforts: Charles G. Brown, MD, and Cardiopulmonary Resuscitation *Charles G. Brown, MD, Douglas A. Rund, MD* 103	
Chapter 7	Celebration: The Department of Emergency Medicine in the College of Medicine, 1990 *Douglas A. Rund, MD, Richard N. Nelson, MD* 119	

PART II
OVERVIEW
The Department of Emergency Medicine: 1990-2023

Chapter 8	Faculty Growth and the Restructuring of the Residency Program: 1990-2001 *Douglas A. Rund, MD, Richard N. Nelson, MD* 141

Chapter 9   Financial Challenges and Organization: The Costs of a
            New Specialty — "Sink or Swim"
            Douglas A. Rund, MD, Richard N. Nelson, MD **179**

Chapter 10 The Rund Chair Years: 1990-2011
            Douglas A. Rund, MD, Richard N. Nelson, MD **209**

Chapter 11 The Tendrup Chair Years: 2013-2015
            Douglas A. Rund, MD **247**

Chapter 12 The Angelos Chair Years: 2011-2013, 2015-2020
            Mark G. Angelos, MD **263**

Chapter 13 The Caterino Chair Years: 2020-present
            Jeffrey Caterino, MD, MPH **281**

PART III

The Mission Areas:
Clinical Services, Education and Research

Chapter 14 Emergency Medical Services
            Douglas A. Rund, MD, David P. Keseg, MD **299**

Chapter 15 Air Medical Transport
            Howard Werman, MD, Steven Steinberg, MD **323**

Chapter 16 The Columbus Heartmobile: History and Influence
            Craig B. Key, MD, Douglas A. Rund, MD **337**

Chapter 17 The Emergency Department
            Douglas A. Rund, MD, Richard N. Nelson, MD **351**

Chapter 18 Ohio State East Hospital
            *Michael R. Dick, MD, Richard N. Nelson, MD,
            Douglas A. Rund, MD* **401**

Chapter 19 The Fundamentals: Medical Student Education
            *David P. Bahner, MD, Nicholas E. Kman, MD,
            David P. Way, MEd* **427**

Chapter 20 A Tradition of Excellence: The Residency Program
            in Emergency Medicine
            Douglas A. Rund, MD, Diane L. Gorgas, MD **457**

Chapter 21 Subspecialties Indeed: Fellowships
            Douglas A. Rund, MD, David P. Bahner, MD **489**

Chapter 22	Leading the Way: Ultrasound *David P. Bahner, MD, Douglas A. Rund, MD* **523**
Chapter 23	Diversity, Equity and Inclusion *Diane L. Gorgas, MD*. **547**
Chapter 24	Growth of the Department's Research Mission – from Infancy to National Prominence (1991-2021) *Mark G. Angelos, MD* **563**

PART IV

Remembering the Past
and Leading for the Future

Chapter 25	Leadership: Advancing the Specialty *Douglas A. Rund, MD*. **587**
Chapter 26	Recollections *Douglas A. Rund, MD, Richard N. Nelson, MD,* *David P. Bahner, MD,* *Jeffrey M. Caterino, MD, MPH* **607**
Chapter 27	Biographies *Douglas A. Rund, MD, Richard N. Nelson, MD*.... **623**
Chapter 28	The Future and the Ohio State Department of Emergency Medicine *Jeffrey M. Caterino, MD, MPH* **643**

Selected List of Figures **655**

Chapter 1

The Prelude: Beginnings of Emergency Medicine

Douglas A. Rund, MD

The general practitioner was vanishing. The doctor of the first part of the twentieth century who knew each patient well, provided comfort and treated a wide variety of ailments was being crowded out by an increasing number of specialists and generalists with advanced training. These "new" generalists had additional education in specialties that were to become known as "primary care."

Such specialties were primarily pediatrics and general medicine. The general practitioner typically began practice after only one year of internship while specialists had three or more. General practice diagnosis and treatment were provided in the office which was sometimes in the doctor's home or in the patient's own home. Treatments also included some emergencies.[1] In so many ways the general practitioner was truly the "ancestor of the emergency physician."[2]

In Columbus, doctor's offices were numerous, especially in the downtown area and in many if not most of the neighborhoods. They were also easily accessible and typically close to home and even within walking distance. Charles Pavey, MD, a physician whose home and office were located just north of the Ohio State University campus, recalled the presence of a doctor's office on every block of High Street from downtown to Worthington.[3]

The Millis Commission, sponsored by the American Medical Association,[4] issued a report in 1966 called *The Graduate Education of Physicians*. The report outlined the decrease in the number of general practitioners in the first half of the century: In 1931, 84% of all physicians reported themselves to be in a general practice; in 1965, the percentage was 37%. The report noted that "the general practitioner leaves behind a vacuum that organized medicine has not decided how to fill." The authors suggested that the *emergency room* might fill some of the gap. The report stated that one result of the vacuum was that patients "become their own diagnosticians and decide which kind of specialist they should approach …or take their problems to the *hospital emergency room*."

The report noted that most specialist physicians at that time completed at least three years of internship and residency training. The report also suggested that if the separate internship could be included in a single specialty residency program, the duration should be at least three years due to the growing amount of material to be learned. This was in marked contrast to the one-year internship usually completed by a general practitioner. The report concluded that the descendants of the general practitioner, internists, pediatricians, and family physicians should be called "primary care" physicians.[4]

In a follow-up editorial to the Millis Commission report, Ivan J. Fahs reported that the precipitous decline in general practice was not matched by a corresponding shift of physicians into other fields identified with primary care such as internal medicine and pediatrics.[5] The editorial noted the drastic reduction of almost 50% in the ranks of general practitioners, from roughly 110,000 in 1930 to 61,383 in 1967 (Figure 1). Of course, the population had increased in this time period. The decrease in the number of general practitioners per person therefore declined ever more drastically. The vacuum created by the marked decline in general practice was only partially filled by "primary care" specialists; the emergency room filled most of the remaining void. In 1958 there were 18 million emergency room visits; 10 years later in 1968 the number more than doubled to 44 million (Figure 1).[6]

The rise in hospital emergency visits that coincided with the decrease in general practice had several causes. Perhaps the most significant was the rapid advance in medical knowledge and technology. Other causes were in play, however. The population was more mobile. People were moving from farms and small towns to the cities. Job opportunities following the economic expansion after the war provided employment opportunities in larger communities throughout the country. People relocating likely did not have immediate access to a primary care

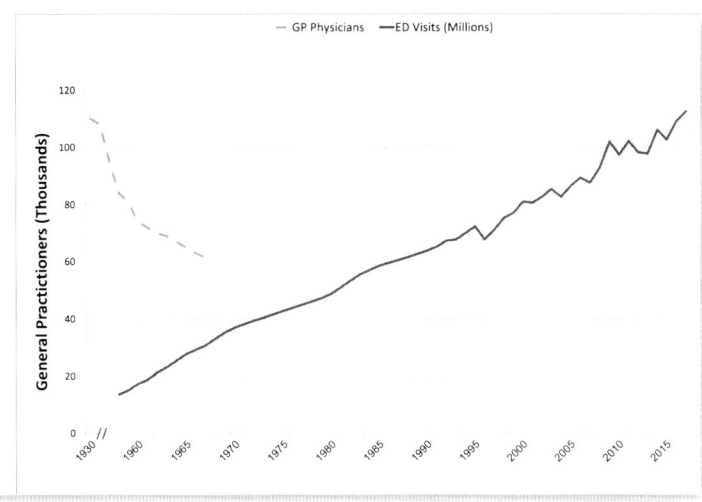

Figure 1: Decline in the number of general practitioners in the United States from 1930 to 1968 (left axis): from Fahs, IJ and Peterson, OL, The Decline of General Practice, *Public Health Reports*. 1968: 83(4):267-270. Increase in emergency department visits from 1958 to 2017 (right axis): from The American College of Emergency Physicians. *Benchmark data study*, Irvine Texas, 2021

physician and resorted to the emergency room (ER) for immediate care.

The population was also aging. The frequency and severity of illness was increasing with advancing age. It was known that a deeper knowledge of the new technologies and procedures was needed. The hospital was often the site where the new procedures and treatments could be provided.

Patients increasingly had health insurance. Private insurance was becoming available partly because labor movements pushed such coverage. One important catalyst for employer-provided insurance occurred during World War II with passage of the 1942 Stabilization Act, which was designed to control inflation by limiting the ability of employers to increase wages.

As a result, in order to compete for scarce workers without increasing wages, employers began offering health benefits instead. This practice caught on and by the end of the war, many large companies were providing employees and their families health coverage and continued to do so after the war. In 1940 only 9% of U.S. citizens had health insurance; by 1966 81% of the population had health insurance.[7] In 1965 Medicare was signed into law and suddenly many seniors had hospitalization coverage.

One of the consequences of the rapid demise of the general practitioner and the office practice in the 1950s and 1960s was a rapid increase in demand for hospital services provided in the emergency room. The solution to the problem of physician staffing, however, had to wait for the time being; but the need was growing for physicians who could care for a wide spectrum of illnesses and emergencies.

In his excellent book on the history of emergency medicine, Brian J. Zink, MD, FACEP, describes the general practitioner as an "ancestor to the emergency physician."[2] Although the need was great, the quality of the care, for the most part, was lacking. ER staffing varied, with interns, residents, moonlighters and hospital attending staff often mandated to cover the ER despite their qualifications—and despite their unfamiliarity with emergency procedures. Nursing staff typically provided continuity and expertise.

Some physicians felt that the situation could not be good for patients with trauma or medical emergencies. In particular, surgeons who had witnessed vast improvements in the quality of care for soldiers with battlefield injuries in World War II and Korea were critical of emergency room service. Robert H. Kennedy, MD, a surgeon, was a passionate advocate for better emergency care for civilians and an ardent critic of the state of the emergency service. In an address to the American College of Surgeons in 1954 he said the following:

> *In the emergency room in your hospital, who examines an injured patient first? May it be the most junior intern, who has never seen a trauma case before, or an indifferently trained foreign physician with language difficulty? Have you prepared and posted a directive which will give these junior men an idea of what instances require the immediate notification of a surgical resident? Will the attending notified be at the most junior level or a senior man with experience? Do you know from personal inspection what goes on in your emergency room in the middle of the night or do you stay away due to a subconscious fear of what you might see? There is little doubt in my mind that the weakest link in the chain of hospital care in most hospitals in this country is the emergency room's attention to the injured.*[8]

The "weakest link" reference was cited in *The New England Journal of Medicine* in 1958 in an article by Shortliffe, et al.[9] He and his colleagues were concerned about the quality of care in the ER at Hartford Hospital. A survey of hospital emergency rooms was prompted by "rising apprehensions about the adequacy of physical facilities and supervision of the clinical work performed in the emergency unit."[9] The authors were also aware that the quality of care performed in the emergency room was a vital factor in public relations. The authors noted the dramatic rise in ER visits at Hartford Hospital from 1945 to 1955 in the 10-year period—3,000 per year in 1945 to 18,000 per year in 1955.

Their report recalled that in 1945 the unit was referred to as the "accident unit", seeing a relatively small number of patients (roughly 10 or fewer per day). The authors surveyed 90 other hospitals in the Midwest and the Atlantic seaboard; the results showed a 400% increase in emergency visits from 1945 to 1955. The authors predicted an annual increase of 15% going forward.

Interestingly enough, the paper used four different terms to describe the ER: emergency room, emergency unit, accident unit and emergency facility. Unfortunately, the report did not envision separate, unique residency training or establishment of a new specialty, but only recommended that local medical groups should "provide improved medical emergency coverage." Despite calls for change, little seemed to be happening to address "the weakest link" in the chain, especially for trauma.

In 1966 the National Academy of Sciences published "Accidental Death and Disability: The Neglected Disease of Modern Society". The report was prepared by the academy's Committee on Trauma and the Committee on Shock. The introduction called accidental injuries a "neglected epidemic of modern society."[10] Impairing 400,000 citizens permanently, trauma was the leading cause of death in the first half of life's span.

Citing numerous areas needing improvement the report described emergency departments in some hospitals as "overcrowded and archaic." The report confirmed:

> *For decades the "emergency facilities" of most hospitals have consisted only of "accident rooms", poorly equipped, inadequately*

> *manned, and ordinarily used for limited numbers of seriously ill persons or for charity victims of disease or injury. Very few hospitals…. have met the needs for vast expansion of facilities, equipment, and personnel demanded by society…. for off-hour treatment of non-emergency conditions and the steadily increasing numbers of accidental injuries… Minimal standards call from around-the-clock staffing by permanently assigned physicians…. trained in all aspects of the care of trauma.*[10]

The report also noted that:

> *The number of physicians experienced in the treatment of multiple injuries is very limited…the need is to now recognize the need for special training in immediate care and in the overall direction of emergency departments of a caliber commensurate with that attained by individuals in active military field units caring for combat casualties. Medical undergraduate and residency training programs are generally inadequate in traumatology and mass casualty care.*[10]

The report enumerated the magnitude of the epidemic of "neglected disease": deaths, disability, costs and medical load. The committee recommended the following: first aid training for lay population, preparation of educational materials for first responders and EMS providers, improved access to ambulance services by the public, consideration of physician staffed ambulances, pilot programs in helicopter evacuation, improved radio communication, categorization of levels of regional emergency care, development of trauma registries, improved rehabilitation programs and improved research in trauma. Strangely absent in retrospect was a recommendation that training programs for emergency medicine be established to meet the growing staffing needs.

Interestingly in discussing research, the report also commended the Ohio State University Disaster Research Center for its extensive studies on the stresses imposed by unexpected disasters.

The Committee on Trauma and concerned surgeons were taking the lead in trying to improve treatment of patients in the academic emergency department. Nationally, surgeons were taking the lead in the direction of emergency rooms, especially at academic centers. Surgeons formed the University Association for Emergency Medical Services (UA/EMS) in 1968.

Despite the calls for change, academic institutions were slow to respond and private practice was moving faster than academic centers to create designated emergency physicians. In 1961 the physician group founded by James Mills, MD, became independent contractors with the Alexandria Hospital in Virginia. The physicians received a stipend from the hospital for professional services (largely for indigent care) and were allowed to also bill for private patients. The hospital provided billing services for 15% of collections. This arrangement became known as the *Alexandria Plan*.

In Pontiac, Michigan, a group of physicians formed a corporation that billed for physician services and paid the physicians an hourly rate (10 dollars per hour initially). The venture was successful financially and patient volumes grew rapidly in the emergency department. This became known as the *Pontiac Plan*.

In the same timeframe, physicians who devoted their practice to care in the emergency room were beginning to organize. They would create educational opportunities for physicians in practice and meet to discuss common issues and developments. John Wiegenstein, MD, and others created the American College of Emergency Physicians (ACEP) and held their first meeting in 1968.

Origins of specialized emergency medicine practice in Columbus

While groups of physicians were slowly forming to staff emergency rooms in this country, Columbus was still staffing in the traditional way in 1969: interns, residents, medical staff of all specialties and part-time help. Two visionary innovative physicians in Columbus who led the way of change were T. William Evans, DDS, MD, FACS and Samuel J. Kiehl, MD.

T. WILLIAM EVANS, DDS, MD, FACS: MAXILLOFACIAL AND FACIAL AESTHETIC SURGEON AND EMERGENCY MEDICINE PIONEER

In Columbus T. William Evans, MD, MSc, DDS, MD, FACS, established the first emergency medicine group in 1969. Evans was born in Youngstown, Ohio, and later in his youth moved to Massillon and then Akron. His father was a football and track coach at Massillon High School (under Paul Brown) and later served as head coach at the University of Akron.

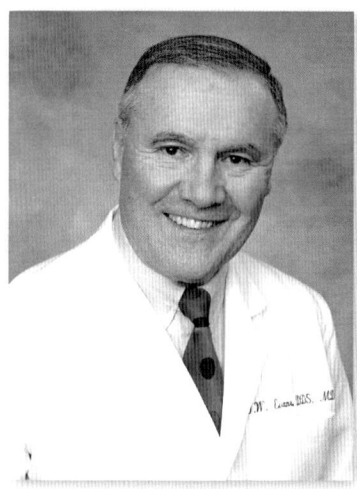

Figure 2: T. William Evans, DDS, MD, FACS. Founder of the first emergency medicine group in Columbus, Emergency Medical Associates, Inc. (EMAI). Founder and first President of the Ohio Chapter of the American College of Emergency Physicians, Columbus, Ohio, 1971-1972.

Evans was an outstanding athlete in high school, receiving all-state honors in both football and track. He attended the College of Wooster where he majored in chemistry and graduated in three years with honors. He then entered the College of Dentistry at The Ohio State University and graduated Summa Cum Laude in 1963. During his years at dental school, he worked as an intravenous technician from 1961 to 1963 at Grant Hospital, in Columbus. He would work the 6 p.m. to 11 p.m. shift as a technician and return to dental school the following morning.

Following graduation, he entered the residency program in Oral and Maxillofacial Surgery at Ohio State. During his residency, he completed graduate work in anatomy of the head and neck and received a master's degree in the anatomy (MSc). He also completed one year in anesthesiology.

During his residency and during medical school, he continued to work part-time at Ohio State Hospital as a surgical assistant for Arthur James, MD. James was a leading surgeon in cancers of the head and neck. James became most impressed with Evans and his surgical skills and encouraged him to enter medical school with the eventual goal of becoming a specialist in cancers of the head and neck. The plan was for Evans to eventually enter practice with James and become his partner.

Evans entered medical school at Ohio State in 1966 and completed the curriculum in three years, graduating in 1969. During his years in medical school, he also practiced part-time with a leading oral and maxillofacial surgeon in Columbus performing outpatient surgery, general anesthesia and hospital trauma calls throughout Columbus for cases with maxillofacial injuries.

Evans began his internship in Internal Medicine at Grant Hospital in 1969. He chose Grant in part because he wanted to study with a leading internist there who had a special interest in cardiology, Jack Stevens, MD. Stevens had a large practice at Grant and was frequently on call for the emergency room. He tended to make his patient rounds starting at 10 p.m. By the time of his internship Evans was already an experienced head and neck surgeon who had worked at Grant in one capacity or another since his second year of dental school. He was often the physician the nurses called for difficult emergency cases. One day Evans received a call that ultimately started his career in emergency medicine. He recalled it this way:

> *It was obvious to the nurses around the hospital that I had more knowledge and experience than a typical intern would have and, it also became apparent to the nurses in the emergency room because the emergency room was being covered by three doctors that could not speak English well and one who had addiction problem. When they had a critical patient come in, the ER nurses started calling me to come down to take care of the critical patient because they didn't have confidence in the four doctors that were working there. I was getting the same things on the floors as I was not a typical intern so if they had a problem, they called me. They called me as well from the ICU. In fact, my sleeping room was actually in the ICU. One day I had been up about 20 hours working and I finally got to bed in my private bedroom in the ICU and I got a call from the emergency room that said they had a patient down here with a knife stuck in his chest. So, I got up after about a half an hour sleep and went to the emergency room and took care of the guy with the knife. As I was examining him, I looked over to my left in another cubicle and*

the emergency room doctor was sewing up an arm not paying any attention to the knife guy. This was not unusual. Things like this happened all the time. But at this time, I was not in a good mood and took care of the guy with the knife and just walked out of the emergency room and walked over to the hospital administrator's office who was Warren G. Harding II, MD and ventilated for about five minutes. Dr. Harding just sat behind his desk, listened to me, and didn't say a word. After I was finished, he got up, took me by the arm, walked me to the emergency room and told the nurses and the doctors that I was going to run the emergency room from then on. And he dismissed immediately the doctor that was there and told him that he and the other doctors were not welcome in Grant's emergency room. So, I immediately took over the emergency room but I was pretty tired so I called one of the other interns to come down to help out so I could get a little sleep. The bottom line is that I met with all the interns, organized all the interns to work in the emergency room and the next day I met with the administrator, Dr. Harding, and worked out a plan that he would pay me $18 per hour and I would pay the doctors that were working $16 per hour. This was in November 1969 and I believe we were the first pure emergency doctors in Ohio. All of the 15 doctors, including myself finished the one-year internship. Six of the doctors decided to go with me and work full time in the emergency room at Grant Hospital. We covered the emergency room as well as the house, as well as the ICU, so we always had two of our doctors in the hospital at all times.[11]

Evans and his group went on to create Emergency Medical Associates, Inc. (EMAI), which gradually expanded to cover other emergency medicine sites in Ohio and Pennsylvania. Evans became a charter member of ACEP and founded the first ACEP chapter in Ohio. He became its first president in 1971. By 1972 the Grant emergency room was covered by seven full-time physicians; all were physician employees of EMAI.

In 1979 Evans and Larry Carey, MD, a surgeon, convinced the Grant Hospital CEO to consider having a helicopter on site in order to bring critical patients from outlying communities to Grant Medical Center. This was accomplished in 1980 and was the first medical helicopter in

Columbus. Evans was also instrumental in helping to develop Grant Medical Center into a Level I trauma center.

Evans eventually left emergency medicine to become a full-time maxillofacial surgeon with expertise in facial aesthetic surgery, for which he became internationally famous. Evans appears later in this chapter with his contributions in recruiting a director of emergency services at Ohio State (Figure 2).

SAMUEL J. KIEHL, MD, AND RIVERSIDE METHODIST HOSPITAL

At Riverside Methodist Hospital, William L. Hall, MD, and George Millay, MD, previously family physicians in private practice, began their exclusive emergency practice as hospital employees in 1970. Hall became President of the Ohio Chapter of ACEP in 1974 and Millay succeeded him in 1975. Samuel Kiehl, MD, joined the Riverside group in 1974. He graduated from the Ohio State College of Medicine in 1971 and completed an internship at York Hospital in Pennsylvania. He chose

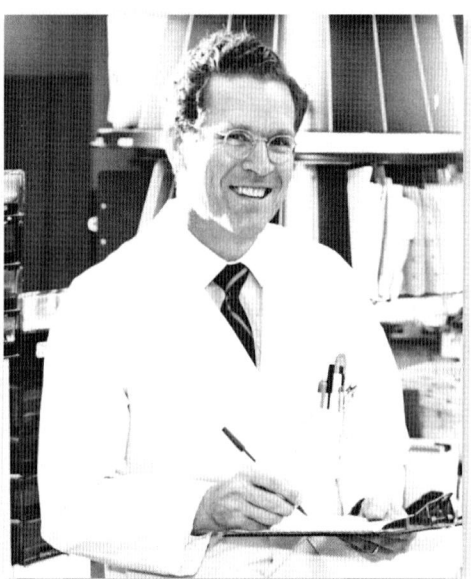

Figure 3: Samuel J. Kiehl, MD, Director Emergency Services, Riverside Methodist Hospital, 1980-1998

York because one of the faculty there was a highly regarded physician teaching family practice, which Kiehl thought he wanted for a career. He had had an intensive experience as a medical officer in the United States Navy following his internship and, on his return to Columbus in 1974, he thought that he would enjoy a family practice and began exploring options in those early years:

We looked for a family practice and we found some guy who was selling his practice in Delaware County. We looked at it and he had an old house and he had his office right there in his house which was really quaint but it didn't really look so good after all...My mother-in-law came home and she said, "Well Sam, why don't you call Riverside and see if they need any help there." So I called the emergency room and told them what I wanted and they put me through to Bill Hall. I talked to Bill and he said, "Well, we are having a group meeting tomorrow in my home. Why don't you come up and meet the guys?" So, I did. He lived in Upper Arlington and I drove up and I met the other members of the group and he offered me a job. I got home in early July of 1974 and I started working at Riverside the first week in August and I loved Riverside.[12]

Kiehl recalled the beginnings of the group and the maturing of his own concepts regarding an emergency medicine group practice:

Bill and George were the founders. Up until then, the staff at Riverside took turns manning the emergency room. It was a small facility and the staff hated it. Imagine having a dermatologist down in the emergency room taking care of heart attacks. That doesn't work so hot. So, they hated it and they elected to hire Bill and George to put together a program to take care of the emergency room. They would hire people and be dedicated to the emergency room. That is what they did and I was the eighth in the group. We were salaried and we had a fixed schedule and we would rotate through this schedule. One of the things that I learned was if you wanted to goof off you could because there was no incentive to really push. It was more like it was in the military. If you weren't self-motivated, then things didn't get done. We had one guy that every time he was assigned to a Saturday and Sunday night shift... he was sick. Every time! I don't think he ever worked that [shift] in the whole time. It only happened about every 8 weeks and yet every time he was sick. I was hungry at the time and I picked up a lot of those shifts. We got paid overtime for those shifts and so anyway, one of the things that stuck in my mind was that this was not a way to run a group. I just stuck that in the back of my mind. I enjoyed it, I had a good time and I liked working with some guys more than others. Some guys were like me and were self-motivated and interested in taking care

> *of patients and you know, working with the staff. We were liked by the staff and others were not liked by the staff and they weren't liked by the other physicians that much either. That was an interesting thing.*[12]

Kiehl was selected to be the director of the emergency room at Riverside in 1980. The hospital wanted him to form an independent group which he did.

> *The hospital in 1980 decided they wanted to change things… I was asked to apply for the job of director… There were some big names of people that applied and I applied for it. I wasn't expecting to be chosen. I went ahead and applied and then they chose me. They also said they did not want to employ us. They said we don't want you to be employed by the hospital, we want you to be independent so you are going to have to go ahead and set up a structure. I told the guys 'Look we are not going to continue on as salaried physicians, we are going to start eating what we kill; we are going to fee for service.' I also invited them to be a part of the ownership if they wanted to. They could be a part of the financing of the receivables, which was a significant thing and they could be a part of the ownership structure. We never got to that because nobody wanted to do it. I think none of them thought I could make this work. I don't know that for sure, but nobody wanted to step up, so I went ahead and the hospital introduced me to the Huntington Bank president and they took me to lunch with them. They told me what was happening. Dr. Kiehl needs a line of credit so he can finance the receivables, pay his doctors, pay any other expenses he has until he starts getting cash in the door.*[12]

Kiehl was remarkably successful and went on to help create the emergency medicine residency. He ultimately joined the faculty at Ohio State, received numerous teaching awards and endowed the first Chair in Emergency Medicine at Ohio State (Figure 3).

Creating the Division of Emergency Medicine at Ohio State

THOMAS WILLIAMS MD, FACS, AND THE OHIO STATE UNIVERSITY EMERGENCY ROOM

Progress in creating effective physician staffing at The Ohio State University Hospital was moving at a slower rate than in the community hospitals. The main advances were in pre-hospital emergency care. Stu Roberts, MD, a surgeon with experience in Vietnam, pioneered helicopter evacuations in the 1960s and 1970s and James V. Warren, MD, created the "Heartmobile" program, the first advanced life support unit in the country in 1969.

The emergency room was staffed by the house staff, primarily the interns. There was also occasional coverage by residents with one year of additional training. The interns were expected to contact more senior level residents for the more serious cases. There were no faculty attending staff on duty. Diane Zinzer, RN, was a nurse in the emergency room in the 1960s. She remembers it as follows:

> *If we had a head injury, like a car accident which had an obvious head injury, we would call for the chief surgical resident. We hardly ever saw attendings. I would say about five times in a year we would see an attending. We didn't see attendings there. If we saw an attending it was because Governor Rhodes came in… or the football coach, Woody Hayes. Those times if a VIP came in, we would see an attending. Other than that, it would be a surgical resident. If it was something bad it would be a head surgical resident, or if we had an arrest, we would call overhead "Code Blue."*[13]

Following the customary pattern at university hospitals throughout the country, Ohio State appointed young surgeons to be the directors of the emergency room. In 1973, Thomas E. "Tom" Williams Jr., MD, was a new assistant professor in cardiothoracic surgery when he was appointed director. Williams received his undergraduate degree from Princeton in 1957 and his MD degree from the Ohio State College of Medicine in 1963. He completed his surgical residency and fellowship in cardiovascular surgery at Ohio State. During that time, he also completed a fellowship at Northwestern University, where he earned his PhD in Industrial Engineering. He joined the faculty as an Assistant Professor in 1970 (Figure 4).

Williams served as Assistant Medical Director of Emergency Services from 1972 to 1976. He was appointed by Richard Rupert, MD, who was the medical director for patient services from 1972 to 1974. Eventually Rupert left Ohio State to become Chancellor for Health Affairs at the Ohio Board of Regents from 1974 to 1977 and went on to become the President of the Medical College of Toledo, where he concluded his career.

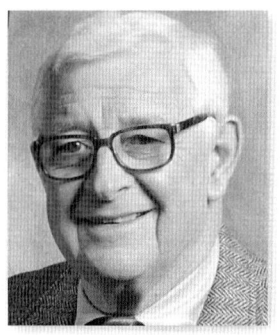

Figure 4: Thomas E. Williams, Jr., MD, PhD, FACS

Rupert and Williams noted the steadily increasing numbers of patients and the increasing limitations of the emergency room. The entire facility consisted of 12 beds: two four bed wards (separated by curtains), a trauma room, a cast room, an ENT/dental room, an Ob/Gyn treatment area and an X-ray room. Staffing was provided by first-year medical interns and a surgical resident. Williams described the coverage pattern as somewhat "helter skelter".

Kathleen "Kate" Bullock, RN, remembers the emergency room layout as follows:

There was a long counter in the hallway on the side of radiology. Room 1, the first bed, was reserved for resuscitation or respiratory distress, because that was the first on in sight. There were four beds in that room separated by curtains. There was a crash cart in Room 2, which also had four beds just like Room 1. Next to that was Room 3, which was the trauma room. It was a single bed and all the emergency equipment was lining the walls Then there was a long counter and Room 4 was dedicated to ENT patients. There was one bed in there and there was a dental chair and this was all separated by a metal partition that rolled around on wheels. And there were a couple of chairs in there if we just had "strep throat" kind of patients that didn't need to lie down. Going around the corner there was Room 5 and there were two beds there. There were two beds on opposite sides of the small room separated also by a metal partition. That is where we did female exams. There were always stirrups available. Room 6 was similar. That was also dedicated as overflow room.[15]

Williams was conscientious in his direction of the emergency room, but also had a busy practice in cardio-thoracic surgery. Realizing the dilemma presented by the emergency room, Williams, Rupert and the hospital leadership at that time invited Erwin Thal, MD, for a consultation. Williams described the situation in this way:

> I thought I can't do this and full-time cardiac surgery both, and so I called Erwin Thal, who led the best emergency room in the nation at that time, and said, "Erwin, can you consult with me?" He said, "What do you need, Tom?" I said, "I need to have somebody else do this job." I said "It's the third weekend in November, can you come up for the Michigan game?"[14]

Thal was the Director of the Surgical Emergency Room at Parkland Memorial Hospital of the University of Texas Southwest Medical Center in Dallas. The surgical service at Parkland was considered one of the best in the nation and, indeed, was the hospital for President Kennedy when he was tragically shot in 1963.

Thal was born in Columbus, Ohio, in 1936. He was an enthusiastic graduate of Ohio State, where he was the manager of the baseball, basketball and two national championship football teams. He received his medical degree from the Ohio State College of Medicine in 1962. He completed his surgical internship and residency at Dallas Parkland from 1963 to 1969 and was appointed director of the surgical emergency room in 1970. Eventually he was considered one of the "Giants" in the history of Surgery at Parkland.

Thal visited Williams and Ohio State on the third weekend in November in 1974 for a consultation. Williams knew of Thal's enthusiasm for Ohio State sports and wisely invited Thal to join him at the Ohio State-Michigan game, one of the greatest football rivalries in the nation. Thal followed up. He wrote a report to Rupert strongly advising the recruitment of full-time director. A search committee was formed with Williams as the chair.

To its credit, the search committee invited several of the most prominent academic leaders in academic emergency medicine to Ohio State to interview for the position of director.

Ronald Krome, MD, was one of those interviewed. Krome was born in 1936 in Baltimore, Maryland. He graduated from the University of Maryland where one of his professors was R. Adams Crowley, who invented the Shock Trauma Center in Baltimore. Krome graduated from the Wayne State Surgery residency in 1969 and, typical of the time in academic centers, he was the choice of young surgical faculty to be the staff member providing oversight for the Detroit General Hospital Emergency Room.

His appointment followed the hospital's realization that staffing solely by interns and residents was inadequate. Following the Detroit riots in 1967, the need to provide enhanced medical oversight for interns and junior house staff was clear. By the 1970s, Krome had begun to develop an emergency physician staff that practiced emergency medicine exclusively in the emergency department.

Under his leadership, the Emergency Department also began to become a formal part of the hospital's administrative structure. Krome became recognized as one of the most active academic emergency physicians in the country. From 1974 to 1980 he was the editor of the *Journal of the American College of Emergency Physicians.* Krome stayed as editor when the journal became the *Annals of Emergency Medicine* in 1980. He also authored the Study Guide in Emergency Medicine, which became one of the most influential textbooks in the specialty. He also wrote *The Floater's Log*, a book about his experiences in the emergency department. He was eventually one of the primary leaders in the specialty's quest for establishing a certifying board. Krome's visit influenced the leaders at Ohio State when he interviewed for the director position but, in the end, he decided to not move to Columbus but remain in Detroit.

Peter Rosen, MD, was another candidate. Rosen was born in Brooklyn in 1935 and received his MD degree in 1960 from Washington University in St. Louis. He completed surgical training at Highland Hospital in Oakland, California, in 1965. Following graduation, he entered surgical practice in Wyoming and was the only board-certified surgeon in the state. He worked long hours, driving from town to town without sleep. While on the road one night, he developed chest pains—he was having a myocardial infarction at age 35.

Rosen remembered that he had "stunningly poor" care in a local emergency department.[17] At the time of his infarction, he recalled, "care was provided in emergency rooms staffed by physicians without formal training. Emergency care was viewed by hospitals as a necessary evil and assigned in academic centers to the most junior house staff, usually without supervision.

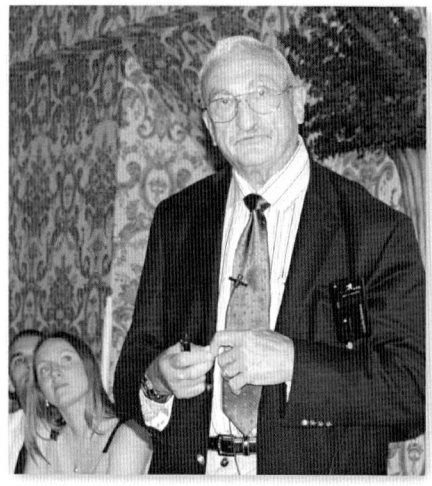

Figure 5: Peter Rosen, MD, speaks to faculty, residents and staff at the retirement celebration for Douglas Rund, MD, at the Worthington Inn, Worthington, Ohio, on Tuesday, May 24, 2011. Rosen was interviewed by Ohio State in the mid 1970s for the position of Division Director of Emergency Medicine but he declined.

Following his recovery, Rosen returned to his undergraduate and internship alma mater, the University of Chicago to become director of the emergency room, thinking that he was heading into a less stressful career. He remained in this position from 1971 to 1977, when he moved to Colorado to become Director of the Division of Emergency Medicine at the Denver General Hospital (Figure 5).

Both Krome and Rosen interviewed at Ohio State for the Emergency Room Director position. No official documents of the interviews can be found, but Williams recalls that both leaders favored an academic division of emergency medicine with qualified faculty and ultimately a residency training program. Evans remembers his involvement with the interview process and with Williams. He also recalls that the proposed salary for a director was too low to attract the national leaders:

> *Tom was a friend of mine, so he knew that I was involved in emergency medicine so he called me and had me put out all the feelers out that we were looking for a chairman of a new Department of Emergency Medicine at Ohio State University. I had them call me and set up the interviews and we would find somebody to do it. I had five doctors call me and I scheduled appointments with them; I interviewed Dr. Krome and Dr. Rosen in my office. I also inter-*

viewed three others but can't remember their names. They were all interested, however the amount of money that was going to be paid was not anywhere near what they expected as Chairman at Ohio State University and so we drew a blank there.[11]

MANUEL TZAGOURNIS, MD, AND THE RECRUITMENT OF A DIRECTOR OF EMERGENCY MEDICINE AT OHIO STATE

Manuel "Manny" Tzagournis, MD, resumed the search when he took the place of Rupert as hospital medical director in 1974. Tzagournis was born in Youngstown in 1934. He graduated from Ohio State with a bachelor's degree in 1956 and his MD in 1960. He completed his internship in internal medicine at Philadelphia General Hospital, where he became particularly interested in diabetes mellitus. He completed his residency in internal medicine at Ohio State, followed by a fellowship in endocrinology.

Tzagournis rose quickly through the ranks of leadership. He held numerous positions at Ohio State, including Assistant Dean for Research and Continuing Medical Education, Secretary of the Faculty of the College of Medicine, Associate Dean, Medical Director for Ohio State Hospitals (1974), and Acting Dean (1980). He also went on to serve as Dean (1981-1995), Vice President for Health Sciences (1994-2002) and Vice President and President of the university's managed care system.

At one-point, Tzagournis was one of the longest serving deans in the nation. The eight-story medical research facility on 11th Avenue was named for Tzagournis.

Eventually, Tzagournis became the undisputed leader at the medical center, rising to the level of Vice President for Health Sciences from 1995 to 2002. But in 1977 as the hospital's medical director, he was looking for a physician to take charge of the emergency room. He had been turned down by national leaders to date.

Evans recalled his conversation with Tzagournis:

I went to Manny Tzagournis and said we are going to have a difficult time getting an emergency physician that is going to be a chair-

man of a department without paying them more. Manny said, "They can't pay any more." So, I said, "I have a physician that is working with our group (EMAI) who is an excellent physician, is interested in teaching and I think he would answer the call."[11]

Tzagournis had to be frugal. The hospital was charging a $24 flat fee for emergency room services, which included care by the house staff, and the fixed salaries he was offering for director and attending staff were far below the market at that time. Nevertheless, patient volumes and acuities were rising in the ER at Ohio State and the national and local trends were favoring full-time groups of dedicated physicians. Acting on the suggestion by Evans, Tzagournis met with Douglas Rund, MD, in 1977.

DOUGLAS A. RUND, MD: THE FIRST FULL-TIME EMERGENCY ROOM DIRECTOR

Douglas Rund, MD, grew up in Columbus and left to attend college at Yale, where he earned his bachelor of arts degree in history in 1967 (Figure 6). He then attended and graduated from the Stanford School of Medicine with his MD degree in 1971. Rund completed a medicine clerkship after his first year as part of an experiment in the effect of early clinical experience on learning.

He also completed what was then a 5-year curriculum in 4 years and graduated as a member of Alpha Omega Alpha. During medical school he became interested in medical education in part because his learning had been so accelerated by his early clinical experience. He created his own student-taught course in physical diagnosis and worked closely with the Chairman of Medicine, Halstead Holman, MD, to introduce early clinical experiences into the curriculum.

Rund's efforts were similar to those of Sam Kiehl, MD, in that he had an interest in a broad-based practice similar to a general practice of earlier times. Rund completed an internship in internal medicine at the University of California-San Francisco, followed by two years of general surgery residency at Stanford, which included rotations in orthopedics, neurosurgery and cardiac surgery.

He left the surgery program to became one of the first Johnson Foun-

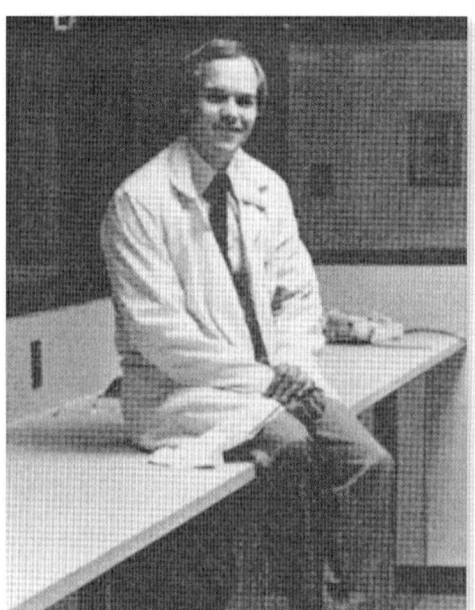

Figure 6: Douglas Rund, MD, Chief of Emergency Medicine Services, The Ohio State University, 1977 to 2011. Photo taken upon the opening of the new emergency department in 1979.

dation Clinical Scholars in the country at Stanford in 1974. He used his fellowship time to try to create innovations in medical education and explore alternate ways of delivering medical care. He and Holman developed the Mid-Peninsula Health Service, which was a patient-owned health cooperative informally affiliated with Stanford. He became the first Medical Director.

While a fellow, Rund created additional residency experiences for himself in anesthesiology and obstetrics and gynecology. He also worked after hours in emergency rooms in the Bay area and did the after-hours scheduling for the San Mateo General Hospital. In retrospect, he was creating his own residency experience in emergency medicine. Following completion of his fellowship, he joined the faculty at Stanford, trying to help develop a nascent Family and Community Medicine Department.

He moved back to Columbus in 1976 and joined William Evans' group at Emergency Medical Associates (EMAI) on what Rund believed would be somewhat temporary basis as he expected to return to California at some point. He also joined the newly created Department of Family Medicine at Ohio State on a part-time basis. The department was headed by its first Chair, Tennyson Williams, MD.

One day in 1977, he was scheduled to meet with Tzagournis, the medical director of the University Hospital. He met with Tzagournis in the hospital's administrative suite. Tzagournis offered him the position of director of the emergency room. Rund accepted immediately and outlined his vision for emergency medicine, including a distinct academic unit (division), a faculty of scholar clinicians and a residency program in emergency medicine.

He was unaware of the previous search for a director at that time. Had he known, he might have negotiated for higher salaries for the faculty to be recruited. Nevertheless, he saw this as an opportunity to create a new program at Ohio State and participate in the development of an entirely new medical specialty. From then on, the Emergency Room became the Emergency Department and a new hospital unit was created: The *Division of Emergency Medicine* (Figure 6).

References

1. Paul Tennyson Williams, MD, personal communication
   Note: Dr. Tennyson "Tenny" Williams (1925-2021) was the first Professor and Chair of Family Medicine at Ohio State. The department began as a Division of Preventive Medicine in 1974. He graduated from Case Western Reserve School of Medicine in 1951 and, after an internship, began his general practice in Delaware, Ohio. He managed many patients in their homes. For example, he used a portable ECG machine, an intravenous line and a transvenous administration of a cardiac glycoside to control the heart rhythm in atrial fibrillation, a treatment that would most certainly be performed in the hospital today. Williams had a very successful private practice and was an outstanding educator and role model to his students and residents in the Department of Family Medicine.

2. Zink, BJ. *Anyone, Anything, Anytime: A History of Emergency Medicine.* Philadelphia PA: Mosby Elsevier; 2006.

3. Charles W. Pavey MD, personal communication.
   Note: Charles Pavey, MD (1906-2004), remembered that there was a doctor's office on every block from downtown Columbus to Worthington. He was an obstetrician who spent most of his career as a member of the Ohio State faculty in the Department of Obstetrics

and Gynecology. He also lived and practiced in two lovely Victorian houses on High Street just north of the Ohio State campus. His family was in the horse raising business. Columbus was known as the "buggy capital" of the county due to the large number of horse-drawn buggies manufactured in Columbus around the turn of the 20th century. He remembered horses grazing in the fields on the East side of High Street where Northwood is today. His family sold horses to the allies in World War I. Most of the horses were kept in the Pavey barn on Kenny Road. He graduated from medical school in 1928. At the time of his death in 2004, he held the record for being the youngest man to ever graduate from The Ohio State University College of Medicine. During his practice years, he delivered more than 25,000 babies.[18]

4. Millis JS. The graduate education of physicians, The American Medical Association. Chicago, 1966.

5. Fahs IJ and Peterson OL. The Decline of General Practice, *Public Health Reports*. 1968: 83(4):267-270.

6. The American College of Emergency Physicians. *Benchmark data study*, Irvine, Texas. 2021

7. Stephens R. *American Medicine and the Public Interest: A History of Specialization*. Berkeley: University of California Press; 1998.

8. Kennedy RH. Our fashionable killer: The oration on trauma. *Bull Amer Coll Surg*.1955: 40:73-81.

9. Shortliffe EC, et.al. The emergency room and the changing pattern of medical care. *N Engl J Med*. 1958; 258(1): 20-25.

10. Committee on Trauma and Committee on Shock, Division of Medical Sciences, National Academy of Sciences, National Research Council: *Accidental death and disability: the neglected disease of modern society*. National Academy of Sciences. Washington, DC. 1966, National Academy of Sciences.

11. Evans, TW. Interview with T. William Evans, DDS, MD, FACS. by Douglas Rund. 2021: Columbus, OH.

12. Kiehl, SJ: Interview with Samuel J. Kiehl, MD, by Douglas Rund. 2021: Columbus, OH.

13. Zinzer, D: Interview with Diane Zinzer, RN, by Douglas Rund. 2021: Columbus, OH.

14. Williams, T: Interview with Thomas Williams MD, PhD, by Douglas Rund. 2021: Columbus, OH.

15. Bullock, K: Interview with Kate Bullock, RN, by Douglas Rund. 2021: Columbus, OH.

16. UT Southwestern News Room, In Memoriam: Dr. Erwin Thal: Trauma expert, outstanding surgical educator. January 19, 2015. https://utsouthwestern.edu>memoriam>erwin>thal

17. Wolfe R. and Faust JS. In memory of Dr. Peter Rosen, a founder of emergency medicine, *ACEP now*, Dec 10, 2019. www.acepnow.com>peter>rosen

18. Paulson GW. Charles William Pavey (1906-2001) In pursuit of excellence: the *Ohio State University Medical Center* from 1834 to 2010. Columbus OH: Lesher Printers; 2010: 138-140.

Chapter 2

Early Struggles: The Division of Emergency Medicine

Douglas A. Rund, MD
Richard N. Nelson, MD

Near the end of 1977, *Columbus Monthly* magazine featured a story with the cover line, "Emergency Rooms: When Your Life Depends on It, How Good Are They?" The cover displayed a photograph of the trauma room at the Ohio State University Hospital with the new Director of the Division of Emergency Medicine, Douglas A. Rund, MD, and veteran emergency department (ED) nurse John Sigafoos, RN (Figure 1).[1]

The story is interesting because it gives a snapshot of emergency medicine in Columbus in 1977 (Table 1). At that time, Riverside Methodist Hospital had the largest patient volume at 60,000 patients per year. Children's Hospital had the next highest followed by Mount Carmel East. The Ohio State University Hospital had the sixth highest volume: 28,000 patients per year.

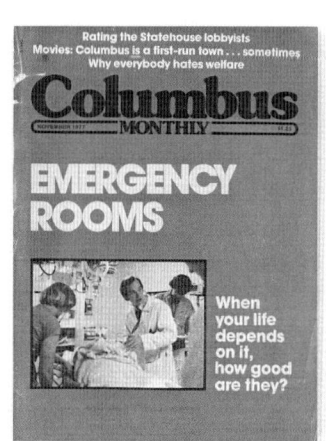

Emergency department visits to all hospitals in Columbus totaled nearly 350,000. The article noted the steady increase in visits resulting from fewer doctor house calls and "the proliferation of insurance policies which cover emergency room (ER) treatment but not a trip to the family doctor." Due to the growing need, hospitals were forced to increase the size of

Figure 1: The cover of the November 1977 *Columbus Monthly* magazine featured Douglas Rund, MD, and John Sigafoos, RN, as they cared for a patient in the trauma room in the Ohio State University Hospital.

Table 1. Columbus Emergency Rooms at a Glance: 1977

HOSPITAL	ER BEDS	ER PATIENTS SEEN/YEAR	CRITICAL PATIENTS	EMERGENCY ROOM STAFF	BILLING AND PAYMENT	ANNUAL BUDGET (DIRECT-EXPENSES)	MINIMUM COST PER PATIENT	SPECIAL FEATURES
Children's Hospital (301 beds)	27	50,000	5%	Dr. Jerome Foster medical director, appointed May, 1976; two full time physicians added July, 1977, one more to be added November, 1977; two supplementary pediatricians hired part time; three house staff rotate each month	Physicians on fixed salary with "straight employer-employee" relationship; hospital sends one bill to patient, which includes room and physician fees	$727,700	Under new billing system, charge for room and physician is determined by cost of delivering the specific service required.	New ER within new part of hospital completed in 1976 at total cost of $10 million; uses helicopter transport; volunteer service to waiting patients.
Doctors Hospital North (330 beds)	20	26,000	5-10%	Until July, 1977, ER covered by house staff; Dr. William Scott, director; contracted in July with Physicians Emergency Medical Services Inc.; Dr. Richard Esler, director	Hospital bills for room fee; corporation bills for physician fee	$702,00 for both hospitals	$21 for room; $20 for physician	Osteopathic
Doctors Hospital West (201 beds)	10	22,000	5-10%	Contracted with Physicians Emergency Medical Services Inc, October, 1976 with Dr. Richard Esler, director	Hospital bills for room fee; corporation bills for physician fee	$702,00 for both hospitals	$21 for room; $20 for physician	Osteopathic
Grant Hospital (598 beds)	16	29,000	20-25%	Contracted with Emergency Medical Associates, Inc., January, 1970; Dr. T. William Evans, administrator	Hospital bills for room fee; corporation bills for physician fee	$435,000	$23 for room $12 for physician	Small section designed for ambulatory patients.
Mercy Hospital (197 beds)	10	12,000	1%	Contracted with Emergency Room Physicians, late 1971; Dr. Cahit Palantekim, director.	Physicians on hourly salary; hospital sends two bills – one for room and one for physician	$158,000	$16 for room; $15 for physician	

Hospital							
Mount Carmel East (233 beds)	14	37,600	10%	Contracted with Emergency Services, Inc., February, 1973; Dr. Don Everett, director	Hospital bills for room fee; corporation bills for physician fee	$1,900,000 for both hospitals	Base room fees; $16 minor; $23 moderate; $27 major; physician fee is $20	Scribe system. Triage system since July, 1977.
Mount Carmel Medical Center (504 beds)	20	33,500	12%	Contracted with Emergency Services, Inc., February, 1973; Dr. Don Everett, director	Hospital bills for room fee; corporation bills for physician fee	$1,900,000 for both hospitals	Base room fees; $16 minor; $23 moderate; $27 major; physician fee is $20	New 4-story building off main hospital houses new ER constructed 1976, costing $8 million.
Riverside Methodist Hospital (870 beds)	21	60,000	5-8%	Individually contracted with full time physicians, July, 1970; Dr. William Hall, director; added 10th physician to staff in July, 1977.	Physicians receive fixed salary from hospital. Hospital sends one bill broken into physician and room components	$2,000,000	Base room fees; $14 minor; $20 intermediate; $35 admission; $75 resuscitation. Physician charge based on "units of care" each unit $3	New ER completed January, 1977 at cost of $1.3 million. Patient service representative in waiting room; treatment areas designed for privacy
St. Anthony Hospital (254 beds)	12	23,000	5%	Contracted with Emergency Medical Associates, Inc., March 1, 1975, Dr. T. Williams Evans, administrator	Hospital bills for room fee; corporation bills for physician fee	$278,643	$18 for room; $12 for physician	ER relocated into new tower completed in 1971.
University Hospital (955 beds)	14	28,000	5%	Individually contracted with three faculty staff physicians, July, 1977; Dr. Douglas Rund, director.	Physicians on fixed salary. Hospital sends one bill which includes room fee and physician fee	$600,000	$24 for room and physician	Triage system; new ER to be completed March, 1979; burn unit staff treats serious burns in ER; uses helicopter transport.

Adapted from Columbus Monthly Magazine, November, 1977

their emergency departments. Both the Riverside expansion and the anticipated University expansion would quadruple the size of their departments.

Physician staffing also needed to change. Prior to 1969 all hospitals in Columbus were staffed by house staff, medical staff members or moonlighters. Starting in 1969 at Grant, and soon thereafter at Riverside, organized physician groups were created to staff the ED. Ohio State was coming relatively late to the game: A new division with three faculty physicians was just coming into being. Still, interns and residents provided most of the care. The article summarizes the thoughts of several physicians interviewed about the emergency rooms of the past:

> *Most hospital personnel looking back to the days of intern staffed ERs, now concede that they were playing Russian roulette with their emergency patients. Of 10 patients nine might be treated by interns competent to handle their problems. For the unfortunate 10th patient an intern's inexperience or indecision might be fatal.*[1]

When interviewed years later Sigafoos, who was photographed in the *Columbus Monthly* article, recalled this about the days of staffing with interns:

> *Every year in July it was incredibly stressful. The new interns on July 1st were fresh out of medical school. So, in July and August we were trying to help the interns take care of patients in a crisis situation. You had to rely on the nurses to provide the good care. You strongly suggested to the intern or resident who was in charge what we ought to be doing during codes because they were as scared as anybody. I don't think they knew how to take charge in a situation, to be honest with you. They were new at it. It wasn't a negative statement; they just weren't experienced and so we, the nurses, had to step in and strongly recommend that maybe you want a little more bicarb here and epi here and things like that. We tried to do it as tactfully as we could, some more than others, but we had to take care of the patients.*[2]

Sigafoos was Assistant Head Nurse on the 3 to 11 shift at the time of the photograph. He later went on to become a leader in emergency medical services (EMS) and hospital administration. He established the Associate Degree Program in EMS at Columbus State Community College and later became the director of the mobile ICU program at Riverside Methodist Hospital. He obtained his MBA degree and ultimately became the Assistant Vice President for Nursing at Riverside.

In the *Columbus Monthly* article, physicians and hospital administrators were noting a wide variation in patient acuity. Some patients were seriously ill or injured while others had far less acute conditions. William Hall, MD, founder of the Riverside physician group felt that "40% of the hospital's patients could be treated in other places if these places were available. At University Hospital, Rund felt that "a lot of patients were using the emergency room as an ambulatory facility. If they don't have a physician or if their physician is unavailable. Often their condition is not life-threatening and sometimes it is a mild illness that would be self-limiting."[1]

Of course, there were critical patients who needed immediate treatment. The photo of the care of the injured patient in the trauma room at Ohio State featured as part of the article on Emergency Rooms was taken in the single bed trauma room of the "old ER" located on the ground floor of University Hospital. Sigafoos recalled this about the trauma room:

> *In reference to the photo that we were in our famous one room trauma room, that was about wide enough that you could fit one person on each side of the cot. That is where we were and that is what our trauma room was like. It was very crowded. Trauma care wasn't what it is today. It kind of showed how compressed everything was in that one room in that picture alone.*[2]

In 1977 care of the trauma patient was managed almost exclusively by surgical residents as it had been since the beginning. In the foreground of the photo is E. Christopher "Chris" Ellison, MD, who was a second-year surgical resident. (Figure 2). Years later Ellison remembered this about trauma care at that time:

> *It brings backs some great memories and also some scary memories. For trauma it was "first person up," so if you were on call that night and your beeper went off, and the chief resident was in the operating room, you went to the emergency room and tried to stabilize the patient, find out as much information as you could*

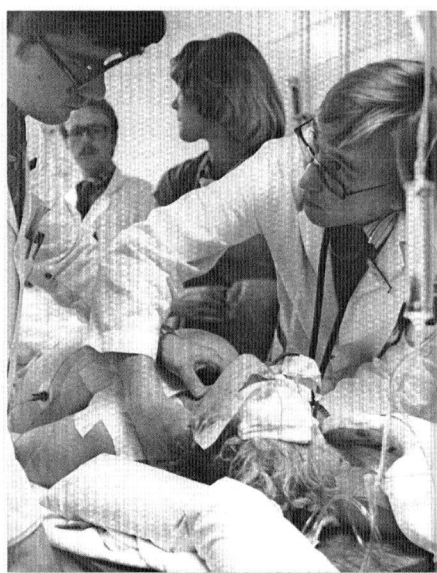

Figure 2: This trauma resuscitation was led by E. Christopher Ellison, MD, a second-year surgery resident at the time who went on to become an internationally renowned surgeon and academic medical leader.

and then get the patient admitted and appropriately cared for. It was really like a triage system. As I think as you can see from that photograph the setting was relatively confined and in 1977 it was a second-year surgery resident, the ER nurse, and an ER attending physician. That was the response team. Our trauma rooms today are very large and when you have a Level 1 trauma called, you might have a response of 10 people, including a pharmacist, nurses, emergency room physicians, surgeons, anesthesia. Things have changed for the better in many, many ways. Fortunately, we now have a trauma system in the state of Ohio that is well organized and has standards for all of the participating hospitals. All the care is coordinated through the emergency department associations as well as the American College of Surgeons and interacts very well with anesthesia societies as well, as well as nursing organizations. I think we are much more organized today and it is really good.[3]

Ellison went on to have an exceptional career of university and national leadership. He became the Chief of General Surgery, Chair of the Department of Surgery, Interim Dean of The Ohio State University College of Medicine and Chief Executive Officer (CEO) of the Ohio State University Physician (OSUP) group practice. On a national level he was elected Chair of the American Board of Surgery, the President of the American Surgical Association and the President of the American College of Surgeons.

Given the wide variations in acuity in patients presenting for treatment, there was a need to create a system to differentiate the sick from the not so sick and assign treatment priorities—a sorting technique known as triage. The medical triage process had been widely used in battlefield conditions since the first world war. Due to increasing patient volumes, triage systems were a hot topic in the 70s. The emergency medicine staffs (nursing and physician) at Ohio State published one of the first textbooks on triage which laid out guidelines for emergency department triage in this nation's hospitals (Figure 3).[4] The book was co-authored by Tondra S. "Toni" Rausch, RN, who was the department's long-standing head nurse and expert in nearly all activities in the department: "If Toni doesn't know it, nobody does.'

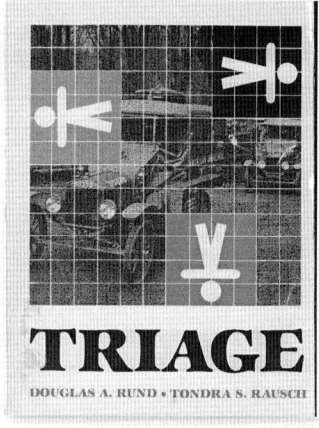

Figure 3: The first textbook published by the Department of Emergency Medicine faculty at Ohio State was a collaborative effort between medicine and nursing.

Physician salary arrangements

The needs for changes in the staffing of emergency departments were great but so were the challenges. At University Hospital and Children's Hospital, physicians were paid a fixed salary by the hospital. At Ohio State, such salaries were low for the market. The low academic salaries prevented the leaders of emergency medicine from providing a competitive wage to recruit physicians by billing patients for physician services.

The situation had not changed at all from that recognized earlier during the failed attempts to recruit a director of emergency services. The Ohio State College of Medicine and hospital leadership at that time also strictly forbade emergency physicians from rendering a bill for professional services despite repeated pleas from the faculty. The rationale was never fully explained but may have been to keep prices as low as possible for patients. Nevertheless, the ban on physician billing was clear.

In the *Columbus Monthly* article, the fixed salary model was criticized by physician leaders in Columbus who were members of the Ohio State faculty. James W "Jim" Killman, MD, an Ohio State cardiac surgeon and president of the Franklin County Academy of Medicine, took umbrage at the idea that physicians would be salaried by a hospital:

> *I object to entering a partnership for the practice of medicine with any person or institution other than a fellow physician. Where did our pioneer spirit of rugged individualism that made our present private system of medical care the best in the world go?*[1]

Killman, who was Chief of Cardiac Surgery at Ohio State from 1976 to 1980, would soon convince the emergency physicians to join the practice plan lawsuit against the University with the anticipated result that they would finally be able to bill for services and recruit the best physicians with a competitive wage.

Ronald B. Berggren, MD, Chief of Plastic Surgery Ohio State and Chairman of the Franklin County Academy of Medicine ethics committee, also opposed the salary arrangement:

> *When physicians are on fixed salaries, you are very close to an institution practicing medicine.*[1]

Riverside physicians were also paid a fixed salary but it was considerably higher than that paid to Ohio State emergency physicians. Nearly all other hospitals in Columbus contracted with physician corporations which billed separately for physician services as shown in Table 1. Seeing successful physician practices in Columbus and throughout the country, the Ohio State emergency physicians wanted to create their own physician practices, bill for emergency physician services separately from the hospital charge and recruit the best physicians for the faculty.

Recruiting, however, was difficult. In his private journal, Rund chronicled his frustration with the prohibition on billing:

> **6/15/1977:** *I am having trouble recruiting physicians because of the low salaries. The people I do interview turn out to have serious flaws.*

7/7/1977: Each day, I try to decide if I have accomplished anything or not. Today I must say I don't know...another set back from the Dean's office and the hospital. Still, I am not done yet.

8/19/1977: The emergency department has not vanquished me.

9/3/1977: Worked the entire day in the ED. A university emergency room filled with people, patients and paper records... and confusion. It goes on and on...24 hours a day.

The fixed salary arrangement would not be abolished until 1979 at the end of the end of what came to be known as the practice plan lawsuit. Killman and Berggren were two of the physician leaders involved.

Creation of a vision for the future of emergency medicine: national and local trends

In 1977, emergency medicine was becoming the fastest growing specialty in medicine.[5] There were already 31 emergency medicine residency programs in 1977. The first was in Cincinnati in 1970 with Bruce Janiak, MD. The next programs to be established were at Los Angeles County/University of Southern California Medical Center (1971), the Medical College of Pennsylvania (1972), the University of Chicago (1972) and the University of Louisville (1973).

The road to specialty recognition was particularly challenging. A provisional Section Council in emergency medicine was established in the AMA House of Delegates in 1973 and became permanent in 1975. Also in 1975, the Liaison Residency Endorsement Committee (LREC), the forerunner to the Residency Review Committee for Emergency Medicine (RRC/EM) was created by the American College of Emergency Physicians (ACEP) to review and accredit residency programs in Emergency Medicine. Nationally, the need for well-trained and certified emergency physicians was great.

In 1977, only 28% of physicians practicing in emergency departments were *certified by any specialty board at all.*[5] The American Board of Emergency Medicine was incorporated in 1976. In 1977 the board was actively developing a new criterion-referenced board examination.[6] The small division faculty at Ohio State aimed to create a residency program as early as possible.

Although the creation of an emergency medicine residency program was an early priority, a more important immediate priority was the recruitment of the highest quality faculty to ensure excellent patient care and teaching for students and house staff. Richard Nelson, MD, a medical student in 1977, recalled his student experience in the emergency room before the arrival of full-time emergency medicine attending physicians:

> *To OSU medical students, the emergency room at University Hospital was a seldom-seen small and crowded area on the ground floor of the west side of what is now Doan Hall, adjacent to the loading docks. A student would only go the ER if they were picking up a newly admitted patient while on call. More commonly, the student would wait for the patient to be transferred to their hospital bed on the floor before commencing with the workup. A medical student could do a final year elective in emergency medicine, but never at University Hospital. There were no faculty assigned to the ER and therefore no one to provide a curriculum, lectures, bedside teaching, or evaluations. Physician staffing was primarily by medical and surgical interns with some backup from residents in their second or higher years. These more experienced residents would have to leave their floor assignments whenever they were called to the ER.*
>
> *One of my most memorable experiences occurred while on call during a neurosurgery rotation, Dr. Stephen Hill (first year neurosurgery resident) and I received a call to the emergency room to take care of a young man who had been brought in from a bar after getting shot in the face at point-blank range. Expecting to see an unconscious, decerebrate patient on a cart, we were surprised instead to see an intoxicated man who was trying to escape the confines of his cart and go home. He seemed oblivious to the bullet hole and powder burns adjacent to his nose. The ER intern had already obtained a posterior-anterior (PA) and lateral skull film. Computerized tomography (CT) scans were not yet available. The lateral view showed a bullet tract extending back to the pharynx*

and then terminating, but no bullet was seen. Dr. Hill astutely ordered an abdominal x-ray, which showed a bullet in the region of the stomach. The bullet had apparently been swallowed after coursing back to the pharynx. This so-called "swallowed bullet syndrome" has since been described in the literature by others. Not suspecting any brain or spine involvement in the shooting, Dr. Hill recommended the ER staff obtain an ENT consult before we both retreated back to the call quarters. To the best of my knowledge, the patient did fine, though it's hard to fathom such a patient presenting to the ER today and being managed exclusively by medical and surgical interns and junior residents, with no attendings, advanced imaging, or trauma alerts.

The need to recruit excellent faculty to staff the emergency department and provide supervision for students and residents was crucial. To some wags of the day the opportunity for a new leader was exceptional because "it can't get worse than it is now." Also, the fledgling faculty were being watched closely by physicians and leaders in the hospitals. The emergency room staff were operating in a veritable "fish bowl" where it seemed as if their every movement could be easily seen by all.

DAVID E. ROBERTS, MD

The first new faculty member recruited was David E. Roberts, MD. He was an Ohio native who had an outstanding education. He graduated from Miami University in Oxford, Ohio, with an A.B. degree in 1968. He completed medical school at Ohio State and received his MD degree in 1972. He entered the Ohio State residency program in internal medicine which he completed in 1975. He then completed his cardiology fellowship, also at Ohio State in 1977 (Figure 4).

In 1977 Roberts was undecided about his next career steps when he learned about Ohio State's pressing need for faculty to join a division of emergency medicine. He may

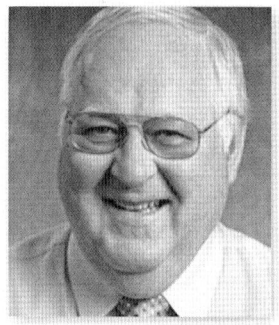

Figure 4: David E. Roberts, MD, graduated from his cardiology fellowship and became the first full-time emergency physician to be hired by the new director of the Department of Emergency Medicine.

well have been influenced by James Warren, MD, Chair of the Department of Medicine, who was an innovator in emergency medical services. Warren, a cardiologist, was the creator of the "Heartmobile" a mobile coronary care unit and the progenitor of advanced life support systems throughout the world.

The cooperative venture with the City of Columbus Division of Fire in 1969 resulted in the creation of specially trained firefighters who could start intravenous lines, administer lifesaving medications, defibrillate the heart and intubate patients—they were the first "paramedics" in the country. They were educated and trained in the "Heartshack", a temporary garage structure located just outside the doors of the Ohio State emergency room.

Roberts was highly recommended by Warren and he was exactly the kind of person the budding division needed: an exceptionally talented and well-trained physician with a five-star Ohio State pedigree. He had all the "stamps of approval" from one of the most powerful departments in the College: The Department of Medicine. Roberts met with Rund and agreed to help start the division of emergency medicine "on a temporary basis"; he remained a predominant figure in the department for the next 15 years.

Roberts and Rund began providing supervision in direct patient care in the emergency department on a part-time basis in 1977. They were each a member of an *academic* department: Roberts was an Assistant Professor in the Department of Medicine; Rund was an Assistant Professor in the Department of Family Medicine. Initially they provided coverage from 10 a.m. to 10 p.m. Each worked approximately three or four 12-hour shifts per week. Both physicians also worked at other facilities because of the small university salaries. At 10 p.m. each night the faculty attending physicians would depart.

They left and returned patient care back to the interns and residents as it had been since the beginning of the hospital. Rund would admonish the house staff to call for upper-level resident help "right away" for very sick or injured patients and to immediately "call anesthesia" for cardiac arrest or any problems with difficulty breathing.

By late 1977 Rund and Roberts had been able to recruit a third physician, Kevyn Deal, MD, a highly respected internist, to their group. With her addition, physicians were able to cover up to 16 hours per day on most days.

The Ohio State University Medical Practice Plan

In 1977 a storm was on the horizon. The controversy about what was to become the medical practice plan of Ohio State University was beginning. For years University administrators had been claiming that Ohio State doctors were billing patients for physician services provided in university facilities—and the doctors were receiving this professional income in addition to the university salaries.

This private practice arrangement for practicing physicians at academic institutions dated back decades as a way to supplement doctors' incomes to make up for the historically low university salaries. The *medical schools* needed gifted teachers for the students; the *hospitals* needed capable teachers and supervisors for residents. Because revenue from student tuition and hospital fees were not nearly sufficient to provide anything close to market physician salaries, professional fee income was needed to attract the best physicians.

Such professional fee collections by faculty provided enough income to bring academic salaries somewhat closer to those obtained in private practice and enabled universities to hire the best people and fulfil their academic and patient care obligations.

At Ohio State, physicians in most departments billed patients for professional services and many physicians paid for some or even most of their departmental expenses with such revenue. In the early 1970s, however, university President Harold Enarson and other administrators began questioning whether or not doctors should reimburse the university for facilities, supplies and equipment they used in their private medical practices.

In 1977, *The Columbus Dispatch* began running a series of articles written by reporter Graydon Hambrick on the issue. The first article published on February 18 of that year reported that President Harold Enarson had sent a letter to Henry Cramblett, Dean of the College of Medicine, urging the institution of a uniform practice plan:

> *The plan should not only require the reimbursement of the college for all direct support services related to the generation of physician fee income, but also the provision for faculty enrichment programs at both the department and college level.*[7]

Some faculty members voiced concern, saying that they already had departmental plans supporting academic enrichment and salaries within their own department.

On September 9, 1977 Enarson instructed the Ohio State Board of Trustees to develop a draft practice plan. The board created a committee to do so. As envisioned, the plan would force the 200 or so Ohio State doctors in practice to contribute to a central practice plan. The doctors, through their medical staff organization and other routes, pushed back with many objections to the loss of control over what they viewed as departmental resources needed to fulfill their departmental missions.

Over the next several months, the Board of Trustees seemed to try to modify the practice plan proposal by giving more control to the college and affected departments, but also adding more complications such as the potential to reduce the already small university salaries paid to the physicians.

On March 3, 1978, the Ohio State Board of Trustees approved the medical practice plan they had created. The plan set out requirements for how doctors were to spend practice income to improve academic programs of the College of Medicine and how they would reimburse Ohio State for costs associated with their practices. The plan was to become effective on July 1, 1979.[8]

On March 31, 1978, two law suits were filed by 139 physician members of the medical staff: one filed in the Franklin County Common Pleas Court and one filed in U.S. District Court. The suits sought injunctive relief from the practice plan.

Rund and Roberts were plaintiffs in the law suit. Their objectives were *not to prevent* the taxation of their income but to *be allowed to begin billing* for their services in the first place. In their estimation, the future for Ohio State emergency medicine would be bleak indeed if they could never bill their professional fees as did other successful ED groups. If initial physician salaries remained low, recruiting would suffer and the residency program could never be established without qualified faculty. The "dominoes" would never fall properly in line to create a first-rate program in emergency medicine.

The lawsuit had negative consequences for the medical center. Most of the faculty members in the Department of Anesthesiology quit over the issue. Many surgeons left because they could not operate without anesthesiologists and they opposed the idea of a central practice plan.

An editorial published in *The Columbus Dispatch* on February 8, 1979, urged a prompt realistic settlement of the controversy surrounding the practice plan:

> *Last year when university trustees approved an administration plan to regulate the income of faculty physicians there were predictions the initiative would disrupt University Hospital, hamper medical recruiting and damage the University. All this is occurred. The anesthesiology department, which is key to all types of surgery, has lost 11 members. As a result, seven of the 13 operating rooms at University Hospital are closed. This turmoil, which is only the tip of the iceberg, stems from the decision of university administration to impose a medical practice plan unaccepted to university doctors. It is imperative that OSU administrators and trustees take a fresh look at the ill-advised medical practice plan and negotiate a settlement better suited to the public interest. The University, the medical College and the central Ohio community will all suffer if the dispute ends in a bitter fight in open court.*[9]

During the months before the settlement there were depositions, meetings and counter proposals. Rund recalled walking to attend his discovery deposition in downtown Columbus:

> *I was standing at the corner of Broad and High Streets with two of the most prominent attorneys in Columbus: Earl Morris and Robert Nordstrom. Morris was a senior partner in the firm, Porter, Wright, Morris and Arthur. Nordstrom was a former OSU law*

> *professor and senior member of the Porter firm. I was about to be deposed by the university's attorneys from the Vorys, Sater, Seymour and Pease firm. I thought "what am I doing here at age 33? I just want to hire great physicians to start the emergency medicine program at OSU."*

Finally, on March 13, 1979, federal judge Joseph Kinneary approved a settlement between physicians and the university that ended the lawsuit.

For emergency medicine, the outcome was excellent. A Medical Research and Development Fund (MRDF) was created with a portion of professional revenues from all physicians. The fund would ultimately fund educational programs for students and residents and even resident salaries. Startup funds for researchers could also be provided. Now that a sizable portion of practice revenues were to be used support the teaching and research missions, the ban on professional billing by the college was lifted.

The college would benefit financially. Full scale recruitment could now begin. The lawsuit had a secondary benefit for the emergency physicians: All the plaintiff doctors were all on the same side against a common threat. There was mutual recognition and colleagueship among fellow physicians of all specialties that might not have been possible without the collective experience. Faculty in Emergency Medicine were now more than ever, accepted, respected and considered equals by the medical staff.

The turmoil created by physician resignations and limited surgical capability persisted after the lawsuit. On occasion the emergency department needed to transfer patients whose condition demanded immediate surgery. One such patient was transferred by ambulance to Grant hospital with one of the best Ohio State surgeons accompanying the patient in the ambulance.[10] Rund remembers going into his new office and hearing the phone ringing:

> *We were just moving into the new emergency department. In my future office there was no one and no furniture: just a telephone on the floor. The phone rang and for some reason I picked up the receiver. The caller was Carol Lease from the Dispatch newspaper.*

She asked about the patient who had been transferred to Grant Hospital during the practice plan crisis and had died weeks later. I said something about we would look into it if needed. The next morning the headline "above the fold" was: "Hospital Begins Probe in Wake of Injured Man's Death." I stayed home from work that day resolving to never pick up the receiver again. From then on if ever speaking to a reporter I would answer "let me get back to you" and immediately contact public relations.

Many elective surgeries had been cancelled due to the small number of functioning operating rooms and surgeons began applying to other hospitals for surgical privileges. Several surgeons, including Tom Williams, MD, who initially drove the search for the emergency medicine directorship, moved their practices to Grant Hospital and other locations in the community. It took years for the university to recover from this, but those efforts allowed emergency medicine to plan for growth.

References

1. Ruben LS. Emergency Room. When your life depends on it, how good are they? *Columbus Monthly*. November 1977.

2. Sigafoos J: Interview with John Sigafoos, RN, MBA, by Douglas Rund. 2022: Columbus, OH.

3. Ellison EC: Interview with E. Christopher "Chris" Ellison, MD, by Douglas Rund. 2022: Columbus, OH.

4. Rund DA and Rausch TS. *Triage*. St. Louis, MO: Mosby; 1981.

5. The American College of Physicians twenty-five years of front line. ACEP, Dallas, TX: 1993.

6. Maatsch JL, Munger BS, Podgorny G. On the reliability and validity of the board examination in emergency medicine. In: Wolcott BA, Rund DA, eds. *Emergency Medicine Annual: Nineteen Eighty-Two*. Norwalk, CT: Appleton-Century-Crofts; 1982:183-222.

7. Hambrick, G. Doctors at OSU see their own patients. *The Columbus Dispatch*. July 27, 1977.

8. Hambrick, G. OSU trustees announce medical plan. *The Columbus Dispatch*. March 4, 1978.

9. Editorial Page. Medical plan turmoil. *The Columbus Dispatch*. February 8, 1979.

10. Lease, CA. Hospital begins probe in wake of injured man's death. *The Columbus Dispatch*. July 9, 1979.

Chapter 3

The Division of Emergency Medicine in the Department of Preventive Medicine

Douglas A. Rund, MD

The tiny division of emergency medicine at The Ohio State University composed of faculty members David Roberts, MD, and Douglas Rund, MD, was formed in 1977 as a hospital division, but the unit had no academic home. A proper academic home would be in one of the existing academic departments in the Ohio State College of Medicine.

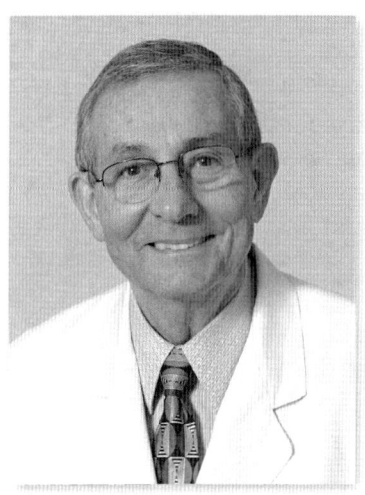

Figure 1: Manuel Tzagournis, MD, was Dean and Vice President for Health Sciences, at The Ohio State University College of Medicine. Tzagournis was Associate Dean and Medical Director for Ohio State University Hospitals from 1976 to 1980 during the formative years of the Division of Emergency Medicine. He remained an advocate and supporter of the specialty until his retirement in 2002.

In the language of the university, such departments were called tenure initiating units, places where faculty members could begin their quests for promotion and the ultimate grail: the awarding of tenure. A tenured faculty member held a permanent academic position.

Many discussions were held with college leadership, including with Manuel Tzagournis, MD, Associate Dean of the College and Medical Director of the hospital (Figure 1). There could have been rationale for locating the division in a clinical department, such as the Department of Medicine or the Department of Surgery, but the unstated reality was that neither of the two departments wanted to give the other department control of the emergency room. An often-repeated mantra among the more perceptive leaders in the hospital was that "medicine doesn't want surgery to have it and surgery doesn't want medicine to have it."

In fact, the emergency medicine faculty set their own goal of becoming a full academic department and strongly doubted the possibility of an easy release from either one of the two powerful departments. The solution emerged with the option to join the Department of Preventive Medicine. The chairman, Martin David Keller, MD, PhD, was enthusiastic about the new addition to his department.

Keller, a Brooklyn native, had five academic degrees. He received his A.B. degree from Yeshiva University in New York in 1944. He received his MS degree from New York University in 1946 and his MD degree from Cornell University in 1957. He received his PhD degree from New York University in 1953 and his MPH from Columbia University in 1958. He completed his internship in pediatrics and residency in internal medicine in New York. After his extensive graduate education, he began fulfilling his service requirement/military obligation with an enlistment in the United States Public Health Service.

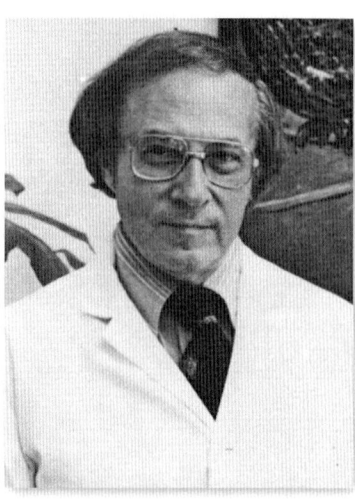

Figure 2: Martin D. Keller, MD, PhD, was Chairman of the Department of Preventive Medicine from 1978 to 1988. Keller agreed to establish the Division of Emergency Medicine in the Department of Preventive Medicine where it could grow in a nurturing environment to become a full academic department.

He was assigned to the Ohio Department of Health and did much of his work in southern Ohio and the poorest area in the state: Vinton County. Following his public health commitment, he served in various roles in the Ohio Department of Health, including acting Chief of Communicable Diseases and also Chronic Diseases. He held both Instructor and Assistant Professor positions in the Department of Preventive Medicine from 1954 to 1960 (Figure 2).

In these roles, he established an excellent reputation and connections with leaders in preventive medicine and public health in Ohio. The connections would eventually bring him back to Ohio for the remainder of his career. In 1960 he and his family moved to Boston where he was appointed the Director of Clinical Affairs at the Beth Israel Hospital and Assistant Professor at the Harvard Medical School.

In 1962 he was recruited back to Columbus and Ohio State to join the Department of Preventive Medicine with the offer of an appointment as Associate Professor with Tenure and a significant increase in salary.[1] Soon after his appointment, he became the director of the community medicine section of Preventive Medicine, then was appointed Chair in 1978.

The Department of Preventive Medicine was established in 1948 as a somewhat eclectic mix of public health, industrial medicine and nutrition. Over the next 20 years, the department was reconfigured to consist of community health, aerospace/aviation medicine and occupational medicine. The nutrition program was eventually transferred to the School of Allied Medical Professions.

Community medicine included a research design and analysis unit (the biometrics laboratory), epidemiology and international health. For many years aerospace/aviation was a dominant force in the department that operated and aerospace laboratory and vibration laboratory.

In his history of the Ohio State College of Medicine, George W. Paulson, MD, stated that "between 1956 and 1977, OSU was the leading medical academic center in civil aviation and space medicine."[2] At that time, all criteria seemed in place to establish a Civil Aviation Medical Institute. In fact, the Chair immediately preceding Keller's tenure was Colonel Harold V. Ellingson, MD, MPH, PhD, who had served as Commander of the United States Airforce School of Aerospace Medicine.[3] Aerospace Medicine gradually faded in significance. Emergency Medicine was to grow in its place.

In 1974, the Preventive Medicine department became the temporary academic home for the newly created Division of Family Medicine, which the Ohio General Assembly mandated for universities receiving state funds. Family Medicine grew under the protective arrangement and soon separated to become a full academic department in 1975. There was precedent, therefore, for preventive medicine to function as a home for units that wished to become full departments. Keller termed this role "an incubator" for new divisions that needed to be nurtured in a protective environment until mature enough to stand on their own. Keller enthusiastically welcomed the task of "incubating" emergency medicine in his department.

In Paulson's excellent book, *In Pursuit of Excellence: The Ohio State University Medical Center From 1834 to 2010*, he recognized the department's role in protecting Family Medicine and Emergency Medicine. He wrote the following regarding Keller:

> *It was Keller who opened the doors of the Department of Preventive Medicine to shelter the formal effort in emergency care as it began. There cannot be many who have had to who had a chance to be Godfather for two major units.*[2]

No other emergency medicine division in the country was begun in a department of preventive medicine. The choice was a most fortuitous one for several reasons.

First, Keller and his wife, Geraldine Keller, PhD, had been studying emergency medical services (EMS) for several years. At that time they were considered experts in aspects of pre-hospital emergency medicine, including medical dispatch. They had both been actively engaged in studying the functions and outcomes of the "Heartmobile" started by Ohio State and the new EMS demonstration projects in Southeastern Ohio in the early 1970s.

Second, Keller was a seasoned academic with exceptional faculty credentials from Harvard and Ohio State. He understood the importance of faculty scholarship. It was particularly important at a university such as Ohio State because creative inquiry and publication were essential for promotion and tenure. A stable faculty could not be developed without tenured faculty because if a faculty member was not promoted by the seventh year of service, there would be no renewal of appointment for the eighth year and the faculty member would have to move on. It was not until much later in the University's history that many non-tenured "clinical" appointments would be available to provide adequate faculty for expanded patient care requirements.

Third, Keller understood the importance of creating new, unique knowledge specific for the specialty. He would often say that emergency medicine could not continue to borrow content from specialties. Textbooks about emergency medicine in that era were written by specialists, not emergency physicians. Trauma content was developed solely by surgeons; cardiology content was developed by cardiologists.

Years earlier, the importance of developing a new body of knowledge—i.e., content—as a first step in the development of a specialty had been diagrammed by Ralston R. Hannas, MD, ("R Squared") who was a pioneering emergency physician who outlined a stepwise progression for a specialty (Figure 3).[3] This diagram showing the pathway to specialty status was considered dogma among the new leaders of emergency medicine in the 1970s and helped guide all decisions presented to leaders of aspiring academic departments.

The evolution of the new specialty required a clear definition of content specific to emergency medicine, which would eventually be developed by emergency medicine researchers. Once the content was established, graduate training programs (residencies) could be established, followed by medical school recognition of emergency medicine as a separate entity—and the eventual establishment of full academic departments. The evolution continued with the creation of specialty boards, certification examinations, continuing education and, completing the circle: research.

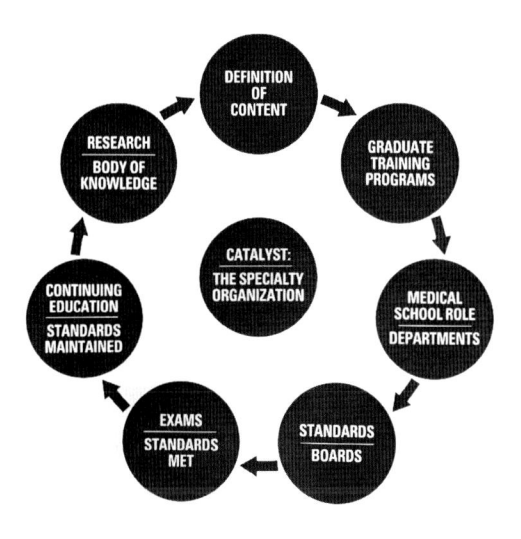

Figure 3: Hannas RR. Diagram outlining steps leading to the full development of a specialty. This was a commonly accepted pathway guiding academic emergency medicine leaders throughout the early years of the specialty. From *The American College of Physicians Twenty-Five years of Front Line*. ACEP, Dallas, TX; 1993.

This road map guided the early leaders of the specialty nationally, and Rund and Keller locally: Establish content through research and publication, create a residency program, become a separate academic department, provide leadership to the certifying board and develop as strong a research program as possible.

During 1978, significant effort was expended to recruit and retain qualified faculty. Second to Roberts, the next faculty member was Kevyn Deal, MD, who was an outstanding physician and educator. Deal was highly recommended by Department of Medicine leadership and particularly by Vice Chair Earl Metz, MD, a hematologist and widely respected clinician and teacher.

Tragically, Deal had a very serious medical condition and died in November, 1979. She was undoubtedly one of the most stoic individuals in the history of emergency medicine. On more than one occasion, she would see her patients even while attached to an intravenous line providing fluids and medication.

Nancy Thrlik, MD, also provided tremendous clinical expertise in the department. Thrlik completed her residency in internal medicine at Riverside Methodist Hospital in 1975 and began her practice there in the emergency department. When the Ohio State Division of Emergency Medicine was created, she worked at both Riverside and Ohio State.

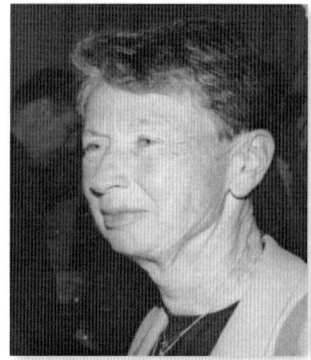

Figure 4: Nancy Thrlik, MD, at the 25th anniversary celebration of the founding of emergency medicine at Ohio State. Thrlik was an early part-time faculty member in the department. Her full-time practice was at Riverside Methodist Hospital. She was instrumental in bridging Ohio State and Riverside in the early development of the residency program.

Thrlik was an outstanding physician and educator. Her internal medicine credentials added immensely to the reputation of the emergency medicine faculty. Later when the time came to develop the residency, she helped provide a communication "bridge" between the faculty at Ohio State and the faculty at Riverside, adding greatly to mutual understanding and cooperation (Figure 4).

By the end of the academic year 1979 three additional faculty members had been recruited: Richard "Rick" Cline, MD; Theophil T. "Tom" Sutton, MD, and John Gaeuman, MD (Figure 5). Cline had just finished his residency in internal medicine. He joined the faculty in June of 1979 and remained until 1981, when he joined the fellowship in gastroenterology and left the emergency department. He eventually practiced as a gastroenterologist in Maryville, Tennessee.

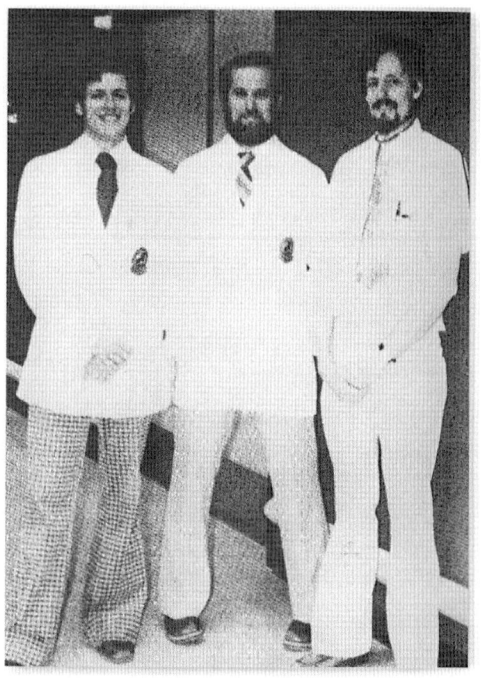

Figure 5: Early full-time emergency medicine faculty members. From left, Theophil T. "Tom" Sutton, MD, Richard "Rick" Cline, MD, and John Gaeuman, MD.

Sutton completed his internship in internal medicine at Ohio State when he joined the faculty in 1978. At the time, being hired to work in an ER after only completing an internship was not that unusual, particularly in parts of the country where there were no EM residency programs. Sutton eventually became an occupational medicine physician in Florida.

Gaeuman was an internist who had completed a residency in aerospace medicine in 1962 and had worked in the aviation industry for years before he joined the faculty in Preventive Medicine, and was the last of the aviation medicine faculty. With the addition of these three physicians, plus Rund, Roberts and Thrlik, there finally were enough faculty members to cover the department 24 hours a day and provide teaching for students and off-service residents.

At that time, the American Board of Emergency Medicine was just fighting for recognition and approval from the American Board of Medical Specialties. Residency-trained emergency physicians were highly desirable, but the small number of residencies in existence had too few graduates to staff most hospitals. Although none of the original faculty had completed a residency in emergency medicine, there were enough in numbers to begin the preparation of the application for approval of the residency program.

Student teaching, long absent in the emergency room, needed to begin. Deal had been working closely with Franklin "Frank" Banks, PhD, in preventive medicine to integrate the didactic teaching in the emergency department with the overall teaching goals of the Department of Preventive Medicine. This included teaching emergency medicine with a broad view of community health systems and epidemiology.

Student demand for emergency medicine was high and the division needed to show more than six faculty members in their department when applying for approval of a residency. Thus, the department arranged for students to take emergency department electives at major hospitals throughout the city, including Riverside Methodist Hospital, Grant Hospital, St Anthony, Mount Carmel East and Mount Carmel West. Voluntary clinical faculty were appointed at Riverside, Children's Hospital and Grant.

At Riverside, the primary faculty members were Nancy Thrlik, MD, and Samuel Kiehl, MD. Penelope Tokarski, MD, was at Children's Hospital and Lewis Seeder, MD, John Cunningham, MD, and Richard Clary, MD, were the primary faculty at Grant. Years later Clary remembered this about the student rotations at Grant:

> *One of the things I remember about the students was that everyone was kind of excited about being in the ER. You go from long periods of boredom to periods of insanity over a short period of time. It was always busy and they had a lot of patient contact. If it wasn't something critical, they would see the patient and present it to you, and then talk about it. Sometimes they had one on one with us. I'm not sure they got much of that at OSU. But they certainly did seem to enjoy it. I remember the medical students thinking the ER was really interesting and exciting and that you saw so many different things. I think that's what really draws everybody's attention. You know if the student was there and there was a code or something; back then they didn't have Code Blue teams and all that, so the stu-*

> dent got to take more of an active part in everything that we were doing. They seemed to certainly enjoy that and appreciate that.[5]

Emergency medicine was working hard to expand its clinical teaching to medical students and joined the new program of Primary Care Emphasis Selectives to expand student opportunities. Department faculty taught in the trauma module for third-year students. A seminar in emergency medicine was developed for fourth-year students. The instructional program for the students included an introduction to cardiac arrest. The department also instituted a faculty lecture series emphasizing topics unique to emergency medicine. Richard Clary, MD, was one of the faculty members (Grant Hospital) who lectured. He remembered this about the experience years later:

> The one subject I remember giving lectures on was ectopic pregnancy. I had several of those cases and reading up on it and how difficult it could be to diagnose. If your list of differential diagnoses didn't include ectopic pregnancy, the symptoms the patient presented with are not going to point to that necessarily. It was a hard diagnosis to make. I can remember giving lectures on that. That's the one thing I can remember for sure I gave lectures on. I can't recall if I gave lectures on anything else or not. I went over to OSU for that. I think all these students that were at these other hospitals came back to OSU for these clinical lectures and so forth. Back then there was no PowerPoint. It was more like sitting around and having a discussion and the students asking questions and so forth. Nobody fell asleep because the PowerPoint wasn't any good. It was better that way.[5]

The lecture series for students also had a preventive medicine flavor, including topics such as a broad overview of the EMS system and the place of EMS in the overall health delivery system. The student experiences included riding as observers with the emergency units of the Columbus Division of Fire and the Fire and EMS Dispatch Center.

Creation of a residency program in emergency medicine was uppermost in the minds of the faculty. Preparations were underway to complete a residency application and also a grant application for federal funding to support the residency program. The ultimate goal was to begin the residency program in emergency medicine in 1981.

Development of a quality research program was also a key part of the vision for emergency medicine. In many ways this was also the most difficult goal. The early faculty leaders took advantage of the resources of the Department of Preventive Medicine to at least attempt the start of a program. They explored potential new epidemiologic studies in emergency medicine and created a new clinical chart with an emphasis on data collection.

Another project focused on the use of clinical laboratory data in emergency medicine decision making using a new tool: the computer.

New Emergency Department June 28, 1979

In the summer of 1979, the Emergency Department relocated to its vastly expanded space on the ground floor of the new Rhodes Hall. The emergency unit had been located in the ground floor of University Hospital since its opening in 1951 and had never expanded until this move.

The new emergency department encompassed 28 separate rooms in 17,000 square feet of space. A significant feature of the new department was the separation into a "medicine" side and a "surgery" side. The attending physician covered both sides and patients could be placed into either side if need be. The 7-bed medicine room included the gynecology treatment area. The 4-bed surgical area was used for minor wounds and minor trauma.

In the center of the department were two large rooms, each holding two beds that were used for major resuscitation and major trauma. These rooms were large and accommodated the equipment used for such major resuscitations. In addition to these areas were an orthopedic room, psychiatric seclusion room (the legendary E4), two X-ray suites, isolation room (E6), and a radiation and chemical decontamination room.

A unit for prison inmates who were patients (known as "the cage") was located on what was then known as the "east corridor", and though it was designed for prison inmates, it pre-dated Ohio State's longstanding relationship with the Ohio Department of Rehabilitation and Corrections by a number of years and thus was rarely used for prisoners. Other rooms on the east corridor included an ENT room, complete with slit-lamp for eye exams, and a dental room, which was mainly staffed in the evenings by oral surgery residents supervised by a College of Dentistry faculty member.

Another small room on the east corridor which was a holdover of academic medicine practices of the '60s and '70s was a small lab to be used by attendings, residents and medical students. Clinicians could perform dipstick and microscopic urinalyses with the help of both a centrifuge and microscope. Nurses would routinely "spin down" the urines, which were almost never sent to the hospital lab, a practice that did not end until the Clinical Laboratory Improvements Amendments in 1988.

An alcohol lamp and reagents were also available for gram stains, often used to examine sputum samples for pneumococci, spinal fluids for bacterial meningitis, and urethral discharges for gonococci. Finally, stool guaiac testing, using the three reagents in separate bottles complete with eyedroppers, could be used to rule out GI bleeds in this pre-guaiac-card era. Other common tests included vaginal wet prep and stool microscopic exams, and urine pregnancy tests, accurate at about six weeks gestation.

Ambulances and patients were protected under a covered entryway when arriving and unloading. The new unit provided far greater capability than the old unit and served the division well until the next major revision in 1995.

In many ways, the new clinical space was part of an introduction to a new era: the creation of a residency program and deliberate steps to become a full academic department. It was time for Ohio State Emergency Medicine to begin the journey—to take its place among the foremost programs in the country.

References

1. Schlan, M. Columbus Jewish Historical Society. Columbus, OH. August 13, 2007.

2. Paulson, GW. The Ohio State University College of Medicine, Vol. 3. The Ohio State University; 1998.

3. Shillito FH. History of the College of Medicine 1959-1968, Chapter 18. Department of Preventive Medicine, The Ohio State University. Centennial Histories; 1958.

4. The American College of Physicians. Twenty-Five years of Front Line. ACEP, Dallas, TX; 1993.

5. Clary R: Interview with Richard "Dick" Clary, MD, by Douglas Rund. 2022: Columbus, OH.

Chapter 4

The Push to Begin: The Residency Program in Emergency Medicine

Richard Nelson, MD
Douglas A. Rund, MD

The practice plan settlement ushered in a new era for emergency medicine. Faculty could now bill for professional services provided to patients. Enhanced income allowed sustained recruitment of the best physicians. The billing arrangements were excellent for the emergency medicine faculty. The hospital billed on behalf of emergency physicians who would then be credited with 70% of their charges. Physicians coded their own charts subject to review and audit. A portion of the practice income was returned to the department for academic enrichment as part of the settlement approved by the federal court decision.

The long-term plan had always been to recruit excellent faculty first and develop the residency program second. In 1979 it was time to plan the anticipated residency program and apply for approval. A Residency Review Committee (RRC) of the Accreditation Council for Graduate Medical Education (ACGME) was years away. The American Board of Emergency Medicine (ABEM) had just been approved by the American Board of Medical Specialties (ABMS) in 1979 as a "modified conjoint" board. The board (ABEM) had to include representatives from seven other specialty boards on its own board of directors.

The newness of ABEM meant that a formal RRC was yet to be formed by the ACGME. In its place the specialty had formed an interim accreditation body called the Liaison Residency Endorsement Committee (LREC). Its offices were located at the headquarters of the American College of Emergency Medicine (ACEP) in Lansing, Michigan.

The LREC was formed by Robert Dailey, MD, and other leaders of the American College of Emergency Physicians (ACEP) in 1975. Initially the Committee included representatives from ACEP and the University Association for Emergency Medicine (UAEM). When the ABEM was incorporated in 1976, three additional members from ABEM were added. The new specialty had been establishing new residency training programs for the past five years at that point. It was recognized that a national standardized review process of some kind was needed. The LREC began reviewing all established programs and all proposed new training programs for emergency medicine specialists. At minimum programs were required to offer two years of training, on site faculty supervision and at least half of the rotations in the emergency department.[1]

Brian Zink, MD, has written an excellent history of emergency medicine entitled *Anything, Anyone, Anytime: A History of Emergency Medicine*.[1] A prominent feature of his book is his presentation of recorded transcripts of interviews with the earliest founders and leaders of the new specialty. Regarding the LREC, he writes the following about its early work:

> *It was very active...visiting and approving more than 30 emergency medicine residency programs in its first 2 years.*

The initial reviews during this early period were not always especially rigorous, however. Site visitors were often friends and colleagues of the residency program leaders and they would socialize and dine together at the directors' homes during the review. Deficiencies were sometimes minimized or overlooked. He writes further:

> *Programs could receive full endorsement, provisional endorsement or no endorsement. Provisional endorsement was for programs that had been in existence less than two years or for programs that had "serious but correctable weaknesses," and would be reviewed in a year. In the first three years of LREC reviews all programs were given full or provisional endorsement.*[1]

In 1979, Judith Tintinalli, MD, MS, FACEP, Emergency Medicine Program Director at Wayne State/Detroit Receiving Hospital, took over as Chair of the LREC from the founder, Robert Dailey, MD. Under Tintinalli, the review process became much more rigorous. The organizational structure was tightened significantly and the site surveyors were required to be much more objective in their assessments. It was to this much *stricter* and more *scrupulous* LREC that Ohio State Emergency Medicine now applied. So much for timing!

On January 14, 1980, the Division of Emergency Medicine submitted its application for approval of its residency program to Tintinalli. The application requested approval of a program with only *one resident per year*. In the cover letter to Tintinalli, Douglas Rund, MD, Director of the Division of Emergency Medicine, stated the following:

> *It is our intent to establish an integrated residency program using the clinical resources at the Ohio State University Hospitals and Riverside Methodist Hospital. It is our ultimate hope that Children's Hospital will become formally integrated with this program by the time of its inception in 1981...we are very strongly committed to developing a highly academic program with the clear-cut goal of educating future teachers, scholars, and leaders in emergency medicine (Figure 1).*

The initial application fee was $200. Several options were available to a new program: independent (conducted within a single institution); affiliated (two or more institutions develop formal agreements and conjoint responsibilities); and integrated (when a single program director assumes the responsibility for the residency program which involves more than one institution).

The Ohio State application requested the *integrated* option. In this option, the single program director (Rund) was responsible for all resident and faculty appointments. Resident salaries were listed at $12,180 for first-year residents and $13,380 for third-year residents. The application asked about the location of the emergency department (ED) in the organizational structure. The word "department" was being strongly encouraged by the specialty in emergency medicine organizations at that time to distinguish it from a "room," which denoted lower status and suggested a mere triage and minor care area. The application, therefore, emphatically pointed out that the emergency unit was a separate hospital *department* even though the corresponding medical school unit was the *Division* of Emergency Medicine in the Department of Preventive Medicine.

```
                    The Ohio State University        University Hospitals
  OSU                                                410 West 10th Avenue
                                                     Columbus, Ohio 43210


January 14, 1980


Judith Tintinalli, M.D.
Chairman
Liaison Residency Endorsement Committee
American College of Emergency Physicians
3900 Capital City Blvd.,
Lansing, MI 48906

Dear Dr. Tintinalli:

Enclosed please find our application to establish a residency program in
emergency medicine at the Ohio State University.

It is our intent to establish an integrated residency program using the clinical
resources at the Ohio State University Hospitals and Riverside Methodist Hospital.
It is our ultimate hope that Children's Hospital will become formally integrated
with this program by the time of it's inception in 1981.

We are very strongly committed to developing a highly academic program with the
clear-cut goal of educating future teachers, scholars, and leaders in emergency
medicine.

Enclosed also please find the required two-hundred dollar application fee.

Many thanks for your consideration in this matter. We will look forward to
hearing from you when your review of our application is completed.

Sincerely yours,


Douglas A. Rund, M.D.
Director, Division of
Emergency Medicine and
Emergency Medical Services
The Ohio State University
(614) 422-8605

DAR:cad

Enclosures




          Dodd Hall / Means Hall / Rhodes Hall University Hospital / Starling Loving Hall /
          University Hospitals Clinic / Upham Hall / Wiseman Hall
```

Figure 1: First letter seeking accreditation for the Ohio State University emergency medicine residency program—from the Liaison Residency Endorsement Committee, 1980.

At the time of application in 1980, the department had an annual census of 33,000. The breakdown was as follows: medicine 43%; surgery 24%; Ob-Gyn 16%; pediatrics 5%; and "other" 12%. Seventeen percent of the patients were admitted to the hospital. Oral surgery and dental patients were seen in the emergency department by oral surgery residents. There had always been a struggle between oral surgery and plastic surgery to treat patients with facial injuries. Oral surgery was always in-house after hours and cared for patients with dental and other complaints.

The oral surgeons were a constant and important presence in the emergency department from its inception. There was always a dental chair in the department and the oral surgeons were occasionally called to help care for other kinds of emergency patients, especially those requiring suturing, particularly in times of departmental overload, usually from raucous student celebrations on Saturday nights following Ohio State football victories. One such example was "mud volleyball", where mud, broken glass and alcohol combined to ensure a steady flow of patients with complex and contaminated wounds.

At the time of the application the monthly house staff assignments were as follows: three first-year medical interns and one first-year surgical resident. The medical interns worked 54 hours per week. Each shift was eight to 16 hours in length (8 a.m. to 12 a.m., 12 a.m. to 8 a.m.). A single first-year surgery resident worked 8-hour shifts, six days a week. Only first-year residents worked regular shifts in the emergency department. More senior residents in medicine, surgery and all major specialties and subspecialties were always available for consults and patient admissions to the hospital. In 1979 the Ohio State University Hospital offered 344 residency positions, but only 301 were filled. The majority of the vacancies were in Family Medicine and Psychiatry. Thirty-two of the positions were filled by foreign medical graduates.

The block rotations outlined in the initial application seem to reflect thinking about emergency medicine that was typical of the time, but it was outmoded compared with the future academic development of the specialty with its own content and residency educated faculty. The proposed block rotations, including the number of months assigned, were as follows:

Year I: Medicine-4; General surgery-2; Anesthesiology-2; Ob-gyn-2; emergency medicine-2

Year II: Advanced cardiology-2; Neurosurgery-2; Pediatric emergency medicine-2; Orthopedics-2; Ophthalmology-1; ENT-1; Emergency medicine-2

Year III: Psychiatry-1; Radiology-1; Elective or research-3; Emergency medicine administration-3; Emergency medicine-4

In its most generous interpretation, the program only offered 13 months of emergency medicine—less than the 18 months deemed desirable. The thought that elements of emergency medicine needed to be taught by non-emergency physicians such as cardiologists or surgeons was prominent at the time and eventually led to the quest for emergency medicine to develop its own content and be taught largely by emergency physicians. The obvious need for the specialty to create its own body of knowledge required research programs. In addition, universities needed to recruit and support academically-oriented faculty who could study clinical emergency medicine critically with an eye to knowledge development and specialized education for students and residents.

There was also a thought at the time that the internship or first year was equivalent to a "rotating" internship, followed by specialty education. At that time some programs in the country offered two years of emergency medicine following a rotating internship consisting of month-long experiences in medicine, surgery and other disciplines.

The decision to proceed with the application listing only one resident per year was difficult. During one of the seemingly endless conversations with Manuel Tzagournis, MD, about starting the residency program, he finally agreed to proceed. He told the faculty, "Let's start with one resident." Thinking that one was better than no residents at all, the faculty agreed. The first application requested permission to create a program with one resident per year for a total of three residents in the entire program!

Tzagournis was the undisputed decision maker in the hospital at that time and there was no choice but to proceed with his decision. It was not clear why there was initial reluctance to approve additional residents, but there may have been the thought among other departments that creating emergency medicine resident slots may have diminished the possibility of expanding their own programs even though over 40 residency positions at Ohio State remained unfilled.

On April 15, 1980, Brooks Bock, MD, conducted a site visit. Bock had been the first emergency medicine program director at the Detroit Receiving Hospital, which was affiliated with Wayne State University. Emergency medicine had progressed rapidly in Detroit since the riots of 1967. The need for greater organization in the Detroit hospital had led to intensive recruitment of faculty and residents. The new vision had been led by Ronald Krome, MD, the young surgeon director of the emergency department mentioned earlier in connection with his unsuccessful recruitment to Ohio State in 1975. Bock eventually became Chairman of the Department of Emergency Medicine at Wayne State and President of the American College of Emergency Medicine and later President of the American Board of Emergency Medicine.

Soon after the site visit, the Ohio State program was informed that it would not be endorsed by the LREC. The main criticism was that one resident per year was simply not enough. Other criticisms were that the program site had too few patients and that the block rotations did not offer enough experience in the emergency department. Other criticisms regarded a lack of journal club, the absence of a patient follow-up process and the need for more education about emergency department administration. Years later Bock was interviewed about the site visit. He remembered visiting the program. He did not recall all the details, but opined the following:

> *It does make sense that the LREC rejected the request to train one resident per year. I suspect that may have helped your institution get more funded slots for EM.*[2]

The rejection galvanized emergency medicine leadership. One resident per year was clearly not enough. The specialty was becoming popular with medical students, so a more robust program with four residents per year could certainly be expected to be filled with high quality students from U.S. medical schools. This seemed all the more reasonable considering the number of residency positions at Ohio State left unfilled each year. The months following the rejection of the approval were focused on finding a way to substantially expand the program. New funds would be needed to pay for resident salaries and additional clinical opportunities for the residents might be found which would improve the overall education.

It was time to meet again with Riverside!

The key emergency physicians at Riverside Methodist Hospital were Samuel Kiehl, MD, and Nancy Trhlik, MD, who had also been working occasionally in the Ohio State Emergency Department. Kiehl immediately recognized the opportunity. The general idea was that the program would be one in which Ohio State and Riverside each would have half the resident time and each would pay for half the residents. Combining the program with Riverside would carry other advantages: The volume of ED patients at Riverside was approximately double that of Ohio State, and Riverside had a sizable emergency medicine attending staff. Years later, Kiehl remembered the conversation with Rund in this way:

> *We talked about the residency: that you had applied and been rejected, because of not having enough resident positions, clinical experience or sufficient dedicated staff. So, you came over and explained to me what you wanted to do. I said that sounded wonderful, we would love to participate. We were eager and willing and able partners.*[3]

Meetings were quickly arranged with the leadership at Riverside. One key individual was Donald J. Vincent, MD, Director of Medical Education. Vincent was born in Portsmouth, Ohio, in 1912. He received his BA and MD degrees from Ohio State in 1937. He then interned at White Cross Hospital, the forerunner of Riverside Methodist Hospital; following that, Vincent became a general practitioner in Utica, Ohio, for several years.

"Realizing he needed more education, and discovering he had no time to even glance at medical journals while practicing in Utica, Vincent took additional training in internal medicine at the St. Joseph's Infirmary in Louisville, Kentucky."[4] He then began a successful practice in internal medicine at Riverside for many years. He was the Director of Medical Education from 1969 to 1984. Vincent engineered or enhanced affiliations for Riverside with Ohio State residency programs in urology, neurology and neurosurgery. He also established independent residency training programs in internal medicine, general surgery and obstetrics-gynecology. He won many teaching awards in his career.

According to George Paulson, MD, prominent Ohio State and Riverside neurologist, Vincent was an excellent bedside teacher, always insisting on a complete physical examination of the patient, "which meant always including a rectal examination. Paulson goes on to quote the Osler aphorism: 'one finger in the throat and one in the rectum make a good diagnostician.'"[4]

Given Vincent's passion for building residency programs with Ohio State, he was enthusiastic about the possibility of sharing the emergency medicine residency. He agreed with the arrangement in which up to two residents per year would be employees of Riverside Methodist Hospital and two would be employees of the Ohio State University Hospitals, and that the number of months spent at each institution would be roughly equal. Both hospitals would support resident salaries while they were on duty at Children's Hospital. In addition, there was always the very real possibility that, if this couldn't be worked out, Riverside would consider starting a program of its own.

Facing a very real deadline in order to begin the residency program in 1981, the Ohio State leadership agreed to the proposal and a new request was sent to the LREC. On August 21, 1980, the site visit was conducted by Harvey Meislin, MD, who at the time was in transition. He had been teaching and practicing at the University of California in Los Angeles until August of 1980 and moved to the University of Arizona in September, 1980. He became Section Chief of the Emergency Medicine, Associate Chair of Surgery and, finally, Chair of the Department of Emergency Medicine at Arizona when the department was finally was established in 2001.

Meislin later went on to become the President of the American Board of Emergency Medicine and the Chair of the American Board of Medical Specialties (ABMS). He was the first emergency physician to hold the leadership position at ABMS, representing tremendous progress since 1979, a time when ABEM was held in such high suspicion that it had to be created with a board containing representatives from seven other boards. Interestingly, Meislin completed the emergency medicine residency at the University of Chicago where Peter Rosen, MD, was the head of the department. This was the same year that Rosen visited Ohio State to consider the position of Director of Emergency Services.

In later years Meislin remembered this about the site visit:

> *It was a very pleasant visit with the leaders of the program and the institution. I do not have any negative memories about the Ohio State residency. In that regard, my assumption is that the program, at that stage of development, was meeting or exceeding all objective criteria we were asked to evaluate.*[5]

The Ohio State EM residency program was approved shortly after the site visit, allowing plenty of time to interview residency candidates who would ultimately begin the new three-year program on July 1, 1981.

RICHARD N. NELSON, MD

At the same time the new residency began, a new physician, Richard N. "Rick" Nelson, MD, joined the faculty (Figure 2). Nelson graduated from the Ohio State University College of Medicine in 1978 and completed a residency in emergency medicine at Akron City Hospital in 1981. The Akron program was among the first in the nation, having been established in 1975. During his third year of residency in Akron, Nelson heard of the new program starting at Ohio State the following summer. He had always been interested in resident education and indeed had given a number of well-received lectures for his fellow residents and attendings during their Tuesday and Thursday morning lectures. In December 1980, during a coronary care unit rotation, he called the Ohio State emergency department to inquire about a position.

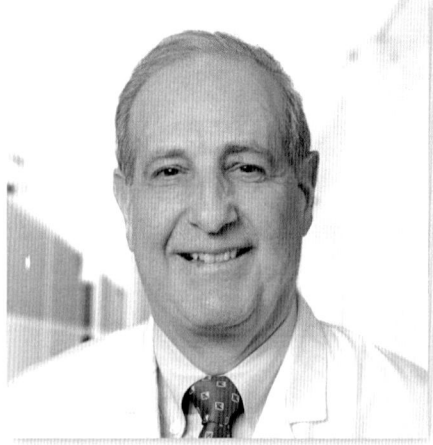

Figure 2: Richard N. Nelson, MD, was the first physician in central Ohio to have completed an Emergency Medicine residency. He joined the Ohio State faculty in 1981 and designed the first residency curriculum. He went on to become Vice Chair for Clinical Affairs and President of the American Board of Emergency Medicine.

The department's medical director, Douglas Rund, MD, spoke with him, confirming the department was looking to recruit faculty for the new residency program. A few weeks later, Nelson drove down to Columbus for an interview. There he met with Rund, Chris Dailey, the department administrator, and a number of other physicians, including Martin "Marty" Keller, MD, Chair of Preventive Medicine (under which Emergency Medicine was a division), Larry Carey, MD, Chief of Surgery, and Calvin Kunin, MD, Chair of Internal Medicine. He also met Riverside's Nancy Trhlik, MD. He recalls being taken to lunch at the Faculty Club where his group stopped at the large table near the second-floor dining room entrance to say hello to then football coach Woody Hayes, who was eating lunch at his usual table that he shared with any other faculty members who would otherwise be eating alone.

Nelson's most vivid memory, though, was his meeting with Kunin, who, like cardiology professor Richard Lewis, MD, a few years before, told him that training in Internal Medicine would have been preferable to training in EM for the job he was applying. It is worth noting, however, that within a few years of this interview and after EM was established at Ohio State, Lewis and Kunin both became avid supporters of the EM residency and of the specialty. Regardless, Nelson was offered and accepted a faculty position at Ohio State. It was the only job for which he applied.

Nelson's official start date was July 1, but he had a number of meetings in June to meet the new residents, help set up the July conference schedule, get oriented and credentialed, and find a place to live. Also, he was surprised to find out that not only he would be the first residency trained emergency physician at Ohio State, he would also be the first such physician in Central Ohio! Because he was the only one to have gone through an emergency medicine (EM) program, he was asked to provide much input in both the clinical and didactic curriculums for the new program. Not surprisingly, his educational experiences at Akron City informed his vision of the curriculum.

Didactic Curriculum

The program's didactic curriculum, called the Lecture Series on Emergency Medicine, included both specific lectures such as "Subarachnoid Hemorrhage," and monthly general topic lectures, such as Radiology, EKG, Toxicology, and Morbidity and Mortality. Lectures would be given by Ohio State EM faculty and residents. Physicians from other specialties and other institutions also presented at these conferences. The monthly radiology conference was given by Charles Mueller, MD, a popular Ohio State radiologist with a special interest in emergency radiology. Most of the monthly toxicology lectures were given by Phil Walson, MD, director of Poison Control at Columbus Children's Hospital.

Another monthly conference, the "Simulated Patient Encounter," was a case-based conference presented in the form of the ABEM oral examination, with a faculty member serving as the "examiner" and a resident the examinee. The purpose of this conference was to familiarize the residents with oral board format and also provide a diagnostic and clinical experience.

Nelson set up the didactic curriculum to reflect the "Core Content in Emergency Medicine," a national document whose purpose was to more or less standardize training across all programs. The Ohio State lecture series was designed to cover the Core Content over two years, and then repeat; this way, all EM residents should have covered the entire Core Content at least once during their training, taking into account some months or weeks they wouldn't be able to attend lectures due to off-service rotations, vacations, illness or other reasons. Similar to the Akron City program, lectures would be given on Tuesday and Thursday from 8 a.m. to 10 a.m., conveniently ending about the same time the ED would start getting busier. In later years, the lecture series would be for four or five hours on Tuesday, and later still, on Wednesday.

In addition, a monthly journal club was established. Initially held at the Faculty Club, it was soon moved to homes of faculty members in deference to more reasonable food and beverage expenses. Attendance was generally quite good and often included Marty Keller and his wife Geraldine "Geri," herself a PhD faculty member with an excellent understanding of research methodology and statistical analysis, though not specific to emergency medicine. Nelson recalls one of the first journal clubs at the Faculty Club in which Marty and Geri participated.

> We were reviewing some articles from the pre-eminent and perhaps only emergency medicine journal at the time, Journal of the American College of Emergency Physicians (JACEP), which would later become Annals of Emergency Medicine. Granted, many of the articles reflected a somewhat primitive version of research methodology and were heavily represented by case reports and observational studies. Nonetheless, this was our journal and our specialty and we discussed each article enthusiastically. Toward the end of the journal club, Geri Keller, who had been somewhat quiet

throughout, finally spoke up. "They really publish this stuff?" she exclaimed, causing us all to reflect on the long journey ahead before this new specialty could claim true academic legitimacy.

The lecture series was created to teach important clinical topics in emergency medicine and to present material unique to the practice of emergency medicine in the constant effort to identify that it was a unique specialty. Sample lecture topics and presenters from the first eight months of the program are as follows:

- Chest Pain – Dave Roberts, MD

- EKG conference – Richard Nelson, MD

- Hypertensive Emergencies – Kendel Kidwell, MD

- Radiology Conference – C-spine – Charles Mueller, MD

- Toxicology Conference – Tricyclics – Richard Nelson, MD

- Morbidity and Mortality – Douglas Rund, MD

- Simulated Patient Encounter – Douglas Rund, MD

- Testicular Pain – Michael Moore, MD

- Approach to Headache – Patrick Hayes, MD

- Trauma Education Conference (held at Riverside)

- Organic versus Functional Psychiatric Disorders – Douglas Rund, MD

- Tylenol and Aspirin Overdose – Richard Nelson, MD

- Reye's Syndrome – Greg Barrett, MD (Pediatrics)

- Alcohol Intoxication – Dennis Bambach, MD

- Research Methods – Martin Keller, MD, PhD

- Hypothermia, Frostbite – Richard Nelson, MD

- Mesenteric Thrombosis – Jeff Fabri, MD (General Surgery)

- PCP and Amphetamines – Phil Walson, MD (Toxicology)

- Skiing Injuries – Robert Behrendt, MD

- Respiratory and Diabetic Emergencies – Nancy Trhlik, MD

- Evaluation of the Impaired Hand – Howard Werman, MD

Clinical Curriculum

The clinical curriculum was also modeled after the Akron City program. In addition to rotations in both Ohio State and Riverside emergency departments, the off-service rotations included internal medicine, cardiology, pediatrics, pediatric EM, toxicology, neurology, hand surgery, orthopedics, critical care, anesthesiology, ob-gyn, and two months at The Maryland Shock Trauma Center in Baltimore, with the department renting an apartment for the residents in Columbia, Maryland.

Nelson also soon became medical director of both Grandview Heights and City of Westerville Fire Department/Emergency Medical Services (EMS) systems. In these capacities, he gave residents the opportunity to work with him and help teach the monthly educational conferences for these departments. Because firefighters, including Emergency Medical Technicians (EMTs), worked 24 hours on and 48 hours off, the monthly educational conferences were repeated on three consecutive days each month for each department so that all EMTs could attend. Over the years a number of residents who worked with Nelson went on to distinguished careers in pre-hospital care, including Howard Werman, MD, Medical Director of Medflight, and Ron Pirrallo, EMS director for the city of Milwaukee and President of the National Association of Emergency Medicine Services Physicians.

Residency Program Administration

The new EM residency program administration was truly a "barebones" operation. Rund served as overall program director. Nelson served as the equivalent of associate program director for University Hospitals, though no such title was conferred. Thrlik served in a similar position with respect to Riverside Hospital. Another important member of the administration team was Christine A. "Chris" Dailey, who functioned as residency coordinator in addition to her other duties as division administrator, financial officer, bookkeeper, scheduler, and anything else that the division or residency needed done.

Finally, Ed Whitehead, a semi-retired military man and former operator with the Preventive Medicine aerospace medicine program, functioned in numerous capacities on an as-needed basis for both the clinical and educational aspects of the division. During the first year of the program, all residency-related activities by the administrators were additional responsibilities not necessarily compensated with additional funding or reduced workload in other areas.

The First Residents

Two residents entered the program with advanced standing: They had completed one year of approved training at another institution. The two residents were Michael Moore, MD, and Kendel "Ken" Kidwell, MD (Figure 3). Moore left the program midway through his first year to pursue training in internal medicine, leaving Kidwell as the sole senior resident. After Kidwell had completed his undergraduate and medical school studies at Ohio State, he chose to enter the emergency medical residency at Geisinger Medical Center in Pennsylvania. He became disenchanted with the program, however, and heard about the new Ohio State program from his older brother, who was a chief resident in internal medicine at the time. Years later Kidwell remembered this about the program:

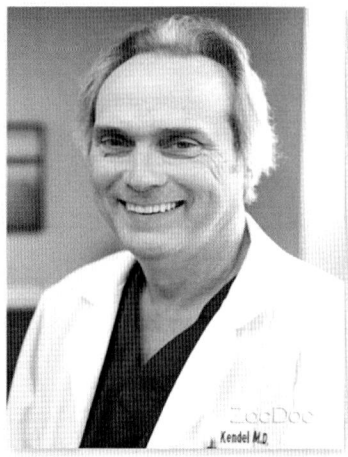

Figure 3: Kendel "Ken" Kidwell, MD, was the first emergency medicine resident at Ohio State.

> *We were pioneering as we went along. I remember us sitting down and going over the curriculum and what you had already struc-*

tured and what you got by input from me and the other residents. I think things went pretty smoothly with this being a new start-up program. I think it was well structured from the stand point of having two sites, which I don't think was all that common at that time...having the university hospital...as well a large community teaching hospital and Riverside and faculty at both sites. Their attendings were good and their volume was a little higher at the time. It was a teaching hospital but not the pure academics of Ohio State. I think things were very smooth. Everyone was eager to teach us and I think we were eager to learn at the same time.[6]

Kidwell finished his residency and ultimately moved to Abington, Pennsylvania, where he became chief of emergency medicine at Abington Hospital. Later in his career he founded an urgent care center, Patient Care Now, in Fairless Hills, Pennsylvania.

In addition to the two second-year residents there were four first-year residents who were scheduled to complete the full three years of the program. Two were employees of Riverside and two were employees of Ohio State. Robert Behrendt, MD, who was an Ohio State medical school graduate, later recalled his impressions of the program:

We were pathfinders to an extent. It wasn't entirely clear at that time that the program was even going to succeed. The sort of initial situation was that other residents were co-signing our orders on certain rotations; and there was just a lot of apprehension about what emergency medicine was about and who these folks were. There was a lot of responsibility or seeming responsibility on our residents to prove ourselves. We were carrying the banner if you will. We all took it seriously and I think we did everything we could to advance. It wasn't certain to be a successful endeavor. Emergency Medicine had been established in certain areas, but it hadn't been

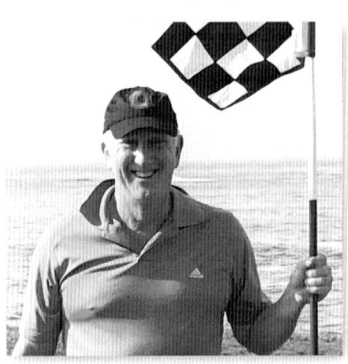

Figure 4: Robert "Bob" Behrendt, MD, was in the first full class of graduating residents in emergency medicine at Ohio State. Here he is years later finishing with a "birdie" on the 7th hole at Pebble Beach Golf Links in California.

established at Ohio State.[7]

Behrendt completed the program in 1984 and went on to practice in Hawaii where he established a popular Ohio State EM third-year rotation at the Kaiser Permanente Medical Center in Honolulu. (Figure 4)

Michael Kelley, MD, University of Cincinnati medical school graduate, was also one of the first-year residents in 1981. Kelley later remembered this about the program:

> *We suggested some different changes. One of the things I know that we had influence in changing was the orthopedic rotation. Based on our input, we did one month of adult orthopedics, one month of pediatric orthopedics and one month of hand. I think the hand rotation was one of the very best rotations that we had at that time. There are a lot of hand injuries that occur. One of the attending hand surgeons thought that every person who came into the emergency room had a hand injury!*[8]

Kelley completed the program in 1984 and became a full-time faculty member. He later completed a fellowship in Medical Toxicology and enjoyed a successful career in Toxicology and Occupational Medicine (Figure 5).

Howard "Howie" Werman, MD, was another one of the first residents. Werman grew in Long Island, New York, graduated from Duke University and enrolled in medical school at the State University of New York in Buffalo. During his senior year in November 1980, Werman completed an elective rotation in emergency medicine at the Akron City Hospital, living with his grandfather who had graduated from Ohio State in 1926 in the College of Pharmacy.

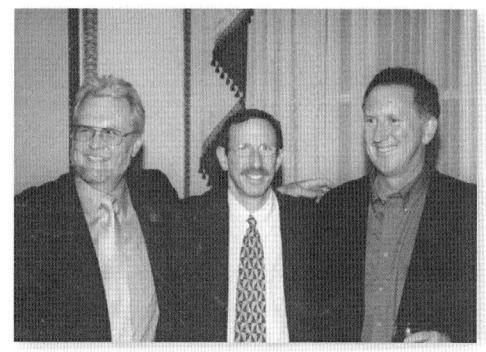

Figure 5: Three of the original four residents in emergency medicine 19 years later. From left: Michael Kelley MD, Howard Werman, MD, and Robert Behrendt, MD. Photo taken at the 25-anniversary celebration of Ohio State Emergency Medicine in 2003

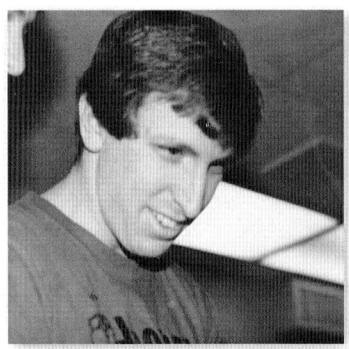

Figure 6: Howard A. "Howie" Werman, MD, as a medical student reviewing match results that showed him to be a member of the first full class of residents in emergency medicine at Ohio State

He interviewed at Ohio State and was impressed with the proposed program. Additionally, physicians at Akron City informed him that one of their senior residents, Richard Nelson, MD, had expressed an interest in joining the faculty of the Columbus program. As fate would have it, Werman matched at Ohio State and started his residency on July 1, 1981 (Figure 6). Werman recalls how challenging the early days of his residency were at Ohio State:

Dealing with other medical specialties who didn't understand or respect Emergency Medicine presented some difficult situations. In one particular instance, Dr. Behrendt was seen pushing a cart onto an elevator with a medical resident trying to resist, insisting that his workup needed to be completed despite the fact that the bed was needed for a more critical patient. Additionally, with only four residents each year, the idea of graded responsibility was difficult to institute. On the other hand, we were fortunate to have great role models, including our first faculty member, Dr. Nelson. He challenged us to have a strong depth and breadth of knowledge and skills so that we would be able to prove our worth on the services on which we rotated. Acceptance did eventually come over time. On the other hand, as new residents, we were provided a great opportunity to provide input into the program rotations, thanks to the openness of our program faculty.[9]

Werman completed the program in 1984 and did an EM research fellowship at Ohio State under Charles Brown, MD, before his long and successful career at Ohio State.

Rounding out the first class of EM interns who began together in 1981 was Dennis Bambach, MD. Bambach graduated in 1984 and went on to a successful career in EM at Riverside Methodist Hospital/OhioHealth.

Early Speculation on the Acceptance of a New Residency and a New Specialty by an Established Academic Medical Center and Beyond

Martin D. Keller, MD, the Chairman of Preventive Medicine introduced in Chapter 2 was a true visionary (Figure 7). Though an expert in epidemiology and public health, he was quite knowledgeable about emergency medicine and emergency medical services. He was always deeply involved in the development of the Division of Emergency Medicine. He worked hard with the emergency medicine faculty to prepare the first application for a residency program to the Liaison Residency Endorsement Committee. He was most insightful and even *prescient* in his assessment of how emergency medicine should develop. *Was this indeed a specialty?* He included the following essay in the first residency application in 1980.

Some Thoughts Regarding the Content of a Residency Program in Emergency Medicine

Martin D. Keller, MD, PhD

One of the key problems facing the establishment of a residency program in emergency medicine arises from the understandable question, "In what way is this indeed a specialty?" This is of particular importance to us in considering the establishment of a residency in an academic institution such as the Ohio State University College of Medicine. Unless we can convince ourselves and our colleagues in other departments that this specialty area can take its place along with other established specialty areas, it is doomed to remain a program assigned, at best, second class status.

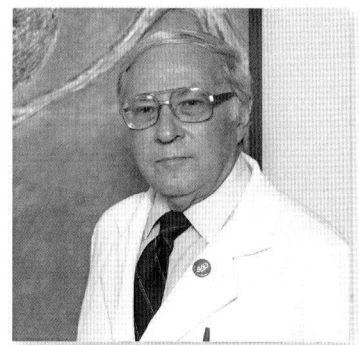

Figure 7: Martin D. "Marty" Keller, MD, Chairman of the Department of Preventive Medicine who accepted emergency medicine into his department as a division. Dr. Keller was a visionary who posited several answers to the question, "in what way is this indeed a specialty?".

The question before us is, in essence, how can we structure a residency in emergency medicine so that it may have sufficient academic strength to be recognized as worthy in the academic community and yet have as its specific aim the education of leadership in the field of emergency medicine. This is clearly a prerequisite to justification of the investment of our resources and energies in the development of such a residency in this setting.

1. **The structure of the community health care system, with special emphasis on emergency medical services:** It is necessary for the potential leader in emergency medicine to understand the history and development of emergency medical services in the setting of the overall community health care system. Against this background it is possible to examine the changing organization and role of emergency medical care in our society and to gain some insight into future trends.

2. **Current issues in the delivery and financing of health care with specific emphasis on emergency medical services:** This should include a review of key items of legislation affecting the organization of health care delivery and financing mechanisms involving third party payment, prepaid systems, etc.

3. **Medicolegal issues of particular interest to emergency medical care:** This includes an understanding of the key providers, varieties of personnel, services, licensure/certification, and issues of responsibility and liability.

4. **The principles of epidemiology as applied to the study of emergency medical problems:** This involves an examination of the causes of major emergency medical problems, approaches to prevention, and alternative methods of delivering emergency care. Epidemiology concerns itself with the distribution and determinants of specific medical problems and with their natural history. One of the shortcomings of the emergency medical specialty has been a lack of attention to the antecedents of the cases seen by the providers of emergency care and the follow-up of subsequent care, complications, and outcomes. The importance of understanding the medical spectrum of the key conditions, from cause to onset to acute event to emergency and subsequent care to outcome, cannot

be overstressed in building this specialty. Only through such means can the clinical information be dovetailed with medical science to generate research, develop effective and appropriate "rounds" in emergency medicine and lend academic content to the overall specialty area.

5. Research methods in emergency medical care: Such methods are at present being developed in a number of medical centers. They include attention to all phases of the emergency case, as noted in the above paragraph. Residents must have some experience in collecting and analyzing relevant research data. It is my feeling that in the course of a three-year residency, every resident should be given at least one opportunity to carry out or collaborate in a worthy research endeavor.

6. Evaluation of emergency medical services: This is closely related to research methodology, involving the assessment of the structure, process, outcome and impact of specifically defined elements in the emergency health care delivery system. Such evaluation studies can be based in an emergency department, in a set of such departments, or in the community at large.

7. Management and administration of emergency medical services: This deals with regional and local systems as well as the hospital emergency departments per se. It should include the matter of hospital emergency department categorization, triage mechanisms in pre-hospital care, and in the emergency department, staffing and the division of activities and responsibilities. Attention should also be given to the physical structure of an emergency department, patterns of patient flow, information systems and varieties of emergency department equipment and linkage with labs.

8. Training of persons involved in pre-hospital emergency care: It is important for the resident to understand the role of public action in emergencies, the nature of first responders, the training and responsibilities of emergency medical technicians, the role of the community physician and the nature and operation of emergency communication systems. There has been enormous growth in the sophistication of communication systems and it is important for potential leaders in the field of emergency medicine to understand the problems of interaction between the public and the system and the concept of the base hospital for online consultation to pre-hospital care.

9. Social and behavioral aspects of emergency medical service utilization: This is important for an understanding for both the pre-hospital and the in-hospital utilization of emergency services. It includes an understanding of the knowledge, attitudes and practices of consumers and providers; how these are rooted in the culture of the region; the history of the emergency services; and the contemporary scene of a given community and the country-at-large.

10. The emergency medical record: This is a key element in many of the items mentioned above, including the pre-hospital record, the emergency department record and special forms provided for case follow-up. They are crucial for the development of effective case studies to be used in the development of hypotheses for research, for the development of emergency medical rounds and for the education of the residents and other physicians and paramedical personnel in the academic institution and in the community.

11. Data collection and processing: This concerns basic statistical methods for monitoring and evaluating emergency services and is essential for the effective management of an emergency department and for advising and guiding community emergency medical service systems. It also serves the case study and the research efforts.

12. Participation in programs of education in emergency medical care: Residents should have experience in understanding of educational programs for the public, for emergency medical technicians, for medical and allied medical students and trainees and for managers and administrators. There should also be some attention to the information needs of public officials and legislators, with emphasis on the emergency medical specialist as a spokesman for the specialty area.

13. The interfaces between EMS and primary medical care and the relationship to other medical specialties: A large and complex academic institution with affiliated hospitals offers an ideal situation for this aspect of the program. The residents should be given the opportunity to interact with community physicians as well as hospital based and academic personnel.

14. The relationship of EMS to other community health agencies and facilities: This should also be extended beyond hospitals and clinics to an understanding of the basic relationship of EMS to such general community factors as communication, transportation, political jurisdiction, public safety programs, disaster control, etc. Arrangements can be made for residents to spend some time as participant-observers in the appropriate public agencies.

15. Comparative emergency medical services: This may include regional, national and international systems, in the developed and in the less developed countries. It is important for individuals who will take leadership roles in emergency medicine to have some understanding of the varieties of organization and staffing of emergency medical care programs in different parts of the world.

16. Sources and uses of data relating to emergency medical problems and emergency medical services: The ability to obtain and utilize compilations of data relating to emergency medicine form the background for many academic and practical enterprises that may be undertaken by specialists and leaders in this field. The residents should have some understanding of what data exists and how to get into this material.

17. Key literature in emergency medicine and current clinical and research reports: It is unfortunate that many residency programs in the medical specialties do not cultivate the habit of staying in touch with key literature and current advances in the field. Through the mechanisms of journal clubs and special seminars it is important to assure that the residents have a thorough acquaintance with the literature and develop a pattern of keeping up with it.

18. Attendance at selected meetings and conferences: It is important for residents to become active on the local and national scenes while they are still in the residency programs. Arrangements should be made for appropriate memberships and participation in all years of the residency sequence.[10]

References

1. Zink, BJ. *Anyone, Anything, Anytime: A History of Emergency Medicine.* Philadelphia, PA: Mosby Elsevier; 2006.

2. Bock, B.: Interview of Brooks Bock, MD, by Douglas Rund, MD. 2022: Columbus, OH.

3. Kiehl, SJ.: Interview of Samuel J. Kiehl, MD, by Douglas Rund, MD. 2021: Columbus, OH.

4. Paulson, GW. In Pursuit of Excellence: The Ohio State University Medical Center from 1834 to 2010. Fremont, OH: Lesher Printers; pp: 255-257

5. Meislin H.: Interview of Harvey Meislin, MD, by Douglas Rund. 2021: MD, Columbus, OH.

6. Kidwell, K.: Interview of Kendel Kidwell, MD, by Douglas Rund, MD. 2022: Columbus, OH.

7. Behrendt, R.: Interview of Robert Behrendt MD, by Douglas Rund, MD. 2022: Columbus, OH.

8. Kelley MT.: Interview of Michael Kelley MD, by Douglas Rund, MD. 2022: Columbus, OH.

9. Werman HA.: Interview of Howard Werman MD, by Douglas Rund, MD. 2022: Columbus, OH.

10. Keller MD. Some thoughts regarding the content of a residency program in emergency medicine. From the first residency application from the Division of Emergency Medicine to the Liaison Residency Endorsement Committee, 1980.

Chapter 5

A Specialty Indeed: The Road to Department Status – 1981 to 1988

Douglas A. Rund, MD
Richard Nelson, MD

The plan for the future of the Division of Emergency Medicine was always to become a full academic department. The department would be the equal of other full departments in the Ohio State College of Medicine. The faculty would participate in leadership discussions and have a full vote in bodies such as the Council of Chairs and the Medical Center Executive Committee.

The location of the division in the Department of Preventive Medicine had a purpose: to be nurtured and protected in an academic environment and eventually be able to emerge as a full academic department when ready. The University designated such departments as Tenure Initiating Units. Becoming an academic department in universities was a major goal of academic emergency medicine leaders throughout the country.

In its beginning, in 1977, Emergency Medicine was an infant and there was the very real worry that becoming part of a dominant department such as Medicine or Surgery would make it difficult or impossible to separate at some point. Emergency medicine units in other medical schools faced that very same problem and thus remained in these powerful departments for many years. As it turned out, years later, the Chair of the Department of Surgery was the only member of the Council of Chairs who voted against elevating Emergency Medicine to department status in 1990. When asked later why she voted this way, she replied: "I think you belong in the Department of Surgery."

The choice of Preventive Medicine was optimal for other reasons. In Preventive Medicine, the Division of Emergency Medicine was the predominant *clinical* unit. Physicians were actively seeing and treating patients. In the past, the Department of Preventive Medicine had been home to a few clinical faculty in aviation medicine and occupational medicine. With time, however, emergency medicine faculty eventually outnumbered the rest of the faculty in the department.

Martin Keller MD, PhD, the department Chair, and the rest of the preventive medicine faculty were also incredibly supportive of emergency medicine. Unlike other departments, they were never looking to keep the division forever and worked hard to teach the faculty about the teaching, scholarly activity and research expectations of a university faculty member. Preventive Medicine leaders also had eyes on another goal: to eventually morph into a School of Public Health within the University.

Emergency Medicine faced big challenges, however, when it came to the politics of becoming a full academic department within the university. In the existing departments there was the worry that the establishment of a new department would reduce their own resources. A secondary worry was that good teaching cases in the emergency department might not be available to residents in medicine and surgery after the installation of emergency medicine faculty and residents.

These two concerns created real obstacles at nearly every medical school in the country. The more prestigious the institution, the more resistance to establishment of a department of emergency medicine in the medical school. Although there were real major issues related to turf, money and teaching for medical and surgical residents, one of the most publicly declared arguments against designation of emergency medicine as an independent specialty was this: *Is emergency medicine really a specialty?* Or do emergency room doctors just take what they know from publications and textbooks of real specialists such as cardiologists or surgeons?

In a 1978 a panel presentation about emergency physicians and university teaching hospitals included three emergency department directors: Ronald Krome, MD, David Wagner, MD, and Joseph Moylan MD. Krome and Wagner were emergency physician pioneers who had initially been trained as surgeons. Moylan was a surgeon at Duke University given responsibility for the emergency department. The dialog was published in the *Archives of Surgery* in 1978. The discussion seems anachronistic today but was highly relevant at that time when emergency rooms at teaching hospitals were usually staffed only by interns and residents, and surgeons were the directors.

The comments from emergency physicians seem tepid in retrospect. Krome argued for full-time emergency faculty to ensure proper student teaching. He opined that "every medical student should be adequately trained in the provision of basic emergency medical care. Most medical students in the United States are not even trained to the level of emergency medical technicians." He also argued the following:

> *The provision of emergency medicine faculty overseeing the activities of residents both in emergency medicine and in other specialties hopefully ensures improved patient care, as well as a consistent educational program.*[1]

Focusing on the student education piece was also a strategy used in the early days of emergency medicine at Ohio State. The area seemed to be "neutral ground" since education was presumably the justification for the existence of a medical school in the first place.

Both Wagner and Krome strongly agreed that residency programs to train emergency physicians were an obligation to the community and were important to ensure that qualified physicians staffed the emergency department. Wagner further opined that such training should be done in a university:

> *To allow the responsibility for educating health professionals whose role in the university is still evolving to pass to non-university sites would be an abdication of basic responsibility and an invitation to further perfusion of nonrelevant teaching activities.*[1]

Presumably the "nonrelevant teaching" was that provided by the traditional specialties, which may or may not directly relate to the realities of emergency medicine.

In response to the dialog, one of the journal editors, Ben Eiseman, MD, the Chair of the Department of Surgery at the University of Colorado, wrote an editorial comment summarizing the most common argument by academic physicians opposing emergency medicine: Is it truly a specialty? Eiseman wrote the following:

> *No dispassionate critic can doubt that the emergency room is a busy money-making place that serves an important clinical service. To me, this clearly qualifies it for hospital departmental status. But this does not equate with a university or medical school department. Emergency medical services must answer some critical questions to qualify for university departmental status. Service and ability to generate income are not enough. To thus qualify as a serious identifiable new discipline and area of scholarly pursuit, these leaders in emergency medical services should answer such questions as these:*
>
> *1. Identify the intellectual discipline and body of basic knowledge in which the emergency medical service clearly is more expert than any other existing specialty.*
>
> *2. Define the specific area of emergency service research. Is it not primarily a system analysis approach to find better methods of applying knowledge and techniques discovered and more thoroughly understood by others? Is such purely applied "research" really worthy of university or academic departmental status?*
>
> *3. In medical student or resident teaching, where can the emergency medical service be more expert in instruction concerning any one disease than the physicians who specialize in that discipline? Does not emergency service teaching primarily consist of skimming off a horizontal slice of the identification and treatment of the early stages of disease that true specialists know about in depth?* [2]

Eiseman was a constant critic of Peter Rosen, MD, during Rosen's tenure in Denver. Rosen, who had turned down an offer from Ohio State in 1975, had moved on to become Chief of Emergency Medical Services at Denver General Hospital in 1977. Eiseman blocked the appointment of Rosen and the emergency physicians from faculty appointments at the University of Colorado. Rosen and the faculty eventually were forced to create a relationship with the Oregon Health Sciences University where they finally obtained faculty appointments.

Still, the message articulated by Eiseman was clear: Emergency medicine must develop its own specialized body of knowledge and conduct meaningful research to create and enlarge this knowledge. The specialty must also offer unique, valuable education to residents and students.

The earliest specialties were Ophthalmology (1916) and Otolaryngology (1924). In an article marking the 75th anniversary of the American Board of Otolaryngology, two authors wrote the following about a specialty:

> *Specialization within medicine follows the creation of knowledge and the growth of science and technology. It typically occurs as a result of advances in a clinical field or the development of diagnostic or therapeutic technology. As physicians gain expertise in a given area, they begin to exchange information with others interested in the field. Subsequently they form an organization, meet formally to share ideas and advances and publish their work. As interested peers learn of the organization, membership in the organization becomes a mark of distinction, more interested physicians join and a specialty is born.*[3]

As far back as the early part of the 20th century, both ophthalmology and otolaryngology were so specialized that they were justified in having their own specialty board, residency program and academic departments. There was too much unique knowledge in skill required to be mastered by the general surgeon.

In 1977, however, to most of the outside medical world, emergency medicine did not have a distinct, specialized body of knowledge. As a consequence, perhaps, there were only three academic departments of emergency medicine in the country. The leaders of emergency medicine at Ohio State and other universities realized that they must develop all the trappings of an academic specialty: textbooks, journals, several courses for medical students, residency programs, subspecialties and fellowships, certifying boards, specialty examinations and national organizations with meetings and scientific presentations.

This was a big challenge for the faculty, which was quite small throughout the 1980s. Although various other faculty members served for short periods of time in that era, the core faculty members were Howard A. Werman, MD; Charles G. Brown, MD; David E. Roberts,

MD; Thomas Bullock, MD; Douglas A. Rund, MD; and Richard N. Nelson MD (Figure 1).

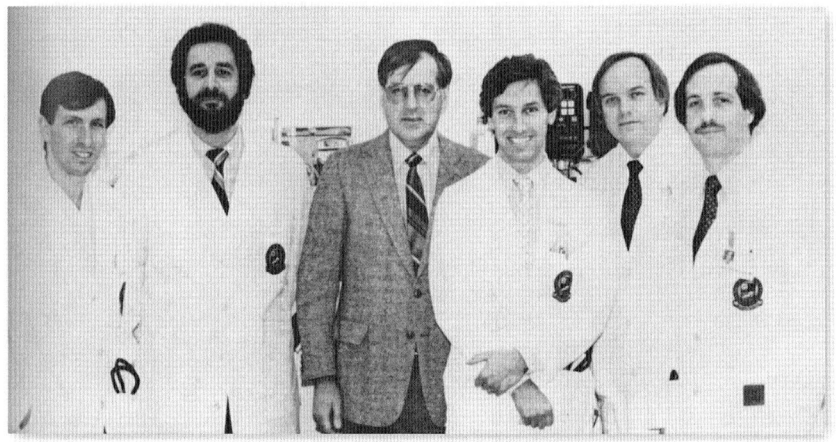

Figure 1: Core faculty members in the Division of Emergency Medicine in the mid-1980s. From left: Howard A. Werman, MD; Charles G. Brown, MD; David E. Roberts, MD; Thomas Bullock, MD; Douglas A. Rund, MD; and Richard N. Nelson, MD. Source: Ohio State College of Medicine, The Caducean, 1986.

Characteristics of Established Medical Specialties

Textbooks

In 1977 there was no textbook of emergency medicine written by emergency physicians. As Zink described the situation:

> *Few of the early leaders of emergency medicine had the academic training or position to be able to embark on a textbook and their time was consumed with fighting the political battles for specialty recognition.*[4]

The first American textbook of emergency medicine was *Emergency Treatment and Management*, written by Thomas Flint, MD, in 1954. In his preface, Flint was probably the first author to use the term "emergency physician":

> *Many excellent texts are available covering first-aid procedures and surgical and medical care in acute conditions. The following pages, however, have a much more limited objective—the presentation of the treatment and management of the patient by the Emergency Physician from the first examination until disposition for definitive treatment can be arranged.*[5]

Flint defined the emergency physician in the following way:

> *the physician in charge of the patient in the emergency room, department or private office. In large hospitals this physician may be on a full-time basis; in smaller units he may have numerous other duties, or be on part-time emergency call. Too often he is an intern, resident or general practitioner of very limited experience in the management and treatment of acute conditions.*[5]

Two other textbooks were *Principles and Practice of Emergency Medicine*, edited by George Schwartz, MD, and published in 1979, and the *MGH Textbook of Emergency Medicine*, published in 1978 and edited by Earle W. Wilkins, Jr. MD, a Harvard surgeon. Both were collections of chapters written by specialists in medicine or surgery, not by emergency physicians. This was symbolic of the lack of identity as a separate specialty at that time.

The closest emergency medicine came to having its own textbook was *The Study Guide in Emergency Medicine*, written in 1979. This book was a large loose-leaf binder with hole-punched chapters that could be removed easily. The thought at the time was that each chapter could be replaced or added to as new information became available. The editors were Ronald Krome, MD, who had also turned down Ohio State's directorship offer in 1975, and Judith Tintinalli, MD. Both were educators at the Detroit Receiving Hospital. The study guide was developed initially from worksheets used to create the first emergency medicine board examination, held in 1980.

Rosen edited the first well-referenced comprehensive textbook of emergency medicine by and for emergency physicians titled *Emergency Medicine: Concepts and Clinical Practice*, which was published in 1983.

Essentials of Emergency Medicine

Douglas Rund, MD, Chief of Emergency Medicine at Ohio State, who had accepted the offer of directorship, wrote the first *single author* textbook of Emergency Medicine titled *Essentials of Emergency Medicine*, which was published in 1982. The book was written primarily for students who elected to take a one-month clerkship in emergency medicine and emergency physicians wanting a quick review in common clinical situations. It was written in a style and length that could be completed quickly in the early part of a clerkship to give quick overview and orientation to clinical emergency medicine.

The text was originally written by hand on yellow legal pads and laboriously transcribed by Christine A. "Chris" Dailey using the comparatively primitive techniques of the day—a typewriter, carbon paper, whiteout and the retyping of major revisions. Dailey was an essential individual within emergency medicine from its inception. She served consummately as secretary, division administrator, residency coordinator, financial officer, bookkeeper, scheduler and took care of any other needed tasks. She was an exceptionally talented individual who played an indispensable role in the ultimate success of the division and the department. The book was also published in Spanish. A second edition was published in 1986 (Figure 2).[6]

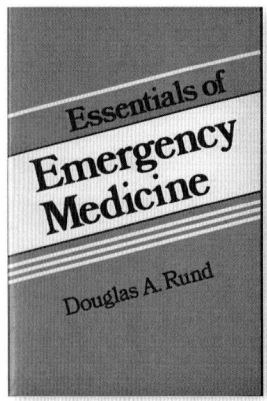
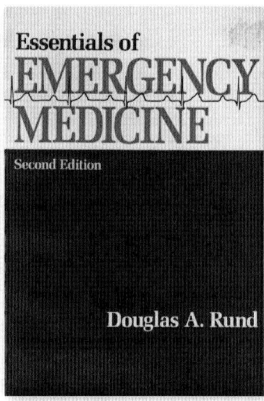
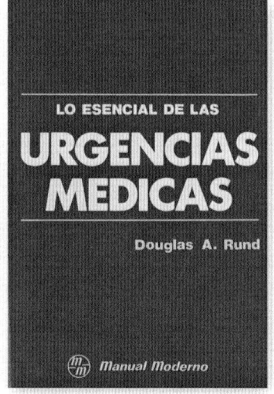

Figure 2: Second textbook in emergency medicine, *Essentials of Emergency Medicine*, written by an Ohio State Emergency Medicine faculty member, 1st edition, 1982

Figure 2: *Essentials of Emergency Medicine*, 2nd edition, 1986

Figure 2: *Essentials of Emergency Medicine*, Spanish Edition, 1985

Years later, the Executive Director of the American Board of Emergency Medicine, Earl J. Reisdorff, MD, wrote this about the book:

> *To this day, there is a dog-eared, sun-bleached copy of the* Essentials *within arm's reach of my desk. It's part of the legacy of our specialty. Dr. Rund's book was the launching point for many medical students interested in Emergency Medicine. It was the book to read when completing a rotation in the emergency department. The conceptual framework for the book mirrored the specialty—it was pragmatic, concise, and focused on treatment.*[7]

Writing the book created a text that was useful to students and physicians seeking a quick review of clinical topics common to emergency practice. But it had another, more pragmatic, purpose: to involve university medical leaders to participate in a scholarly educational endeavor that showed that emergency medicine was indeed becoming a distinct specialty. Rund wrote each chapter single handedly but asked prominent leaders at Ohio State to review the chapters associated with their specialty. The tactic had two objectives: Involve important faculty leaders in an academic emergency medicine project and foster the sense that emergency medicine was growing to become a distinct academic discipline.

Medical leaders at Ohio State were eager to help. The Chairman of Medicine, James V. Warren, MD, a cardiologist, reviewed the chapter on myocardial infarction. The Chairman of Surgery, Larry C. Carey, MD, reviewed the chapter on shock. The Dean of the College, Manuel Tzagournis, MD, an endocrinologist, reviewed the chapter on diabetic emergencies. The Chairman of Ophthalmology, William Havener, MD, reviewed the chapter on eye emergencies.

The Chairman of Otolaryngology, William H. Saunders, MD, reviewed the chapter on eye, ear, nose and throat emergencies, and the Chairman of Obstetrics and Gynecology, Frederick Zuspan, MD, reviewed the chapter on obstetrics and gynecologic emergencies. In total, there were 28 faculty reviewers from Ohio State.

The wording of the preface revealed elements of Rund's search for the essence of the specialty:

> **1.** Many of the conditions discussed represent potential or actual life-threatening emergencies where prompt care is necessary.

2. The clinical situations discussed occur with enough frequency that the emergency physician will be required to recognize and manage them at sometime early in his experience.

3. The emergency physician is expected to institute proper and accepted therapy in these conditions prior to the arrival of a specialist or the patient's primary care physician.[6]

Other characteristics of the specialty suggested in that early period were the need to understand causes and treatments of a wide variety of conditions (breadth of knowledge about many conditions) and to be able to quickly tease out elements of a patient assessment that signaled a serious condition that needed quick and efficient attention. The emergency physician must also have a comprehensive knowledge of the direst life-threatening emergencies that need immediate expert treatment (depth of knowledge about the most acute conditions).

Emergency Radiology and Emergency Psychiatry

Six additional textbooks were authored, co-authored or edited by emergency medicine faculty between 1980 and 1990: *Emergency Radiology: Self-Assessment* (Mueller and Rund) (Figure 3); *Emergency Psychiatry* (Rund and Hutzler) (Figure 4); *Environmental Emergencies* (Nelson,

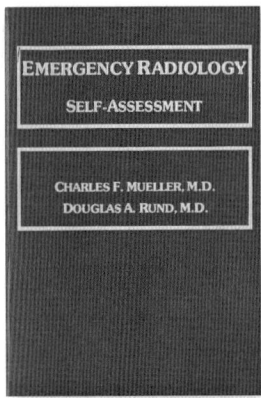
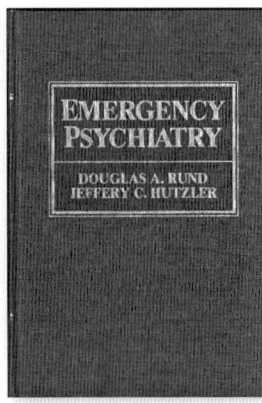
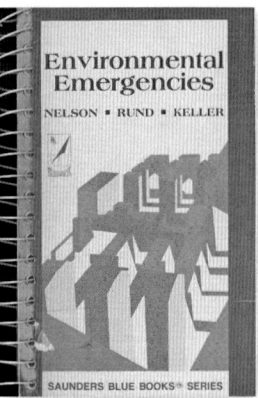

Figure 3: *Emergency Radiology: Self-Assessment*, by Charles F. Mueller, MD, and Douglas A. Rund, MD (Williams and Wilkins, Baltimore, MD, 1982)

Figure 4: *Emergency Psychiatry*, by Douglas A. Rund, MD, and Jeffery C. Hutzler, MD (Mosby, St. Louis, MO, 1983)

Figure 5: *Environmental Emergencies* by Richard N. Nelson, MD, Douglas A. Rund, MD, and Martin D. Keller, MD (W. B. Saunders, Philadelphia, PA, 1985)

Rund and Keller) (Figure 5); and three volumes of the *Emergency Medicine Annual* (1982-1984).

Emergency Radiology was written by Charles F. Mueller, MD, and Douglas Rund, MD. Mueller was a Professor of Radiology and Director of the Diagnostic Radiology Resident Training Program. An exceptional radiologist, Mueller developed a passion for interpreting radiographic studies taken in the emergency department. He led radiology teaching conferences for emergency medicine residents from the very beginning of the program.

He also spent time in the emergency department helping to teach residents, an unusual practice for radiologists of that era. He continued to be a dominant advocate of emergency medicine throughout the rest of his career. The *Emergency Radiology* book was written to meet the following objective:

> *This book is intended to present the radiology of emergency medicine in a way which is probably most effective for the clinician; the material is presented in the context of individual case studies. By viewing the radiograph as it applies to a specific clinical problem, the clinician enters into an activity of interpreting x-rays as they apply to real patients with real medical problems.*[9]

As with the *Essentials* book, *Emergency Radiology* involved a senior, respected faculty leader in a well-established department. The project was a scholarly educational endeavor. The goal was effective teaching, not turf or revenue. Writing the book, however, implied that *emergency physicians could interpret radiographs for their patients* (especially after hours) and reinforced the idea that this specialized skill was a unique part of a specialty that was different from other specialties.

It is interesting to note in retrospect that the book was written before the advent of digital radiology and computerized medical records. The images were, therefore, photographs of films reproduced as faithfully as possible on the pages of the book. There were no computerized tomography scans as they were just then coming into clinical use. Mueller became a champion for emergency medicine when the time came for the vote to establish the department.

Emergency Psychiatry was written by Rund and Jeffery C. Hutzler, MD, who was Assistant Professor and Chief of the Consultation-Liaison Service of the Department of Psychiatry. The objective of the book was the following:

> *To make emergency physicians as comfortable and adept with psychiatric disorders as they are with medical or surgical disorders and to ultimately improve the care of the psychiatrically-impaired patient in the emergency department.*[9]

Rund always had an interest in psychiatry and felt that it was one of the things omitted in his self-created five-year training program for emergency medicine at Stanford. Over the years he authored chapters dealing with psychiatric issues in all of the major textbooks. He also presented lectures in emergency psychiatry at national meetings. He always noted that attendance at his lectures fell off at meetings of the American College of Emergency Physicians if the lecture in the adjoining room dealt with billing and reimbursement, perhaps reflecting priorities in the minds of the early emergency physicians.

Environmental Emergencies

Environmental Emergencies was created and edited primarily by Richard N. Nelson, MD. The text was one of the Blue Book series published by W. B. Saunders Company in 1985. This series addressed a wide range of clinical areas and the volumes were published in spiral bound, pocket-sized books. As the publisher noted, the books "give ready access to the facts which form the foundation upon which sound health care practice is based…and help clinicians remain current. Each is a valuable clinical tool—as important to patient care as a stethoscope or blood pressure cuff."[10]

Nelson attended medical school at Ohio State and then completed three years of residency training in the new specialty of Emergency Medicine at Akron City Hospital. During the course of his education, he was often disturbed by both the unintentional and intentional references used by others to describe his chosen specialty. Even during his student years at Ohio State, faculty members who he greatly respected advised him to pursue residency training in Internal Medicine. They reasoned that a well-trained internist could supposedly practice in any setting, including the emergency room.

Residents from other specialties at Akron City Hospital often derided emergency physicians as "Jacks-of-all-Trades and Masters of None" or "glorified triage officers" who knew little about definitive care beyond the emergency department. This perception was made all the worse when calls from the ED were made in the middle of the night to overworked and underpaid "floor" residents who always assumed that this meant bad news and more work. Their only solace was the realization it was up to *them* to definitively diagnose and manage such patients, and along the way complain about the mismanagement and misdiagnosis that occurred in the emergency department. Even friends and family members would ask Nelson when and where he would open his medical practice and in what specialty. He came to the realization early on that for emergency physicians to achieve respect and legitimacy in the hospital let alone the house of medicine, they would have to become the acknowledged experts in specific areas of medicine. To him, environmental emergencies represented one such area.

During his resident years at Akron City, Nelson was often called upon to give lectures as part of the department's educational program. The topics frequently were left up to the speaker, and Nelson found himself gravitating to subjects he perceived as more in the realm of the emergency physician's areas of expertise, such as "environmental emergencies," rather than those "owned" by other specialties. His first such lecture was "Drowning and Near Drowning," inspired by an excellent review article published in the *Journal of the American College of Emergency Physicians* (JACEP) by Robert Knopp, MD, in 1978.

Another lecture was "Cyanide Poisoning," presented shortly after the tragic 1978 Jonestown Cult Massacre. During this presentation Nelson served up grape Kool-Aid and almonds, the latter in recognition of the supposed smell of cyanide (bitter almonds) and the former the delivery vehicle used in the mass killing. This prompted one of his faculty members to compliment him on the lecture, but also suggest that he was "warped". Other lectures Nelson gave included "Hypothermia," "Frostbite" and "Heat Related Illnesses."

Such topics were part of a broader range of subject matter referred to as "environmental emergencies" and were so listed in its own category in the recently published *Core Content of Emergency Medicine*. Nelson thought emergency physicians were among the few physicians who actually diagnosed and treated such conditions, often providing life-saving and even definitive care. Therefore, environmental emergencies seemed to represent at least one area of medicine where emergency physicians were the acknowledged experts and thus could contribute to the legitimacy of the specialty.

Nelson continued his interest in environmental emergencies as he began his faculty position at Ohio State. He not only lectured on these subjects to residents but also presented a lecture on environmental emergencies to medical students. In many cases, this was the only educational exposure medical students had to this group of conditions. He also arranged for a visit by renowned expert on animal venoms, Findlay E. Russell, MD, PhD, of the University of Arizona, whom Nelson had heard speak at national conferences.

The visit, which occurred on January 13, 1983, was arranged in coordination with the Department of Surgery and was referred to as "Emergency Medicine/Surgery Grand Rounds." Russell's first lecture was "Management of Snake Bites"; his second was "Arthropod and Marine Bites." The snake bite lecture was of particular interest to the surgeons, who at the time were taught that fasciotomy was often the appropriate management strategy to prevent compartment syndrome following severe envenomation. Russell strenuously disagreed with that approach, sometimes with near-religious zeal. The lectures were well-attended and well-received, likely enhancing the profile of emergency medicine at the medical center.

In 1983, W. B. Saunders approached Nelson, Rund and Keller about contributing to the company's "Blue Book" series of medical texts. Saunders regarded them as portable clinical tools. This new book was to focus on environmental emergencies. Given his interest in these subjects, Nelson was offered the role of lead editor with co-editors Rund and Keller.

Over the next two years, Nelson, Rund, Keller and contributing writers worked on *Environmental Emergencies*, which came out in 1985. Chapters included "Accidental Hypothermia," "Peripheral Cold Injuries," "Heat Illness," "Drowning and Near-Drowning," "Hypobaric Disorders,"

"Compressed Air Diving Accidents," "Radiation Emergencies," "Animal Bites," "Insect Bites and Stings," "Venomous Marine Animals," "Venomous Reptile Bites," "Botanical Allergens and Toxins," "Inhalation Injuries," "Mass Hysteria," "Lightning Injuries," "Sunburn," "Disaster Management," and "Medical Air Evacuation."

Outside contributors included Ken Kizer, MD, former Navy compressed diving expert and former Undersecretary for Health in the U.S. Department of Veterans Affairs, and Donald Kunkel, snakebite expert from St. Luke's Medical Center in Phoenix, Arizona. The book was well-received and remained in publication for a number of years.

The Emergency Medicine Annual

The *Emergency Medicine Annual* was a "publication of international scope with scholarly articles of use to the academicians, students and practitioners of emergency medicine...including broad concepts unifying management of patient with diverse diseases, and research data the clinical applications of which lie in the future." All the texts were clearly exploring ways in which emergency medicine could claim its distinct identity as a specialty. The third edition stressed the "critical relationship of emergency medicine to basic clinical sciences." (Figures 6a, 6b and 6c)

The specialty was recognizing the need to create its own knowledge

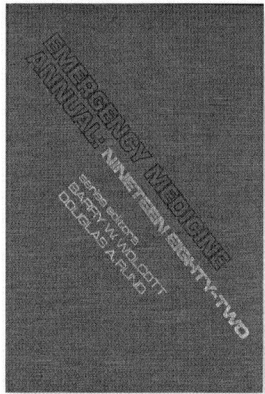
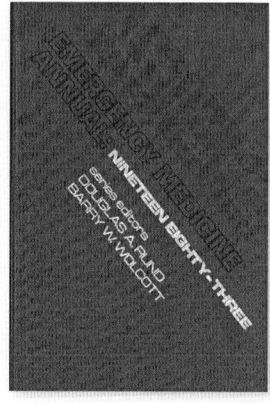
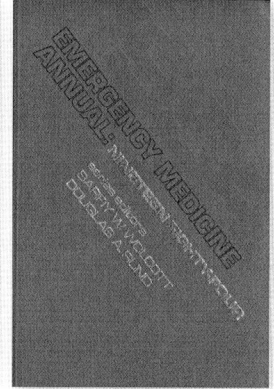

Figure 6a: *Emergency Medicine Annual Series 1982* (Appleton Century Crofts, Norwalk, CT, 1982-84)

Figure 6b: *Emergency Medicine Annual Series* (Appleton Century Crofts, Norwalk, CT, 1982-84)

Figure 6c: *Emergency Medicine Annual Series* (Appleton Century Crofts, Norwalk, CT, 1982-84)

through its own research. One of the initial articles was a comprehensive report of the development of the board examination which was never published in depth in any other publication.

Multiple Media: The Ohio State Series in Emergency Medicine

The technique of involving faculty leaders in the relatively non-controversial area of medical education was successful in broadening the acceptance of emergency medicine. A second effort was a project called Famous Teachings in Modern Medicine: *The Ohio State Series in Emergency Medicine* (Figure 7). The series was in the form of illustrated slide lectures and published by MEDCOM.

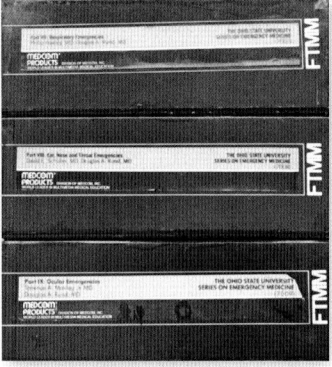

Figure 7: The Ohio State University Series on Emergency Medicine, slides and audio tapes: *Famous Teachings in Modern Medicine* (MEDCOM, Inc., 1980-1986)

At that time PowerPoint was unknown. Lectures were illustrated by 35 mm photographic slides displayed by a projector on a screen. The Ohio State Series presented 12 separate lectures with slides in carousels from the personal collections of the most influential and effective professors in the College of Medicine. A cassette tape reproduced the audio portion of the lecture. College Dean Tzagournis often remarked that once he was the commencement speaker at a medical school and the students presented that institution with a gift of the Ohio State series. He often said that he was filled with pride by the quality of the series.

Journals

In the 1970s it was clear to the founders of the specialty that a journal about emergency medicine was needed. A privately owned journal, *Emergency Medicine* was a "throw away" journal containing clinical articles written by a variety of authors not necessarily a part of the specialty. In 1972 the American College of Emergency Physicians (ACEP) published the *Journal of the American College of Emergency Physicians* (JACEP). The journal contained review articles about clinical topics, but little in the way of rigorous peer reviewed research. The journal was a start in the slow progress toward specialty recognition but was certainly not of the same caliber as other specialty journals in medicine or surgery.

That journal became the *Annals of Emergency Medicine* in 1980 and the editor, Ronald Krome, MD, was interviewed years earlier for the Ohio State position. Under Krome's leadership the journal improved its scientific content and credibility. Later, as the specialty developed, many more excellent journals would be published in the field of emergency medicine and its subspecialties.

The Emergency Medicine Survey

The first emergency medicine journal produced by Ohio State faculty was the *Emergency Medicine Survey*, published by Williams and Wilkins from 1982 to 1984 (Figure 8). The Editor-in-Chief was Martin D. Keller, MD, and the co-editors were Geraldine Keller, PhD, and Douglas A. Rund, MD (Figure 9). The journal included summaries of the major articles published in the year's literature regarding emergency medicine as well as a "think piece," which was written by an Ohio State faculty member or a nationally known emergency physician on a major topic in emergency medicine.

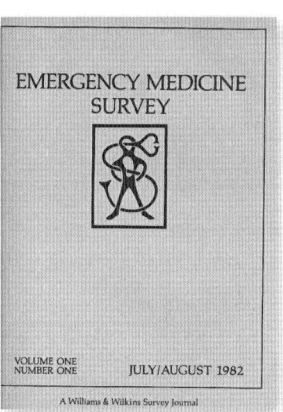

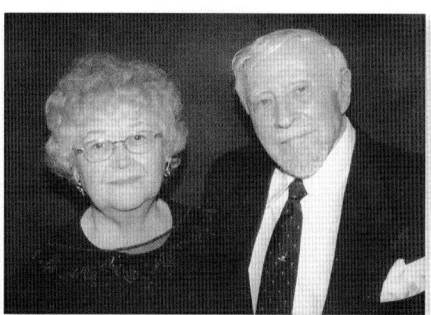

Figure 8: *Emergency Medicine Survey*, by Martin D. Keller, MD, Geraldine B. Keller, PhD, and Douglas A. Rund, MD (Williams and Wilkins, Baltimore, MD, 1982-1984)

Figure 9: Geraldine "Geri" Keller, PhD, and Martin D. Keller MD, PhD

Journal Articles and Sections

From 1985 to 1986 the faculty produced a monthly Journal Club section in the *American Journal of Emergency Medicine* and contributed a regular series of articles to the *Physician and Sports Medicine.* Charles G. Brown, MD, joined the faculty in 1983 and began a program of basic science in resuscitation that resulted in many scientific publications outlined in Brown's chapter on early research efforts.

Textbook Chapters

Howard A. Werman, MD, was the lead author of a chapter on ileitis and colitis in the first edition of the Tintinalli textbook *Emergency Medicine: A Comprehensive Study Guide*, published in 1985. He remained the author through all nine editions of the textbook.

Research

In seeking recognition of its unique specialty status, it was clear to academic leaders that rigorous research addressing real problems in emergency medicine was vitally needed. Only in this way, it was believed, could the specialty truly develop its own *intellectual discipline and body of basic knowledge*. Keller had an outstanding sense of humor. He often quipped:

> "Without research you are not an academic specialty. You are really just dispensary workers."

Historically the term "dispensary" referred to the most basic of medical services such as company medical office, perhaps staffed by a nurse dispensing only the most rudimentary services, something far inferior to what the doctor's office and certainly the hospital provided. The quote, however always got the attention of the emergency medicine faculty members who knew that excellent clinical service and even superb teaching would never be enough to bring academic recognition, respect and the status of a full department in the university.

At Ohio State the constant focus had to be directed toward research, especially basic scientific research. This had to be the aim even in the face of unrelenting demand for patient care and the natural inclination of doctors entering the specialty for its "action." Most emergency physicians chose the specialty because they were attracted to its full-tilt pace, case variety and a real chance to intervene immediately in acute life-threatening injury or illness.

In the early days of the specialty, by contrast, physicians choosing research were typically more likely to select traditional paths with well-known mentors that included the probability of grant funding and promotion within an established department. In the early days of the specialty, conducting a credible research program was an uphill battle while recruiting residents and stimulating student interest were easy endeavors.

The recruitment of Charles G. Brown, MD, and the subsequent success of his basic and clinical research in cardiac arrest brought the Division of Emergency Medicine at Ohio State exceptional national recognition. Ohio State faculty members believed so strongly that research was essential to their success that they devoted practice-generated dollars to the research mission and not to their salaries.

Teaching

- **Student Teaching**

    The *sine qua non* of an academic department in a university is student teaching. At Ohio State two opportunities presented themselves early in the division's existence: a course for first-year medical students providing basic instruction for dealing with emergencies (i.e., first responder) and a required senior rotation in emergency medicine.

    In the 1978 panel discussion previously described, Ronald Krome noted the following:

    > *Currently, the presentation of emergency medical care to the undergraduate in most medical schools is in a disjointed fashion. The management of cardiac arrests is discussed on one service, splinting of fractures on another and control of bleeding on a third. In this disjointed*

fashion, there is no goal direction ensuring that every medical student is adequately trained in the provision of basic emergency medical care.

The solution to this problem meant involving full-time academic emergency physicians in student education and curriculum development. This would further solidify the argument that emergency medicine faculty were full-fledged academic partners participating significantly in the medical school curriculum.

The first course developed was the fourth-year clerkship in emergency medicine. Prior to the creation of a division with supervising faculty, there was no student rotation in the Ohio State emergency room. Students on an inpatient service such as medicine would, on occasion, accompany the resident to admit a patient to the hospital. Because there were no faculty attending physicians on duty, there was no one to supervise the student.

Beginning with a 4th year clerkship, the emergency medicine division gradually convinced the College of Medicine to require a senior rotation in the emergency department. This was initially a requirement to obtain training in "critical care." The division had to move cautiously and always gather allies in other departments along the way. Critical care was a good compromise. Over time emergency medicine became a required rotation. Students had supervised clinical experience at Ohio State University hospitals, Grant Hospital, Riverside Methodist Hospital and the Mount Carmel hospitals. The student lecture series took place at Ohio State with lecturers from the participating hospitals.

The second course was *Special Victim Care* for first-year students. The course was essentially a first responder course with additional elements from a basic emergency medicine technician (EMT) course. The concept was appealing to medical students who saw only courses in anatomy, pharmacology, physiology and other basic sciences in the first year. One of the course's selling points was that students could often experience being considered the "expert" in cases of illness or injury. The course covered cardiac arrest, respiratory emergencies, medical emergencies, bleeding and soft tissue injuries, injuries to muscles and bones—including splinting and bandaging—emergency childbirth and use of the EMS system. The course was limited to 20 students and was always oversubscribed from the first day.

- **Resident Teaching**

  Following the definition of the specialty's content, the second step in the establishing an academic department was the creation of "graduate training programs" (see Chapter 3). Such programs were initially the residency programs, but eventually included fellowships and other doctoral programs.

  The Ohio State emergency medicine residency program that began with its first class in 1981 consisted of four residents per year: two were Ohio State employees and two were Riverside employees. This arrangement continued for the first seven years of the program. By 1988, however, it was becoming apparent that residents were spending considerable time in rotations outside the emergency department and the total number of residents was insufficient to adequately staff the emergency departments of the two main teaching hospitals.

  In the 1988, the Program Information Form submitted to the Residency Review Committee reported that emergency medicine residents spent only seven months of their entire three years in the Ohio State emergency department, and that they only saw, at most, 25% of patients. The rest were treated by faculty and residents from other departments. Seven months were spent in the Riverside emergency department and only one month in the Children's Hospital emergency department. In addition, residents spent two months of their final year at the Shock Trauma Center of the University of Maryland in Baltimore.

  Members of the Residency Review Committee had several concerns. They felt that trainees were not given enough time at a single hospital with a structure that gave them graduated responsibility as they progressed through the program. They also felt there was not a "critical mass" of residents at any one site to ensure optimal didactic and clinical teaching. In response, the residency program would change over the next two years, coinciding with the creation of the academic department of emergency medicine.

Contributions and Leadership in Emergency Medicine Organizations

- **The American Board of Emergency Medicine**

Nelson and Rund devoted considerable effort to the examination process of the American Board of Emergency Medicine (ABEM). Rund became an examiner in 1980 and Nelson became an examiner in 1983. Nelson became an item writer in 1987 and at one point was the longest serving item writer in the history of the Board. Rund became a member of the scenario development panel in 1981 and a member of the ABEM Board of Directors in 1988. He became President of the Board in 1995; Nelson became President of the Board in 2011.

Rund served on two test committees for the National Board of Medical Examiners from 1982 to 1986. He served as Chairman of the Committee on Publications for the University Association for Emergency Medicine in 1985.

- **International**

Marty and Geri Keller were cosmopolitan in their interests. In their work with the United States Agency for International Development, they collaborated with other countries in developing emergency medical services (EMS). There was a close affiliation with an organization founded in 1980 called the International Society of Emergency Medical Services. The purpose of the society was to develop, promote and improve EMS throughout the world. The founding members came from 16 nations and represented such regions as Africa, the Americas, Europe and the Middle East.

- **The International Research Institute for Emergency Medicine**

On the national level during that time period, there was discontent about the amount of funding the ACEP was directing toward research. Academic leaders who advocated for emergency medicine recognized the critical need for research to ensure the specialty's ultimate success, but they believed that ACEP was dominated by large private emergency medicine groups with funding that enhanced the organization's ascendancy. John Wiegenstein, MD, founder and first President of ACEP, was disturbed at the ACEP's relative inattention to scientific research in the specialty. To address this disparity, he and Rund formed the International Research Institute for Emergency Medicine in 1986.

Rund became the President of the Institute and The Ohio State University became the organization's headquarters. The institute received financial support from various state chapters and private donors throughout the country. Rund was also a member of ACEP's research committee at the time and discussed with the organization how he and Wiegenstein had created a research institute that was competing for funding. Wiegenstein and Rund worked both within and outside ACEP to convince the organization to substantially increase funding for emergency medicine research. Their efforts were eventually so successful, the institute disbanded in 1989 and the remaining funds were donated to ACEP to fund research.

References

1. Johnson G, Krome RL, Moylan JA, Wagner DK. The emergency department physician and university teaching hospitals. *Arch Surg*. 1978; 113: 678-683.

2. Eiseman B. Editorial comment. *Arch Surg*. 1978; 113:683.

3. Cantrell RW, Goldstein JC. The American Board of Otolaryngology, 1924-1999: 75 years of excellence. *Arch Otolaryngology Head Neck Surg*. 1999(Oct);125(10):1071-9.

4. Zink, BJ. *Anyone, Anything, Anytime: A History of Emergency Medicine*. Philadelphia, PA: Mosby Elsevier; 2006.

5. Flint T. *Emergency Treatment and Management*. Philadelphia, PA: W. B. Saunders; 1954.

6. Rund DA. *Essentials of Emergency Medicine*. New York, NY: Appleton Century Crofts; 1982.

7. Reisdorff EJ. Personal communication. May 2022.

8. Mueller CF and Rund DA. *Emergency Radiology: Self-Assessment*. Baltimore, MD: Williams and Wilkins; 1982.

9. Rund DA and Hutzler J. *Emergency Psychiatry*. St. Louis, MO: Mosby; 1983.

10. Nelson RN, Rund DA and Keller MD. *Environmental Emergencies*. Philadelphia, PA: W. B. Saunders; 1985.

Chapter 6

Early Research Efforts: Charles G. Brown, MD, and Cardiopulmonary Resuscitation

Charles G. Brown, MD
Douglas A. Rund, MD

The initial priorities of the Division of Emergency Medicine at Ohio State were first, to provide excellent, state-of-the-art patient care, and second, to develop a residency program in emergency medicine. The next goal was to demonstrate that emergency medicine was *indeed a specialty,* and that the division was worthy of stature as a full academic department within the university. This clearly required the development of a *research program* focused on areas that were essential in emergency medicine practice. In addition, it was felt that the research had to be of high quality and excellent enough to be published in the most prestigious medical and scientific journals.

Emergency medicine in the early 1980s was still a budding specialty, and its advocates believed there were definitely research opportunities available to study in the areas of patient care that were unique to emergency medicine. This collective understanding led to the search for physicians and clinicians in emergency medicine who wanted to dedicate part of their career to improving patient care through both basic science and clinical research. Moreover, it was this combination of basic science and clinical research that created a composite picture that the early leaders of emergency medicine felt mirrored the best academic departments nationally.

Thus, there was a strong need to develop a research program in emergency medicine at Ohio State. In this regard, Douglas A. Rund, MD, Director of Emergency Medicine at Ohio State, recruited Charles G.

Brown, MD, to join the faculty in 1983. At the time Brown was working and teaching at the emergency department and emergency medicine residency program at The Johns Hopkins University (Figure 1).

CHARLES G. "CHUCK" BROWN, MD

During medical school at Georgetown University (1974-1978), Brown studied and completed a clinical rotation with the world renown cardiologist, Watkins Proctor Harvey, MD. Thinking that he was going to pursue a career in internal medicine and cardiology, Brown welcomed Harvey's suggestion that he spend an additional month of internal medicine on cardiology training at Grady Hospital in Atlanta with another renowned cardiologist, Nanette Wenger, MD, at Emory University. During his one-month rotation at Grady Hospital, Brown often "volunteered" to work in the emergency department on the nights he was not on call, thinking that this would help him secure an internal medicine residency program position.

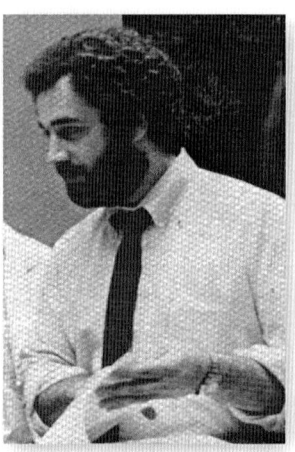

Figure 1: Charles G. "Chuck" Brown, MD, teaching at Johns Hopkins Hospital in 1982.

His plan was to follow the residency training with additional training in cardiology. After several shifts in the emergency department, he realized that those physicians who were capable of providing immediate care for patients with acute medical and surgical emergencies were, in his opinion, the most well-rounded physicians. Emergency medicine, looked like a potentially interesting and rewarding career choice.

When the time came to apply for residency programs, he learned that in 1978 there were only a few three-year programs in emergency medicine. Most emergency medicine residency programs were two-year programs that accepted applicants after they completed one year of an internal medicine or surgery internship. Wanting to stay on the East Coast, he decided to hedge his bets, and he applied to Hershey Medical Center, which was a part of Pennsylvania State University, one of the three-year emergency medicine residency programs on the East Coast. He also applied to several internal medicine residency programs.

Thinking he might not be accepted into a three-year emergency medicine residency program, Brown decided that a "one-year" residency in internal medicine would give him the opportunity to make a decision on an emergency medicine or internal medicine path at the end of his first year of internal medicine residency. In March 1978, he was accepted to Hershey/Pennsylvania State University Emergency Medicine Residency. Since the first year of emergency medicine training was broad-based, and it included internal medicine and the coronary care unit, he felt that he could switch after one year if emergency medicine wasn't a fit.

Brown's first year at Hershey/Pennsylvania State University emergency medicine was excellent: He learned to perform endotracheal intubation, place central lines, repair lacerations, splint, cast, stabilize and treat critically ill patients, and to think more acutely and broadly about differential diagnoses. While the experience was rewarding, Brown was concerned that it looked like many of the approaches to the care of emergency patients were being 'borrowed' from other disciplines. He wondered if emergency physicians could diagnose and treat such patients better, and whether there were other questions and issues unique to emergency medicine that were either poorly addressed or not addressed, and that needed to be investigated. He began keeping a list of these clinical questions.

While there was no opportunity for research during his residency program, Brown knew then that he wanted to pursue an academic career that would combine both clinical care and research in emergency medicine. He wondered where he could find such a career path in 1981 after the completion of his residency. He took a position as an assistant professor in the emergency medicine program at Johns Hopkins Hospital. While Brown found the clinical work and clinical teaching rewarding, and that he had time to pursue research, there was no seed money available or little mentorship provided for aspiring emergency medicine faculty researchers.

After two years at Johns Hopkins, he interviewed at several residency programs across the country to see if there were opportunities for both clinical practice and research. In time, Brown connected with Rund at Ohio State, where Rund offered him dedicated research time, opportunities for research seed money, mentorship and research collaboration opportunities.

Emergency Medicine Research in the Early 1980s

In the early 1980s, emergency departments in the United States were still primarily developing their clinical, administrative and residency training programs. A perusal of emergency medicine journals at that time showed that the majority of publications were focused on administrative, teaching and educational issues. Papers that tried to address clinical questions suffered from methodological problems, and usually had little applicability to clinical practice. Within a few months of coming to Ohio State, however, it was clear to Brown that the opportunity for a research and clinical practice career was possible. Seed money was available, and interdisciplinary opportunities for research presented themselves.

Given the long list of potential research questions that he wanted to address, Brown thought it most important to select an area of research that was unique to emergency medicine. Such areas would, ideally, help to avoid any turf wars, but even more compelling was the effort to begin to develop interventions that were needed to address the unique issues of emergency medicine patients. In this regard, he thought of addressing clinical issues that were occurring in the out-of-hospital environment, and specifically, in the management of out-of-hospital cardiac arrest.

What made this research area unique to emergency medicine versus in-hospital cardiac arrests, he surmised, was that clinicians rarely observed out-of-hospital cardiac arrests. In cases of unwitnessed cardiopulmonary arrest, cardiopulmonary resuscitation (CPR) was often delayed, sometimes for long periods. Thus, in cases of cardiac arrest occurring outside the hospital, a more prolonged ischemia time (low or no blood flow to vital organs) was occurring compared to that observed with cardiac arrests that occurred within the hospital. Patients in the hospital typically received CPR earlier than those not hospitalized. The question that arose, therefore, was the following: Were current therapeutic interventions recommended for hospital in-patients also appropriate for patients having an out-of-hospital cardiac arrest?

With this in mind, the first clinical question Brown wanted to address was that of prolonged cardiac arrest in patients not receiving CPR in a timely fashion: Given that the duration of arrest (ischemia time) before CPR was started was longer in the out-of-hospital setting versus in-hospital setting, were the medications, doses of such medications, and sequence of interventions currently being employed appropriate for out-of-hospital cardiac arrests? In addition, most of the cardiac arrest animal models that were previously used to assess cardiac arrest interventions used animals that were dissimilar to humans in several respects. Differences in thoracic anatomy was one example. The configuration of the animal chest could have an effect on the mechanics of the CPR being performed. Another difference was the use of cardiac arrest models with short ischemia times, or induced cardiac arrest by asphyxia (preventing the animals from breathing properly), which did not generally simulate the out-of-hospital cardiac arrest scenario, which typically resulted from cardiac disease/coronary artery occlusion.

At this time, Brown met with John Stang, MD, who was a cardiologist at Ohio State and Medical Director of Emergency Medical Services (EMS) within the Columbus Division of Fire (Figure 2). Stang was in charge of EMS training and education in Columbus, Ohio. Brown explained his ideas for research to Stang, specifically looking at varying doses of adrenergic agonists in out-of-hospital cardiac arrest. He explained that his research and literature review showed that the 1 milligram (mg) dose of epinephrine that was currently recommended

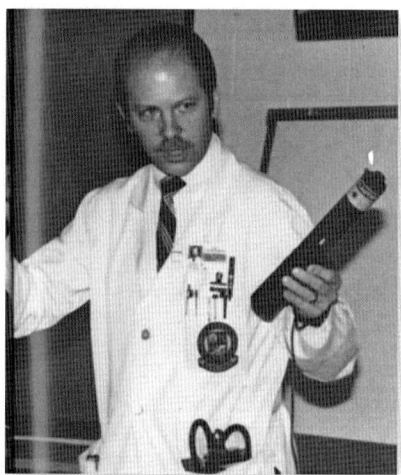

Figure 2: John M. Stang, MD, a cardiologist at Ohio State, was tremendously supportive of emergency medicine and the department's research efforts. Stang was medical director of the Columbus Division of Fire from 1981 to 1984.

for patients with cardiac arrest, could be traced back to a single study in small dogs done in 1906.[1] When this dose was extrapolated to a 70-kilogram (kg) adult, it would equate to approximately 0.2 mg per kg, and not 0.01-0.02 mg per kg, which was the currently recommended dose for patients with cardiac arrest during CPR.

Stang suggested that Brown also work with Robert Hamlin, DVM, PhD, in the Department of Biosciences at the Ohio State College of Veterinary Medicine, where Hamlin had a research interest in cardiology and ran a basic science animal laboratory. Hamlin was an internationally renowned veterinarian and investigator focusing on cardiovascular physiology and pharmacology, and an expert in clinical veterinary cardiology (Figure 3). Hamlin's basic science laboratory was funded by the National Institutes of Health (NIH). He published over 300 scientific papers, received numerous academic awards, and became an excellent mentor for and collaborator with Brown.

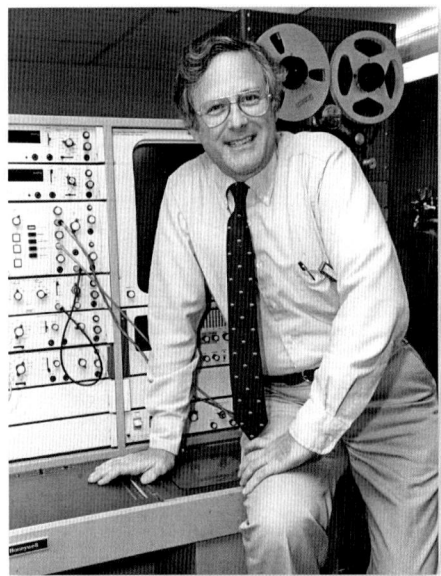

Figure 3: Robert Hamlin, DVM, PhD, was a renowned veterinary investigator whose expertise in veterinary cardiology aided CPR research by Charles G. Brown, MD. *(photo courtesy of Oho State Archives)*

After meeting and discussing these ideas for CPR research with Hamlin, Brown devised what he felt was a more relevant animal model for conducting this research. The model used swine, whose thoracic anatomy was more similar to humans than previous animal models of cardiac arrest that used canines. The research animals would undergo electrically induced ventricular fibrillation (VF), which was the most common heart rhythm abnormality in patients suffering a cardiac arrest, and a 10-minute ischemia time before the researchers started closed chest cardiac massage and ventilation (assisted breathing) with a mechanical CPR device called a "thumper" (CC-CPR). After three minutes of CC-CPR, an adrenergic agonist medication such as epinephrine, norepinephrine, methoxamine or phenylephrine, of varying doses was delivered through a peripheral vein. These medications were employed in an effort to improve blood flow to the heart and brain during CPR. Cerebral (brain) and myocardial (heart) blood flow were measured using a radio-labelled microsphere technique during three separate periods: first during normal sinus rhythm (NSR) before cardiac arrest; second during CC-CPR after 10 minutes of cardiac arrest; and finally, during CC-CPR following adrenergic agonist drug administration.

After these blood flow measurements had been performed, defibrillation was attempted to determine if the animals could be successfully defibrillated with return of a pulse and blood pressure, also known as the return of spontaneous circulation (ROSC). Hamlin provided the expertise for radio-labelled microsphere measurements of blood flow. Preliminary funding for these studies came from various seed grants from Ohio State and subsequently from the Emergency Medicine Foundation.

Results from the studies using epinephrine and norepinephrine in the swine model of out-of-hospital cardiac arrest appeared to be more beneficial in improving myocardial and cerebral blood flow during CC-CPR versus other adrenergic agonists such as phenylephrine and methoxamine. Also, the 0.2 mg/kg dose of epinephrine provided better cerebral and myocardial blood flows and ROSC rates than 0.02 mg/kg of epinephrine.[2]

There were clearly several short-comings with this research, however. The research did not examine any doses of epinephrine between 0.02 mg/kg and 0.2 mg/kg, and no assessments of neurological status were done post-resuscitation. Of note, while norepinephrine provided better blood flows than epinephrine, post-resuscitation, norepinephrine appeared quite arrhythmogenic. Thus, if a clinical trial was to be performed, epinephrine appeared to be a reasonable candidate at a dose of 0.2 mg/kg.

In addition, given these findings with various adrenergic agonists, Brown and his colleagues first began looking at the structure activity relationships of these medications to see if they could develop a new adrenergic agonist that had the peripheral vasoconstrictive properties of norepinephrine without its potential to cause a heart rhythm disturbance and cause a secondary cardiac arrest. Brown and his team hypothesized that constricting the peripheral blood vessels with an adrenergic agonist during CPR would help improve blood flow to the heart and brain. The team decided to collaborate on this effort with Duane Miller, PhD, in the Ohio State Department of Medicinal Chemistry.

Miller joined the faculty in 1969 and became Chairman of the Division of Medicinal Chemistry and Pharmacognosy in 1982. He had a highly synergistic collaboration with his colleagues, including Brown. Miller's work included, in part, elucidating steric interactions of catecholamines with adrenoreceptors. In particular he studied dopamine and norepinephrine with leading investigators in the field. Miller had a highly successful career at Ohio State and at the University of Tennessee, where he moved in 1992. He eventually secured over 100 patents for novel pharmaceutical drugs.

Second, it was Brown's clinical observation that the VF waveform observed prior to defibrillation looked different in animals that were successfully defibrillated with subsequent ROSC than the animals that were not successfully defibrillated. This led to a collaboration with Roger Dzwonczyk, MSBME, an electrical engineer in the Department of Anesthesiology, to look more critically at an analysis of the VF waveform. Dzwonczyk was also interested in other aspects of cardiac arrest and resuscitation, including the use of supplemental oxygen during cardiac resuscitation.

While there were clearly limitations of these studies of adrenergic agonists in this swine model—given the dismal resuscitation and hospital discharge rates for out-of-hospital cardiac patients that were initially found with the heart rhythm disturbances of asystole and electrical mechanical dissociation (EMD)/pulseless idioventricular rhythm (PIVR), and in patients who failed to have ROSC following up to three defibrillation attempts in VF— Brown proposed an out-of-hospital cardiac arrest study comparing 0.02 mg/kg versus 0.2 mg/kg of epinephrine, in asystole, EMD/PIVR and defibrillation failure of VF following up to three countershock attempts. The outcomes measured included ROSC rates and rates of hospital discharge.

Brown received funding from Abbott Laboratories who made the calibrated blinded epinephrine syringes for the clinical study. The syringes allowed paramedics to estimate the weight of the patient and administer the 'appropriate' dosage of epinephrine (0.02 or 0.20, mg/kg), based on the patient's estimated weight. In addition, given the clinical differences that the research group wanted to detect in this study, a sample size of more than 1,200 patients would be required. To support a larger patient sample, Brown developed collaborative research ties with five additional EMS centers besides Columbus: Syracuse, Richmond, Houston, Milwaukee and Seattle. Training and standardized data collection was provided for all EMS centers.

While Brown and his co-investigators were successful in forming the first large scale, multi-center study of out-of-hospital cardiac arrest, the results of the study were disappointing. There was no difference in rates of ROSC, rates of hospital discharge, or the percentage of patients who were conscious at hospital discharge between the two treatment groups. The study was published in the *New England Journal of Medicine*.[3] This was, in a way, the epitome of accomplishment for the department of emergency medicine and the specialty.

While the study did not demonstrate any benefit from this higher dose of epinephrine, it raised the question of whether epinephrine was of any value at all in out-of-hospital cardiac arrest. Of note: *Endogenous* epinephrine levels were measured during CPR prior to drug administration and were found to be extremely elevated in cardiac arrest. Thus, the team began to question how much a 0.02 mg/kg or even a 0.20 mg/kg dose of *exogeneous* epinephrine actually contributed to the *total* epinephrine levels.

Although they never completed or published any of this work, the investigative team had a new question they wanted to address: Would altering the environment (i.e., pH) be beneficial? Another question was whether or not using an adrenergic agonist that only stimulated peripheral post-synaptic alpha-2 receptors, could have less arrhythmogenic potential, and thus could be more beneficial in this setting, since it was hypothesized that stimulation of the post-synaptic alpha-2 receptor was potentially responsible for the beneficial effects of adrenergic agonists (improving cerebral and myocardial blood flow), and stimulation of other adrenergic receptors could be arrhythmogenic.

Although the team developed several novel compounds in this regard in collaboration with Miller in Medicinal Chemistry, the few compounds tested were not successful in improving blood flood in their animal model. Unfortunately, while they still had available a number of additional compounds proposed that they hoped could help deduce the optimal structure-activity relationship, the investigators were unable to secure any funding to continue the research and development of these novel compounds.

As noted above, concurrent with these research efforts, in collaboration with Dzwonczyk, Brown began to analyze the VF waveform, both from the animal studies and from out-of-hospital cardiac arrests. Since several EMS centers had automated external defibrillators (AED) that recorded both the ECG, the defibrillation, the ambient sounds, and in addition, had the out-of-hospital medical records, Brown and his colleagues were able to analyze the VF waveform using fast-Fourier transform analysis (FFTA) to see if there was a correlation between various VF frequency parameters, as determined by FFTA, and successful defibrillation leading to ROSC. Their understanding at the time was that most AED algorithms for determining VF versus other cardiac arrest rhythms, was in part, based on the amplitude of the VF waveform.

Given all the factors that could affect VF *amplitude*, they hypothesized that looking at *frequency* parameters instead of just amplitude could eliminate the variable effects of amplitude, and provide a more accurate approach to the recognition and defibrillation of VF. As a result, they embarked on an analysis of VF waveforms from all of their animal studies, as well as from the out-of-hospital setting. Again, the goal was to see whether they could find any correlation between various VF frequency parameters and successful ROSC. Using FFTA, they began to focus on several frequency parameters. While several parameters looked predictive,[4,5] it also began to raise the question of how VF was being defined, and whether all VF should be defibrillated.

In fact, what the team was beginning to explore was whether an analysis of the VF waveform should be done initially in cardiac arrest patients using FFTA, and depending on the VF parameter, defibrillation would be attempted only when the "optimal" value of the VF parameter was noted. If this was not carried out, other interventions (i.e., CPR, medications) should be given first in an effort to improve the VF parameter prior to defibrillation. Thus, defibrillation may not be the first intervention in VF. Unfortunately, despite their efforts to continue with this research, it was being done at a time when several organizations were promoting early defibrillation of VF. Thus, it was impossible to garner any funding or enthusiasm for the research, so Brown and colleagues abandoned this line of research as well.

Emergency Medicine Fellows and the Stanley J. Sarnoff Medical Student Research Fellowship: Mentoring Next Generation Emergency Medicine Researchers

Brown's contributions to the development of emergency medicine at Ohio State cannot be over emphasized. He added a vital element in the creation of the specialty and the department: research and the development of the next generation of emergency medicine researchers. This led to the establishment of the full academic department in 1990. One of his most innovative accomplishments was the identification of exceptional scientific collaborators within the immense Ohio State campus. During approximately 13 years of conducting research at Ohio State, the research team led by Brown started research training programs for graduating residents in emergency medicine.

Although emergency medicine research was still in its infancy, Brown made significant collaborations with established investigators both inside and outside the university. The combination of the research team's own growth and the interdisciplinary collaborations that were developed led Brown to establish an Emergency Medicine Research Fellowship in 1984. While the focus of the laboratory and clinical research was on CPR, the goals of the fellowship were to introduce and foster critical research skills so clinicians would be able to conduct their own research, as well as critically analyze the biomedical literature. In this regard, from 1984 through 1992, the department had eight research fellows and one Stanley J. Sarnoff Medical Student Research Fellowship recipient. (Table 1)

One of Brown's protégés was Robert W. Neumar, MD, PhD, who was a

Sarnoff Medical School Research Fellow from 1988 to 1989 following his third year of medical school at the University of Pittsburgh (Figure 4). Neumar eventually became Professor and Chair of the Department of Emergency Medicine at the University of Michigan. Years later Neumar recalled his experiences in Brown's laboratory:

That was a very early formative time in my career. My plan was to do family medicine and after finishing my training, to go home and be a family doctor back in my hometown of Johnstown, PA. Within the first couple of months of medical school, I was growingly frustrated about the fact that the professors didn't have the answers to questions that I had; and I realized that there is a lot more that we don't know about medicine than we do about medicine. So, I decided at that time that I needed to be able to have the tools and skills to be able to answer questions that were important that nobody knew the answer to; so that's what drew me to research. I interviewed for a number of different labs, including, Hopkins and Duke and found out about this guy in emergency medicine – Chuck Brown who was doing very innovative work in catecholamines during CPR with swine model. As a medical student the idea of being able to do actual large animal experiments was really exciting so I went out to visit Chuck and learn what he was doing and ended up at Ohio State to go and do research. It was just great experience in terms of working on that physiology of CPR and learning a ton about how CPR actually works and ways in which we can augment blood flow to the heart and brain through catecholamines or other strategies to improve spontaneous circulation in survival. That

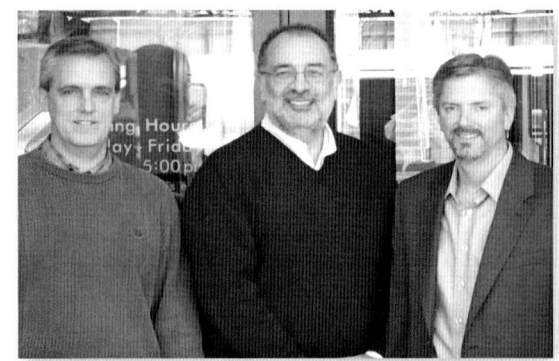

Figure 4: Robert W. Neumar, MD, PhD (far left), Charles G. Brown, MD (center) and Kevin Ward, MD. Neumar was a Sarnoff fellow under Brown. He ultimately became Professor and Chair of the Department of Emergency Medicine at the University of Michigan. Brown began the basic science research program at Ohio State, bringing national recognition to the department. Ward was a research fellow in 1992 and joined the faculty at Ohio State following his fellowship.

work basically launched my career to this day to where I continue to do research and have NIH grants focused on cardiac arrest and resuscitation, both in animal models and humans.

Also, it is what hooked me on emergency medicine. I think if I would have gone to any other labs I interviewed at, I would have been a cardiologist because they were cardiology mentors. I certainly attribute Chuck's mentorship into bringing me into the specialty of emergency medicine as well. Chuck was very involved nationally and internationally and introduced me to a great network of investigators

The work that I did with Chuck was very much involved in ventricular fibrillation and cardiac arrest. We did work on catecholamine doses and different kinds of catecholamines to increase coronary perfusion pressure during CPR, but we also studied myocardial metabolism during ventricular fibrillation. One study we did was we took these serial biopsies of the defibrillating ventricle of a pig and then did chromatography on that to study the metabolism of adenine nucleotides, and how that deteriorated over time to the point to where it defined when injury was likely to be irreversible. So that was very much laboratory-based work that I presented at my first meeting of the Society for Academic Emergency Medicine (SAEM) in 1989 and got the best oral basic science presentation award as a medical student.

One thing that I would really like to emphasize, because I tell this a lot. As a specialty, as in any specialty is, you have an obligation to create new knowledge that improves the care and outcomes of our patients. Emergency medicine is no exception to that. We made tremendous progress in advancing the science of emergency medicine and growing the number of investigators doing emergency medicine, but we also have a long way to go. Opportunities like I had as a medical student to work with Chuck Brown, an emergency medicine principal investigator launched my research career and my clinical career. These are things that we really need to find ways to provide for more and more people. It gets harder and harder with all the pressures of the finances of academic medicine and the ED crowding, every year it becomes worse and worse, and it is really hard to carve out bandwidth and effort to focus on the bigger academic missions. [6,7]

As department chair at the University of Michigan Neumar went on to create the Weil Institute for Critical Care Research and Innovation, a multi discipline endowed and well-funded research institute.

In general, the research fellows went on to make significant contributions to academic emergency medicine. Table 1 lists the research fellows, the Sarnoff Medical Student Research Fellowship award recipient, and their most recent positions or roles in emergency medicine.

Career Change

In addition to his work with research fellows, Brown was an advisor to the Landcare Society from 1990 to 1992. The society was an organization promoting medical student research at the Ohio State College of Medicine. One of his responsibilities was to help select a guest lecturer to speak at "Landacre Day Medical Grand Rounds". While the guest lecturer was typically a physician, Brown and the student research group decided one year to invite Gertrude Elion, PhD, who in 1988, received the Nobel Prize in Medicine for her work on several discoveries while working at Burroughs Wellcome/GlaxoSmithKline Pharmaceutical company. Elion's discoveries included 6-mercaptopurine, the first treatment for leukemia; azathioprine, the first immuno-suppressive for organ transplantation; allopurinol for gout; pyrimethamine for malaria; trimethoprim for urinary and respiratory tract infections; and acyclovir for herpes infections. As a result of lengthy conversations with Elion, Brown began to consider a possible alternative plan, which could include conducting clinical research in the pharmaceutical industry.

In 1996 Brown decided to leave Ohio State. It was a difficult decision, but given the relative lack of funding for emergency medicine research and the opportunities open for clinical research in the pharmaceutical and medical device industries, he decided to move back East, and began work in the pharmaceutical industry while continuing to work part-time clinically.

Brown returned to Ohio State for Emergency Medicine Grand Rounds in 2011, and noted the following (see page 118):

Table 1.
Research fellows studying with Charles Brown, MD, from 1984 to 1992

EMERGENCY MEDICINE RESEARCH FELLOW	YEAR OF FELLOWSHIP	MOST RECENT ROLE IN EMERGENCY MEDICINE
Howard Werman, MD	1984	Professor, Department of Emergency Medicine, The Ohio State University
Eric Davis, MD	1985	Formerly Professor of Emergency Medicine, University of Rochester School of Medicine and Dentistry (Deceased 2020)
Ronald Taylor, MD	1986	Emergency Physician, Columbus, Ohio
James Jenkins, DO	1987	
Peter Van Ligten, MD, JD	1988	Attorney, Columbus, Ohio
Robert Griffith, MD	1989	President of Emergency Services, Inc. (Mt. Carmel); retired
Charles Little, DO	1990-1992	Medical Director of the Mountain Plains Regional Disaster Health Response System; Chief Medical Officer of the Federal Disaster Medical Assistance Team (DMAT CO-2) and Medical Director of Emergency Preparedness, University of Colorado Hospital, Professor, Department of Emergency Medicine, University of Colorado
David Persse, MD	1992	Professor of Medicine and Surgery, Baylor University Director of Emergency Medical Services City of Houston

STANLEY J SARNOFF MEDICAL STUDENT RESEARCH FELLOW	YEAR OF FELLOWSHIP	CURRENT POSITION/ CURRENT ROLE IN EMERGENCY MEDICINE
Robert Neumar, MD, PhD	1989	Professor and Chair, Department of Emergency Medicine University of Michigan

The broad clinical training that physicians receive in emergency medicine and the ability to do a differential diagnosis on a wide variety of clinical signs and symptoms, gives emergency physicians a unique advantage in conducting and analyzing pharmaceutical and medical device research.

As importantly, it has been a rewarding career to practice emergency medicine, to contribute to the development of emergency medicine clinicians and researchers, and to have helped in the development of several new medications while conducting clinical research in the pharmaceutical industry.

References

1. Crile G, Dolley DH. An experimental research into the resuscitation of dogs killed by anesthetics and asphyxia. *JEM*. 1906;8(6):713-725.

2. Brown CG, Werman HA. Adrenergic agonists curing cardiopulmonary resuscitation. *Resuscitation*. 1990;19:1-16.

3. Brown CG, et al. A comparison of standard-dose and high-dose epinephrine in cardiac arrest outside the hospital. *N. Engl. J. Med.* 1992;327:1051-1055.

4. Brown CG, et al. Estimating the duration of ventricular fibrillation. *Ann Emerg Med.* 1989;18:1181-1185.

5. Dzwonczyk R, Brown CG, et al. The median frequency of the ECG during ventricular fibrillation: its use in an algorithm for estimating the duration of cardiac arrest. *IEEE Trans on Biomed Eng.* 1990;37:640-646.

6. Neumar, RW: Interview with Robert W. Neumar, MD, PhD, by Douglas Rund. 2022: Columbus, Ohio.

7. Neumar, RW, et al. Emergency medicine research: 2030 strategic goals. *Acad Emerg Med.* 2021;29(2):241-251.

Chapter 7

A Celebration: The Department of Emergency Medicine in the College of Medicine, 1990

Douglas A. Rund, MD

There was shouting from the rooftops and the celebration bells were ringing. On May 3, 1990, The Ohio State University Board of Trustees approved Resolution Number 90-110 establishing the Department of Emergency Medicine in the College of Medicine to be effective July 1, 1990 (Figure 1).

The division faculty had been working steadily since the division's creation in 1977 to convince the university that department status was warranted. As the trustees noted: "Emergency Medicine had been a specialty area since the late 1970s and has a body of knowledge distinct from Preventive Medicine."

Proof of these elements had been the objective from the start. First, the faculty had to show beyond a doubt that the existence of clinical content that was new and unique to emergency medicine to be a *specialty*. Second, the *distinct body of knowledge* argument would be more difficult to demonstrate in a department of medicine or surgery, hence the wisdom of location in the Department of Preventive Medicine in the first place. In addition, the faculty of Preventive Medicine approved the creation of the department.

The trustees noted that creation of academic departments was a trend throughout the country. This was true, but at the time of the approval only 15 other academic departments had been established. The trustees also accepted the faculty's argument that recruitment of students and residents would be enhanced by department status.

A critical feature of the application for departmental status regarded

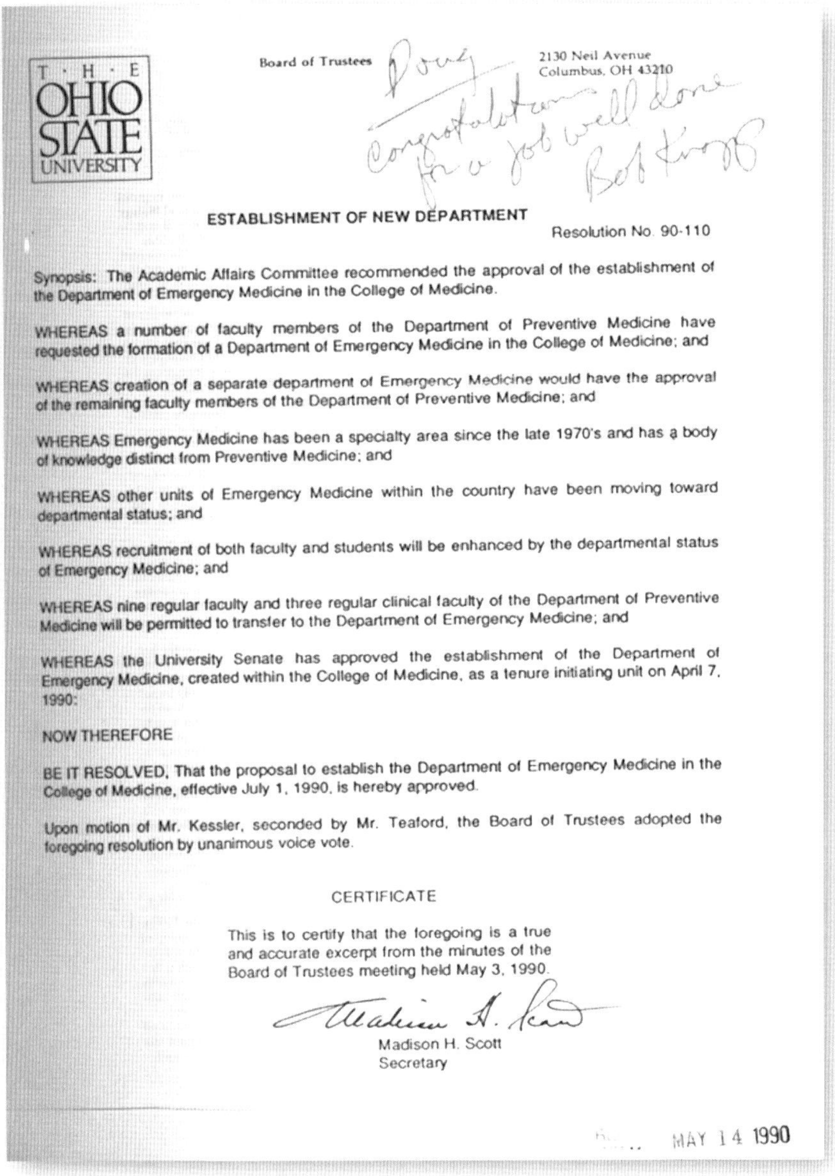

Figure 1: Resolution of the Ohio State University Board of Trustees, May 3, 1990, establishing the new Department of Emergency Medicine

the separate designations of "regular" faculty and "clinical" faculty. At the time of approval, university rules required that no more than one-third of the faculty could hold regular clinical appointments. Regular faculty were on the tenure track. Such faculty had six years to demonstrate worthiness for promotion to the rank of Associate Professor, which was nearly always associated with the granting of tenure: an academic position for life.

Faculty promoted to the rank of Associate Professor had to demonstrate excellence in scholarship, which typically required high quality research and, better yet, external grant support. At the time of the application, nine faculty members were on the tenure track and three were on the regular clinical track. The clinical track faculty held time limited appointments and no possibility of tenure. Over time these rules would change to allow for more clinicians to care for greater numbers of patients in the university hospitals.

Ohio State emergency medicine faculty could not wait to spread the word of the trustees' action and the text of the resolution itself. There was great cheering in the emergency medicine academic community. Congratulations came pouring in from national leaders of the specialty, including those who had been involved in the growth of the division since its inception.

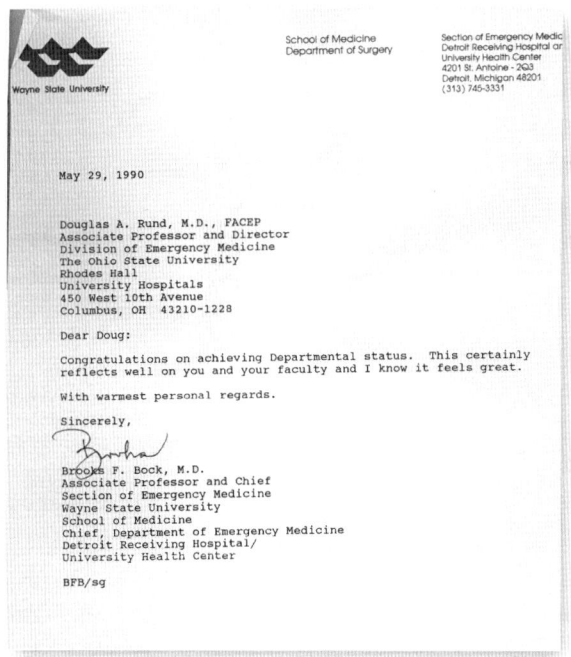

Figure 2: Letter of congratulation from Brooks Bock, MD, who conducted the first accreditation site visit of the division in 1980.

Brooks Bock, MD, conducted the first site visit of the residency program in 1980. In 1990 he was the Chief of the Section of Emergency Medicine at Wayne State University. He wrote congratulations to the faculty and enthused, "I know it feels great" (Figure 2). Harvey Meislin, MD, did the second site visit in 1980 and 10 years later wrote, "I am going to be sending my dean the announcement

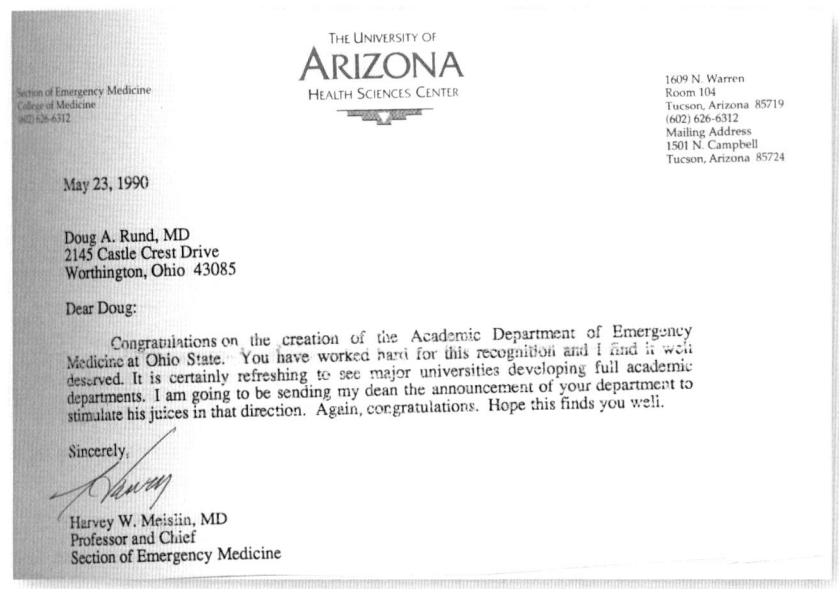

Figure 3: Letter from Harvey Meislin, MD. Meislin conducted the second site visit which led to the approval of the residency program in 1980.

Figure 4: Letter from Ronald Krome, MD, on the establishment of the department. Krome turned down Ohio State's offer to direct the division in 1975. At the time of his letter, he was the Editor of the *Annals of Emergency Medicine* and the popular textbook, *Emergency Medicine: a Comprehensive Study*.

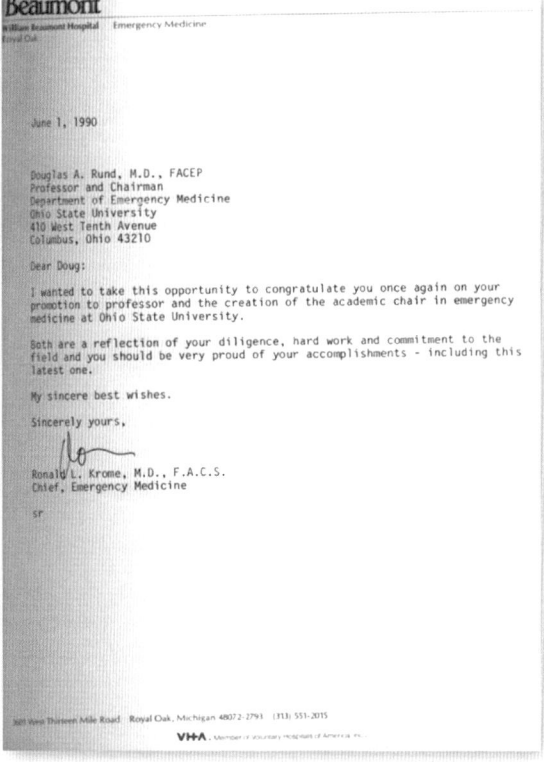

of your department to *stimulate his juices in that direction*" (Figure 3). He was the Chief of the Section of Emergency Medicine at the University of Arizona at the time. The section was in the Department of Surgery. Meislin later became Vice Chair of the Department of Surgery and eventually Chair of the Department of Emergency Medicine when the academic department was created in 2001.

Richard M. Nowak, MD, Chairman of the Department of Emergency Medicine at the Henry Ford Hospital in Detroit wrote:

> *Congratulations on the establishment of a full Department of Emergency Medicine in the College of Medicine at Ohio State University... With further academic department development, I believe the specialty will rightfully take its place in the house of academic medicine.*[1]

Ronald Krome, MD, who was initially recruited to be the director of the Ohio State Emergency Department in 1975 wrote a letter of congratulations praising the "diligence, hard work and commitment to this field" (Figure 4).

In 1978 Krome was part of the panel discussion published in *The Archives of Surgery* (see Chapter 5) regarding the specialty of emergency medicine. David Wagner, MD. who was also a part of the discussion wrote an enthusiastic hand written note: "Yeah!! Everything comes to the person who waits...and PRODUCES. Congratulations."

Wagner, like Krome, was one of the founders of emergency medicine. He started the Department of Emergency Medicine at the Medical College of Pennsylvania where he was Chairman. The College eventually became a department in Drexel University and he served as Chair. Initially trained as a surgeon, Wagner became an icon in the world of academic emergency medicine. Always calm and thoughtful, he served as President of American Board of Emergency Medicine and the Society for Academic Emergency Medicine; he also served as a Chair of the Residency Review Committee for Emergency Medicine (Figure 5).

The developments leading up to the creation of the department at Ohio State began with the original plan in 1977. The pace and intensity of this effort ramped up considerably, however, in July 1988 when Martin D. "Marty" Keller, MD, PhD, stepped down as the Chair of Preventive Medicine due to a university age restriction for chairmen that

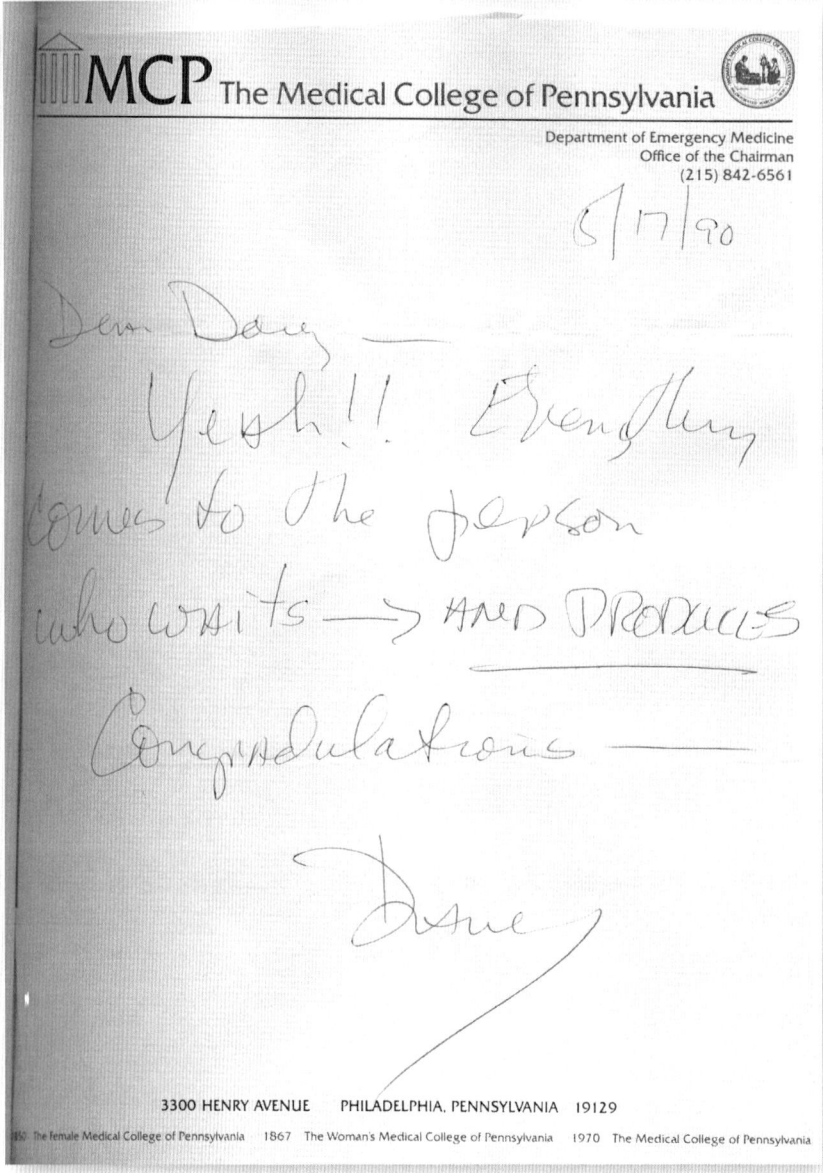

Figure 5: Letter from David Wagner, MD, who was among the top echelon of leaders in academic emergency medicine in the early days of the formation of the specialty.

existed at that time. Douglas Rund, MD, was then appointed Interim Chair of the Department of Preventive Medicine. As Interim Chair he had additional resources and help from the College of Medicine to create the separate department while the college began the search for a new leader for Preventive Medicine. Keller continued his teaching and research in the department as a professor and never stopped supporting emergency medicine.

As Interim Chair Rund had the opportunity to tout emergency medicine to a wider audience including respected faculty leaders such as the illustrious Robert M. Zollinger, MD, considered a giant of American surgery: onetime president of all major surgical organizations in the United States and former Professor and Chairman of the Department of Surgery.

Just prior to his appointment as Interim Chair of Preventive Medicine, Rund elected to begin his six-month sabbatical leave at the University of Edinburgh. He became a post-graduate Fellow in the Department of Community Medicine. His curriculum included courses in epidemiology and public health. His research work addressed trauma prevention and exploring the differences in public demand for emergency services in the United Kingdom and the United States.

Dr. Zollinger: On Board
By Douglas Rund, MD

One morning in 1988, at 8:00—surgeon's time—Dr. Robert Zollinger called me and asked for a meeting. He said, "Is this a good time?" I was thinking, "Are you kidding? Of course, I have time to meet the most legendary surgeon at Ohio State."

When we met, he asked me, "What is this emergency medicine anyway? Surgeons aren't doing their job are they?"

I explained that we were about more than surgery and trauma. Patients were coming in for all sorts of problems and we had to train doctors to take care of all comers everywhere, especially in smaller communities that may not even have a surgeon available at all times. I explained that we had patients with medical, obstetric, pediatric and psychiatric problems, that we needed to train specialists in the early care of an incredibly wide range of problems and be really good at things that needed immediate care like cardiac arrest.

He got it right away. We had a great conversation. It lasted at least an hour and he was so very helpful in talking about leadership and faculty development—how to encourage people, make opportunities available and create an environment where they can be successful. He was a supporter from then on.

THOMAS R. BULLOCK, MD

In 1987 during Rund's absence, Thomas R. Bullock, MD, became the Interim Director of the Division. Bullock grew up in Ohio. He graduated from Kenyon College and enrolled in the George Washington University School of Medicine. He graduated with his MD degree in 1979 and completed his residency training in emergency medicine at the St. Vincent Hospital/Toledo Hospital program in 1982. He joined the faculty at Ohio State in July of 1982.

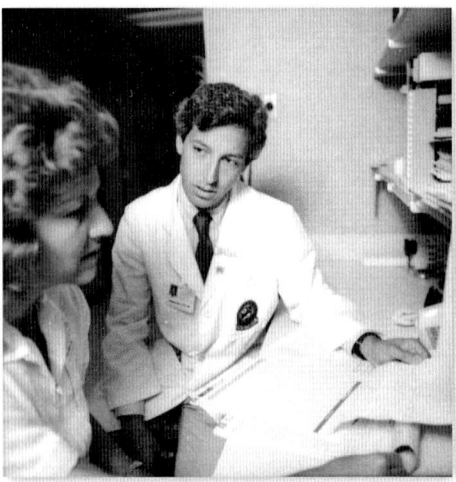

Figure 6: Thomas R. Bullock, MD, teaching in the emergency department. Photo shows the paper charts of that era.

Bullock was an outstanding clinician and educator (Figure 6). Compassionate and thoughtful, he was an excellent role model for students and residents. Years later Bullock reflected upon his early years at Ohio State. In a glaring omission, the orientation process for new faculty members in the early days was startlingly nonexistent. Many years later he recalled his first shift at Ohio State:

> *At the beginning of my first shift in the emergency department, I met Polly Hansplant, RN. She was excellent. I worked an evening shift. At that time, we didn't do things where you would shadow somebody for weeks, so the time to get oriented in a place it was just "trial by fire". I went in and she thought I was one of the new interns and within minutes I was doing a central line.*[2]

Bullock further remembered the early days in the department:

> *We were working really hard and there were only five of us. We covered all the hours and our schedule at that time, was going nights, evening, days and covering all the weekends. It was a lot of work. We ran back and forth from the medicine side to the surgical side, and the first-year grads or interns in surgery and medicine had a lot more autonomy those days than they do now. We did have a full*

> *second-year class of emergency medicine interns. I remember that it was always so awesome to be working with an actual emergency medicine house staff member, but there were so few of them and they had so many other things to do that we only got to work with them once in a while. It made life a whole different when we were working with one of them.*[2]

During Rund's sabbatical, Bullock became Interim Director of the Division of Emergency Medicine. He recalled part of his experience years later:

> *I was attending meetings that you would have gone to and we were still attached to Preventive Medicine and that was an interesting experience as my first experience going to faculty meetings and I was often surprised at how much acrimony there was. I was taken aback by that. Those guys didn't hold back at all. I also remember from just talking with you that how wise we were, [being] placed in the care of Preventive Medicine and Marty Keller because it probably saved the department from being taken over by medicine or surgery, and helped you become autonomous.*[2]

Bullock began working with the hospital administration to develop quality assurance programs. At that time such programs were just coming into existence. A crisis developed when two attending physicians, a married couple, abruptly decided to quit and move on. Bullock began recruiting in earnest and eventually convinced Michael T. Kelley, MD, to return to Ohio State from California. Kelley was one of the first graduates of the emergency medicine residency program. He remained a member of the faculty until 1997. Over time he began to focus his practice increasingly in the area of his subspecialty: toxicology.

Bullock's recollections of the relatively stressful working environment in the early days were recalled as he remembered the following:

> *I remember leaving the department, which I don't think you would ever do now, to leave in the middle of the night, to get home to my wife, who was in labor. I remember leaving the department in the hands of an intern and running home to Upper Arlington, grabbing her and bringing her in, and then finishing up my shift and running up there and spending the rest of the 24 hours waiting for my first child to be born in October 1982.*[2]

Preparation for the Effort to Become a Full Academic Department

Faculty Recruitment

It was clear that additional faculty members would be needed to accomplish all that needed to be done to convince the university that emergency medicine qualified for department status. In 1988 three additional physicians were recruited to the faculty: James W. Hoekstra, MD, Daniel R. Martin, MD, and Jonathan B. Brooks, MD.

JAMES W. "JIM" HOEKSTRA, MD

The recruitment of Hoekstra in 1988 was a critical step on the path to becoming an academic department. Hoekstra was a much prized "triple threat." In academic medicine that meant that the faculty member was excellent in the three important mission areas: research, patient care and education. These attributes were essential to the success of the division and its ultimate transformation to an academic department. Faculty members like Hoekstra were on the tenure track or appointed as "regular" faculty, in university parlance. The division had to demonstrate that two-thirds of the faculty were on the tenure track and were scholars. The physicians in the hospital needed to have confidence in the clinical skills of the emergency physicians and the division had to demonstrate a range of student courses taught by division faculty.

Hoekstra grew up in Michigan and graduated with his BA degree from Hope College. He completed medical school at the University of Michigan, receiving his MD degree with distinction in 1984. He completed his residency program in emergency medicine at the University of Cincinnati in 1988. His residency program was one of the oldest in the nation and was four years in duration. He completed his residency in 1988 and immediately joined the faculty at Ohio State as an Assistant Professor. He completed residency one day and began his first shift at Ohio State the following day.

He worked with Charles G. Brown, MD, in the area of cardiac resusci-

> ### "Sick" or "Not Sick" *By Douglas Rund, MD*
>
> One of Hoekstra's more famous teaching tactics was to ask the residents to hone their skills in quickly assessing patients. His reasoning was that in practice they could quickly be overwhelmed by a sudden deluge of patients and thus must be adept at taking care of many patients almost simultaneously.
>
> He therefore asked the resident to quickly determine by an immediate and rapid assessment if each patient was in one of two categories: "sick" or "not sick." If the patient was "sick", they needed resuscitation, consultation and hospital admission. If they were "not sick" they needed to be diagnosed, treated properly and, in all likelihood, discharged from the emergency department. The exercise, seemingly simple on the surface, was essential for success in a busy practice following graduation.

tation and co-authored eight publications from laboratory and clinical studies in his first few years. He was an outstanding clinician and teacher, and his four years of residency prepared him well to teach. During the final year of his program in Cincinnati he was Chief Resident with significant responsibilities for resident education.

Hoekstra was an outstanding clinician. In later years Hoekstra remembered his first day as an attending physician in the emergency department (ED):

> *I remember my first day at Ohio State. I was a young, eager, energetic new grad from the University of Cincinnati (UC) emergency medicine residency. My last shift at UC was a Friday evening shift from 3-11 PM. I got home, hit the bed, and dug out early in the morning for Ohio State. I started my first ED shift at Ohio State University Hospital at 11 AM. I was bleary-eyed, but eager to get going.*
>
> *When I arrived in the ED, I was given the typical OSU orientation: "There's a whole bunch of yellow tags here. Go ahead and get started. You're a smart guy. You'll figure it out." I was off and running! Welcome to the ED.*
>
> *Those were the days of paper charts, spread on the counters on clipboards, with no electronic tracking or electronic orders, and no dictation. Everything was done by paper, and every order required a lot of*

continual communication and individual follow through. "Yellow tags" were plastic tags on the clipboard that indicated a patient was waiting to be seen. There were tags for orders and tags for discharge. Needless to say, these processes would easily allow a patient to slip through the cracks.

One of the most infuriating processes was the gathering of "old charts" on any patient with prior admissions or a complex medical history. We would ask the back desk clerk (who was the most valuable person in the ED) to "order up old charts" on a patient. They would call medical records, and have the old paper charts sent to the ED. About an hour later, they would show up, maybe, sometimes on a cart, and often with large pieces missing. Sometimes they were a foot thick. Knowing where to search for meds, discharge instructions and lab studies was an art form. It would be an invaluable lesson for the residents of today, on how good they have it.[3]

Hoekstra was the "de facto" director of student education in the division when he began and continued on in greater and greater leadership positions within the College of Medicine, particularly in the student curriculum long after the establishment of the department. In the accelerated preparation of the application for department status, the faculty felt that the University would require additional course offerings for students. The faculty quickly developed curricula for additional student courses, including a seminar and an individual studies program.

Ohio State had always had a very popular fourth year medical school elective in emergency medicine. The students got more one-on-one faculty teaching, patient variety and direct hands-on care than in any other rotation. The student ratings of the elective were stellar. After becoming a department, the rotation became a medical school requirement as the part of the "Differentiation of Care" "selective" series. Emergency medicine was crucial for teaching the approach to the acute and undifferentiated patient. Rural sites at Marysville and Delaware were added, and eventually a third-year required experience was added to the curriculum.

The department also taught Basic Life Support (BLS) and Advanced Cardiac Life Support (ACLS) to all the students, and emergency medicine faculty were involved in many administrative and leadership roles in the medical school. Education was always a strong point with the Ohio State Department of Emergency Medicine (Figure 7).

In 2003 Hoekstra was recruited to Wake Forest School of Medicine as Professor and Chair of Wake's Department of Emergency Medicine. Over the years he became the driver of the system's expansion and network creation. He became Senior Vice President and Associate Dean, Clinical and Academic Network Development and Professor, Department of Emergency Medicine at the Wake Forest Baptist Medical Center in North Carolina. He also became the President of the Wake Forest Baptist Hospital High Point Medical Center.

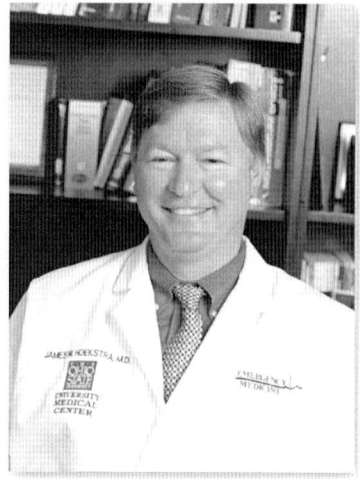

Figure 7: James W. Hoekstra, MD, was recruited to the faculty in 1988. His considerable strengths in clinical care, research and education strengthened the division's application to become a full department. He led the expansion of the student curriculum in the department and the college for years to come.

Bootstraps
By Douglas Rund, MD

I always wondered, in later years, whether or not I made a mistake in claiming that our faculty would support ourselves without college help when we pushed so hard to become a full department in 1990. At that time, one of the major road blocks in getting all other departments to agree was that if a new department was formed, it might take away money and space.

One day, during the negotiations to become an academic department, I was speaking with Dr. Tzagournis, Vice President and Dean, and told him the division simply had to become a full department as soon as possible, and that "it won't cost you anything...we will support ourselves through our patient billings." Tzagournis replied, "Okay but you will have to pull yourselves up by your own bootstraps...it will be either sink or swim." The faculty swam, and did so for many years, paying nearly all our expenses and several resident salaries from patient billings.

DANIEL R. MARTIN, MD, MBA

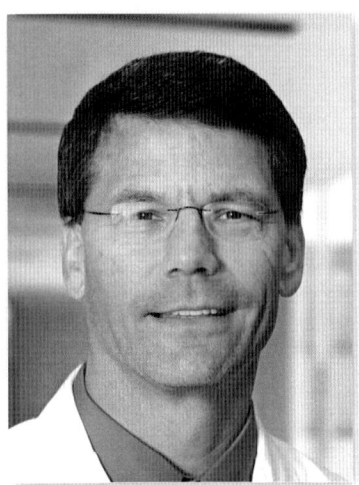

Figure 8: Daniel R. Martin, MD, was recruited in 1988 to join the regular faculty leading up to the application for departmental status. Martin completed residencies in both Internal Medicine and Emergency Medicine, helping to create understanding between the departments.

Like Hoekstra, Daniel R "Dan" Martin, MD, MBA, FACEP, FAAEM, was also a "triple threat." He had completed five years of residency and had research and teaching skills that made him an essential addition to the tenure track scholars in the department. Martin also worked closely with Charles Brown and was the second author on Brown's widely read study about high dose epinephrine in *The New England Journal of Medicine*.[4] His dual education in Emergency Medicine and Internal Medicine also made him an excellent teacher for students and residents in emergency medicine. In two years after his appointment, he took over as the Program Director for the Ohio State University Residency program and served in that role until 2010 when he became Vice Chair for Education (Figure 8).

Martin grew up in Indiana. He received his undergraduate degree from Indiana University and his MD degree from the Indiana University School of Medicine. He completed his Internal Medicine Residency at the University of Iowa Hospitals and Clinics and his Emergency Medicine Residency at the Medical College of Wisconsin. He was Chief Resident during his final year.

One of the most important credentials Martin possessed was his residency training and board certification in internal medicine. He held a dual appointment in both Internal Medicine and Emergency Medicine and functioned as a "bridge" between the departments. His presence on the faculty was important in securing the positive support of the powerful Department of Medicine when the issue of departmental status arose in formal and informal meetings of the leaders of the College. Martin showed that he provided outstanding patient care, teaching at all levels and scholarship. Later in his career, he initiated a Combined Emergency Medicine and Internal Medicine Residency Program which benefited both internal medicine and emergency medicine. Martin remained as the remained the combined program's founder and director.

Early in his career Martin developed expertise in infectious diseases. He lectured and published about all types of infectious diseases, especially those affecting the respiratory system.

JONATHAN B. BROOKS, MD

Jonathan B. Brooks, MD, received his MD from the Medical College of Pennsylvania n 1985 and completed his residency in emergency medicine at Ohio State in 1988. He joined the faculty as an Assistant Professor immediately following graduation. He joined Howard Werman, MD, as one of the first residency graduates to join the faculty. He was an excellent clinician and teacher.

Engagement of the Ohio State College of Medicine

The Ohio State College of Medicine leadership understood that the division was determined to meet all university criteria for full academ-

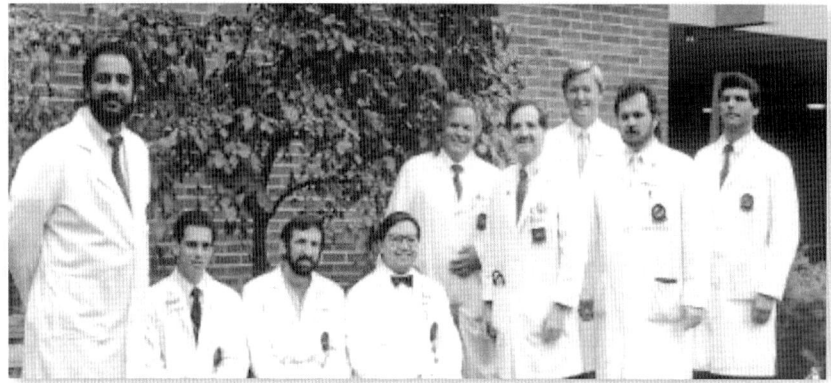

Figure 9: Department of Emergency Medicine faculty after establishment of the academic department. From left to right: Charles G. Brown, MD; Jonathan B. Brooks, MD; Howard A Werman, MD; Peter Van Ligten; Douglas A. Rund, MD; Richard N. Nelson, MD; James W. Hoekstra MD; Michael T. Kelley, MD; and Daniel R. Martin, MD.

ic department status. As noted, the faculty were demonstrating that emergency medicine was indeed a specialty and that original research from the division was contributing greatly to its body of knowledge. Student demand for the clinical experience was high and so were the evaluations of teaching. Teaching materials, including textbooks authored by the faculty, were well-received and the faculty were being recognized for their leadership in national organizations. The residency consistently did well in the match program and always filled with excellent graduates. The division had the correct proportion of regular faculty members and "regular clinical" faculty members, which was two regular members to one regular clinical member (Figure 9). Preventive Medicine supported the application for full academic department status.

DAVID G. CORNWELL, PHD

After intensive urging by the faculty, The College of Medicine agreed to help pursue departmental status assigned a mentor. The Dean gave the task of assisting in the preparation of the application to David G. Cornwell, PhD, Associate Dean for Academic Affairs and Secretary to the Faculty (Figure 10). Cornwell was a biochemist. He earned his BA degree from the College of Wooster in 1951, his MA from Ohio State in 1952 and his PhD in chemistry from Stanford in 1955. After graduation

Cornwell: A Problem Solver Who Thinks "Out of the Box"

By Douglas Rund, MD

According to Paulson, Cornwell found the solution to problems with imaginative approaches. Regarding the matter of informed consent, he avoided the issue by using *his own blood* in his lipoprotein studies. At Harvard and later at Ohio State he would ingest "various lipids and then would have his future wife, skilled at venipuncture, take blood samples from him."[4] Obviously, he was a problem solver not afraid to use novel approaches to problems. This attribute served him well in his future career, and ultimately to the benefit of emergency medicine as the application for approval of the department progressed through the various bureaucratic hoops at the university.

he accepted a National Academy of Sciences fellowship to study lipoprotein chemistry at Harvard Medical School.

Cornwell was a successful investigator funded early on by the National Institutes of Health (NIH). His areas of study included new methods for the identification of lipids, the study of the surfaces of cell membranes and the chemistry and biology of the prostaglandins. In his later years he studied vitamin E, cultural aspects of diet and the "nutritional and dietary

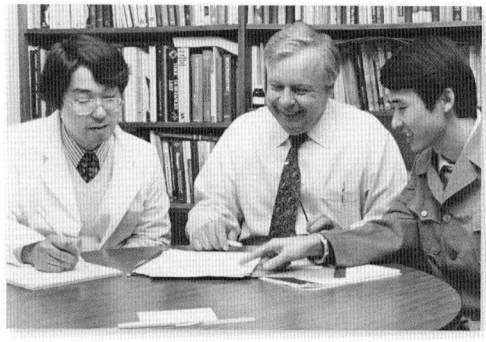

Figure 10: David G. Cornwell, PhD, Associate Dean for Academic Affairs and Secretary to the Faculty in 1990, when Emergency Medicine became a separate academic department in the university. He was invaluable in the process toward approval of the new department.

Rund Appreciates Cornwell   *By Douglas Rund, MD*

I wrote the following in my personal journal on February 21, 1990:

Today the Council of Academic Affairs approved the resolution on the next page. In essence, this clears the way for our departmental proposal to the University Senate. They will meet sometime in April or May to consider this again and again. Dave Cornwell and I will be present. Dave C. has been a great help in this matter...he steps in when I'm in trouble, which is not infrequent. Today, for instance, the question was asked... "if there are only two senior level faculty members, who will serve on the department's promotion and tenure committee?" Dave pointed out that this is not unusual for the college and that they would help as needed.

Later I noted the following:

Dave C. told me that my promotion passed College and University P and T and that they were impressed with my credentials and his letter! He says he specializes in fiction at this time of year...should be a Hemmingway.

By the end of this whole process, I was referring to Dean Cornwell as "Uncle Dave," a highly deserved and affectionate honorific for all the work he did on our behalf.

changes that occurred at the dawn of modern civilization."[5] Cornwell was the Chairman of the Department of Molecular and Cellular Biochemistry prior to taking on his important role as associate dean.

Once Cornwell was sure that the College backed the proposal to establish an academic department of emergency, he warmed considerably to the idea of helping the department and eventually became one of its strongest advocates. He was especially impressed by Chuck Brown and the quality of his research and clinical acumen.

The Race to Become a Department: The University's Hurdles

The Council of Chairs in the College of Medicine

The first step in the process of becoming a department was the approval of the Dean and Vice President of the College of Medicine. The outcome of their approval was the selection of David Cornwell as the guide. The second step was approval by the Council of Chairs in the College. From the beginning, the division faculty worked hard to create support and build alliances within the college toward the day when the vote would be taken to create an academic department. In his undergraduate days, Rund was active in student politics. As the Speaker of the Yale Political Union, he learned early on to create and communicate a vision for others to see; and secure commitments for affirmative votes well in advance of an actual election. In the case of the department vote by the Council of Chairs, he felt secure; he had firm commitments from all the departmental chairs and dean's staff—or so he thought. The early morning discussion about the proposal to establish the department was brief and a few questions answered. Then came the vote. All hands were raised in the affirmative...all but one.

Upon the call for those opposing the motion, one hand slowly went up. Olga Jonasson, MD, Chair of the Department of Surgery, voted against Emergency Medicine. The motion passed with all but one vote and would proceed to the next step in the process. Astounded, Rund asked Jonasson as everyone filed out: "Why did you vote no?" Her reply seemed incongruously almost friendly: "I think you belong in the Department of Surgery." All the years of planning, starting with the decision to grow in the Department of Preventive Medicine were affirmed. In another department, escape would have been difficult indeed.

The Council on Academic Affairs

The next step in the tortuous road was consideration by the Council on Academic Affairs. The council reported to the Office of Academic Affairs led by the provost. On February 21, 1990, Cornwell and Rund presented the following resolution to the Council: that the Department of Emergency Medicine be created within the College of Medicine as a tenure initiating unit, effective July 1, 1990. The resolution included an extensive description of regular clinical faculty who held the title, for example, of assistant professor of clinical emergency medicine. The resolution further stipulated the following:

> *The number of persons holding regular clinical faculty titles in each department or college cannot be greater than one-third the number of persons holding regular faculty titles in that department or college. Individuals appointed to the regular clinical faculty are limited to participation in governance at the departmental and college levels, but may not participate in promotion and tenure matters of regular faculty.*

The issue of regular clinical faculty was a potentially contentious one. Tenured faculty members who held their positions for life did not relish being replaced with faculty members who held "clinical" positions with time limited contracts. Nevertheless, the university recognized that a medical center needed practicing physicians to care for the increasing patient demands. The regular clinical designation only applied to the colleges of optometry, dentistry, veterinary medicine and clinical departments within the College of Medicine. This rule would change over time, but in 1990 emergency medicine had to have as many faculty on the tenure track as possible.

The University Senate

Rund and Cornwell headed to the University Senate. On Saturday morning April 7, 1990 the University Senate of the Ohio State University passed a resolution recommending the establishment of a department of emergency medicine. There was a presentation and very little discussion. The approval was the second to last hurdle for the resolution to establish the Department of Emergency Medicine. The approval meant that the matter would be placed on the agenda of the Ohio State Board of Trustees for its May 3rd meeting. This was essential if the establishment of the department was to take place on July 1, 1990.

The Board of Trustees

Rund and Cornwell were present when the Ohio State Board of Trustees voted to approve the establishment of the new Department of Emergency Medicine. By the time of the meeting, the issue had been thoroughly vetted by the university—through the College of Medicine, university subcommittees, councils, the provost, the university senate, the academic affairs committee of the board and the president's office. The decision was certainly not made without significant scrutiny. The resolution passed unanimously by voice vote.

The Parties

On July 2, 1990, the new department faculty bought trays of food and pizza for everyone working in the emergency department during all shifts. Flowers were sent to the department by the preventive medicine faculty. A few weeks later a gala was scheduled at the home of the Runds in Worthington. Tents, food, bar and the band were set up in the back yard. The mood was incredibly joyous. Thirteen years of work and planning had finally brought results. All emergency medicine faculty members, residents and administrative staff were there.

Faculty from preventive medicine and supportive faculty members from all departments were invited. All members of the dean's staff who were involved in anyway were invited and attended. Just as the party was getting under way, a flash rainstorm drove everyone inside: close and personal. Speeches expressed gratitude from emergency medicine to all for their hard work and congratulations from college leaders to emergency medicine. The rain finally ended and the party moved back outdoors. Two medical students served as "bartenders." Both eventually became full professors of emergency medicine in universities on opposite ends of the country.

The department was off and running. The numbers of patients seeking care was increasing. The department needed to add faculty members and increase the size of the residency program. The research program was growing in prestige and the department's courses were always brimming with students. The challenge was to grow to greater national prominence, secure the department's finances and continue to provide the best possible treatment to patients needing expert care in our department.

References

1. Nowak RM. Personal communication with Douglas Rund. 1990.

2. Bullock TR. Interview with Thomas R. Bullock, MD, by Douglas Rund. 2022: Columbus, Ohio.

3. Hoekstra JW. Personal communication with Douglas Rund. 2022: Columbus, Ohio.

4. Brown CG, Martin DR et al. A comparison of standard-dose and high-dose epinephrine in cardiac arrest outside the hospital. *NEJM.* 1992; 327:1051-1055.

5. Paulson GW. Cornwell GD. *In Pursuit of Excellence: The Ohio State University Medical Center from 1834 to 2010.* 2010:177-179.

Chapter 8

Faculty Growth and the Restructuring of the Residency Program: 1990-2001

Douglas A. Rund, MD
Richard N. Nelson, MD

The establishment of the academic Ohio State University Department of Emergency Medicine in 1990 was the result of the faculty's concentrated and sustained effort, beginning with the division's founding in 1977, a triumph requiring the recruitment of *academically* oriented faculty as early as possible. In those early days, the hiring of faculty members with clinical skills only was not possible: The faculty member *had to have research interests* as well. Clinical appointments were time limited and did not lead to a lifetime appointment unlike tenure track (regular) appointments, which did lead to a lifetime appointment.

In this time period the university requirements limited the number of faculty who could hold regular *clinical* appointments to only one-third of the number of regular faculty. This was done to protect the tenure system, which could be threatened if regular faculty members were gradually replaced by those with five-year contracts, for example. This was a constant restriction to unlimited clinical growth in that era.

During those years it was also vital that faculty members have a high likelihood of promotion. If a faculty member was not promoted by the seventh year of service there would be no eighth year. They would, in effect, be terminated. There was also a need to have all ranks of faculty in a department from assistant professor to professor so that all levels were represented. The department needed tenured associate professors and professors. This required a constant, intentional effort to ensure a stable faculty. It was therefore essential that the division's scarce resources be used to support faculty members with the greatest potential for scholarship.

The need for educators was also increasing due to a blossoming student program, a residency program that was undergoing a restructuring and the need for additional attending faculty members. Starting in 1990 the eventual reorganization of the program required an increase in the number of residents, which meant the experience at Ohio State had begun to change. Residents were constantly present and took care of far more patients. Also, senior residents were present to supervise junior residents and care for the sickest patients with faculty supervision.

Faculty Growth: Research and Scholarship

In 1990 Charles Brown, MD, was the undisputed leader of the research effort in the department. Talented research-oriented physicians joined the faculty first as research fellows and then as regular faculty. It was clear, however, that the search for research faculty had to continue to broaden the research base of the department.

MARK G. ANGELOS, MD

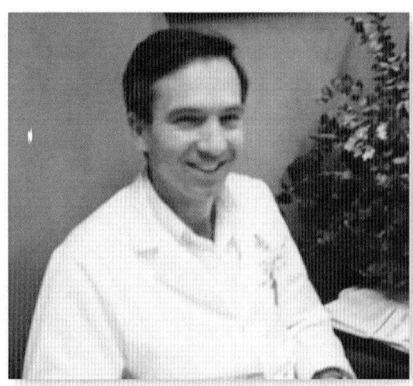

Figure 1: Mark G. Angelos, MD, was trained in emergency medicine and critical care. He joined the faculty in 1991 and continued the research program begun by Charles Brown, MD, and others in the department. He eventually became Chair of the Department of Emergency Medicine.

The recruitment of Mark G. Angelos, MD, in 1991 was an example of such recruitment efforts. He had completed a fellowship in critical care at the University of Pittsburgh with Peter Safar, MD, founder of modern cardiopulmonary resuscitation. Angelos was an Assistant Professor at Wright State University when he was recruited. He immediately began working with Brown and Charles Little, DO, in resuscitation research.

When Brown departed from the faculty, Angelos took over as research leader in the cardiopulmonary resuscitation research effort. He was highly productive during his career and eventually became Professor and Chair of the Department of Emergency Medicine. Through his sustained effort as faculty member and chair, the department grew in stature to become one of the foremost in research in the country (Figure 1).

CHARLES MEDARIS "CHARLIE" LITTLE, DO, FACEP

Charles M. "Charlie" Little, DO, also showed research talent. A resident in emergency medicine at Ohio State from 1988 to 1991, he stayed on as a faculty member and remained a member of the faculty until 1998. A Colorado native, Little received his BA degree from the University of Colorado in 1980, then became a Denver paramedic for the next three years. In 1983 he enrolled in the Des Moines University College of Osteopathic Medicine and graduated with his DO degree in 1987. He completed an internship at the Detroit Osteopathic Hospital and upon completion of his internship joined the emergency medicine residency program at Ohio State in 1988. Having already completed an internship and three years of practice as a paramedic, Little was advanced in his clinical skills, especially early on. He was also a leader and was elected chief resident at the end of his second year (Figure 2).

Following his residency, he completed a 2-year fellowship in resuscitation research methodology in 1993. He then joined the faculty and worked with Brown and Angelos, studying changes in the heart during cardiac arrest and resuscitation as well as novel therapeutic approaches to cardiac arrest. The team also developed highly collaborative relationships with other investigators throughout the university. Years later, Little remembered his research efforts:

> *When I moved on to faculty, I remember being with other core cardiac arrest researchers and we had a shared office with cubicles a floor below the hospital's kitchen. The office would flood occasionally when overflows occurred in the kitchen. It was actually very productive and cooperative because everyone was sitting in there and we could bounce ideas off each other.*

> *Chuck Brown at that time was working on developing kind of novel alpha-adrenergic agents for cardiac arrest. We actually had a lot of success in some early work in the adrenergic realms where I was working for cardiac arrest. Chuck Brown at that time was working on developing novel alpha-adrenergic agents for cardiac arrest. We also put together some proposals for some adrenergic vasopressors. That actually went pretty well. We had some pretty novel stuff where we worked out what we could actually do using the radiolabeled microspheres and some pretty invasive instrumentation on the pig model. We could actually measure myocardial and cerebral blood flow and oxygen delivery and consumption across the organs as well as survival.[1]*

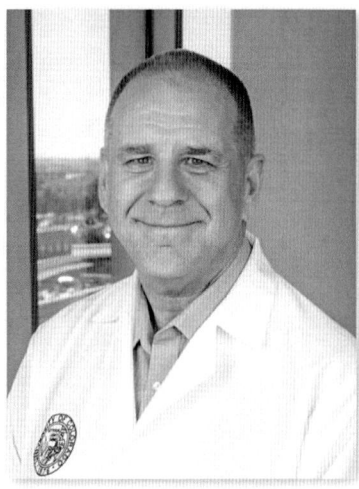

Figure 2: Charles M. Little, DO, worked with Charles Brown, MD, in the area of cardiopulmonary resuscitation in the early 1990s. He was also the incoming Chief Resident when the residency review committee for emergency medicine expanded its scrutiny of the Ohio State residency program in 1990.

Little and Brown's work with a swine model of cardiac arrest involved an intensive care unit for the animals in the basement laboratory. Residents volunteered to staff the unit throughout the night. Little remembered the experience:

> *We brought some lawn chairs into the animal care facility and we would sit there all night long for 12 hours watching the animal. There was also a baboon colony nearby. About 4 o'clock every morning the baboons would start howling. It was really kind of eerie. You would be sitting there listening to your little radio watching the pig and listening to the baboon's howl.[1]*

During his years at Ohio State, Little was extremely productive in resuscitation research and was highly valued by the faculty for his wisdom and leadership skills. He was also a superb clinician. His work was supported by the Emergency Medicine Foundation and other granting agencies.

Little was an Assistant Professor during his fellowship and afterward until 1998 when he returned to his native Colorado and became an Assistant Professor of surgery in the division of emergency medicine. At the University of Colorado, he was promoted to the rank of Associate Professor in the Department of Emergency Medicine, which had eventually emerged from the Department of Surgery. He became full Professor in 2019. At Colorado he had a distinguished career in the area of medical disaster and rescue. He eventually became the Medical Director of the Mountain Plains Regional Disaster Health Response System, Chief Medical Officer of the Federal Disaster Medical Assistance Team (DMAT CO-2) and Medical Director of Emergency Preparedness, University of Colorado Hospital.

JAMES W. HOEKSTRA, MD

James W. Hoekstra, who was recruited in 1988 (Figure 3), had considerable academic potential. He soon joined Brown and Little in their research efforts. At the time that he joined the research group they were using a swine model for their resuscitation experiments. Years later, Hoekstra remembered this about the research:

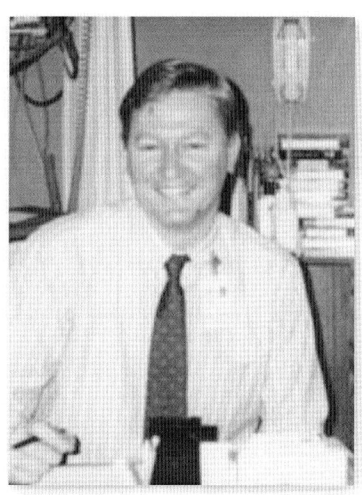

> *When I started at Ohio State, Chuck Brown, Bob Hamlin and Howie Werman were already establishing a national reputation for their work in cardiac resuscitation. They had perfected a pig model of ventricular fibrillation cardiac arrest and resuscitation, and were investigating the effects of high dose epinephrine and norepinephrine in the return of spontaneous circulation. I was placed in an office with Chuck and Howie. It did not take long to get involved.*
>
> *I have great memories of our pig lab experiences. We would start early in*

Figure 3: James Hoekstra was a "triple threat": He was excellent in patient care, teaching and research. He led the educational efforts for both the Department of Emergency Medicine and the College of Medicine at Ohio State.

the morning at the veterinary school, grabbing a 60-pound pig by the back legs, shooting them up with ketamine IM, and letting them go to sleep. This was not a process for the faint of heart. We would intubate the pigs, put them on inhaled nitrous oxide anesthesia, and instrument them for the procedure. We got very good at doing vascular cut-downs, thoracotomies, and even cardiac core biopsies. Sometimes it took a little work to get the smell out of our clothes, however.

Pig research was fun work, with good people. Heading out for beer or golf afterward made it even more fun, and presenting papers at SAEM or ACEP got us our start in EM academia. I remember my first oral presentation at SAEM, as a junior faculty member, on the utility of high dose norepinephrine in the pig model. I did not read the presentation, but my knees were shaking the whole time while I went through the slides.

Doing research was different back then. The paperwork involved in grant writing, ordering supplies, putting together a budget, etc. was daunting. It's amazing how hard it was to get a grant out the door with very basic word processors and secretaries typing everything up for you. Papers would undergo multiple typed revisions by Joyce (Rice), who could type faster than anyone (and she would let you know it!). Writing a paper was a process of actually writing the paper on a legal pad, typing by Joyce, revising, cutting and pasting, and bringing revisions back to Joyce to type all over again.

What takes three hours on a plane now took weeks back then. Even slide production was done in a home-grown shop with a 35mm camera, spotlights, and lots of revisions. We made our own slides and then spread them out on a display rack to coordinate them. We went to the meetings with 35mm slide carousels of slides in our bags. It was "old school" at its best.[2]

ROBERT "ROB" GRIFFITH, MD

Robert "Rob" Griffith, MD, was exposed to research as an undergraduate, synthesizing liquid crystal compounds for experimental purposes at the Liquid Crystal Institute at Kent State University in Ohio in 1978. He completed his MD degree at Washington University in 1982 and his residency training in emergency medicine at the University of Arizona Medical Center in Tucson in 1986. He then entered an internal medicine residency program at Saint Mary Medical Center in Long Beach, California. The hospital was part of the University of California-Los Angelos (UCLA) medical center.

While completing his last year of residency in the program in 1987, Griffith met Robert Simon, MD, who founded the International Medical Corps to aid the people of Afghanistan during the years of Soviet occupation in the 1980s. Immediately following completion of emergency medicine and internal medicine board examinations, Griffith became the Medical Director of the Clinic and Training Center in Peshawar Pakistan (Figure 4). Years later he recalled those formative years:

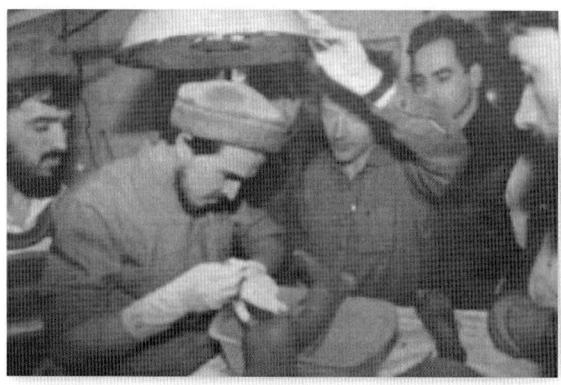

Figure 4: Rob Griffith, MD, watches as a student at the International Medical Corps clinic drains an Afghan refugee's wound.

> *The experience in Peshawar during the war between the Soviet Union and Afghanistan was an amazing combination of culture, language, medical practice and teaching. It rekindled an interest in academic medicine. When I finished there, it left me wondering what would be next.*[3]

Griffith completed his work in Afghanistan in 1988 and returned to his home in Ohio to deal with illness in his family and worked temporary assignments in several states, including North Dakota, with the Indian Health Service. While there he found a listing for the research fellowship at Ohio State. Griffith interviewed in Columbus and was accepted into the position. Years later he recalled this about the experience:

> *I was invited to join the fellowship in July 1989. The Research Director in the department was Dr. Charles G. (Chuck) Brown, an amazing person who combined an intellectual fire for improving delivery of care for our patients who suffered from cardiac arrest with a warm and supportive personality. His animal model used radiolabeled microspheres, small enough to get into different tissues of the heart but large enough that*

they would lodge in the target tissue. Using different radiolabels, it was possible to measure blood flow during CPR with different drug interventions and once spontaneous circulation returned. His work was largely performed in the pig model, as it was physiologically closest to human, and interventions could be compared. The team assembled by Dr. Brown worked incredibly well together and was a wonderful place to learn, participate and be productive.

A typical week in fellowship involved assembling with the team in the lab to perform an experiment, attending course work in statistics and studying related topics. Lab results were analyzed and compiled in papers, applications to present work at research meetings were made, and applications for funding were submitted as future projects were planned.

As busy as we all were, there was great esprit de corps among the team members, with Dr. Brown joining us every week or two for pizza at Flying Pizza or sushi at Restaurant Japan. I remember once flying to Toronto to present at a Canadian meeting. Chuck and I went out in search of a sushi place where we found the unusual situation that the guy bussing tables was also the sushi chef. The tuna had a slight brownish tint and I think we both were glad later that we did not get ill![3]

Griffith worked as an attending physician in the emergency department during and after his fellowship. He recalled this about his experience:

Alternate weekends, I would work two shifts in the Ohio State emergency department. At the time, the ED had single covered attending staffing, and as a fellow, you were considered an attending. There would typically be a second or senior resident who would assist in supervising interns, medical students, and the overall chaos. On Friday or Saturday nights, particularly in the fall, along with all the typical cases in a big city emergency department, we would have Ohio State freshmen discovering the fun that turns bad when excessive alcohol leads to deteriorating mental status and failure to protect their airways. At times, intubation was required. The faculty in the department shared supervisory responsibilities, each bringing his or her own stories and approaches to emergency medicine, strategies in the ED and their own particular research or administrative interests.

After completing two years of fellowship, I joined the faculty of The Ohio

State University Department of Emergency Medicine through 1993. I continued to participate in the academic activities along with increased responsibilities in the department with teaching and patient care. It was an incredible experience and one that I cherish.[3]

Griffith left Ohio State in 1993 and entered private practice at Emergency Services, Inc. (ESI), one of the oldest EM groups in the country, celebrating their 50-year anniversary in 2022 at Mount Carmel Health System in Columbus. At Mount Carmel he became President of ESI and ultimately President of the entire hospital medical staff. After 25 years at ESI, Griffith left the group with plans to share time between two places he loved, Hocking County, Ohio, and Costa Rica.

ROBERT GUTHRIE, MD

Robert Guthrie, MD, joined the Department of Emergency Medicine in 1992. Trained as an internist and family physician, he began his career in the Department of Family Medicine as an Assistant Professor on the tenure track in 1982. While there he became highly productive in research and teaching. He was the Director of the Residency Program in Family Medicine from 1983 to 1990. He was promoted to Associate Professor and awarded tenure in 1989. Guthrie's main research efforts were in the area of pharmacology and he had begun to assist the Department of Pharmacology with its Clinical Pharmacology Research program developing new medications. He also began his own research program testing new pharmaceutical agents with assistance from the Department of Pharmacology.

A dispute with the leadership of his department led to his transfer in 1992 to emergency medicine, which was a great boon to a department needing researchers and scholars. His transfer request was speedily approved and he was warmly welcomed into his new department. For a time, he worked clinically in the Prompt Care fast track area but his main interests were in research.

Seeing a need to evaluate new pharmacological agents in his unique area of interest, primary care, Guthrie began to study and evaluate agents to treat hypertension, high cholesterol and diabetes, among other common problems. Guthrie added considerably to emergency medicine's

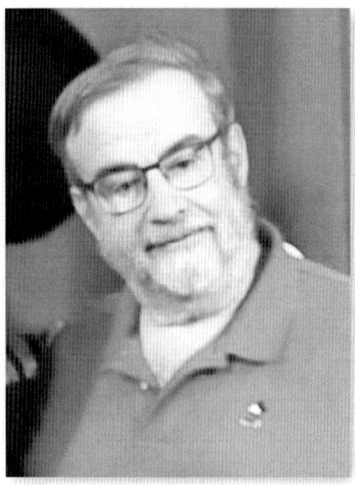

Figure 5: Robert Guthrie, MD, joined the Ohio State Emergency Medicine faculty in 1992. He was a vital addition to a faculty searching for academic scholars.

research portfolio, especially in the early years of the department—and his work provided badly needed income and prestige to the department.

During his distinguished career, Guthrie conducted over 70 pharmaceutical trials for new medication development earning over $2.7 million in grants. He had also assisted the Clinical Pharmacology research program in the Department of Pharmacology in conducting numerous trials for over $40 million in grants. He was also very involved with an investigator, Moon Chen PhD, from the Ohio State School of Public Health in research on health issues in the Asian American community funded by federal grants.

In 2009 Guthrie authored the book, *Hypertension and Dyslipidemia Management Essentials*, published by Jones and Bartlett. During his career, he authored 90 published articles in peer reviewed journals, presented 61 peer reviewed papers at national and international meetings and had 38 peer reviewed abstracts published, along with 44 editor reviewed papers and two book chapters. Guthrie was promoted to full Professor of emergency medicine in 1999. In 2009 Guthrie was awarded the Faculty Researcher of the Year in the Ohio State Department of Emergency Medicine.

From 1990 to 2000 Guthrie served as the Chair of the Family Practice Advisory Panel of the US Pharmacopeial Convention, a national organization overseeing the purity and quality of U.S. pharmaceutical products and the important scientific information about those pharmaceutical products. Guthrie's advisory service was recognized by The Ohio House of Representatives in 1990. A member of the Diagnostic and Therapeutic Advisory Panel (DATTA) of the American Medical Association from 1986 -1998, Guthrie served on the editorial review boards of *The Journal of Clinical Hypertension* and *Vascular Health and Risk Management*.

Guthrie became popular as a speaker regarding his research at Ohio State and attained a national and international reputation. He also served as a regular live air volunteer guest on WOSU Radio's "Open Line" show. He would answer questions from callers in the general public about medical problems and he would also discuss medical issues affecting the general public. He received the Josephine Failer Volunteer Award from WOSU in 1998.

After his retirement in 2012, Guthrie began his current role as the Editor in Chief of *The Physician and Sports Medicine*, an international peer reviewed sports medicine journal published by Taylor & Francis in London. Under his leadership the journal experienced significant growth. In his 10 years of his service, the journal saw a near doubling of its impact factor and more than a doubling of the number of manuscripts submitted for consideration with a 22% acceptance rate (Figure 5).

Faculty Growth: Education

Excellence in Education and Scholarship

Medical Students

Leading up to the application for full department status, student course offerings had to be expanded and included individual studies, a special victim care course for first-year students and the ever popular fourth-year clerkship in emergency medicine with its accompanying lecture series. Years later James Hoekstra reflected back on his early experiences with the student education program:

> *Medical student education in the ED at OSU was always stellar. We were one of the best clinical rotations in the medical school, and everyone knew it. We spent hours with the students in lectures and labs. It was a true team effort. Every faculty member participated.*
>
> *I remember I was in charge for many years of two basic courses: 1. Approach to the ED patient and 2. Wound care. Every month I would steal a bunch of suture materials, plaster, and bandage materials from the ED. We had a box or two full of discarded instruments from the ED as well. I would go down to the Kroger on Neil Avenue and buy a half dozen pigs feet, and bring it all to the wound care lab. We would teach*

medical students how to tie knots, close simple and complex lacerations, apply splints, and generally do wound care on patients in the ED. My hands would smell bad all day. Can you imagine doing that today?? That was the 1990s version today's simulation lab.[2]

DIANE L. GORGAS, MD

Diane L. Gorgas, MD, was a 1990 graduate of Case Western Reserve University School of Medicine. She completed a residency in Emergency Medicine at the University of Cincinnati and was appointed Chief Resident in 1993-94. She joined the faculty at Ohio State in 1994 and quickly became one of the most effective teachers in the department. She was recognized widely for her extensive knowledge of medicine, her exceptional clinical acumen and her ability to pinpoint the most critical features of a patient's condition in her teaching and clinical care.

Gorgas possessed a long-standing interest in and study of educational methods. Her exceptional teaching abilities led to her appointment as the Program Director for the Residency Training Program in emergency medicine at Ohio State, a position she held from 2010 to 2015. She was highly successful. Under her leadership the residency program grew and gained in national recognition for excellence. She was a strong advocate for diversification in the residency program and received university recognition for her efforts

Gorgas continued the Ohio State tradition for leadership of the American Board of Emergency Medicine (ABEM). She was elected to the board in 2018 and served as an item writer, case developer and case administrator. She also served on the Emergency Medicine Review Committee for the Accreditation Council for Graduate Medical Education (ACGME). She serves as Chair of the Test Administration Committee, and Chair of the Becoming Certified Initiative and its Task Force to reimagine and design the future of initial certification in Emergency Medicine. Her research interests include global health, maternal child health care, including obstetrical and neonatal emergencies in low resource settings, emotional intelligence, competency assessment and learning styles.

She serves as the Executive Director of the Office of Global Health/Center for Global Health Studies and Vice Chair of Academic Affairs for the Department of Emergency Medicine. As the Director of Global Health at the Ohio State University College of Medicine, she oversees the graduate interdisciplinary studies program and all international health experiences of medical students, chairs the medical center committee on Global Health Outreach, and is also responsible for the direction of the OSU Greif Neonatal Survival program. This program works to improve the lives of mothers and infants in low-income countries through self-sustaining education and training programs to increase the in-country capacity of health care workers in Haiti, Ethiopia, Eswatini (formerly Swaziland), Kenya, Tanzania and Rwanda. Gorgas received the Ohio State 2018 Distinguished International Engagement Award, honoring her work in neonatal survival.

Gorgas serves the Wexner Medical Center as the co-chair of the Disparities of Care committee as part of the Diversity and Inclusion Council. She was also named as the Emergency Medicine Inaugural member of the Mazzaferri-Ellison Distinguished Clinicians Society for her excellence in diversity, equity and inclusion and her recognized mentorship of residents, students and faculty, and is the inaugural recipient and namesake of the Diane L. Gorgas Endowment in Emergency Medicine Leadership at Ohio State University, which was endowed by a grateful alumnus.

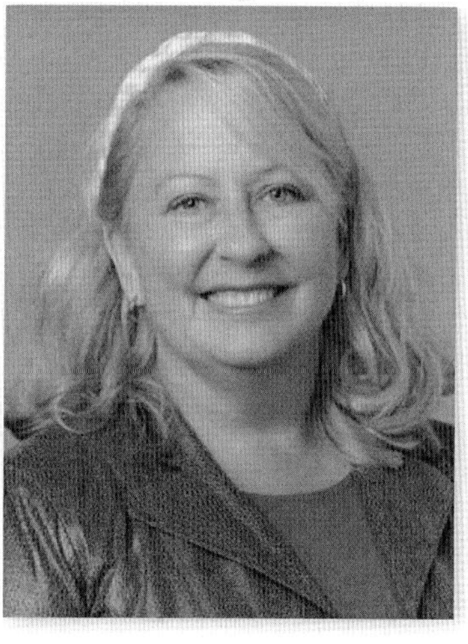

Figure 6: Diane L. Gorgas, MD, was an extraordinary teacher and Program Director of the Residency Program in Emergency Medicine from 2010 to 2015.

She lectures nationally and internationally on training program development, health care equities and challenges to access of care, maternal and child health care, and global health program value in medical education (Figure 6).

MICHAEL WAITE, MD

Michael Waite, MD, completed his undergraduate degree from the University of Pennsylvania School of Engineering and Applied Science and his MD degree from the University of Washington School of Medicine in 1993. He began his residency in emergency medicine at Ohio State, where he showed significant leadership qualities and was selected to be the chief resident from 1995 to 1996 (Figure 7). One of the major attractions of Ohio State for Waite had been the opportunity to pursue Critical Care fellowship training. He knew of the significant efforts of the American Board of Emergency Medicine (ABEM) under the presidency of Douglas Rund, MD, to secure a pathway to certification in critical care and was inspired by the careers of other Ohio State faculty such as Angelos and Michael Dick, MD, who had completed fellowship training in critical care.

Following residency graduation in 1996, Waite entered the Surgical Critical Care fellowship in the Ohio State Department of Anesthesiology under Thomas Reilley, DO. He started the fellowship without an established track to become Board certified in Critical Care, hopeful that with Rund's efforts during his ABEM presidency, a pathway would be approved. As it turned out, he would have to wait another 14 years until the board was able to establish such a pathway under the leadership of another Ohio State ABEM president, Richard Nelson. Following his fellowship Waite served as an Emergency Medicine Research Fellow in Angelos's lab from 1997 to 1998 and was awarded the Departmental Fellow of the Year Award. He also received the Emergency Medicine Specialty Award from the Society of Critical Care Medicine in 1998 for cardiac arrest research conducted in the Angelos lab.

Following completion of his fellowships, Waite joined the Ohio State emergency medicine faculty. He continued to work in the Angelos lab with Holt Murray, MD, and John Younger, MD (from the University of Michigan), and others. He also obtained a university grant to investigate myocardial ischemia-reperfusion injury in an isolated, perfused rat heart model. Options for an emergency medicine trained physician to practice critical care were limited at the time, but in 2001 Waite seized the opportunity to join the critical care practice of Victoria Ruff, MD, at Riverside Methodist Hospital as Herb Rogove, DO, departed for California.

Waite continued to work some shifts in the Ohio State emergency department until 2005, but worked solely in the intensive care unit setting after that time. His critical care practice at Riverside was broad and included attending in the medical, cardiac, surgical and neurocritical critical care units. He continued to work with Ohio State emergency medicine residents on the Riverside medical intensive care unit (MICU) and Neurocritical Care services until they stopped rotating to Riverside in 2020. Waite went on to serve as the hospital's Medical Director of the OhioHealth electronic ICU, Medical Director of Neurocritical Care, and System Medical Chief of Neuroscience Quality.

In 2010, he became certified in Neurocritical Care, and finally in 2012 (with the work that Richard Nelson, MD, championed as ABEM President), he was among the first group who received Board certification in Internal Medicine-Critical Care Medicine from ABEM. Years later, in reflecting on ABEM and critical care, Nelson recalled the following about his days as the President of the American Board of Emergency Medicine who finally secured a pathway for emergency physicians such as Waite to become board certified in critical care:

> *During the negotiations with the American Board of Internal Medicine (ABIM) (and later boards of Anesthesiology and Surgery) the one person who was always forefront in my mind was Mike Waite. Mike was our one graduate who did a two-year fellowship in Critical Care Medicine and was practicing it full time and with great success. Although board certified in EM, there was no pathway for him to achieve certification through an American Board of Medical Specialties board. Given his dedication and intellect, I had no doubt he could easily pass such any such examination that came his way. Indeed, when he became board eligible through ABEM/ABIM, he immediately took the exam and passed it, thus becoming board certified in Critical Care Medicine at long last. In what was undoubtedly a rousing affirmation of the decision to grant board eligibility in critical care to ABEM certified physicians, the pass rate on the critical care boards for emergency physicians that first year was 100%.*

In 2014, Waite was honored with the Ohio State Department of Emergency Medicine Outstanding Contribution Award and in 2016 he was selected as a Champion of Healthcare by *Columbus Business First* for his contributions to Neuroscience at Riverside. In 2021, he was named OhioHealth's Vice President for Quality and Patient Safety and worked his last clinical shift on January 2, 2022.

With his career in medicine, Waite embarked on an uncharted course for emergency physicians who practice critical care medicine, showing emergency medicine residents what was possible—and several followed similar paths.

Years later he remembered the following:

> *I can still hear Jim Hoekstra telling me to "pick up that chart" and order a "five-way"; Dan Martin telling me that we need to "order a VQ scan"; and Doug Rund saying that we should "go to the bedside". I remember working with Howie Werman on his routine weekly night and the snacks he always brought in. The "golden hour" was always a concern as the overnight attending. We always talked about "winning the game" by having no patients on the board but it's uncertain if that ever happened.*[4]

The "five-way" recommended by Hoekstra was a reference to a serving option for Cincinnati chili and included a chest x-ray, electrocardiogram, complete blood count, chemistry panel and urinalysis. The "golden hour" was an hour during the early morning that the department was without residents and the attending physician had to cover the department single handedly.

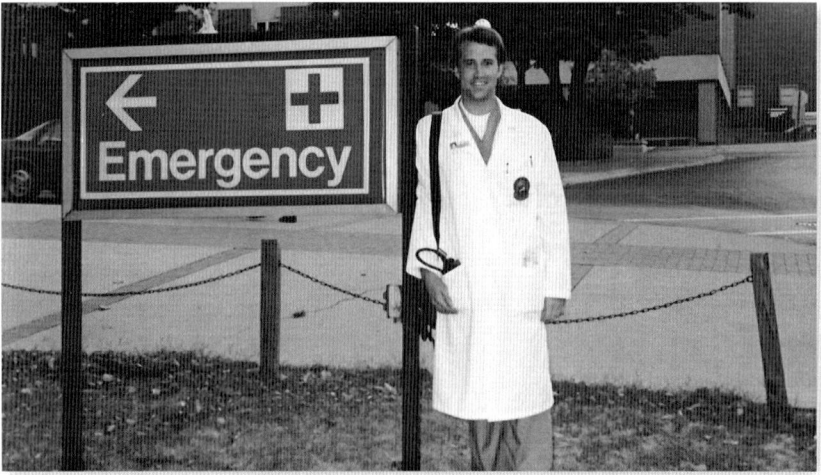

Figure 7: Michael Waite, MD, was an outstanding emergency physician who pioneered in the area of critical care. He is pictured here on his first day of residency at Ohio State.

EMILE EL-SHAMMAA, MD

Emile El-Shammaa, MD, completed his undergraduate studies from 1987-1990 at the University of Maryland, with a major in biology and a minor in chemistry. He earned his doctor of medicine degree from Duke University in 1994. He arrived at Ohio State in June 1994 for his emergency medicine residency. In 1996, he and Michelle Flemmings, MD, were selected as chief residents for the program. After completing his emergency medicine training, El-Shammaa stayed on as part-time faculty while pursuing a fellowship in Pediatric Emergency Medicine at the Columbus Children's Hospital. Upon completion of the program El-Shammaa stepped into a dual-faculty appointment with Emergency Medicine and Pediatrics. Being board-certified in both Emergency Medicine and Pediatric Emergency Medicine, he divided his time between the two sister institutions, and became a key liaison between the two. He provided an essential focus on pediatric preparedness at the adult institution and adult preparedness at the pediatric one (Figure 8).

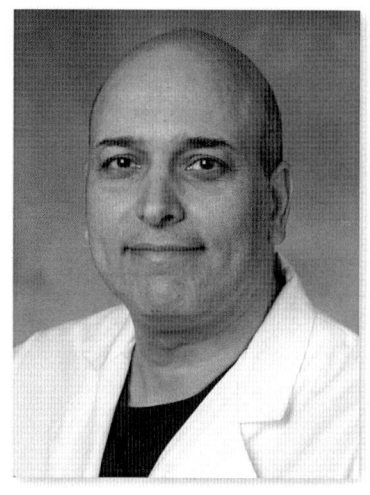

Figure 8: Emile El-Shammaa, MD, a highly esteemed physician with a speciality in emergency medicine and emergency pediatrics.

El-Shammaa's academic interests focused on bedside education and point-of-care ultrasound. He helped start the emergency department point-of-care ultrasound programs, both at Ohio State and Nationwide Children's Hospital (NCH), and became the Associate Ultrasound Director at NCH. His love of bedside clinical education led to many clinical publications, numerous department and College of Medicine teaching awards, as well as the Ohio ACEP Emergency Physician of the Year in 2018.

In 2015, El-Shammaa took an 18-month leave-of-absence to move, with his wife and children, to Queensland, Australia. This exposure provided a different and new perspective, both in health care and culture. He worked as a staff physician at one local access hospital and one regional community hospital, serving a community of about 50,000 in a single-payer, state-run medical system. While in Australia, El-Shammaa gained experience navigating a completely different health care system, negotiating a limited medication formulary, mentoring trainees, exchanging experience with peers, learning about exotic and tropical emergencies, and serving the underserved aboriginal population. He returned in 2016 to share this unique perspective and nuance with his colleagues here in Ohio.

Since then, El-Shammaa has continued in his dual role at both Children's and the University hospitals. He always carried a full clinical workload, and enjoyed teaching and learning from medical students, residents, fellows and peers.

LEO RICHARD "RICH "BOGGS JR., MD

Leo Richard "Rich" Boggs, MD, joined the faculty in 1997. He received his BS degree in biology from Alderson Broaddus College in Phillipi, West Virginia, in 1979. He received his MD degree from Marshall University in 1983 and completed his residency in emergency medicine at Hershey Medical Center of Penn State University in 1986. Prior to joining the faculty at Ohio State, Boggs worked as an emergency physician at hospitals in West Virginia and Columbus. He left Ohio State in 2003 for the University of Kentucky Medical Center until 2006, when he began working as a traveling physician for US Acute Care Solutions. His position was known as a "firefighter," which meant that he "traveled a lot" (Figure 9). He returned to Ohio State in 2014. Years later he reflected upon his career:

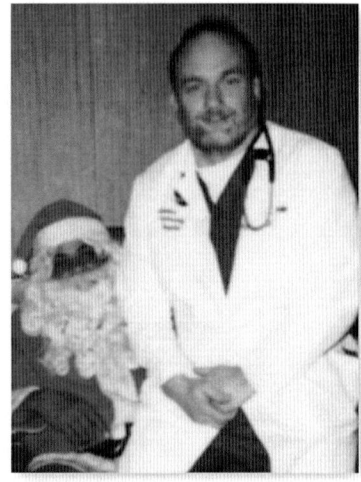

Figure 9: Leo Richard "Rich" Boggs Jr., MD, worked at hospitals in Columbus and West Virginia before joining Ohio State as a faculty member in the Department of Emergency Medicine.

My name is "Rich," unless you are Dan Martin or one of the newer docs, then I'm known as "Leo," to which I may not always answer as that was my dad's name. I've been practicing Emergency Medicine for a really long time, with a large chunk of that time at OSU. I practiced community medicine for the first 10+ years of my career, plus eight years in the middle of my academic career. When I graduated from my residency, I obviously was not the brightest egg in the carton, but I never stopped learning from those I worked with and reading "the literature." In 1996, Dr. Jim Hoekstra approached me about working at OSU and introduced me to Dr. Rund. My academic career began with much trepidation on my part. Still, I approached it as an opportunity to continue learning from the staff physicians there and realized that I could also learn from the residents. To this day, I still try to learn from those I work with—physicians, residents, nurses, etc.—and share what I think I know with them. As I approach the twilight of my career, I want to thank Dr. Rund for taking a chance on a community physician. I may not have made his job any easier, but he helped make me a better doctor and educator.

DAVID P. BAHNER, MD

David Paul Bahner, MD, joined the faculty as an Assistant Professor in 1998. He received his undergraduate degree from Clemson University and his MD degree from the University of Cincinnati. He completed his residency in emergency medicine at Ohio State and immediately joined the faculty (Figure 10). Highly regarded as a teacher and an innovator, Bahner soon became interested in emergency ultrasound, which was regarded as an imaging tool for radiologists at that time.

The emergency department had acquired a complex ultrasound machine primarily for use in obstetrical and gynecological emergencies and Bahner quickly learned how to operate the machine, completing an ultrasound-in-trauma course at Grant Hospital in 1996. He began to read and practice ultrasound, independently using this machine in his spare time. Bahner soon realized the potential for use of ultrasound in emergency patients and began to teach the use of ultrasound. He soon acquired additional training and certifications, obtaining his Registered Diagnostic Medical Sonographer (RDMS) certification in January 2000.

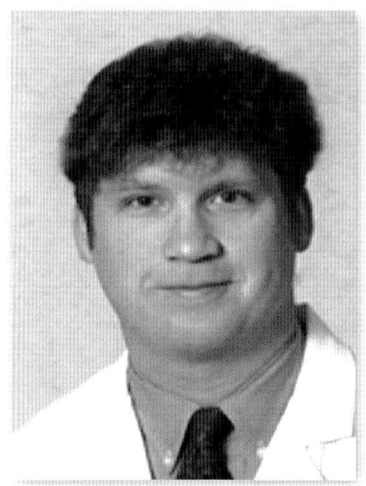

Figure 10: David P. Bahner, MD, RDMS, began the specialty of emergency ultrasound in the department. He became internationally famous for his work.

Bahner was innovative and passionate about using ultrasound in emergency patients. His efforts, however, started to push against the turf boundaries of other specialties. On one occasion, a cardiologist who routinely performed detailed cardiac ultrasound studies complained to Rund after hearing that Bahner had performed cardiac ultrasound in the emergency department. Wanting to investigate, Rund asked Bahner about the procedure. Bahner quickly replied: "The patient had an arrow through the chest!"

Bahner was a diplomat and eventually found common ground with radiologists through tact, professional respect and the offer to provide needed patient care imaging after hours. At Ohio State, Bahner was an advocate for medical student and resident teaching and became involved in all levels of medical education. His work with beginning medical students in his novel Evidence-Based Learning (EBL) program, along with his development of the honors ultrasound fourth-year longitudinal elective, was instrumental in providing leadership development for students with an aptitude in what would become known as point-of-care ultrasound, or POCUS.

Bahner was named the Professor of the Year in 2010 by the fourth-year graduating medical students. This was the first time an emergency physician had won this prestigious College of Medicine award. Eventually Bahner began an ultrasound division and a fellowship program, which acquired an international reputation for excellence. His efforts are covered in greater detail in the chapters about ultrasound.

SORABH KHANDELWAL, MD

Sorabh Khandelwal, MD, joined the faculty at Ohio State in 1998 after completing his residency in emergency medicine at MetroHealth Medical Center in Cleveland, Ohio. A lifelong Buckeye, Khandelwal received his undergraduate degree in Biochemistry and his medical degree from Ohio State. Shortly after coming to Ohio State, he took over the leadership of the Emergency Medicine Clerkship from Jim Hoekstra, MD. During his tenure as clerkship director, he lobbied successfully to have emergency medicine (EM) be a required clerkship for all fourth-year medical students. At the time, it was only an option for an Undifferentiated Care rotation. He always remembered having a few "heated" discussions during that time.

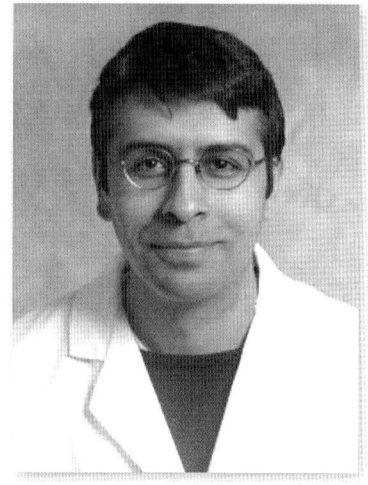

Figure 11: Sorabh Khandelwal, MD, is known as a leader in education at Ohio State. He eventually became the Program Director of the Residency Program in emergency medicine.

He led the development of Advanced Topics in EM (ATEM), a longitudinal advanced emergency medicine elective which was replicated by many other specialties over the next several years (Figure 11).

Nationally, he was part of the core group of educators responsible for the formation of Clerkship Directors in EM (CDEM), the national voice for medical student educators. After leading the EM Clerkship for several years, he transitioned to an Assistant Dean position in the College of Medicine, where he helped develop and implement the Lead. Serve. Inspire medical school curriculum.

In 2015 he transitioned to Program Director of the EM Residency Program, taking over the helm from Diane Gorgas. He helped lead the efforts of transitioning the program from what was considered a "hybrid community and academic" program to one that embraced the real distinction of the Ohio State program— a top academic program in the country. He and his team successfully recruited applicants from top medical schools across the country like Harvard, UCLA, Vanderbilt and University of Washington. Under his leadership, close to 50% of the residents went into fellowships or directly into academics. The residents were leaders in the Emergency Medicine Residents association

(EMRA), ACEP and SAEM. Years later Khandelwal recalled this about his accomplishments:

> Now this was not all my doing; this was a department effort. Our department changed. We grew. We developed numerous fellowships. We recruited many talented faculty who joined our existing pool of amazing faculty. Our residency program increased from 16 to 18 residents per year, two of whom came from a partnership with the United States Air Force. I helped secure, along with Dr. Mark Angelos, a one-million-dollar endowment from Dr. Sam Kiehl, matched by the department, earmarked to help foster resident well-being.
>
> Nationally, I served as an item writer and oral examiner for ABEM, was President of the Clerkship Directors in Emergency Medicine (CDEM), served on numerous committees for USMLE and was on the Advisory Council for the National Board of Medical Examiners (NBME) Board of Directors.
>
> Teaching has been my passion. My learners fuel me. I have been involved in the education of college students through the development of two undergraduate courses at Ohio State, medical students, residents and faculty through numerous national presentations and publications over the course of my career. What I remember most fondly are the personal connections I have made over the years. I am grateful to have received numerous EM Teacher of the Year Awards, the ACEP National Teaching Award, CDEM Distinguished Faculty Award, Master Teacher designation from Ohio State, and the Douglas A. Rund, MD Distinguished Emergency Medicine Faculty Award. I hope that I have made some difference in the lives of people, to Ohio State, and to the field of EM.
>
> One final story... I was very close to joining a private group in Columbus when my Residency Director, Dr. Rita Cydulka, called Dr. Doug Rund and told him that she had a resident who should be in academics. Dr. Rund took the chance and hired me. Amazing how that one phone call changed my career.

THOMAS J. GAVIN, MD

Originally from Philadelphia, Thomas J. Gavin, MD, graduated from medical school at Thomas Jefferson University. Years later he remembered his return to Philadelphia after his interview at Ohio State for his emergency medicine residency:

> *After interviewing I spent the night and was driving home the following day. I should have known that day that I would be destined to match at Ohio State based on the adventure of my travels. I woke to mild snow falling in the Columbus area but being young and stupid felt that I would be fine. The trip home was slow but I was making steady progress.... until the mountains of PA! In driving snow and pitch-black night, the truck in front of me slid causing me to do the same and ended up in a ditch. There was no movement on the highway in either direction. After about 30 minutes there was a beacon of flashing yellow in the form of a tow truck and then the best phrase ever—"for 20 bucks I'll tow you to the top of the hill." I had $28 in my wallet! He towed me to the top of the hill, I got off the next exit, spent the night and drove home the next morning in bright sunshine and dry roads. Even prior to starting residency, Ohio State was teaching me life lessons: Don't try to drive through mountains, at night, in the snow, in a Mustang!*[5]

Gavin was accepted into the residency program and finished as Chief Resident with Carol Clinton, MD. After completing his residency, Gavin accepted a position at Cleveland Metro Health as a Flight Physician, working part-time in the ED. This lasted about a year and a half when he decided to head home to Philadelphia to take a position at Hahnemann University Hospital working in the ED and as the medical director of the hospital's helicopter flight program, University Medevac, the same program he grew up with when working as a paramedic in an earlier career.

As medical director, he was again working in EMS with many previous friends. It was an ideal job for Gavin and lasted five years until the hospital system went bankrupt. His wife, Karen, was working as a nurse in another hospital within the system so they both faced the potential for their unemployment to the point that they would check the news in the morning to see if they still had a job. Soon the market for physicians and nurses in Philadelphia collapsed around them. So, the couple made the decision to return to Columbus, which was Karen's hometown.

Gavin remembered this about his return to Columbus:

After a very pleasant dinner with Doug and Sue Rund, I graciously accepted a position within the Department of Emergency Medicine as an Assistant Professor. I have a strong EMS background so was tasked with teaching and co-leading the EMS training program with Doug at Columbus State Community College, developing an EMS section with Dr. Craig Key who came on board shortly after I arrived and staffing OSU East, which was just recently acquired. My time working in the department was wonderful with the ability to interact, teach and learn from so many colleagues and residents. I was not always the guy who could quote articles about topics, but I have a keen sense for people and the ability to teach "practical" emergency medicine. Dividing my time between the academic world of main campus with the underserved of the eastside gave me the best of both worlds. I had the opportunity to share those eastside experiences to residents to help prepare them for life after residency in the "real world". But alas, academia was not my true calling and I left OSU in 2007 to join MidOhio Emergency Services working with OhioHealth primarily at Riverside.[5]

Eventually Gavin became the Regional Medical Director for the network of freestanding OhioHealth Emergency Departments. When he trained, the concept of a "freestanding ED" was unheard of, but they became very realistic alternative to hospital based EDs. Gavin served in a number of administrative roles within OhioHealth, including being president of the medical staff at Grant Medical Center. Throughout the COVID pandemic response, he served as the lead emergency physician working with the command center to assist in planning for surges and aiding in the rolling out of testing strategies and treatment modalities as physicians learned more about the disease.

Residency was a very enjoyable and notable experience, but none other than meeting my wife, Karen. She was, and still is, a nurse in the Emergency Department of Children's Hospital. We started dating during internship and were married shortly after completing residency. We have two boys, Sean, 24, and Kyle, 21 (Figure 12). Sean has an interest in following my footsteps despite all the horror stories and will be applying to medical school this year. Kyle is smarter and plans to stay far from medicine and is studying Supply Chain Management at the University of Akron with the desire to work in the aeronautical industry. We have always been a hockey-focused family with the boys playing since a young age up to and including currently in college. I still "strap 'em on" and play weekly despite several injuries!

There are too many memories from residency to be able to list in a short narrative. Wednesday and Thursday night shifts with Howie Werman listening to REM, eating pizza in the call room with Karen at RMH at midnight when on call, interviewing and touring prospective residents during interview season, running B-side by yourself with only a dental resident, Roger M having his beloved truck stolen on the night he picked it up, white water rafting and camping trips, or stopping by Riverside on the way home for free food since I was too tired to cook and the "Wheel of Death" (what we called the Ohio State cafeteria) was too scary to try, midnight runs to Wendy's when it finally opened and Adriatico's mammoth Buckeye pizza are some of the thoughts that immediately come to mind. But overall, we were a family–residents and attendings alike, all working together to educate, learn and have fun. Going to work, even as an attending when I worked for OSU, was never difficult. It's the people you work with that make a stressful, challenging profession like Emergency Medicine enjoyable and I was fortunate to train with and work with some of the best![5]

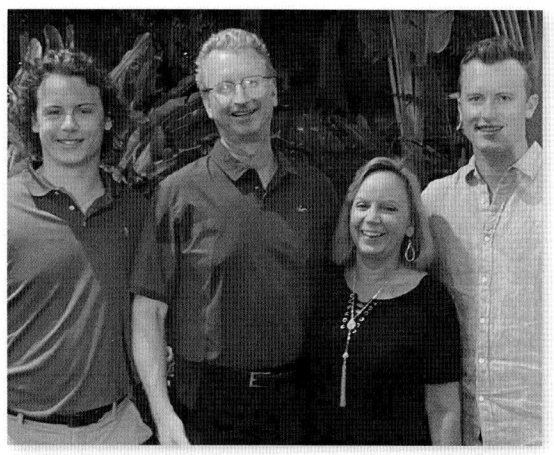

Figure 12: Thomas Gavin, MD, with his family. From left: Kyle, Tom, Karen and Sean Gavin.

The "Wheel of Death" was an ill-conceived apparatus that featured a giant disk containing servings of food that rotated endlessly throughout the day. The older food turning around on the wheel was in little demand since the time of its original preparation was highly uncertain. The effect was a concern for preventive medicine specialists and gastroenterologists who claimed that merely observing the wheel had the effect of "drying up" all gastric secretions. In fact, Howie Werman, MD, referred to the device as "The Desiccator".

CRAIG B. KEY, MD

Craig B. Key, MD, obtained a degree in electrical engineering from The Ohio State University. After graduation he received his medical degree from The Medical College of Ohio, which is now the University of Toledo Medical School. Following medical school, he completed a residency in emergency medicine at the Orlando Regional Medical Center in Florida. He then traveled to Houston to participate in an emergency medical services (EMS) fellowship under the direction of Dr. Paul Pepe and remained there for five years as associate medical director of the Houston Fire Department. He was one of the first physicians in the country to complete a fellowship in emergency medical services.

He joined the faculty in emergency medicine at Ohio State in 2000. As one of the first fellowship trained EMS physicians in the country, he became interested in creating the Center for Emergency Medical Services, which had been proposed in 1991 but was never established or funded by Ohio State. He "dusted off" the 10-year-old proposal, rewrote it and presented it to the university; this time it was accepted and funded. He became the center's first director and it grew under his leadership.

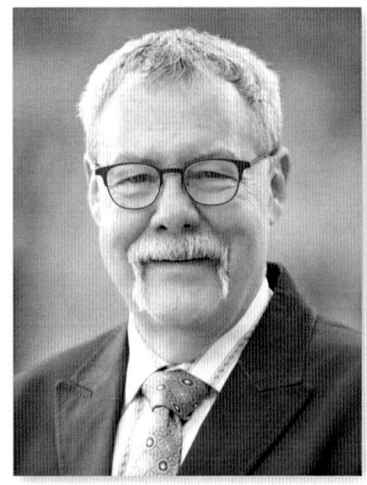

Figure 13: Craig Key, MD, was a leader in emergency medical services and developed the Center for Emergency Medical Services at Ohio State.

Key always enjoyed teaching residents and students. For years he led EMS agencies in central Ohio as medical director. Among his academic activities, he authored or contributed to many publications and professional presentations concerning the subject of out-of-hospital cardiac care and the need for early recognition, response and treatment of heart attacks. He also developed and implemented research concerning the subject of out-of-hospital resuscitation and emergency medical dispatch.

Key's undergraduate education in electrical engineering and his skill in technology led to considerable innovations in the application of technology to medicine and EMS. He developed numerous websites and iPhone apps dealing with teaching and practicing medicine. He created the website for the Department of Emergency Medicine.

COLIN G. KAIDE, MD

As a native of Chicago, Illinois, Colin G. Kaide, MD, completed his undergraduate studies and medical school at the University of Illinois, Urbana/Champaign. He completed a residency in emergency medicine at The Ohio State University in 1996. After residency, he served as the Assistant Director of Emergency Department in Lima, Ohio, for three years while serving as part-time faculty member at Ohio State. In 2000, he joined the Department of Emergency Medicine at Ohio State as a full-time faculty member. He became board certified in emergency medicine in 1997 and hyperbaric medicine in 2007. In addition to emergency medicine and hyperbaric medicine, he completed advanced training in wound care and was certified by the Council for Medical Education and Testing in 2001.

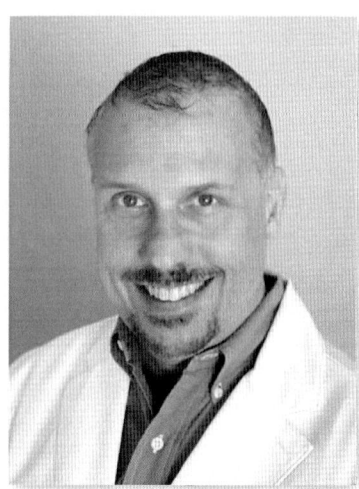

Figure 14: Colin G. Kaide, MD, established a reputation as an excellent clinician and teacher, particularly in the area of resident education and management of the difficult airway.

Kaide was a superb educator who progressed through the faculty ranks to become Professor of Emergency Medicine. He was a core faculty member in the residency program from the beginning. His academic interests always included medical education, rapid-sequence intubation and the advanced management of the difficult airway, hematological and oncological disorders, anticoagulation and its reversal, procedural sedation, and hyperbaric medicine.

He was honored as Teacher of the Year for the Department of Emergency Medicine in 2008. He received the College of Medicine's Excellence in Teaching Award in 2004. He also received the Outstanding Teaching Award in 2008. At the 2017 American College of Emergency Physicians Scientific Assembly, he was presented with the 2016-17 Outstanding Speaker of the Year Award. This award was designed to recognize a single faculty member who has consistently demonstrated teaching excellence through performance, versatility and dependability during ACEP educational meetings throughout the year. In March of 2020, he was awarded the Ohio Chapter of The American College of Emergency Physicians' Educator of the Year.

Kaide made numerous contributions to academic emergency medicine. Such contributions include 27 journal publications and 38 textbook chapters, including some with electronic format. His chapters are included in the major textbooks of the specialty, including Rosen's Emergency Medicine, Tintinalli's Emergency Medicine and Roberts' and Hedges' Clinical Procedures in Emergency Medicine. He has been guest editor of Oncologic Emergencies published in the Emergency Medicine Clinics of North America. In addition, he created, edited and published, in conjunction with a colleague, a book called LEARNing *Rounds: Case Studies in Emergency Medicine*, a 68-chapter, 650-plus page book that addresses uncommon, yet important case presentations to the emergency department.

In addition, Kaide has given countless invited local, regional, national and international lectures on various topics in emergency medicine. He has participated in over 30 enduring content Podcasts and recorded lectures. He developed an emergency medicine curriculum for Ohio Dominican University's Physician Assistant program and lectures for about 8 hours per year in that program.

His contributions to the Department of Emergency Medicine Residency Program have been exceptional. He developed and implemented the airway management and difficult airway portion of the resident curriculum in 2000, and continues to teach in this essential program. He extended this training to attending physicians to standardize the approach to airway and difficult airway management. He has created multiple hospital guidelines that serve to help standardize the approach to management of various conditions, including anticoagulation reversal, headache, subarachnoid hemorrhage, evaluation of pulmonary embolism and others. He has created many small group modules and unique immersive exercises to teach basic emergency medicine topics. He regularly provides grand rounds lectures to residents and he regularly precepts residents during their clinical rotations in the emergency department.

Kaide has made substantial contributions to students within the College of Medicine. He has participated in the Longitudinal Practice Preceptorship since its inception and regularly works with two new students per year and has taught multiple lecture topics for medical students at all levels of training. Considered one of the most effective and inspiring teachers in the College, he actively precepts medical students during their emergency medicine rotations.

Kaide has also been a principal developer and chief medical editor for a medical software company named Callibra, Inc. The company produces a computer-based electronic medical record product that creates computerized ED and inpatient discharge instructions, prescriptions and work excuses with over 800 hospitals using the software and instructions. The medical record product is called Discharge 1, 2, 3.

Leadership and Innovation in Clinical Services

Prompt Care and the University Health Connection

In 1990 clinical care was provided primarily in the emergency department at the university hospital and in a clinic for more minor conditions. The clinic was called Prompt Care. In the late 1980s it was determined that the department should develop a "fast track" site to efficiently care for patients with comparatively minor medical issues not thought to require the complete range of services in the emergency department. Rund was just returning from his sabbatical leave in Edinburgh, Scotland, and gave what he thought might be a British twist to the name of such a place: Prompt Care. The clinic was located across the driveway from the emergency department in the Cramblett Hall Ambulatory Center.

The physician hired initially to staff the clinic was William Hall, MD, who had started the emergency medicine group at Riverside Hospital in 1970. Hall's father had been a general practitioner in the Columbus suburb, Upper Arlington, with an office in the busy Five Points area. Hall joined his father after medical school and took over the busy general practice. In those days general practitioners had a wide range of clinical skills and his practice included obstetrics and deliveries at all hours of the day and night. In the late 1960s Hall closed his general practice and began the pioneering work of developing emergency medicine. He began a full-time practice in emergency medicine at Riverside Methodist Hospital and served as President of the Ohio Chapter of the American College of Emergency Physicians (ACEP) from 1974 to 1975. When he left Riverside and transitioned to Prompt Care at Ohio State, he was exceptionally well suited to provide medical care for patients in an urgent care setting. He could completely and professionally manage patients with less acute symptoms and quickly transfer patients with emergency conditions. Upon Hall's retirement, Stephanie Cook, DO, took on the leadership of the Prompt Care clinic.

STEPHANIE COOK, DO

Stephanie Cook, DO, joined the emergency medicine faculty in 1992. She graduated from the Texas College of Osteopathic Medicine in 1985 and completed her residency in Family Medicine at Ohio State in 1989. Cook began working in the Prompt Care Clinic in 1992. An exceptional clinician who received the highest respect and gratitude from her patients, Cook over time developed an extraordinary clinical concept: a primary care practice with onsite support services located in the College of Pharmacy. The innovative service, called the University Health Connection, included onsite consults with an academic pharmacist, onsite patient prescriptions and in-depth patient education

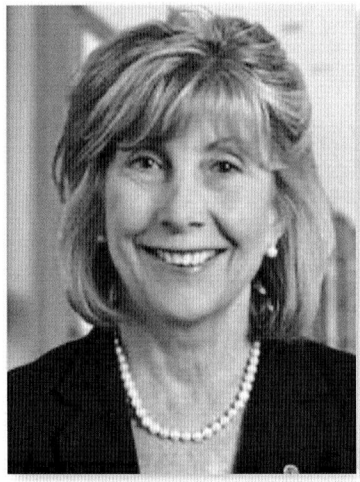

Figure 15: Stephanie Cook, DO, was a visionary leader in primary care. Her innovative University Health Connection provided medical and pharmaceutical services in the same location at the time of the patient visit. The service provided exceptional patient care and patient education.

about their condition and their medication.

Cook and her pharmacy colleagues were able to conduct clinical research and report their successes with the novel clinical approach.

The Restructuring of the Residency Program

In 1990 the residency program was facing its most serious challenge since the failed initial application to start a program with only one resident per year in 1980. Just as the leadership of the department was preparing the application for department status to the university, the residency program, was coming under the intense scrutiny of the Residency Review Committee for emergency medicine (RRC EM).

From the beginning in 1981, there was always a concern about the number of residents in the program for the number of clinical sites: The Ohio State University Hospital, Riverside Methodist Hospital and Columbus Children's Hospital. As noted, the first application to begin the program with one resident per year had been quickly rejected.

In 1989 the RRC EM began its periodic evaluation of the program. As usual, the program information form listed four residents per year for the 3-year program. Two were paid by Riverside and two were paid by Ohio State. The structure of the program rested heavily on a base of "off service" rotations, such as orthopedics and neurosurgery, for what was deemed to be the best preparation for a broad-based clinical education. The residents spent only seven months during their 36-month program in each emergency department, Riverside and Ohio State.

The RRC reviewed the program with close scrutiny, with its final analysis determining that the number of residents in the training program was simply inadequate for the number of sites. In correspondence with Douglas Rund, MD, the director of the program at that time, the RRC requested a full review of the program, including a serious look at the issue of the insufficient number of residents in one location. The RRC felt that residents were not a consistent presence in the busy emergency departments of either Riverside or Ohio State. Further, there were rarely senior and junior level residents in either place at the same time so graduated responsibility from year to year could not occur. The same was true for resident-to-resident teaching.

Rund tried hard to provide a response and perhaps gloss over the issue about the number of residents and clinical sites; the RRC did not buy it. In a letter to Rund Dated March 23, 1990, the RRC responded:

The Committee gratefully acknowledged receipt of the program director's progress report dated December 11, 1989, but considered it largely unresponsive to the Committee's previously identified concerns. Accordingly, the program director is asked to submit another progress report in triplicate by June 1, 1990 on the following topics:

1. *The Committee wishes to see a completed, current, comprehensive curriculum of the program.*

2. *The Committee wishes to see a comprehensive description of the reorganized experience in emergency pediatrics.*

3. *The number of residents training in the program is insufficient for the number of training sites. It is noted that emergency medicine residents spend only 7 of 36 months in the Ohio State emergency department. This results in insufficient graded responsibility and insufficient impact in the emergency department to foster a sense of a residency program and departmental identity.*

4. *The department is asked to document precisely the exact number of trauma resuscitations directed by emergency medicine residents at University Hospital.*[6]

It was definitely time for action. The program was in trouble with the accrediting body. Something had to be done to bring the residents back to the university. Expanding the program to add more residents was not a possibility since any extra residents at Ohio State would have to be funded from practice dollars that were already stretched thin. The university would not provide additional support.

Rund felt the stress. For a start, he needed input from the residents. On one afternoon he and Charlie Little, the incoming chief resident walked the length and breadth of the Ohio State campus, from the Olentangy River to High Street for hours mulling over the scenarios to improve the program and respond to the RRC. The more they walked and talked, the more they realized that they would have to pull back from Riverside to provide the coverage at Ohio State demanded by the RRC. Years later Little remembered the difficult years around the time that the residency review committee demanded a return of most rotations to Ohio State:

> *I remember we walked all over campus for quite a while. We walked... up by the faculty club, got into the central heart of campus. We were... discussing in general how to re-do things and how to pull people over and everything.*[1]

Next was the difficult discussion with the Riverside leadership. After all, it was the physician group at Riverside that added the additional funding and clinical experience so badly needed by the residents when the program was first turned down for accreditation in 1980. The patient census in the Riverside emergency department was always high and resident rotations on services such as emergency medicine, neurosurgery and orthopedics were excellent.

Nevertheless, the RRC demanded that more resident rotations be done at Ohio State—the "mother ship," to use the words of one of the reviewers—and it was time to begin difficult discussions. The leaders at Riverside were taken somewhat by surprise and pondered their next steps if resident months were withdrawn. There was talk of Riverside starting its own residency program in emergency medicine.

Columbus Children's Hospital and Grant Morrow, MD

The program needed to increase the number of months in the Ohio State emergency department and also find a way to pay for them. It was time to ask for help from Columbus Children's Hospital. Rund scheduled a meeting with Grant C. Morrow, III, MD.

Morrow had become the medical director of Children's Hospital and the Chair of the Department of Pediatrics at Ohio State in 1978 (the year of the practice plan turmoil). He graduated from Haverford College and the University of Pennsylvania Medical School. His residency in pediatrics neonatal fellowship was completed at the Children's Hospital of Philadelphia. He joined the pediatrics faculty at the University of Arizona before being recruited to Ohio State to lead pediatrics. Soon after arriving he was placed in charge of a committee looking at the faculty practice plans.

When the RRC demanded a change in the emergency medicine residency program Rund met with Morrow and asked for his help. Rund outlined the issue: Residents must spend more time at Ohio State but the university would provide no additional salary support. Rund also emphasized how important the Children's rotations were to the program since both Ohio State and Riverside were predominantly adult hospitals. Morrow listened carefully and acknowledged the excellent clinical skills of the Ohio State residents.

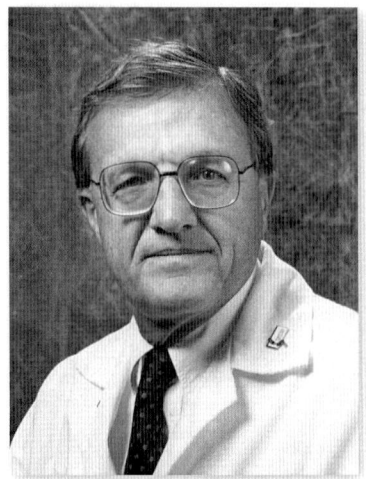

Figure 16: Grant Morrow, MD, was the Medical Director of the Columbus Children's Hospital and the Chair of the Department of Pediatrics at Ohio State when he approved additional funding for resident salaries and an enhanced presence for emergency medicine residents in the pediatric emergency department in 1990.

By the end of the meeting, Morrow essentially agreed to pay emergency medicine resident salaries and benefits for the months spent at the Children's. Rund determined that at least two months of every year of training should be spent in pediatrics: The program could now be funded and the residents would learn how to take care of sick children, which was one of the most stressful parts of an emergency physician's life. Morrow pledged to review the arrangement with his staff and, in the end, the arrangement went into effect.

Expanding the Residency Program

The residency program needed to expand but growth was always constrained by lack of funding. Until the breakthrough agreement with Children's Hospital, all additional residents on the Ohio State side needed to be paid for by patient billing revenues. Despite this restriction, the department added residents. This occurred because of an arrangement with the United States Navy in which officers wishing to obtain specialty training in emergency medicine could be assigned to civilian programs and their entire support would be funded by the military. In 1988 the program grew to six per year. In 1989 the program matched seven per year, including a naval officer. In 1989, the year of the RRC pressure, the program expanded to eight per year, including two additional military officers in the program.

After an extensive reorganization effort, more resident months were to be spent in the Ohio State emergency department and the presence of more junior and senior residents in the department would allow for resident-to-resident teaching and graded responsibility. More complex cases would be assigned to more senior level residents and senior level residents could provide supervision to students and junior level residents.

The prospects of expanding the program and increasing EM resident presence at Ohio State and Children's Hospitals with a corresponding decrease at Riverside did not go over especially well with the Riverside leadership, particularly with the brief time to implementation. The relationship changed in order to comply with the mandate of the RRC. Resident months would be added at Ohio State and decreased at Riverside. Major decisions about the program would be made by the Ohio State program director. Over the ensuing years the relationship continued to become more distant.

Riverside continued to reimburse Ohio State for resident salaries but only for the portion of resident months assigned to that hospital. Because the time spent at Riverside was reduced, the reimbursement was considerably reduced. As noted, Riverside also contemplated establishing a separate residency program. The Residency Review Committee decided to continue the full accreditation of the Ohio State program. In a letter to Douglas Rund, program director, dated October 5, 1990, the RRC wrote the following:

> *The Committee gratefully acknowledged receipt of the program director's progress report dated May 29, 1990, and found it responsive to their previously cited concerns. Another progress report is requested in triplicate by December 1, 1990, in which the program discusses the impact of an emergency medicine residency at Riverside General Hospital [sic]*

on the rotations, curriculum, and financial support for the residency. The program director is also asked to discuss the program's anticipated relationship to Riverside General Hospital [sic]in the future under both scenarios—if the new program is accredited and if its accreditation is withheld.[7]

In the end, Riverside did not establish a new program in emergency medicine but the relationship continued in an entirely new format. With the significantly reduced contribution from Riverside, funding had to be found elsewhere. Ohio State's emergency medicine faculty practice group, Emergency Care Associates, Inc, elected to fund Riverside's portion of EM residency support with income from the practice plan. The amount was somewhat reduced given the new support from Children's Hospital, the military, and a small amount of additional institutional support from Ohio State. To do this the clinical hours for faculty would need to be reduced and the money saved would need to go towards resident salaries.

Thus, beginning August 1, 1990, attending coverage in Ohio State's emergency department went back to three 8-hour shifts, single coverage, from what had been four 8-hours shifts, with 2 p.m. to 10 p.m. double covered. At the same time the number of residents assigned to the emergency department increased. The added resident presence, particularly at the second- and third-year levels, would ensure adequate coverage with the premise that residents would see almost all patients primarily and the attending faculty physician would function in a supervisory role though still required to see and write notes on all patients, and of course, teach.

It was a relatively tumultuous period. All the changes added significant fluidity and complexity to the scheduling process for the residents. In later years, Charlie Little summarized the difficulty of being the chief resident at the time:

> *We wanted to be able to cover for trauma and we were currently on ten-hour shifts and so we put it out to the entire group of residents to vote on whether they wanted to go to eight-hour or twelve-hour shifts and everybody except for one person voted for twelve hours. The twelve-hour shifts were brutal. The thing is that you didn't really get anything to eat or drink. In theory you could leave, but when you came back everyone*

was so behind it didn't seem worth it to go eat.

We had a little early version of scheduling software that was hooked up to a dot matrix printer in a little office. Because all these rotations were brand new, we had to juggle people around and move them. So, whenever a schedule got released, it was updated and printed off on the dot matrix printer and given out to everyone. I think we were soon well up into the low teens of official releases, and then after we got pretty well about halfway through the year, we started moving people around with a pen on the schedules so we could tell where people were actually assigned and we had given up on doing formal re-writes of the schedule, because there were a lot of changes over the first few months.[1]

At his graduation ceremony Little was given a framed sheet from his dot matrix printer covered with arrows, scratch outs and handwritten changes throughout reflecting the turbulence of the period.

References

1. Little CM. Interview with Charles M. Little, MD, by Douglas Rund. 2022: Columbus, Ohio.

2. Hoekstra JW. Personal communication with Douglas Rund. 2022: Columbus, Ohio.

3. Griffith R: Personal communication with Douglas Rund. 2022: Columbus, Ohio.

4. Waite M. Personal communication with Douglas Rund. 2022: Columbus, Ohio.

5. Gavin T. Personal communication with Douglas Rund. 2022: Columbus, Ohio.

6. Residency Review Committee for Emergency Medicine: Letter to Douglas A. Rund, MD. March 23, 1990.

7. Residency Review Committee for Emergency Medicine: Letter to Douglas A. Rund, MD. October 5, 1990.

Chapter 9

Financial Challenges and Organization: The Costs of a New Specialty – "Sink or Swim"

Richard N. Nelson, MD
Douglas A. Rund, MD

The College of Medicine at Ohio State never received anywhere near adequate funding from the State of Ohio to pay competitive salaries for full-time physician faculty members. Adjunct faculty who taught medical students on a part-time basis in community offices and hospitals were volunteer non-salaried physicians. These physicians needed a teaching appointment *of some kind* to teach and evaluate medical students.

This was true from the very early days. Paulson writes of an interview with a faculty member of the 1930s and 40s who was the *only full-time faculty member* in the entire College:

> *In those days men of the faculty were part-time, you know and sometimes they came to lecture and sometimes they didn't. Well, I was at the university hospital so if they didn't come in, I would give the lecture. I would show a patient often. So, I taught medicine and lectured three times a week. I took care of university hospital in the forenoon, then I went to the State Street Dispensary in the afternoon. We got our clinical patients from the Dispensary.*[1]

Clearly such volunteer faculty members always served a critical function in the education of medical students. Even as full-time physicians were gradually added to the faculty in subsequent years, there was a need for additional clinical sites and additional teachers outside the Ohio State system to provide adequate education for all students in the traditionally large classes.

In the 1970s when emergency medicine was first forming as a division, the full-time faculty in emergency medicine received a single salary from the College of Medicine. The salary was low and the division had difficulty attracting faculty members. For unclear reasons division faculty were not allowed by the dean to bill for their professional services in 1977. This was the original impetus for the two emergency physicians who were present at that time to join the practice plan lawsuit against the university. When the lawsuit was settled in 1979 all were exhausted by the brutal struggle and the restriction was lifted. The dean advised, "go ahead and do what you want to with billing."

In other departments from conception, however, physicians were always permitted to bill patients for professional services and supplement the low salaries. There were many permutations. In some departments, a practice corporation billed professional fees and compensated the physician faculty members with salary and benefits. In other departments salaries were relatively fixed; in still other departments the salary amount varied according to the amount of professional revenue collected for the physician's services. Research grant "release time" could be used to replace the salary of physicians to provide time to conduct their scientific research.

In some of the medical school departments each *individual* physician had a separate professional corporation. The individual's corporation paid for benefits, malpractice coverage and a retirement plan. Some retirement plans were rumored to contain rather dubious assets such as race horses. At the time of the practice plan controversy in 1978, there were thought to be well over 100 different physician practice corporations associated with the Ohio State clinical departments.

The first effort to unify and standardize faculty salary, benefits and department funding began in the 1970s when the university president and board of trustees began to push for a way to recoup money that was paid by the university to support clinical facilities. The reasoning was that the university paid for practice overhead and the doctors reaped the rewards without giving back.

The doctors pushed back in court, and the disagreement led to the practice plan lawsuit in 1978. When the lawsuit was finally settled in federal court in 1979, the University Practice Plan was established. The plan required that physicians disclose their professional fee income to the department chair and contribute to a departmental fund that supported research and education. This plan still allowed quite a bit of autonomy and variability between departments, but it did establish a mechanism by which a certain percentage of patient care revenue had to flow back into each department as well as the college.

One of the disruptive results of the lawsuit was the nearly wholesale resignation of the Department of Anesthesiology faculty, an event that essentially shut down surgical services at the medical center for almost a year, and the migration of many surgical faculty members to the medical staffs of other area hospitals where they could operate on their patients and continue their practices. This was the environment in which the new Division of Emergency Medicine (EM), established in the Department of Preventive Medicine, found itself in 1979.

Richard "Rick" Nelson, MD, the first residency-trained emergency medicine faculty member, arrived at Ohio State in July 1981. His "official" salary was roughly $32,000 per year plus health benefits. While still a third-year resident in the Akron City Hospital program, he had heard rumors about this new emergency medicine program starting at Ohio State and that the starting faculty salary was closer to what a resident would earn—far from what an attending physician would earn. This may have helped explain why there were so few applicants for faculty positions.

The relatively small salary represented a combination of so-called A1 funding (which was funding that came directly from the university and the state of Ohio) and the Medical Research and Development Fund (MRDF), which was part of the college practice plan and consisted of patient care revenue funds redirected back to the division. The A1 and MRDF funding, while meager, also allowed the faculty member to be eligible to participate in the State Teachers Retirement System (STRS), a traditionally popular and well-managed retirement system for Ohio teachers.

When the practice plan lawsuit was finally settled in 1979 and the college dean permitted patient billing, the physicians formed a partnership: Emergency Care Associates. Now, in addition to the small fixed salary from state funds, there was additional funding from patient revenue through the department's practice plan. The physicians had two employers: the university and the partnership. They received two paychecks, one from each employer.

Initially the hospital performed the billing on behalf of the physicians. Each physician received 70 percent of their monthly billed charges, minus a contribution to the practice plan. The amount would be paid to the doctor the following month. The patient records were paper charts. Faculty members working in the emergency department had to individually code every patient chart by hand. This meant that the doctors had to memorize common service codes or have a reference for each code for both levels of service and procedures. To the physicians, the codes were critical because they were used to calculate a monthly payment: The greater the value of the codes, the greater the income. Each physician would earn approximately 70 percent of whatever that month's coding yielded, and as a result, each physician's earnings would change from month to month.

The most astute physicians would comprehensively treat the patient and document in great detail to ensure any outside scrutiny would support the billable codes. Also, all possible applicable billing codes were used especially regarding procedures. The patient care income varied widely from physician to physician according to the value of the codes; some were paid more and some were paid less. Physicians less meticulous in their coding were paid less. Physicians were also incentivized to work shifts with higher numbers of patients and procedures.

Still, under the new system, the overall individual incomes could be substantial and more comparable to what emergency physicians in the private sector could earn. The university appointment and component of the salary included health insurance and membership in the STRS. Partnership income from physician billing paid for professional liability insurance, disability insurance and a retirement plan. Some of these items were purchased individually. Each doctor had an individual disability policy. It was not unusual for physicians in the same department to use different malpractice carriers.

To try to provide some structure to all of this, Richard A Nelson, MD, approached an attorney friend of his, Chuck Koenig, for advice on how to navigate this new world of public-private employment. Koenig explained that, for all intents and purposes, Nelson's employment was that of an independent contractor. As such, it would benefit him to individually set up a limited liability corporation with Nelson as the sole member. In addition, he would have to figure out a way to pay state and federal taxes. Since income varied from month to month and no withholdings occurred, there could be a substantial tax bill at the end of the year. In 1981 federal tax rates were as high as 70%.

Prior to 1982, hospital and physician billings were fairly straight-forward: Insured patients would be seen by physicians, physicians would submit bills to insurers, and insurers would pay physicians what they billed or what they contracted to be paid. Hospitals operated under a similar arrangement, the so-called cost-based system of billing and reimbursement. In the case of emergency physicians at Ohio State, the hospital submitted both the hospital component and the physician component and likely got paid a fairly high percentage of billed charges for each. Some emergency physician groups took it upon themselves to bill insurers on their own, separate from the hospital. The advantage to doing it on their own was that they could charge higher fees, raise or lower fees as needed (though lowering fees was rare), and negotiate with insurers separate from the hospital. Some of the more entrepreneurial of these groups and some individual physicians set up billing companies of their own and billed not just for their own physicians but for other physician groups in other hospitals, often for specialties other than emergency medicine.

This all changed in 1982 when the Tax Equity and Fiscal Responsibility Act (TEFRA) went into effect. Passed in 1981, TEFRA was a response to congressional concern about a growing federal budget deficit that was worsening due to reduction in tax receipts and an ongoing recession. The act did a number of things to reduce tax loopholes and increase enforcement of tax rules, targeting health care expenditures in particular. Concepts such as utilization review, the diagnostic related group coding system (DRGs), and special provisions for health maintenance organizations (HMOs) were new features included in TEFRA. Hospitals had to justify their charges, particularly with Medicare and Medicaid patients, and penalties for noncompliance were increased.

By 1982, it became apparent that the "70% of billed charges" physician payment arrangement was problematic for the hospital given the new federal requirements. Also, including physicians in the cost side of the equation effectively reduced what could ultimately be charged for the facility. Therefore, in mid-1982 the hospital notified division director Douglas Rund, MD, that emergency physicians would, in *two weeks henceforth*, be totally responsible for their own billing and collections. This created an obvious crisis within the new division. First, neither the physicians nor the departmental administrative staff, which consisted of one person, knew anything about physician billing. Second, and more important, cutting off this revenue flow amounted to the immediate reduction of physician salaries by 80% or more, with no guarantee this revenue could be recouped.

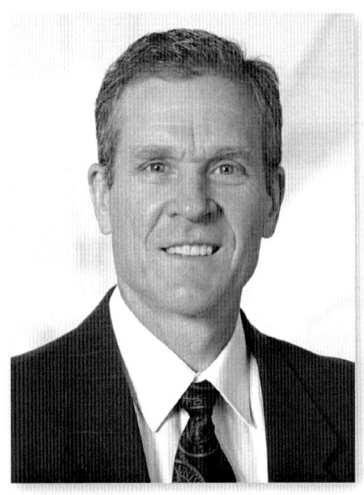

Figure 1: Samuel J. Kiehl, MD, had established his own billing company to bill patients for services of emergency physicians at Riverside. His billing company came to the rescue in 1982 when Ohio State abruptly discontinued its billing services for its emergency physicians.

Rund approached Sam Kiehl, MD, director of the emergency department at Riverside Methodist Hospital, for help (Figure 1). Kiehl owned a billing company, Physicians Professional Management Corporation (PPMC), which provided physician billing services for his own group at Riverside as well as other groups. He agreed to take over billing for the Ohio State group for a percentage of collections. While this move prevented any interruption in patient billings, it did create a major problem in that cash flow back to the group from insurance companies, Medicare, Medicaid and self-paying patients would take weeks if not months to occur. Therefore, for a few months in 1982, Ohio State emergency physicians' salaries consisted of their university salaries and little else. In essence they went without a paycheck.

This process of PPMC's billing for Ohio State emergency physicians went on for a few years and worked out reasonably well. Although the collection rates were not nearly the 70% of billed charges as they were before the change, employing professional coders and increasing physician charges made up much of the difference. The obvious and most visible problem was that any new faculty member would receive minimal income until their billed charges were paid, which usually took a few months to reach a steady state of cash flow.

A less visible but just as critical problem was that if a physician left the practice, they owned their accounts receivables. Any ensuing payments to that physician were paid to the departed physician, leaving no extra funds for new hires. This problem turned into a crisis when a physician husband and wife who were hired in July 1986 both left the practice in October 1987, taking with them close to 25% of the division's billing revenue. This was a drain that continued monthly in gradually decreasing amounts over the next three years as their accounts receivable came in.

After the departure of the two faculty members (along with their rightful revenue), the division was left with the problem of paying not only current faculty members but also recruiting replacement faculty because the ED was now understaffed. Recognizing all these problems that would soon be upon them with the departure of the two physicians, the five full-time faculty at the time, Drs. Rund, Nelson, Michael Kelley, Howard Werman and David Roberts, held a pivotal meeting at Rund's house in Worthington in September of 1987.

Four important decisions were reached at this meeting. First, all clinical income would be pooled into one revenue stream and distributed as salaries that would be similar if not the same for faculty, except for the university component of the salary which would typically increase with academic promotion and longevity. Second, newly hired physicians would be paid a salary from day one of their employment and their accounts receivables would belong to the group and not to the individual physicians.

Third, physicians involved in administrative service within the division such as residency director, medical director and division chief would be granted a yet-to-be calculated reduction in clinical time to allow for their administrative duties while keeping their salaries on par with the other physicians. This so-called "shift reduction" method of compensation was distinct from the prior system in which those doing administrative activities could request less clinical time, but would earn less income since revenue was linked directly to clinical time.

Fourth and finally, in recognizing a shortage of physicians to staff the

ED, all five agreed that, at least temporarily, the schedule would be reduced from four 8-hour shifts to three 12-hour shifts: 7 am – 7 pm, noon – midnight, and 7 pm – 7 am. Such a schedule would allow for fewer, though longer monthly, shifts per faculty. It also provided 12 hours per day of double attending coverage, which was desperately needed in the setting of increasing patient volumes.

Emergency Care Associates, Incorporated

By the end of 1987, Emergency Care Associates, Inc. (ECAI) was registered in the state of Ohio as a professional corporation, taking the trade name Rund previously registered for the partnership on June 19, 1979. The 1979 organization had been a general partnership initially consisting of Rund, Roberts and Richard Cline. Cline had joined the faculty in 1979 when he finished his internal medicine residency and left in 1982 when he began a fellowship in gastroenterology. In the new corporation (that replaced the partnership) the sole shareholders and Board of Directors were the five physicians who attended the Worthington meeting three months before. Richard Nelson became President (Figure 2); Chris Dailey continued as business manager. Emergency Care Associates, Inc. ultimately existed until 2004 when the group reorganized as OSU Emergency Medicine LLC and became a part of the Ohio State University Physicians, Inc. Emergency Care Associates, Incorporated, then merged out of existence.

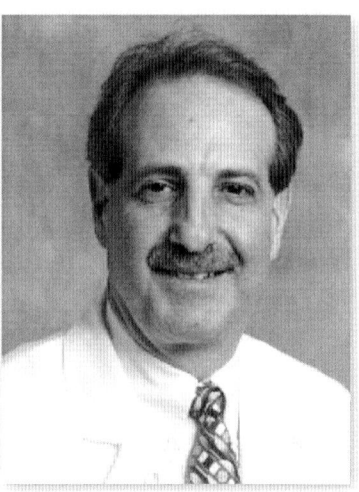

Figure 2: Richard N. Nelson MD, was the President of Emergency Care Associates from 1987 to 2004.

CHRISTINE A. "CHRIS" DAILEY

Christine A. "Chris" Dailey became an indispensable part of emergency medicine when she was initially hired by the university as the

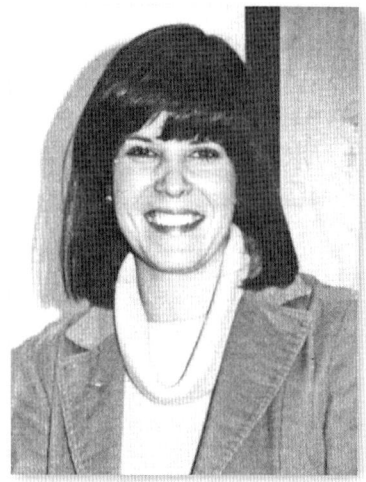

Figure 3: Christine A. "Chris" Dailey was among the few responsible for the early success of emergency medicine at Ohio State. Among other vital roles, she was the business manager of Emergency Care Associates for many years while managing the administration of the academic department.

division secretary in 1979 (Figure 3). Over the following years she was among the handful of pioneers who were most responsible for the department's ultimate success. As the sole division administrator for many years, Dailey was assigned all organizational tasks for emergency medicine. She managed such tasks creatively and diligently all throughout the formative years of the division and afterward for the new department of emergency medicine.

In all phases of faculty practice organization that evolved from partnership to corporation to integration into the large group practice, Dailey also managed the business side of the department. She assisted with preparing the work schedules and keeping track of each individual's work hours.

Her complex tasks included keeping all financial records of the corporation, maintaining the checkbook, preparing financial statements, preparing and retaining all other corporate records, including meeting minutes, preparing materials for tax returns and responsibilities associated with patient billing. At one time she hand-delivered paper records for coding every evening to the coder who lived away from campus. She personally issued all patient refunds.

For many years Dailey handled all the business aspects singlehandedly, doing the work of two or more people. Over time, additional staff members were added to manage the business aspects of the practice, but Dailey was always the "go to" person for all questions.

Moving Forward

Once ECAI was established, the division was able to function less as a group of individual physicians and more as an interdependent team of professionals. With the help of a line of credit, new faculty members coming into the group would have a contract and would receive their full salaries from day one rather than having to wait until their patient billing payments came in.

A number of other positive changes occurred. A governance structure allowed the group to manage its finances and administration in a democratic manner. Group malpractice insurance was provided at more favorable rates than previously available to individuals. A pension and profit-sharing plan was established that allowed physicians to plan and fund their retirements beyond what the university offered which was limited to the State Teachers Retirement System (STRS) and an optional 403B plan. A bonus plan was established to provide financial rewards and incentives. Finally, the group was now able to allocate funds for educational and research activities, including the hiring and support of additional residents beyond what the sponsoring institutions were capable of funding.

However, there remained some issues that would eventually need to be resolved. Physicians received two paychecks per month, one from ECAI, Inc. and one from Ohio State; physicians essentially had two employers. Also, STRS contributions and benefits were based on the university portion of the salary and varied greatly from physician to physician, though their total salaries were similar. Finally, all risk, financial and otherwise, was carried by ECAI and if billing income fell short for a given month, not paying physicians their full salary was always a possibility. Fortunately, this never occurred.

One of the challenges the new group faced was how to fairly compensate the five physicians who did not get paid when the billing system transferred from the hospital to PPMC in 1982. The founding physicians assumed they would eventually get paid their lost income either when they retired or when they left the group; they assumed, as in the past, that they still owned their individual accounts receivables. However, one of the principles in establishing ECAI was that new physicians would get paid from day one. Individual physicians would no longer own their accounts receivables, thus eliminating the possibility of reduced cash flow whenever a physician left the group.

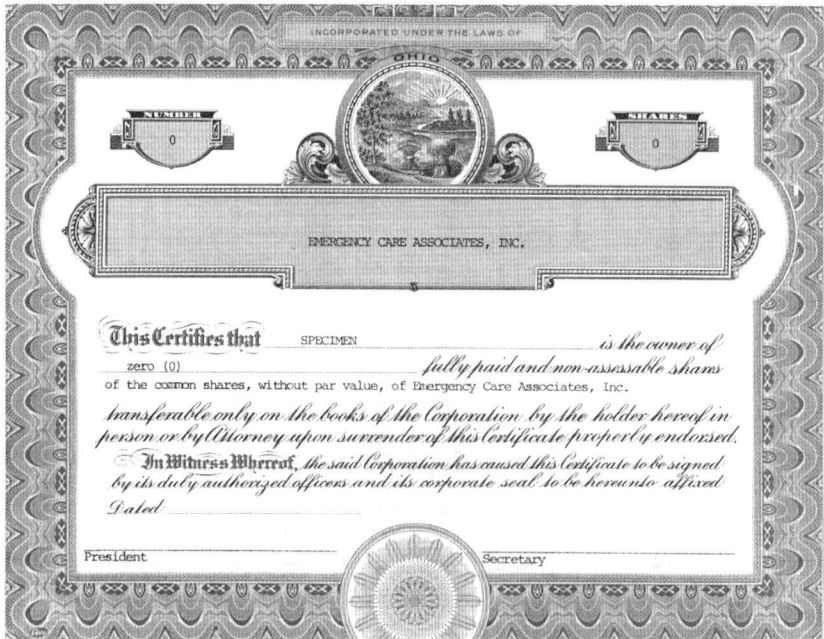

Figure 4: Sample stock certificate issued to founding physicians who were owed revenue from the period when patient care revenues had been disrupted. The stock could be sold at retirement or leaving the group. Newer faculty members could purchase shares of stock if they wished.

This problem was solved when attorney Chuck Koenig proposed a plan to issue shares of stock to each of the founding five that would be paid out at the time each retired or left the group. Newer physicians would be offered the option of becoming equal partners in ECAI by purchasing shares of stock equal to that of the founders after they had been in the division for three years. Purchase price for the six shares required for partnership was approximately $30,000 and could be purchased over time (Figure 4).

Costs of the Department of Emergency Medicine

Leading up to the decision by the college to pursue full departmental status, the division had to agree that no additional university funds would be required. The dean advised the division leaders that, under those circumstances, they had to "sink or swim." With this understanding, the college and university moved ahead and by 1990, the division had become the Department of Emergency Medicine and under the hybrid academic/corporate model, finances were reasonably stable and allowed for growth and expansion of most programs. Still, faculty salaries were on the low side compared to what emergency physicians could make in the private sector.

Also, the College of Medicine had a limited amount of funds it could disperse to departments that in turn would disperse to faculty. With a growing number of departments, competition for these limited dollars was fierce and often favored the older and more established academic departments. With the heavily siloed structures within the medical

Table 1. Academic Departments of Emergency Medicine in U.S. Allopathic Medical Schools, established 1971 to 1990

	UNIVERSITY	YEAR
1.	University of Southern California	1971
2.	University of Louisville	1971
3.	University of Missouri-Kansas	1972
4.	East Carolina University	1980
5.	Wright State University	1980
6.	University of Kentucky	1983
7.	George Washington University	1984
8.	Loma Linda University	1984
9.	Medical College of Pennsylvania	1984
10.	University of Cincinnati	1984
11.	Albany Medical Center	1986
12.	Summa/Northeastern Ohio University	1986
13.	Wake Forest University	1989
14.	State University of New York, Buffalo	1989
15.	Texas Tech University	1989
16.	**The Ohio State University**	**1990**

Table 1: The Ohio State Emergency Medicine Department was the 16th academic department of emergency medicine in the country. The department had to pledge to support itself financially to attain departmental status in the university. (Adapted from Zink B. *Anyone, Anything, Anytime.* Mosby, 2006)

center and the College of Medicine, there was no interest among departments to share what little non-clinical salary support they received with other departments, let alone upstarts like emergency medicine whose legitimacy at the time was questioned anyway.

Emergency Medicine faculty were thrilled being in their own department, the 16th academic department of emergency medicine in the country, and arguably among the first in one of the largest medical schools (Table 1). However, the granting of department status did not include a substantial increase in university funding. As a result, the fledgling department established a culture of carefully managing its finances and being prudent with any choices requiring added expenses. This good stewardship of resources ultimately resulted in fiscal strength and relative independence in plotting its course.

By the time the department merged with the Ohio State University Physicians, Inc, it had the strongest balance sheet in the College of Medicine. Nonetheless, being in one's own department did not negate the fact that emergency medicine faculty at Ohio State were paid less than their emergency physician colleagues in other settings, making recruiting new faculty challenging. As a result, the ECAI Board and individual physicians were always on the lookout for ways to supplement their incomes, ideally in ways that would also benefit the department and its mission.

Finding Ways to Earn Revenue

Medical Services at the Rehabilitation Center

One of the first such faculty endeavors to earn additional revenue began around 1987 and involved the J. Leonard Camera Center. This facility was built in 1986 by the Ohio Bureau of Workers Compensation (BWC) to serve as a residential rehabilitation facility for injured workers. The center included an 11-story residential tower, a three-story medical building, and parking garage. Besides rehabilitation, the center also provided medical services. Daniel R. Martin, MD, joined the EM faculty in 1988 and was trained and board certified in both emergency medicine and internal medicine. The bureau was looking for physicians and approached the medical center, which in turn approached the Department of Emergency Medicine. Martin, Rund, and Rob Griffith, MD (an EM faculty member also dual trained and certified), began working shifts at the Camera Center, getting paid an hourly equivalent, but probably generating more income for the department than comparable time in the ED. Years later Martin, recalled his experience:

> *I started working there about a half day a week but this grew over the next several years to the point that I worked a couple eight-hour shifts per week there and occasionally more. At one point they paid me a stipend to be the director of internal medicine there and even the medical director of the center.*
>
> *The upside was that the cases were bread and butter internal medicine cases and we performed many cardiac stress tests for patients with risk factors. We managed chronic obstructive pulmonary diseases, hypertension and diabetes. We occasionally made some interesting diagnoses like thyroid disease, Cushing's disease and porphyria. The biggest upside was that I was paid as though these were ED hours and our collection rate from BWC was 100%. Three stress tests an hour netted nearly $1000. One of our early (ECAI) corporation meetings that I attended was very memorable when we were all looking at our finances for ECAI during a particularly low revenue period and Mike Kelley looked at me from the head of the table and said, "Dan, you're keeping us afloat."[2]*

Unfortunately, the state of Ohio got out of the residential rehabilitation business and the center closed in 2001. The building was converted to an Ohio State outpatient center now called Martha Morehouse Medical Plaza.

Hyperbaric Medicine

Another important revenue stream for the department was hyperbaric medicine. In the early 1990s, there were few hyperbaric oxygen facilities in Ohio but none in Central Ohio. By 1991 a number of EM faculty, including Richard Nelson, were interested in establishing hyperbaric medicine at Ohio State. Interestingly enough, the hospital previously had a large multi-place unit as part of its aerospace institute in the 1960s. Ed Whitehead, a sergeant major in the army reserves who worked in Preventive Medicine and EM administration, actually operated the unit.

As an aerospace chamber, it was used more for high-altitude and thus *hypo*-baric research than *hyper*-baric, and was rarely if ever used therapeutically on patients. The chamber was housed in Wiseman Hall on 12th Ave. and was eventually sold when the institute closed. The hospital agreed to establish a hyperbaric program, which was to be under the departments of Emergency Medicine, Anesthesiology and Respiratory Therapy. Nelson was one of the co-directors. He and a number of other physicians and nurses obtained their initial hyperbaric training at St. Luke's Hospital in Milwaukee, Wisconsin. Other emergency physicians trained included Howard Werman, Jim Hoekstra, Peter Van Ligten, Jonathon Brooks and Linda Robinson.

The program opened in 1991 with two Sechrist monoplace chambers located in the east corridor of the emergency department. This location was a point of contention with Anesthesiology, who wanted the chambers in the Surgical Intensive Care Unit. The ED won out owing to the anticipated use of the chambers predominantly for outpatient wound care rather than inpatient critical care. This may have contributed to Anesthesiology's decision to abandon the program in 1992, leaving emergency physicians as the only physicians in the medical center providing hyperbaric consults and supervising treatments.

Within a few years, EM had developed a core group of physicians who would do hyperbaric on-call and consult duties, while most of the other emergency physicians were trained and could supervise emergency "dives" at night and after hours, thus allowing the on-call physician to go home after the consult was completed. Over time, the program grew in size and reputation, and three emergency physicians, Angelos, Kaide and Khandelwal, took and passed the Hyperbaric Medicine ABEM subspecialty board exam, thus becoming among the first physicians in the country to become board certified in Hyperbaric Medicine. In addition to enlarging the EM's academic and service profiles, hyperbaric medicine provided some sorely needed revenue for the department.

Other Opportunities

Other areas contributing to added revenue for physicians and the department included work in the Comprehensive Wound Center, serving in medical director roles for local EMS services, software consulting work such as early versions of computerized discharge instructions, expert witness and consultation services, and medical control services for the medical helicopter program (Medflight).

An unusual source of enhanced revenue for the department occurred in 1992 when the hospital was asked to bid on a contract to provide physician and hospital services for city and county prisoners, i.e., those newly under arrest but not yet convicted and transferred to the state prison system (Ohio Department of Rehabilitation and Corrections). Nelson was involved in the negotiations and he realized that no other hospital system in the area was interested in bidding to provide these services. He suggested that Ohio State and the emergency physicians bid to provide the services, but at no less than 100% of billed charges. The county accepted it, probably because there were no other options, and services were provided at this rate for the next year until the decision was made for these prisoners to be taken to the nearest hospital when they needed urgent medical services.

Administrative Compensation

Another source of income for the department involved medical director compensation from the hospital. In 1989, the federal Physician Self-Referral Law, commonly known as the Stark Act after the law's chief sponsor, Sen. Pete Stark, was passed by Congress and made it illegal for physicians to refer patients for certain designated healthcare services to an entity if the physician (or a member of the physician's immediate family) had a financial relationship with the entity. As interpreted by many hospitals, including Ohio State, this meant that emergency physicians could not be paid directly by the hospital for medical services they provided as this would be considered a "kick-back" to these physicians in return for referring or admitting such patients to the hospital. The fact was, however, that, emergency physicians would almost never send a patient to another hospital for admission owing to legal, administrative and time issues. Children transferred to the Children's Hospital were an exception.

However, the Stark law did allow for hospitals to pay physicians stipends for administrative functions. The Department of Emergency Medicine took full advantage of this mechanism. Over the years, emergency physicians received, through their department usually in the form of shift reductions, funding for medical directorships at Ohio State Main and Ohio State East EDs. They were also reimbursed for executive medical leadership for hyperbaric medicine, Emergency Preparedness Chair, J. Leonard Camera Center, Prompt Care, Observation unit, and the University Health Connection.

Fighting to Protect Revenue

Generating revenue from new and existing sources was not the only financial concern for the department. Maintaining existing streams of revenue also became more and more important. Like most if not all clinical departments within the Ohio State College of Medicine, the vast majority of revenue for the new Department of Emergency Medicine came through patient billings. From the onset, billing for emergency department patients was in evolution and not necessarily consistent between practices at different institutions given the newness of the specialty.

The initial billing company, PPMC, and later the department's own billing service would typically bill for x-ray and electrocardiogram (ECG) interpretations performed by attending emergency physicians. Not all payers paid for this charge, however, and some would combine the interpretations into a general lump-sum or bundled payment for all emergency physician services provided for each patient. Other payers, particularly private insurers, would pay for such interpretive services separately, however, item by item for each individual service.

Given the decentralized and specialty-specific billing at Ohio State in the 1980s and early 90s, it is doubtful any department knew what the other departments were doing with regards to billing, even if multiple departments were billing for the same services. Payment would either go to both groups, or more likely to the first group to submit their bill—

the so-called FIFO (first in, first out) standard. This changed around 1994 when the Health Care Finance Administration (HCFA)—predecessor to CMS—cracked down on duplicate billings. The administration recognized that many emergency physician groups billed for x-ray and ECG interpretations, as did radiologists and cardiologists, often for the same patients. They determined that Medicare and Medicaid would only pay for one such bill: the one that was done at the time of the visit. This ruling caught the attention of radiology and later cardiology, which typically performed their services well after the patient ED visit, or the following day if the visit was during the evening or night.

Radiology

In March 1995 the Chair of Radiology, Dimitrios G. Spigos, MD, went to Vice President and Dean of the College of Medicine Manuel Tzagournis, MD, with this issue. Spigos was a highly respected radiologist who had been recruited from the University of Illinois to Ohio State in 1992. He was widely recognized for his work in splenic embolization and percutaneous kidney biopsy under ultrasound guidance. Tzagournis first met with Spigos and Rund and heard the radiology arguments as to why Emergency Medicine should not be sending out bills for x-ray interpretations. Next Tzagournis set up a meeting with Rund and Nelson to hear more about their side and their concern about the lack of after-hours x-ray interpretations. Rund and Nelson explained that their department (and before that their division) had been billing for these services for many years. The revenue generated was an important source of income, and interpreting x-rays while the patient was still in the ED was entirely consistent with HCFA's contemporaneous interpretation standard.

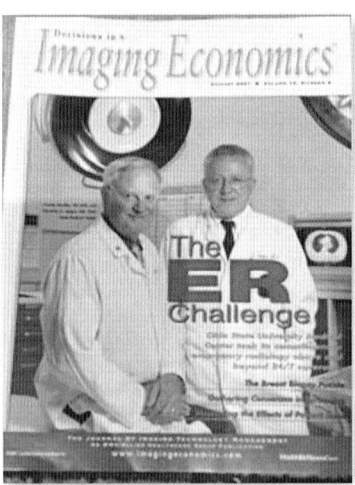

Figure 5: Charles Mueller, MD, and Dimitrios Spigos, MD, featured on the cover of *Imaging Economics* for their innovations in after-hour reading of radiographic images taken in the emergency department.

Tzagournis proposed a compromise: Emergency medicine would cease billing for x-ray interpretations and in return radiology would commit to 24-hour per day x-ray readings. When Nelson commented that it was unlikely the radiologists would provide 24-hour services anytime soon, Tzagournis commented, "You'll just have to hold their feet to the fire," not making it entirely clear what kind of "fire" this fledgling department could exert on mighty Radiology.

X-rays After Dark

By Douglas Rund, MD

From the beginning of the division, emergency physicians interpreted x-rays after dark. The radiologists were usually gone and done reading for the day. They would not return until morning. The meaningful reading was done by the emergency physician, and the patient was treated according to that interpretation. If the "overread" the following day revealed an undetected problem, the patient would have to be called back for another visit to the ED. This was inconvenient for everyone (especially the patient). In the early days, the emergency physicians began charging for films not read by radiology in the nighttime when the patient was still in the department. In the mid-1990s radiology pushed back, insisting that they were the only physicians who should rightfully be compensated for x-ray interpretation. Dimitrios Spigos, MD, Chair of Radiology, demanded a meeting with Manuel Tzagournis, MD, Vice President and Dean, the final decision maker. During the meeting Spigos and I pleaded our cases regarding who should bill for "after hours" x-ray interpretation. In the end the Vice President agreed with radiology and determined that emergency medicine could no longer bill for interpretation of after-hours radiographs. There was also a vague acknowledgement that radiology should read films at all hours. I left the administration building (Meiling Hall) feeling that I had lost the battle. I shook hands with Dimitri, the winner, on the street corner outside the building. I walked back to the office defeated. A fellow chair used to call this kind of despondent journey "the long walk back from Meiling." In the end, however, radiology started reading films in the nighttime and Spigos became a great colleague and friend. It was a victory for all concerned, especially our patients because they would have the benefit of a final reading at all hours, day and night.

In the end Spigos and Charles Mueller, MD, finally convinced their reluctant faculty. They designed a 24-hour radiology coverage system that earned them nationwide recognition.[3] This establishment of continuous radiology coverage and immediate reporting of cases was a radical departure from the modus operandi at that time which was that reports were concluded a day or longer after the study was completed. The 24-hour radiology coverage they pioneered eventually became the accepted standard of care throughout the country (Figure 5).

The real winners were the patients who had a radiologist interpreting their images while they were still being treated in the emergency department.

Cardiology

Electrocardiogram (ECG) interpretations by emergency physicians were met with similar objections by the cardiologists, who generally provided readings the following day. They took a different approach than Radiology. Instead of taking their case to the Dean, Cardiology offered to "certify" emergency physicians in the reading of ECGs, using a course developed by the American College of Cardiology.

Successful completion of the course would allow the "ECG-certified" emergency physician to bill for ECG interpretive services. This idea was politely but firmly rejected by Rund, who was on the American Board of Emergency Medicine, considered the only appropriate body to certify emergency physicians in ECG interpretations or any other functions pertinent to the practice of Emergency Medicine. Cardiology eventually dropped their objection and Emergency Medicine continued to bill for ECG interpretations and continued from then on.

Park Medical Center Becomes Ohio State East

The indirect form of subsidizing department finances and salaries became more direct when the medical center purchased Park Medical Center in 1999, renaming it Ohio State East. The Department of Emergency Medicine almost immediately began providing physician coverage, and the hospital agreed to provide direct subsidies to the department to offset an unfavorable payer mix combined with growing patient volume in the ED.

Towards a Unified Practice Plan

The hospital and some in physician leadership had long wanted a structure that resulted in a mechanism that patients would receive only a single bill for hospital services or, at the very least, physician bills from a single billing entity. Because each department and even divisions within departments were often responsible for their own billing, patients would typically get multiple bills, each with a different design and logo from the various physicians who would see them during their hospital, clinic or ED visits. Depending on the efficiency of the respective billing departments, patients could continue to receive medical bills for months after their visits. This not only was a source of patient dissatisfaction, it was also confusing and probably contributed to low collection rates, particularly among self-paying patients.

This practice changed in the 1990s when the medical center contracted with a long-established medical billing software company that offered IDX, a single billing system. The idea was that all physicians would bill using the IDX system, thus creating uniform *appearing* bills, though not yet a true *single* bill. This created a problem for emergency medicine as PPMC, the department's billing service, did not use IDX, and it was highly unlikely the medical center would allow IDX to be used by an outside billing service. This was particularly true for one such as PPMC with its close affiliation with Riverside Methodist Hospital, a direct and indirect competitor of the Ohio State University Hospital.

The Department of Emergency Medicine was thus forced to end its relationship with PPMC and establish its own billing services using IDX billing software. In 1993 ECAI hired Una Barbee, a practice manager with a local pediatric practice, to set up its billing office. Barbee was able to quickly hire a number of coders and billers, and soon the ECAI billing office was established in a former conference room within the department offices on the ground floor of Means Hall.

The department billing office was successful overall, and billed not just for emergency medicine services, but also other areas in which department physicians were involved, including Hyperbaric Medicine, Prompt Care, Wound Care, Dr. Stephanie Cook's University Health Connection, Robert Guthrie's hypertension and lipid research clinics, and the J. Leonard Camera Center rehabilitation services.

When Barbee left the practice in 1998, Nelson called Jim Coleman, who was President and Chief Operating Officer of PPMC. Nelson had worked closely with Coleman when his company did Ohio State EM's billing. Nelson asked Coleman if he knew of anyone knowledgeable in EM billing who was looking for a position in managing the billing office. Coleman, who as it happened had long been interested in working in an academic EM setting, suggested that he himself would be interested in the position. He was quickly hired and soon became proficient with IDX while running the billing office and serving as ECAI's business manager. He worked to improve billing efficiency, increase revenues and collections and negotiate with payers. At that time, the department offices, including billing, had moved to the basement of the Health Sciences Library, a small space considering the size of the department. Years later Coleman recalled the billing office as "five people working in a sleeping room."[4]

JAMES "JIM" COLEMAN

Jim Coleman was born in Columbus, Ohio, and graduated from Bishop Watterson High School (Figure 6). He went on to attend Columbus International College in Seville, Spain, for two years, followed by classes at Ohio Dominican and Ohio State, earning his finance degree from Ohio Dominican. He took a job in information services at Riverside Methodist Hospital, and owing to his finance background, was eventually offered a position by Sam Kiehl, MD, to set up a billing system for Riverside's emergency physician group. This new company became PPMC and not only provided billing for Riverside's EM physicians, but also did physician billing for groups in other hospitals. He left PPMC to join Emergency Care Associates, Inc. in 1998. In 2001, he co-founded Healthcare Management Associates, a billing service company, with Immediate Health Associates, where he served as Chief Operating Officer and equal partner in the entity. Eventually, Healthcare Management

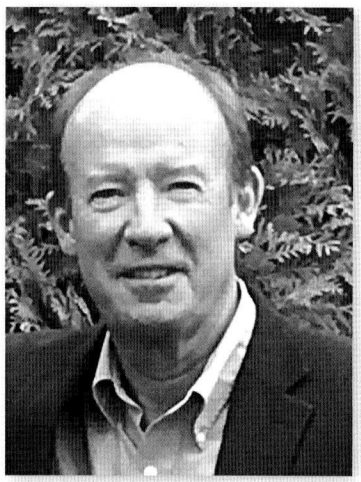

Figure 6: James "Jim" Coleman became the business manager and billing expert for emergency medicine in 1998.

Associates was rolled into Immediate Health Associates, where he served as Director of Billing and Contracting until his retirement in 2016.

When ECAI business manager Coleman announced he would be leaving the group to join another practice, President Rick Nelson began the search process for this critical position. One lead came from a familiar source: Una Barbee, who had set up ECAI's billing office eight years before. She called Nelson and told him about a consultant from the Blue and Company accounting firm who had recently done some financial work for an orthopedics practice for which she was employed. She noted this consultant, Rich Sobieray, had been a paramedic in a previous career and also was a certified public accountant (CPA). She was impressed with his abilities and credentials and suggested ECAI may want to interview him for the position.

Nelson called Sobieray and arranged an interview. The two of them ended up spending the afternoon together at the PGA Memorial Tournament at Muirfield Golf Club in Dublin. Nelson had volunteered at the tournament's first aid trailer earlier in the week and was given two passes which he used for himself and Sobieray. The two of them had a good time watching the tournament and also grew to know each other. Sobieray was hired soon after. In the meantime, there was growing interest at the medical center and College of Medicine to change the practice plan in some major way.

The Clinical Enterprise

In 1995 Bernadine Healy, MD, became Dean of the College of Medicine. Previously Chair of the Cleveland Clinic Lerner Research Institute and the Director of the National Institutes of Health, Healy was very supportive of emergency medicine. In the late 1990s Healy pushed the departments to form a more unified organization, and named the organization the *Clinical Enterprise*. This early organization was a loose one with departments continuing to do their own billing and collections and contract negotiations. Healy felt that a more organized practice organization would benefit the College immensely and also recognized that an exact model to duplicate did not yet exist. As she would famously observe, "If you've seen one academic practice plan, you've seen one academic practice plan."

Healy selected the officers she felt would be most effective in furthering the cause and elections were held in 1998. Ernest Mazzaferri, Sr., MD, Chair of Internal Medicine was elected Chairman of the Board. Ronald Ferguson, MD, Chair of Surgery, was elected Chief Executive Officer and Douglas Rund, MD, Chair of Emergency Medicine, was elected President. The clinical enterprise was the first step toward a unified group practice. When Healy moved on from the dean's position in 1999 to replace Elizabeth Dole as President and CEO of the American Red Cross, a search for a new vice president and dean was begun. The position was filled by Fred Sanfilippo, MD, PhD, a pathologist from Johns Hopkins who served as dean and vice president from 2000 to 2007. Sanfilippo was adamant that the physicians form a unified medical practice corporation and continued pushing hard toward the goal throughout his early tenure.

While a plan for a unified group practice was evolving, Emergency Care Associates continued to do business. In 1999 the corporation included 12 shareholders. Three years later, the shareholders grew to 17 with the new inclusion of the faculty practicing primarily at Ohio State East emergency department. The shareholders in 2002 were the following: Angelos, Bahner, Boggs, Dick, Eiginger, El Shammaa, Gavin, Gorgas, Hoekstra, Kaide, Khandelwal, Martin, Nelson, Neltner, Rund, Waite and Werman.[5]

Ohio State University Physicians, Incorporated

The early 2000s were a time of transition for the practice organizations. Known for his determination, Sanfilippo provided the drive to form a new practice organization. The name of the new organization was to become Ohio State University Physicians, Incorporated (OSUP). The Family Medicine Foundation was created by the Department of Family Medicine in 1995. On September 4, 2002, the Family Medicine Foundation merged with the University Physicians Systems, Incorporated, the Department of Surgery's billing corporation, to create the new corporation: Ohio State University Physicians. Rund was elected president of the new company and remained so until his retirement as chair of the Department of Emergency Medicine in 2011.

The organizational structure of the new corporation was a kind of holding company consisting of departmental limited liability corporations (LLCs). The emergency medicine faculty created such a company and named it OSU Emergency Medicine LLC. The company was incorporated in June of 2003 and Richard Nelson was the statutory agent for the new corporation. In December, 2003, Emergency Care Associates merged with OSU Emergency Medicine LLC and was merged out of existence in 2004.

RICHARD J. SOBIERAY, MHA

In the meantime, Richard Sobieray, who was hired by ECAI in 2001 as practice manager and CFO, oversaw the transition and merger of the organization to OSU Emergency Medicine, LLC. His main job was to ensure the department's finances were strong and the balance sheets favorable. He oversaw a number of improvements in billings and collections, and initiated a bonus structure for faculty members (Figure 7).

Years later Sobieray had the following recollections:

> We increased rates quite significantly with many of the top commercial payers and improved that aspect of our business. I think we remained a rather lean organization from an overhead perspective. I worked closely with Chris [Dailey]. We didn't add any more layers of overhead structure to the group. We kept it relatively lean to ensure that the monies we were earning were being invested in our doctors and what they were doing. That was primarily what we did. We focused on productivity and contract rates when I first came in. Quite frankly the emergency medicine group became financially one of the strongest groups that ultimately ended up

in OSUP – it was strong, and we were generating some really good margins. I believe we were able to give a bonus to the doctors for the first time. I don't remember when they got one previously, but it was a long time. [6]

Still, faculty salaries in the limited liability company remained low—at approximately 25th percentile of AAMC. Sobieray noted:

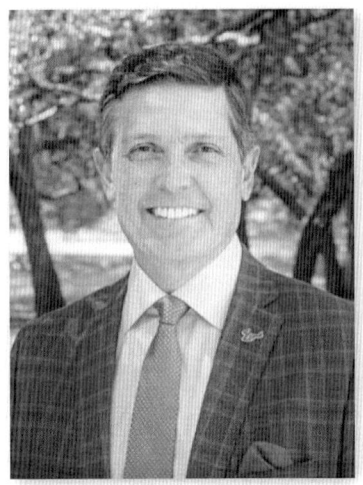

Figure 7: Richard J. Sobieray, MHA, began managing the business affairs of the Department of Emergency Medicine in 2001. He soon transitioned to a major leadership role in OSUP. He later moved to Tampa and became the Chief Financial Officer of the University of South Florida.

We didn't control our payor mix. Quite frankly the emergency medicine group had the worst payer mix within the medical center. We had to go back to the university and to the medical center and state the case that our rates are what they are, we worked hard to improve our rates, but there is still this part of our business that we don't control: that is the medically underserved. We do provide the lion's share of the medically underserved care due to their lack of access to other care, and the medical center stepped up and provided us with the difference between what we negotiating in managed care rates and what we were receiving from the medically underserved. This was, at least, the original calculation. Whether it was Medicaid or even our charity care, we got a sizable increase from them in support of the fact that we were seeing those types of patients." [6]

Prosperity at Last

In the last half of the decade, the finances of emergency medicine improved significantly under Sobieray and Nelson's leadership. At first, most of Sobieray's time was devoted to the LLC, but he soon began to work directly for OSU Physicians, Inc. He noted later:

I was still your CFO with the Emergency Medicine, LLC from 2002-2003, but at the same time I became the Associate Executive Director and Chief Financial Officer for the Practice Plan for OSUP."[6]

He continued to provide important direction for the LLC, however as OSUP expanded, his work as its associate executive director and CFO dominated much of his time. At his suggestion, he left the practice in 2007 to devote his entire position to OSUP, and Kelly Scheiderer became the departmental administrator. Scheiderer had been the administrator for the Ohio State Dental Faculty Practice and came with exceptionally high recommendations from the practice and from the medical center (Figure 8).

KELLY J. SCHEIDERER, RHIA, MHA

Kelly J. Scheiderer, RHIA, MHA, spent her entire professional career at the Ohio State University. She received both her Bachelor of Science in Allied Medial Professions with a certificate in Health Information Management and a Master's Degree in Health Administration from Ohio State. She worked within the university for 36 years, serving in various departments, including Medical Information Management, Quality and Operations Improvement, the College of Dentistry and the Department of Emergency Medicine.

Years later Scheiderer recalled some of her most important efforts:

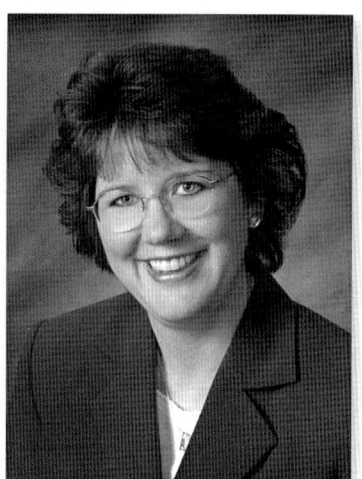

Figure 8: Kelly J. Scheiderer, RHIA, MHA, was the departmental Administrator for the Department of Emergency Medicine from 2007 to 2012. Under her leadership the department grew in reputation and financial strength.

> *When I first started, we realized that we would need an expansion of medical center support in part because we started to see insurance companies deny payment for some different types of emergency department visits. We didn't control who came into the ED and because of the EMTALA laws we had to treat everybody and then the insurance company would say "that wasn't really an emergency" and*

> they would deny payment for that ED visit. So, we were able to go to the hospital leadership, Larry Anstine, and talk to him and show the billing data, and he agreed this model was unsustainable. We were then able to revise a five-year plan so they would support us if we had a deficit in our financials so we would be able to continue to function. We also focused on billing, and we retrained all of the doctors on how to best document in the patient's medical record so we could get the highest level of care and increase our billing to reflect the actual care provided.[7]

Medical center support had also finally come through to support resident salaries. Around the time that Sanfilippo started the Strategic Initiative Program, the practice funds that had supported resident salaries could finally be used for departmental research initiatives and the medical center would finally fund resident salaries and benefits which was, of course, appropriate and long awaited. Additional support for the increasing number of subspecialty fellows came from their medical practice. As Scheiderer recalled:

> When we started getting the Medicare Cost Report Coverage, we were allowed to negotiate total salary support for residents and in programs approved by the Accreditation Council for Graduate Medical Education (ACGME). Some fellowships were not approved by the ACGME such as ultrasound, administration and education. We supported the fellows by giving them a faculty title and appointing the attending physicians with a reduced clinical schedule and salary appropriate for a fellow so they could complete their educational requirements. We also added the emergency medicine/internal medicine residency and that helped us to be able to increase coverage in the two emergency departments. We proposed to open up a free-standing emergency department but we couldn't get the hospital to approve that so we instead pitched the creation of a 20-bed observation unit which then added a new revenue stream.[7]

The fellows also provided much needed clinical coverage of the emergency departments at the Main and East campuses. Many years later the fellows were assigned to other hospitals, including Mount Carmel East and Memorial Hospital in Marysville, Ohio.

Scheiderer recalled other important innovations that led to new found prosperity:

The other thing that we did was what I called a zero-base budget exercise. So, clean slate, you have no money in your budget. Write down everything, all the programing you want to do, other than staff—we took the staff out because we already had the staff—and you had to justify how much you wanted and for what purpose. For example, Dr. Jeff Caterino wanted some training related to research and needed to plan it carefully; and Dr. Diane Gorgas ended up really thinking about what would make the training program so much better. When we added up all the identified expenses, we had actually decreased our expenses by 20% compared to the previous fiscal year. In the end, it made us focus on what we thought really made the biggest impact on our training programs. The academic leaders discussed with the residents and fellows to see what improvements were most important. The reaction from the leaders was, "Oh my gosh, this is much better. We took the time to evaluate what we need to do to make a really great program." That was fun![7]

Scheiderer added financial rigor to the department. As she later recalled:

We were pretty lean and frugal where a lot of places would be, "Oh we need more secretarial support, or we need another billing person, or we need another medical student coordinator." We really did need additional staff but because of our finances we were very frugal in trying to make sure that we didn't just add expense without being able to afford it. We were also the first group to move into the OSU Physicians Group Practice. Doctors would be university employees and covered by the self-insurance fund so that we would not have to pay malpractice insurance premiums directly. We were close to having 90 days cash on hand reserves for operating expensed in case of a shortfall. We had more cash on hand compared to other physician groups. I think that was because Dr. Rund was the leader of OSUP and we were trying to lead by example.[7]

In the annual budget presented to the university medical center in 2010, faculty salaries totaled roughly $2.5 million. Costs of staff and benefits for all other employees totaled an additional $2.5 million. The financial picture was finally looking rosy. A reduction in spending, elimination of the strategic initiatives funding, complete support of resident salaries and benefits and adequate support for the clinical mission at Ohio State Main and East resulted in a small positive balance for 2010. When added to the beginning balance, however, the cash reserve balance was the very positive figure of $701,787.

After 30 years of struggle after the early Dean's warning that "it was sink or swim" the department was finally prosperous and able to support the critical missions of clinical care, education and research.

Still, challenges remained. Faculty salaries were far below the mean for emergency department physicians in academic medical centers and philanthropic support was limited at best. In the coming decade due to the efforts of Mark G. Angelos, MD, and Jeffrey "Jeff" Caterino, MD, faculty salaries would rise to the mean level and the department was finally able to add programs from philanthropy. At the end of the decade in 2010 the department's financial position was finally secure.

References

1. Paulson GW. In Pursuit of Excellence: The Ohio State University Medical Center from 1834 to 2010. George Irving Nelson (1895-1986). Fremont, OH: Lesher Printers; 2010: pp: 109-110.

2. Martin DR. Interview of Daniel R. Martin, by Richard Nelson. 2022: Columbus, Ohio.

3. Reader DW, Spigos DG. The graveyard shift: experience with a night float system. *Emerg. Radiol.* 2002;9:82-87.

4. Coleman J. Interview with James "Jim" Coleman by Richard Nelson. 2022: Columbus, Ohio.

5. Ohio Secretary of State website, *businesssearch.ohiosos.gov*, 2022.

6. Sobieray RJ. Interview with Richard Sobieray, by Douglas Rund. 2011: Columbus, Ohio.

7. Scheiderer KJ. Interview with Kelly Scheiderer, by Douglas Rund. 2022: Columbus, Ohio.

Chapter 10

The Rund Chair Years: 1990-2011

Douglas A. Rund, MD
Richard N. Nelson, MD

On September 11, 2001, the United States was attacked. The World Trade Center in New York was struck by commercial airliners that had been hijacked by terrorists. Brian Hiestand, MD, a resident at the time, remembered the morning of the attack:

> The morning of September 11, 2001, was our weekly block of resident conferences—four hours of emergency focused didactics, with nearly all the trainee physicians attending, as well as whichever faculty had the availability and the interest. I happened to have both that morning, and so was sitting in.
>
> While the precise topic of the 9 a.m. lecture escapes me, I will never forget Dr. Rick Nelson, our department medical director, walking in shortly after the speaker began. In a calm, quiet voice, Dr. Nelson informed us that planes had crashed into the World Trade Center towers, and it seemed to be deliberate. Rick was well known for a very dry sense of humor, and for a second, I wondered if this was a joke I was just not processing. When he went on, though, that disaster management was preparing to receive casualties at our trauma and burn center, though, it became starkly apparent that this was real. The projection system in the lecture hall was re-tuned to local television, and we watched the footage on broadcast with the rest of the nation.
>
> We gradually finished the planned lectures for the morning, although clearly everyone was distracted. Normally, after lectures, people would disperse – residents back to their off-service rotations, or to home if they had a few hours off. Some attendings would head back to the academic offices, or home. Today, we waited. We knew that if there was a wave of

casualties transported out of New York to available trauma centers, we would be part of that necessary response.

We were ready.

We waited.

And no one ever came. The eventual knowledge that the sheer damage was so complete, so massive, that there were no injuries, only fatalities, left such a void of helplessness that I can remember it to this day.[1]

In fact, the lecturer at the 9 a.m. session was Douglas Rund, MD, speaking about administrative issues in emergency medicine. It is not really remarkable that Hiestand forgot the topic since clinical teaching was always in greater demand. Rund remembers that David Bahner, MD, also rushed into the back of the auditorium and announced that the towers collapsed in the deliberate attack. As Hiestand recalls, the faculty and residents quickly tuned to the local channel to watch the news.

BRIAN C. HIESTAND, MD, MPH

Brian C. Hiestand, MD, MPH, received three degrees from Ohio State: a BS in 1994, an MD in 1998 and an MPH in 2007. He joined the faculty as an Assistant Professor following his residency in emergency medicine in 2001. He remained in that position until 2010 when he joined the faculty at Wake Forest University as an Associate Professor. He was promoted to full professor there in 2016, and obtained his board certification in Clinical Informatics in 2018.

Hiestand had an outstanding start to his career at Ohio State. He was one of the first of a growing number of faculty members engaged in clinical research. His studies were primarily in the general area of cardiovascular disease, with a focus on cardiac biomarkers and risk stratification. He was also investigating several new treatments to improve the lives of patients with heart failure, including new assays using biomarkers to enhance the diagnosis and management of heart failure in the emergency setting. He led several clinical trials during his early career. Many of these were sponsored by industry, bringing considerable revenue to the department. In addition, he was a co-investigator with many Ohio State faculty, including Jim Hoekstra, MD, Dan Martin, MD, and Jeff Caterino, MD, MPH.

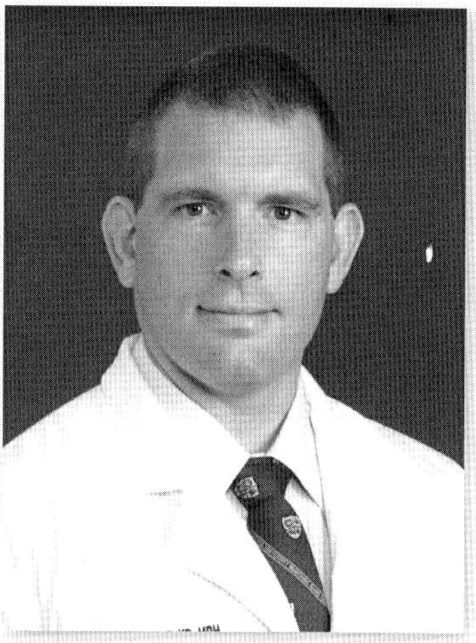

Hiestand was an exceptional physician and leader. His skill and insight were essential in developing the Clinical Decision Unit, focusing on those patients who did not necessarily need a full hospital admission but needed more than the initial ED visit. Hiestand was a leader within the department and the medical center. He served in a variety of roles, including as a member of the Institutional Review Board and several clinical guideline writing committees, and chairing the Medical Center Ethics Committee.

Figure 1: Brian C. Hiestand, MD, MPH, had a long history with Ohio State as a student and faculty member. He was instrumental in developing the Clinical Decision Unit, as well as the Undergraduate Research Associate Program, introducing Ohio State students to both emergency medicine and clinical research.

His long history with Ohio State gave Hiestand the somewhat unique opportunity to observe changes in emergency medicine over the years. In looking back, he recalled the following:

> "Coming up through Ohio State was a different experience at every level – undergraduate, medical school, residency, faculty. I discovered early on in medical school that Emergency Medicine resonated with me, and I was extraordinarily fortunate to meet my lifelong mentor, Jim Hoekstra, as a first-year medical student. Ohio State, housing one of the first full academic departments of Emergency Medicine, provided an outstanding place to train and develop a career. By the time I began, the department had already successfully navigated the growing pains many programs sustained while moving from a division of some other discipline to stand on their own. We had strong relationships with other departments in the hospital, which was instrumental as we developed the Clinical Decision Unit. Most of the patient care protocols we developed relied on active partnerships with the other departments – Cardiology and Neurology in particular. While the technology involved in emergency care went through a number of changes over the years – enhanced CT access,

the growth of point of care ultrasound, the development of novel and improved biomarkers – the core commitment of the people of the department to the tripartite mission never changed.[1]

Research

CARLOS A. TORRES, MD, MPH, PHD

The recruitment of Carlos A. Torres, MD, PhD, was the result of an international mindset that had been embedded in the department from the beginning. This had started with being a part of preventive medicine, which included an emphasis on international health. The department had the lofty ambition to help establish the specialty in other countries. Torres was recruited from Brazil to be a resident in emergency medicine in 1992. At the time there was some concern that the department could recruit a resident from another country but the lure of having the possibility to promote growth of the specialty abroad was too great to pass up. He finished the residency program in 1994, completed course work to receive his MPH degree, then became a research fellow. He returned to Brazil from 1997 to 2002 to help develop emergency medicine there, then returned to Ohio in 2002 and joined the faculty as an Assistant Professor. He continued his research and received his PhD degree as one of the first doctoral students in the department. Torres had completed his undergraduate program at Colejio University and received his MD degree from the Universidade Federal Minas Gerais, both in Brazil.

Years later Torres recalled choosing Ohio State and his career:

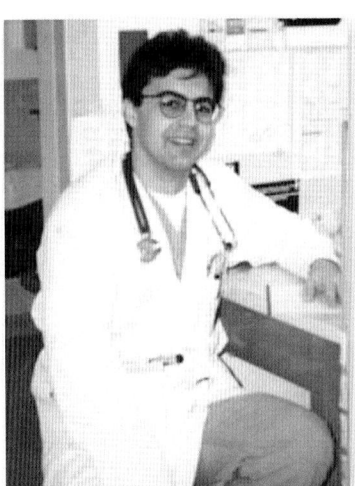

Figure 2: Carlos A. Torres, MD, PhD, was recruited to Ohio State from his native Brazil. He was a collaborator with Dr. Angelos in basic science research focusing on cardiac resuscitation.

My first contact with Dr. Rund was over the phone. In those days (1990) we still communicated through landlines and an international call was a big deal. About a year prior I had been invited to join a select team of physicians interested in developing emergency medicine in Brazil. Not only would I be working with this exceptional group: I had been chosen to be the first Brazilian formally trained in emergency medicine. Imagine, at the young age of 26, fresh out of residency (I had just concluded a cardiology residency in my native Brazil) and being involved in a project of this dimension...I was elated!

I had recently returned from Ohio after having spent two weeks meeting with exponents from the emergency medicine leadership at the time, including then Ohio ACEP president Dr. Edward Charnock. I was very impressed with the state of development of emergency medicine and with the various sites I visited, but mostly with the program at The Ohio State University. Dr. Rund was not in town on the dates I interviewed but I met with several faculty members, including Dr. Richard Nelson, then vice chair of the department of emergency medicine, who was very clear about the enthusiasm that both he and Doug shared for this project.

The phone call came at the end of the afternoon, Brazil time. I had just returned from working at the Heart Hospital (Hospital do Coração) and set a frying pan on the stove. Fried tilapia was going to be the main course as I settled in for dinner at the small bachelor studio I rented on the 10th floor of a downtown building in Curitiba (a city of about 2.5M then and the capital of the state of Paraná in the south of Brazil).

The phone rang a few times and as soon as I picked up, I quickly realized I was on one of the most important phone calls in my life:

"Hello? Dr. Torres this is Chris Dailey. Can you speak with Dr. Rund?"

"YES! I can speak to Dr. Rund!!"

What followed is not as clear: I recall sentences that were barely keeping up with the rush of thoughts on how I would like to join the OSU residency program and get the training and be prepared to contribute to the future development of emergency medicine in Brazil.

I can remember how calm and determined Dr. Rund sounded on the other end of the conversation but also how palpable the enthusiasm was. As we kept on discussing some of the possibilities, including combining the residency with an MPH program focused on EMS systems, I couldn't *stop thinking about the next few months and years.... The smell of burnt oil snapped me back to my immediate reality as a plume of smoke drifted from the kitchen into the living room where I was still mesmerized on the phone call.*

".. Dr. Rund, can you excuse for a minute?"

I placed the phone next to the cradle and stepped into the kitchen: The pan with oil that I had sat on the stove earlier had now caught fire. The hot oil was everywhere and the flames had now spread onto the kitchen cabinets. Running out to the hallway to fetch the extinguisher I remember having the presence to quickly pick up the phone and let Doug know that I would be right back "as soon as I handled the kitchen fire."

I don't know if he had second thoughts on the other end about this crazy Brazilian doctor who had just set fire to his kitchen, what I do know is that when I was finally able to pick up where we left off, he seemed unfazed by the whole incident and confirmed that I would be accepted into the residency program. The rest is history: I went on to complete the residency program, completed the MPH program and a subsequent research fellowship with Dr. Mark Angelos, including a Masters in Medical Sciences before returning to Brazil. For the next five years (from 1997 to 2002) I worked with many brilliant physicians in the house of medicine both in Brazil and in the U.S. to keep the dream of emergency medicine becoming a specialty in Brazil alive.

It would be 25 years from that phone call before Emergency Medicine became recognized as a medical specialty by the Conselho Federal de Medicina (2016) and the dream could finally become reality.

In 1998 Dr. Rund had visited Sao Paulo and helped promote the need for the recognition of emergency medicine as a medical specialty and in 2001 he again played a pivotal role in my career. The department of emergency medicine at OSU was interested in expanding its research program. I was now 40 years old and despite all the excitement with emergency medicine in Brazil I was yearning to return to my research interests. I was welcomed back and for the next 10 years I worked as faculty and researcher and eventually completed my PhD program (in Biophysics).

I am now a consultant in the Emergency Medicine Institute at Cleveland Clinic in the United Arab Emirates. Emergency medicine is a recognized specialty here but still in its infancy. There is much work to do and I often find myself reflecting back to the time I spent at Ohio State as I try to replicate some of those values half way across the world... Go Bucks![2]

JEFFREY M. CATERINO, MD, MPH

Jeffrey M. Caterino, MD, MPH, joined the faculty in 2004. He completed his undergraduate studies with a BA in history at Dartmouth College and attended medical school at the Pennsylvania State University. He then completed a combined emergency medicine/internal medicine residency at Allegheny General Hospital, where he served as chief resident. He completed his MPH in clinical and translational sciences at The Ohio State University.

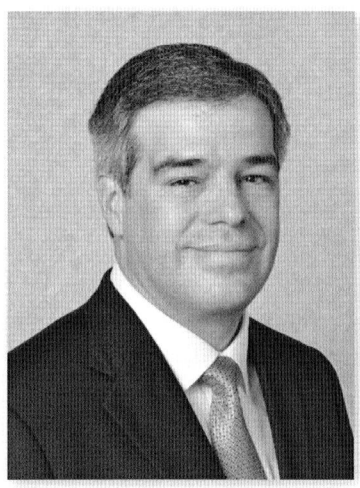

Figure 3: Jeffrey M. Caterino, MD, MPH, was highly successful in building a clinical research program for the department. He ultimately became the Chair of the department.

Caterino was highly successful in research following his recruitment. Soon after his arrival he developed an undergraduate research associate program where students could volunteer in the emergency department to enroll patients in all ED research studies. He also held a joint appointment in the Department of Internal Medicine. He specialized in clinical research relating to the geriatric population and was funded by multiple grants awarded by the National Institutes of Health. Caterino was outstanding in all the missions of the department. He became Chair of the Department of Emergency Medicine in 2020.

MICHAEL R. SAYRE, MD

Michael Sayre, MD, joined the faculty in 2003 as an associate professor. He received his undergraduate degree from Xavier University in Cincinnati and graduated from medical school at the University of Cincinnati in 1984. He obtained residency training in Emergency Medicine at Allegheny General Hospital in Pittsburgh and served as Chief Resident during the final year of training. In 1987, he joined the faculty of the emergency medicine training program at Allegheny General.

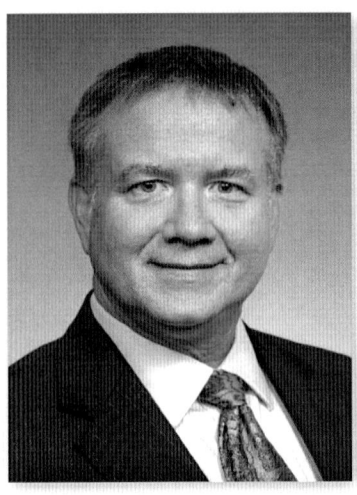

Figure 4: Michael R. Sayre, MD, was an internationally reknown expert in cardiac resuscitation and emergency medical services. He ultimately became the medical director of the highly esteemed Seattle Fire Department.

In 1990, Sayre returned to the University of Cincinnati and became one of the core faculty members in the Department of Emergency Medicine. He was appointed as the medical director for paramedic training in 1990. In 1992, he was appointed medical director for the Cincinnati Fire Department, a position he held until 2000.

In 1990, Sayre founded the emergency medical services fellowship at the University of Cincinnati. The program was a partnership with the UC AirCare program, the Cincinnati Fire Department and the UC Department of Emergency Medicine.

When Sayre joined the faculty of the Department of Emergency Medicine at Ohio State in 2003, he was immediately recognized as an excellent clinician and researcher especially in the area of resuscitation and emergency medical services (EMS). He helped lead a prehospital clinical trial of the AutoPulse CPR device in conjunction with the Columbus Fire Department. The AutoPulse was a squeezing, chest constricting type device that wrapped around the thorax and provided cardiac compression in cases of cardiac arrest. The device was rather widely used by EMS agencies at the time. Due, in part, to Sayre's research the device began to fall out of favor in central Ohio in favor of the LUCAS device, which delivers chest compressions by a battery-powered piston device to the anterior chest in cases of cardiac arrest.

Sayre also was active with the development of guidelines for Cardiopulmonary Resuscitation (CPR) and Emergency Cardiovascular Care with the American Heart Association (AHA) and the International Liaison Committee on Resuscitation (ILCOR). He helped develop and disseminate the AHA's model of "hands only" CPR. Sayre served as the Chair for the AHA ECC committee from 2009 to 2011.

In 2012, Sayre moved to Seattle and joined the faculty of the newly established residency in emergency medicine at the University of Washington (UW). In 2013, he founded the emergency medical services fellowship at the UW. In 2014, he was appointed as the Medical Director for the Seattle Fire Department. He was only the third person to have served in that role since the program was started in 1969.

In addition to that role, Sayre works as an emergency physician at Harborview Medical Center in Seattle and contributes to the Resuscitation Academy and the Global Resuscitation Alliance. He is also the Medical Director for the University of Washington Michael K. Copass Paramedic Training Program and is a Professor of Emergency Medicine at the University of Washington. Sayre contributed to more than 160 peer reviewed articles with an H-index of 61 during his career.

MICHAEL T. CUDNIK, MD, MPH

Michael T. Cudnik, MD, MPH, joined the faculty in 2007. He was engaged in large database analysis for the study of trauma and sudden cardiac arrest in the prehospital setting and developed expertise in economic analysis techniques for effectiveness research. He was the recipient of an AHA grant to investigate the role of geospatial analysis in improving survival after sudden cardiac arrest.

DANIEL P. ZELINSKI, MD, PhD

Daniel P. Zelinski, MD, PhD, joined the faculty in 2008. He received his undergraduate degree from Denison University, where he played on the varsity baseball team. He had a strong interest in science and next enrolled in the doctorate program at Perdue University, looking at proteins on cell surfaces of tumor cells and at the end received his PhD degree. Midway through graduate school he knew that he wanted to be a physician. He applied for admission and was accepted into the Ohio State College of Medicine in 2004. Years later Zelinski remembered that he "defended his thesis one week, and two weeks later was taking anatomy at Ohio State."

Following graduation Zelinski joined the residency program in emergency medicine at Ohio State and finished in 2008. He then began the research fellowship and, as was the custom, began practicing as an attending physician during his fellowship. He remained at Ohio State until 2015 when he began private practice in the Ohio Health system.

Years later, Zelinski recalled the following about his career:

> *I was a typical boy in that I was in science and sports my whole life and quickly realized that "I am not going to make a career in sports," so, science it was. I went to Denison and loved the science. I was working with a lot of professors and researchers there. I think that probably helped push me to start out to get my PhD and thinking of a life in the lab and things like that. But it became pretty clear after a couple of years in the lab it really wasn't the life for me and that I really didn't have the interest or the focus for it but I also knew that I was doing it because I wanted to help people. I think I just realized that I preferred to be closer to the people than to the science part of it.*
>
> *Then eventually talking with some friends I made the decision to go to medical school. It was a really busy last couple of years of my PhD, studying for the MCAT, interviews, and all those things for med school but also finishing up my PhD project, which I was able to do a couple of weeks before I started gross anatomy at OSU. I never really looked back in that I felt that the clinical realm was the place for me.*
>
> *I did do some research at Ohio State, and I really enjoyed it and found it fascinating, but I also felt that it just would take me away from what I really felt I loved, and I was good at: the clinical part, being at the patients' bedside in the emergency department. I love being in the ED and talking to the patients. I just get more hands on at Ohio Health, whereas there are so many students and residents [at Ohio State]. They get to do all the fun stuff in putting in the chest tubes and the lines and spending more time with the patients. I like being at the bedside.*[3]

Continued Progress in Research

There was considerable progress in research during the period from 2001 to 2011. The clinical research program was enhanced by the addition of Jeffrey Caterino, MD, who conducted studies of the older population, including antibiotic prescribing for elders with urinary tract infection, predictors of decompensation after admission in patients with sepsis, balance problems in the elderly and increased mortality in elder trauma patients. Caterino was awarded a Jahnigen Career Development Award by the American Geriatrics Society.

Robert Guthrie, MD, and Brian Hiestand, MD, continued to conduct clinical trials and Mark Angelos, MD, continued with his basic science research related to cardiac resuscitation. He and his graduate students studied the oxidation–reduction mechanisms involved in myocardial reperfusion and functional recovery of the heart following resuscitation. This research, along with investigations into the origins of mitochondrial dysfunction during cardiac arrest, were designed to improve the understanding of cellular reactions during reperfusion to allow physicians to treat patients in a way that maximized recovery of the myocardium following cardiac arrest.

During 2009 eight faculty members submitted 15 grant applications totaling $5,929,403. Revenue from research funding increased almost seven-fold from $224,682 in 2007 to $1,537,310 in 2009. There were four primary research staff associates: Lynn White, MS, CCRP; Michael Hill, RN, Sverre Aune; and Alan Blumberg. White worked closely with Sayre. Aune and Blumberg worked primarily with Angelos and Hill worked with Caterino and Hiestand in clinical research.

Expansion: New Clinical Opportunities and Faculty Growth

At the turn of the century, in 2000, a new era for expansion and prosperity was beginning for Ohio State Emergency Medicine. Patient volumes were increasing, due, to a large extent, the addition of Ohio State University East Hospital on the near east side of Columbus. The original hospital was Saint Anthony Hospital founded in 1890 by the

Poor Sisters of St. Francis (later known as the Franciscan Sisters of the Poor). In 1992 the hospital changed hands when Saint Anthony was purchased by the Quorum Health Group of Tennessee and was renamed Park Medical Center.

Seven years later, in 1999, the Trustees at Ohio State authorized the purchase of Park Medical Center from Quorum for $13 million. The hospital was renamed Ohio State East. One of the thoughts prior to the purchase was that Park had considerable resources, including imaging and operating room capability. Bernadine Healy, MD, who was the College of Medicine Dean at that time, envisioned that the hospital could become similar to the Hospital for Special Services in New York which specializes in orthopedic and rheumatologic conditions.

Coverage of the Emergency Department at the new Ohio State East Hospital was discussed among the faculty. Quorom's purchase of Saint Anthony Hospital in 1992 had resulted in coverage by a physician group that was quite deficient in many ways, and the Park Medical Center ED's reputation plummeted. By 1999 patient volume had declined dramatically to 13,000 visits per year. The College of Medicine leadership at Ohio State realized that the situation could only be repaired if physicians seeing ED patients were outstanding in all respects. They decided that the Department of Emergency Medicine faculty could provide such coverage, but that Ohio State would need to subsidize that effort, as patient collections were insufficient to support the new faculty due to the decreased census that had occurred and an unfavorable payor mix. Ultimately it was decided that the department would staff the ED and that a subsidy would be provided.

In 1999 Michael Dick, MD, was selected to lead the effort. Dick was an Associate Professor who had completed his residency in emergency medicine and critical care fellowship at Ohio State. His mission was to assemble and lead an extremely capable faculty team to staff the ED. An outstanding physician with exceptional clinical skills, Dick soon recruited and hired physicians with proven excellence in the care of emergency patients: Sondra Shellman, MD; Ann Haynes, MD; Brandy Helminiak, MD; Melissa Kerg, MD; Kurt Nelter, MD; and Mark DeBard, MD. This rapid expansion of the faculty required medical center financial support. The new physicians were stunningly successful, providing a remarkable upgrade in medical services to the hospital and the

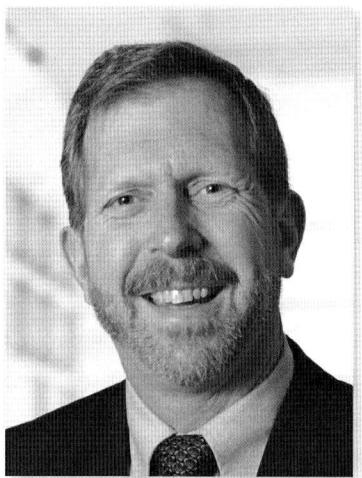

Figure 5: Michael Dick, MD, joined the faculty in 1993. In 1999 he successfully built and led a physician team to care for patients at the newly acquired Ohio State University East Hospital. In addition to his training in emergency medicine, Dick completed a fellowship in critical care medicine at Ohio State.

surrounding community.

Five years after the ED reorganization, the census almost tripled from the low of 13,000 in 1999 to a new high of 35,000 in 2004. In June 2005 a ribbon-cutting ceremony marked the opening of the newly expanded emergency department at Ohio State East. The new department had approximately 15,000 square feet of direct patient care areas and 10,000 square feet of support areas, for a total of 25,000 square feet. There were 26 private examination rooms, two major resuscitation rooms, a dedicated CT scanner and separate entrances for patients and ambulances.

At the main Ohio State campus, the annual patient census was also rising. In 2000 there were 50,403 visits; 10 years later the number had grown to 70,829. Additional faculty members were needed but recruitments were still targeted to enhance all the departmental missions, which consistently emphasized research and scholarship. Teaching and excellent clinical care were a given. Faculty members had to have outstanding patient care skills in a unit as highly visible as the emergency department and the teaching program for students and residents were always robust and excellent. By the end of 2004 the department had grown to 33 faculty members with the additional hiring of several more: Donald Norris, II, MD; Richard Limperos, MD; Samuel Kiehl, MD; Gary Katz, MD; and Mark G. Moseley, MD. By 2009 the number had grown to 38 with the addition of Andrew Wagner, MD; Jillian McGrath, MD; Erika Kube, MD; Ayesha Khan, MD; Miles Hawley, MD; and Aaron Bernard, MD.

Medical Student Education

Ohio State faculty members in emergency medicine were always looking for ways to increase their roles as teachers in the medical school. Prior to 1978, a faculty presence in the emergency room was rare indeed and medical students only saw patients when accompanying a resident to evaluate a patient. A student taking a cardiology rotation, for instance, could go "down" to the emergency room with the resident in consultation.

After 1978, following the creation of the Division of Emergency Medicine in the Department of Preventive Medicine, the development of student electives became a priority. A fourth-year elective in the emergency department with formal lectures seemed the obvious first step. In the early years the lectures were conducted with help from Preventive Medicine faculty and included such topics as "emergency medicine in a community's health" and "the place of emergency medical services in the health system."

Division faculty felt strongly that emergency medicine should be a part of every student's curriculum. The faculty argued that a physician needed to be able to respond capably to an emergency regardless of specialty, so there was a push to make emergency medicine a mandatory course in the fourth year of medical school. The fourth and final year of medical school was called Phase IV at the time. The term "phase" originated at a time when the medical school curriculum was a shortened to three years in length from the customary four. For a short time during the transition in the early 1970s, both third-year and fourth-year students were in medical school at the same time. Eventually the school reverted back to the traditional 4-year curriculum for nearly all students.

In 1980 Rund became the Chairman of the Phase IV Subcommittee on Elective Review and Chairman of the Phase IV Subcommittee on Critical Care Electives. His objective was to make these one-month rotations mandatory and not electives. It should be remembered that only three years earlier there was no clinical rotation in the Ohio State emergency room because there were no faculty present. The division had made considerable progress during the interim. Following the subcommittee's recommendations, the college required that the final year had to include a rotation in either emergency medicine or critical care. This increased the educational requirement that all major emergency departments in Columbus provide a clinical venue for students in order to accommodate the more than 200 students needing the clinical teaching.

Still, challenges remained. Faculty salaries were far below the mean for emergency department physicians in academic medical centers and philanthropic support was limited at best. In the coming decade due to the efforts of Angelos and Caterino, faculty salaries would rise to the mean level and the department was finally able to add programs from philanthropy. At the end of the decade in 2010 the department's financial position was finally secure.

Differentiation of Care (DOC) Clerkships

In 1993 James "Jim" Hoekstra, MD, was appointed to the fourth-year curriculum committee called the Differentiation of Care (DOC) Subcommittee, which was charged with developing a curriculum to provide students with educational experiences in different patient care settings. The DOCs included four "selective" rotations in which students could select the site of their clinical work but would meet one day a week for didactic education. DOC 1 covered care that would be delivered in the acute setting such as emergency medicine. DOC 2 covered care that would be delivered in the ambulatory setting, such as primary care. DOC 3 was about chronic care and the care of special needs populations. And finally, the DOC 4 was a sub-internship. Hoekstra became the director of DOC 1. Over time, additional teaching faculty from emergency medicine—Sorabh Khandelwal, MD, and Nicholas Kman, MD—became the leaders of this new requirement.

NICHOLAS E. KMAN, MD

Nicholas E. "Nick" Kman, MD, joined the faculty in 2007. He completed medical school at Ohio State and his residency in emergency medicine at Wake Forest University, where he served as chief resident. Following his recruitment to Ohio State, he became deeply involved in medical student education and curriculum development. In late 2009, he took charge of the fourth-year medical school clerkship in emergency medicine which was called DOC 1 at that time. He created many innovative improvements in the clerkship, including expanded summative simulation, a National Board of Medical Examiners (NBME) Shelf exam and virtual reality training.

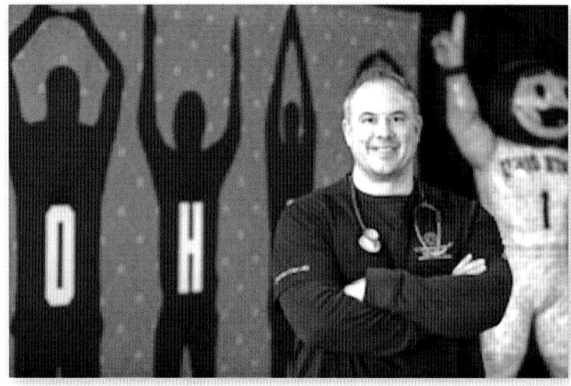

Figure 6: Nicholas E. Kman, MD, became the leader of the emergency medicine education program for students in the College of Medicine and the program director for the entire fourth-year curriculum in 2015.

His teaching and administrative skills quickly became apparent to college leadership and he was appointed the academic program director for the *entire fourth year of medical school* at Ohio State in 2015. Kman's ascension to this key leadership position fulfilled many of the aspirations of the early leaders of emergency medicine who recognized the fundamental importance of student education: There was great confidence that the comprehensive view of clinical medicine required for effective practice in the emergency setting and the innate teaching abilities of academic emergency physicians would ultimately lead to leadership at the highest level in the college. During his tenure as program director, Kman accomplished several innovations, including the following: robust bootcamps and clinical tracks to prepare medical students for residency, expanded simulation and Team Based Learning (TBL) activities on important topics like sexual violence, opioid abuse and end-of-life conversations.

Kman also rose to national prominence as a widely recognized leader and innovator in education. From 2014 to 2015 he served as the President of Clerkship Directors in Emergency Medicine (CDEM). Over the years he has led several programs for the Society of Academic

Emergency Medicine (SAEM), including chairmanship of the medical student symposium and the education research interest group. He was recognized by the Association of American Medical Colleges (AAMC) for his leadership in the Leadership Education and Development (LEAD) Certificate program and the Medical Research Certificate (MERC). Throughout his career Kman has presented his research at virtually all of the relevant education research forums and meetings worldwide.

Kman also established his expertise in disaster response and emergency preparedness. Serving as one of the Medical Managers for Ohio Task Force 1, Ohio's FEMA Urban Search and Rescue team, Kman has deployed to major hurricanes: Harvey (2017), Dorian (2019), Laura (2020), Ida (2021) and Ian (2022). Currently, Kman and the Ohio State Advanced Computing Center for the Arts and Design (ACCAD) received a grant to teach Mass Casualty Triage to First Responders in Virtual Reality. The program uses a virtual reality headset and program to enable the learner to view many casualties simultaneously and work through their sorting process quickly. Learners are required to make rapid clinical assessments, and assign an urgency level guiding treatment and evacuation priority. Lifesaving treatments such as tourniquets are applied immediately if needed during the sorting process.

Additional Student Courses

In addition to DOC-1, medical student course offerings were expanded to include several other courses. Advanced Topics in Emergency Medicine (ATEM) was a 10-month longitudinal honors course designed for students planning to enter an emergency residency. The primary goal was to provide them with advanced skills and knowledge in preparation for the next step in their educational pathway. The course included lectures, skill stations, journal club, preparation of lectures and special emergency medicine clinical shifts. In 2009 the course enrolled 15 students.

Created and led by Aaron Bernard, MD, a new course for third-year students was developed as part of an ambulatory clerkship to provide junior students with exposure to emergency medicine.

AARON W. BERNARD, MD

Aaron W. Bernard, MD, joined the faculty in 2009. He graduated from Stony Brook University Health Sciences Center School of Medicine in 2003 and completed his residency in emergency medicine at the University of Cincinnati in 2007. Bernard created a third-year elective course for medical students interested in emergency medicine. Years later Bernard recalled the impetus to create the course for third-year students:

> *At the time the university was looking to make some more third-year electives available. The students had a two-week block where they could elect to do different things. It was a great experience. We would host a handful of students of each month. It was big enough where it was noticeable, but it was still very intimate. I think it was four to six students per block or month.*
>
> *The goals were a couple of things. One was to let the students get some early exposure to careers they were interested in, and obviously in emergency medicine we wanted to encourage that. Particularly for a student this was really important (if I recall the timeline) because they had a mandatory fourth-year clerkship but they had to decide their career early in fourth year. [This meant that they had to] complete their clerkship in the first two months to be able to decide their career and get everything in order to apply for residency. So, a lot of students entering fourth year would come to the end of fourth year and they had already matched in [various other] specialties and then did their mandatory [emergency medicine] clerkship—and they had some remorse that they didn't know more about emergency medicine earlier.*
>
> *By giving them early exposure, it helped with their career selection and*

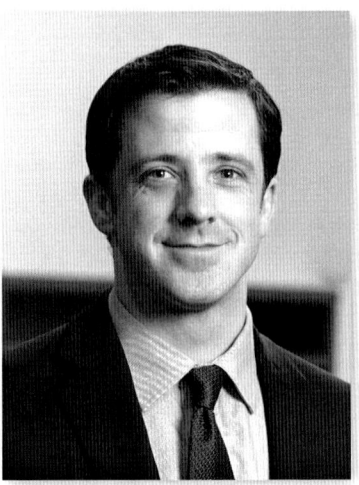

Figure 7: Aaron W. Bernard, MD, created the third-year elective course in emergency medicine for medical students at The Ohio State University College of Medicine. He went on to help found the new Quinnipiac Medical School in Connecticut.

career undertaking and gave them more touch points to see emergency medicine over the course of a medical student career. So, we would have four to six students who had some inkling that emergency medicine was the career for them. For us that was fun because the students who are interested in your career are probably more interesting for the faculty to have because they are more engaged. We tried to make sure the students got to rotate in places where they were supported and with faculty that would mentor them. They rotated with us in the ER. We also did various things with them–we had a day of simulation in the simulation lab, we had a day where we did didactics in the oral board style where they got to work through a case. We had a suturing session. They had a lot of one-on-one faculty time with myself and a lot of other people as well if they decided to go in that career. I remember the culmination of their elective they were asked to do a presentation.

If I recall correctly, we asked them to pick a case that was interesting to them and present it to the faculty. Again, it was fun for us to see the students pick something interesting, present it to us and tell us what they learned. We gave them comments on their presentations in terms of style and substance. It was nice chance for them to be surrounded by faculty and [for us to get to] know them early on and if they decided they wanted to go into our field, they weren't strangers when the time came to ask for letters of recommendation and such.[4]

Bernard left the faculty in 2013 to help found a new medical school in Connecticut: The Frank H. Netter MD School of Medicine at Quinnipiac University. Bernard credited his mentors, including Khandelwal, with helping him join national committees such as the national committee writing Step 2 Clinical Skills examination where students would go to a testing center and have to demonstrate doing history and physical exams on standardized patients.

Years later Bernard remembered this about the preparation for his new role at Quinnipiac:

I was in a great position at my new job at Quinnipiac Medical School to help found a curriculum to ensure the students would have the skills to do really well on that exam. We went 3 or 4 years without having one student fail that national exam. There were some established medical schools with really strong backgrounds having 5-10% failure rate. That was a real moment of pride for myself and I was really happy to contribute that way to the medical school. That wouldn't have happened if I didn't have the supportive faculty and experiences I had at Ohio State.

For the last two years of my time at Quinnipiac I taught the physical diagnosis course for first- and second-year students. I think that was one of the favorite roles I had over the years. I was really mentoring students from the day they walked into the medical school until the time that they entered their clinical rotations on how to be a physician, how to talk to patients, how to do physical exams and care for people. I really liked and enjoyed that. I had a really good stretch in academics. I am really thankful to my time at Ohio State developing and growing there.[4]

Other Courses

An honors ultrasound course was developed under the guidance of David Bahner, MD. The course became extremely popular and expanded to include nearly 20% of the graduation class. The faculty also played an integral role in other courses, including the Clinical Skills Immersion Course for third-year students, and the Learning Community program where faculty and students met once a month to discuss topics not covered elsewhere in the curriculum and to establish a mentorship relation between individual faculty members and students.

DONALD L. NORRIS II, MD

Donald L. Norris II, MD, was an exceptional faculty member who devoted himself to medical student education (Figures 7 and 8). He joined the faculty in July 2003. Originally from Barboursville, West Virginia, he graduated from West Virginia University in 1995 and Marshall University School of Medicine in 2000. He served as chief resident during his final year in residency at East Carolina University before joining the faculty at Ohio State.

With outstanding mentorship from other faculty members, including Diane Gorgas, MD, and Sorabh Khandelwal, MD, Norris advanced his passion for education. He helped develop the simulation curriculum

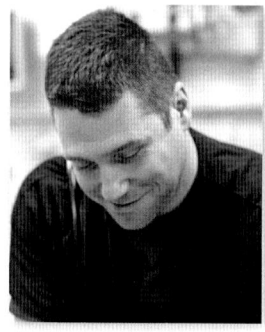

Figure 8: Donald L. Norris II, MD, served on the faculty from 2007 to 2013. He was a leader in medical education.

for the department and his interest in undergraduate medical education led to teaching small groups of second year medical students and serving on the medical school admissions committee.

After leaving Ohio State in 2013, Norris served as medical director and Chair of the Department of Emergency Medicine at Ascension Genesys Regional Medical Center in Grand Blanc, Michigan. There, he went on to develop his leadership skills while also being active in the core faculty for their EM residency program. He went on to help re-establish the EM residency program at Summa Health in Akron. He is currently an Associate Clinical Professor of Emergency Medicine at his alma mater, East Carolina University.

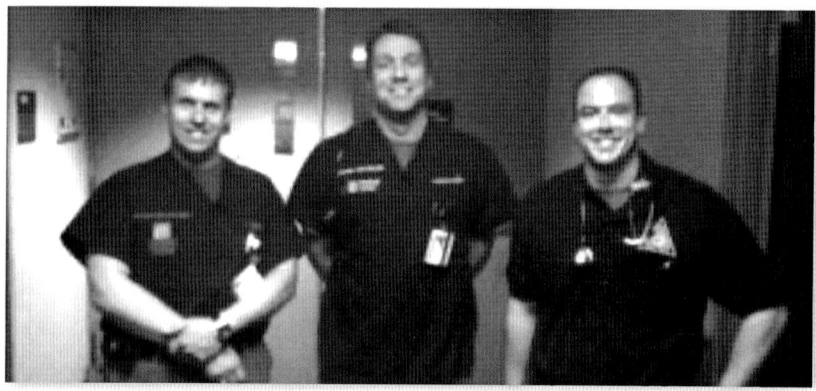

Figure 9: Three top educators in the department of emergency medicine include, from left to right: Colin Kaide, MD; Donald Norris, MD; and Nick Kman, MD.

SAMUEL J. KIEHL, MD

Samuel J. Kiehl, MD, co-founder of the residency program when he led the group at Riverside, joined the Ohio State faculty in 2002. With years of clinical experience, Kiehl quickly became one of the most outstanding clinical teachers in the department. Students and residents highly valued his wise and sensible teachings. He was preferentially sought out for his teaching and he consistently won teaching awards for students and residents. He was also an expert in the business of medicine and presented his experiences in conferences and in person the residents to prepare them to enter the real world of medical practice.

JILLIAN L. MCGRATH, MD

Jillian L. McGrath, MD, joined the faculty in 2008 (Figures 10). She completed her undergraduate education at the University of Wisconsin in 2000 and her received her medical degree (Alpha Omega Alpha) from the University of Wisconsin School of Medicine and Public Health in 2004. She completed one year of an internal medicine residency at Wisconsin from 2004 to 2005, then entered the emergency medicine residency program at Ohio State. Immediately post-residency, she joined the faculty as an assistant professor. She was promoted to Associate Professor in 2017.

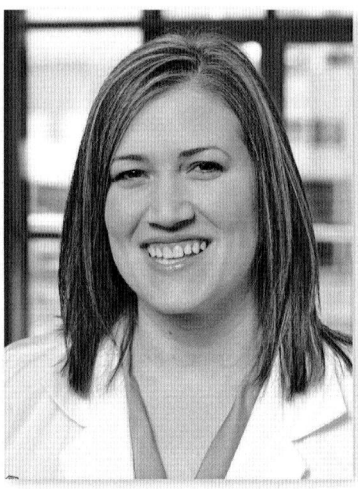

McGrath had a strong interest in graduate medical education. With an outstanding clinical background from both Wisconsin and Ohio State, she was an exceptionally talented resident and physician. She began her highly effective teaching from the moment she joined the faculty. She was the Associate Director of the residency program from 2011 to 2015 and became a highly regarded mentor for the residents. She has a passion for mentorship of female physicians in emergency medicine through curricular innovations and led by example as she integrated a growing family and academic emergency medicine career.

Figure 10: Jillian L. McGrath, MD, excelled in resident education and evaluation throughout her career in emergency medicine at Ohio State.

An expert in clinical skills assessment, McGrath is an oral board examiner for the American Board of Emergency Medicine. Her research focuses on assessment of emergency learner competency using virtual simulation environments. Her current funded research examines the use of virtual reality to teach mass casualty triage to providers at all levels, from paramedics to physicians in all phases of their education.

AYESHA KHAN, MD

Ayesha Khan, MD, joined the faculty at Ohio State as an assistant professor in 2008. She graduated from Wayne State University School of Medicine and completed her residency in Emergency Medicine at Detroit Receiving Hospital. At Ohio State she became interested in global health and searched for fellowship training, which was not available at that time through the department. She opted to begin a fellowship in Global Health at Stanford University School of Medicine. On completion, she joined the faculty at Stanford and began her work focused on two areas of population health: addressing the neglected burden of global emergency disease as a public health concern through projects focused on education and capacity building, and use of the emergency department to create and disseminate public health interventions to subpopulations not touched by other parts of the American health care system.

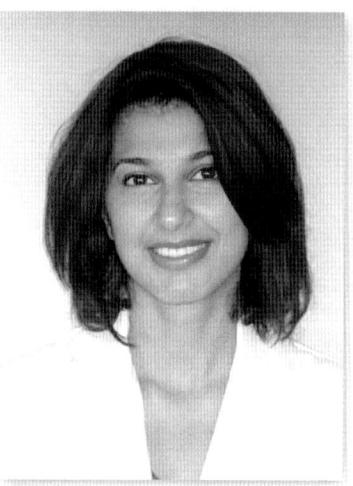

Figure 11: Ayesha Khan, MD, served on the faculty at Ohio State until she became a fellow in global health and joined the faculty at the Stanford School of Medicine.

Passionate about teaching the plumbing and poetry of being a holistic, healthy health care provider, she has delivered over 50 national and international lectures to health care providers on emergency medicine. She has also created curricula and mentored residents through global health and social emergency medicine electives, and started *Announce*, a podcast focused on the emergency department as the clinical home of social medicine and health equity efforts. *Announce* discusses the influence of addiction, opiate use disorders, immigration, human trafficking, race, gun violence, homelessness, malnutrition, and language barriers on patient care and programs and projects that address these issues in community, county and academic emergency departments. Lastly, Khan started and runs a monthly inter-institutional journal club for fellows, faculty, residents and students in Social Emergency Medicine and Health Equity to discuss timely topics and works-in-progress. Participating institutions include: University of Washington, UCLA, Stanford, University of Kansas, Boston University, University of Chicago, Duke and Highland Hospital.

Challenges: Increasing Patient Demand and Overcrowding

The steady increase in the numbers of patients seeking emergency care started in the middle of the 20th century and continued unabated. Beginning with the decline of general practice, an aging population, increased complexity of illness, increases in insurance coverage, increased mobility of the population, demand for immediate care and a desire for all the resources of the hospital, emergency departments and hospitals felt the weight of these patient burdens. The growth never stopped. The onslaught of patients created an obligation that became more daunting as time progressed. By 2007 the overcrowding in emergency departments led to the publication of *Hospital-Based Emergency Care at the Breaking Point* by the Institute of Medicine. At Ohio State long gone were the days of the early 70s when doctors could take naps during the night shift.

One of the nationwide issues facing hospital-based emergency departments was the increasingly limited capacity of inpatient services to admit patients promptly from the department. The orderly flow of patients through the evaluation and treatment process was blocked when an inpatient bed was not available for the patient ready for admission. This began happening with alarming regularity. Admitted patients continued to occupy emergency treatment rooms and new patients had to wait somewhere for their bed. The phenomenon, known as "boarding" became a frightening national problem.

Faced with long waits for care, patients began to leave the hospital without being seen (LWBS). For one month in 2009 the LWBS rate at Ohio State was as high as 7.4%. Faced with an overwhelming load of patients, the hospital had to divert ambulance patients to other hospitals. In July of 2009 the hospital was "on diversion" 78 hours for the remainder of the year, yet the rate fell as low as zero for some months. When all hospitals in Columbus were diverting, a city-wide diversion plan went into effect which distributed the patients to hospitals in rotation. The crowding worsened as time went on.

A proposal was developed to establish a physician-staffed "greet" area. The thinking of the time was that an early session with a physician could result in immediate initiation of orders for lab work and x-rays and perhaps even rapid treatment and discharge for patients with minor conditions. Serious conditions could also be identified early and the patient transferred for more immediate treatment. Unfortunately, the hospital never agreed to fund this program and an opportunity to improve throughput and patient satisfaction was lost.

Surge Capacity

The Ohio State emergency department was becoming overcrowded almost daily and the surging demand for emergency care continued. Wait times to be seen by a physician were increasing ominously. All beds were routinely filled and the ED used beds and chairs in the hallway to get patients evaluated and started in treatment. Faced with rising concerns that there could be no excess capacity at all during a disaster, there was the constant issue of coordinating flow through the entire hospital in the most efficient manner, which required the cooperation of all units and employees. At the time there was an urgent need to communicate the degree of overcrowding in the ED to the rest of the hospital.

In response, the hospital turned to the National Emergency Department Overflow Capacity Score (NEDOCS), a uniform method to measure the ED surge. The score was calculated from the numbers of patients waiting for beds, ED bed occupancy and levels of illness severity, with the score calculated and portrayed as a color for quick reference. Colors ranged from green (not crowded) to black (dangerously overcrowded). The statistics were posted on the front page of the hospital's webpage (OneSource) and updated throughout the day. When scores rose, the hospital surge plan was implemented in stages according to the crowding score. Since all relevant hospital areas were activated (housekeeping, admitting, clinical staff, administration) the idea was that the entire organization should contribute to handling the increased overall capacity. A vastly expanded emergency department was desperately needed, but was years away.

The Clinical Decision Unit (CDU)

In February 2009 the Clinical Decision Unit (CDU) began operation. An observation area of sorts had been implemented years earlier using a few beds off one of the hallways in the department. Finally, new space was found that was immediately adjacent to the emergency department where central sterile supply had been previously. The area was renovated to create 20 beds and a separate staff of nurses and nurse practitioners were hired to staff the unit. The unit was headed by Mark G. Moseley, MD, MHA, who was developing increasing expertise in the clinical and business affairs of the department. Years later Moseley recalled his sense of urgency to add additional patient beds:

> *Both of our EDs were under constant pressure due to rapid expansion of volume and patient complexity, as well as demands from the broader community that wanted access to OSU's inpatient bed capacity. As a result, our EDs were forced to care for many patients in hallways, and to board patients awaiting an inpatient bed, which was very challenging for our teams. We were nearly six years away from the new ED and inpatient capacity opening.*

> *As a result, we focused intensely on efficiency, effectiveness, and patient safety initiatives in the EDs at this time. It was that focus that led us to create the CDU. We decided we had to own the patients that were too sick or complicated to go home but were perceived as not sick or complex enough to need inpatient admission (and utilize scarce inpatient beds). Like the ED doctors, nurses and staff we were, we took matters into our own hands and "announced" that we would care for these patients; we would innovate around care protocols; we would enhance care coordina-*

> ## "Finding" Space for the Clinical Decision Unit
>
> *By Douglas Rund, MD*
>
> I prowled through the areas around the emergency department relentlessly because I was always on the lookout for additional patient care space. We were looking for a place to locate the Observation Unit (which was ultimately named the Clinical Decision Unit). There was a space next to the emergency department which had always been the Central Sterile Supply. The space was vacated when the hospital created the first James Cancer Hospital.
>
> When the Sterile Supply Unit left, I noticed how quickly the empty space became filled with "squatters." The area became a warren of temporary plywood walls and padlocked doors with names like "carpentry" or "plumbing." These fiefdoms just appeared without any authorization or approval from anyone. In addition, there was the seemingly random storage of all sorts of equipment such as hospital beds, gurneys and wheelchairs.
>
> One day at the conclusion of a leadership meeting I invited Jay Kasey, one of the more visionary hospital administrators, to go with me to this "storage" area. I offered the message that this incredibly valuable space was being wasted. I said, "We can convert this space into a clinical decision unit and serve our patients and earn some revenue." Our faculty had already toured observation units throughout the country and learned that patients appreciated the opportunity to rest in a quieter place while their condition was being evaluated over time. Kasey immediately saw the potential for the area and we moved forward with the creation of the unit. We had to get some variances because of the need to use a somewhat atypical enclosed space. The unit added much to the capacity of the emergency department and the comfort of our patients. Kasey eventually became the Senior Vice President for Administration and Planning at Ohio State.

tion; and we would send more patients home after an intense period of observation, diagnostic testing and therapeutic intervention.[5]

Prior to the opening of the Clinical Decision Unit, Moseley and Rund visited the observation unit at the University of Rochester to determine the best practices. The director of the unit was invited to speak at Ohio State and there was an attempt to recruit him to direct the new program. He declined, but provided Moseley and Rund with valuable insights about the management of such an observation service. The initial origin of some units had been an attempt to observe and monitor patients with chest pain who had a low to intermediate probability of acute myocardial infarction (AMI). The thinking was that a period of monitoring and repeated cardiac enzymes would clarify the picture in 24 hours.

Gradually it became clear that many other conditions might also resolve in a 24-hour period such as asthma or heart failure. Initially the Center for Medicare and Medicaid Services reimbursed CDU stays for only three conditions: chest pain, asthma and congestive heart failure. This changed over time as the benefits in terms of cost and efficiency became clear.

The new unit at Ohio State was a great success with patients, who loved the enhanced ability to go home after their ED care. Overall patient flow and capacity improved markedly. The patient satisfaction scores for the CDU physicians ranged from 87% to 92% of patients ranking the physician with the highest possible score.

MARK G. MOSELEY, MD, MHA, CPE, FACEP

Mark G. Moseley, MD, graduated in 2002 as one of Ohio State's first graduates from the combined five-year dual degree MD/MHA program. He completed a residency in emergency medicine at Christiana Care Health System in Wilmington, Delaware, serving as chief resident in his final year of training. Moseley then returned to his Ohio State alma mater in 2005, and began a journey of progressive leadership responsibility over the next 12 years. He served as a residency core academic faculty member, Medical Director of the Emergency Department, Medical Director of the Clinical Decision Unit, and Vice-Chair for Clinical Affairs for the Department of Emergency Medicine.

In 2012, he was asked to take on the role of Assistant Chief Operating Officer for the medical center to help oversee systemwide patient flow management and patient throughput. In 2014 he was selected as the system Medical Director for Case Management, Social Work, and Utilization Management. He left Ohio State in 2017 to become the Chief

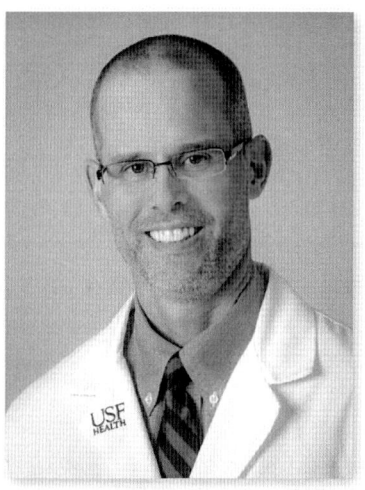

Figure 12: Mark G. Moseley, MD, MHA, held important leadership positions at Ohio State and was instrumental in developing innovative new programs. He was one of the founders of the administration fellowship at Ohio State.

Medical Officer for the University of South Florida (USF) in Tampa, Florida. He subsequently was promoted to the role of Chief Clinical Officer, and served as the chief executive officer of the faculty practice for the USF Health's Morsani College of Medicine. In 2022, he was appointed the Vice-Dean for Clinical Affairs in the medical school, and was selected through a national search process to be the President of the new combined USF and Tampa General Physicians practice corporation. He is a full Professor in the Colleges of Medicine and Public Health at USF.

Years later Moseley remembered some of the experiences at Ohio State that helped him grow to attain his leadership goals:

> *My time at OSU was a crucible that forced me to become a better doctor, a better colleague, and a better, more complete leader. I think it was that way for many of us that started our careers at this pivotal time. Our emergency medicine faculty, regardless of their focus, were frequently asked to solve complex and significant problems that often had no traditional answer. As such, we had to innovate, be creative, and be assertive with "the system." With the supportive senior faculty and leadership of our department, we were encouraged and supported to try new solutions and implement them.*
>
> *For me, regardless of the domain—ED operations, CDU, After-Hours Clinics, Physician Advisor Program, or the ED Administrative Fellowship—there was a sense that our department was going to get the job done on behalf of our patients. The passion and persistence of my colleagues at that time was critical for my development as a senior leader. It showed me what was possible with grit, tenacity and resilience. There is not a day that goes by in my current c-suite roles, that I don't draw from experiences cultivated during this time. I was blessed and fortunate to have been part of OSU Emergency Medicine for certain.*

Developing Leaders and Planning for the Future

Moseley and Gary Katz, MD, studied the administrative and business aspect of emergency medicine. The department encouraged them to learn the best practices of businesses in the service industry to bring them back to Ohio State. Years later Moseley recalled one of the efforts:

> The department sent us to the Disney Institute for Quality Safety and Service, and we developed an entire program for patient experience in the emergency department. At the time, this was a very innovative approach—to learn from other service industries and apply those learnings to the ED. This started a series of "innovations," not only with me, but with other faculty as well. I believe this was because of the environment that Dr. Rund fostered. He was a sophisticated, mature, academic leader who gave us the latitude to experiment and innovate. That wasn't very typical in academia at that time, and still isn't to this day. He was a catalyst for change, and we were the reagents necessary for the reaction. Those reactions fundamentally changed the ED at OSU, and propelled the department to national prominence and reputation.

Moseley, Katz and other faculty leaders closely observed best practices in hospital systems throughout the country and even more closely in central Ohio, the hospitals primary catchment area. The need for free standing emergency departments away from the sometimes-congested university area seemed obvious, and the other major systems in town were rapidly constructing such facilities. The free-standing centers were located in areas closer to homes in the rapidly growing city and offered shorter wait times with the same physicians and capabilities of the main hospital for most conditions. The expertise to develop a free-standing emergency department was available "in house." Gary Katz, MD, MBA was the perfect person to create such a plan.

GARY KATZ MD, MBA

Gary Katz, MD, MBA, joined the faculty at Ohio State in the spring of 2003. He completed his undergraduate medical education at the Medical College of Ohio followed by his residency in Emergency Medicine at Summa Health System in Akron. During residency, Katz was elected to the board of directors of the Emergency Medicine Residents Association (EMRA), where he served as a full member of the Residency Review Committee for Emergency Medicine (RRC-EM). While serving on the RRC-EM, he worked with Douglas Rund, MD, who represented the American Board of Emergency Medicine on the committee.

After residency, Katz joined the faculty at Eastern Virginia Medical School in Norfolk, Virginia. Two years later he returned to Ohio in 2003 to join the Ohio State faculty. He took a strong interest in leadership development and facilitating new growth opportunities for the field of emergency medicine. Completing his MBA studies at The Ohio State University Fisher College of Business, he brought best practices in leadership innovation to the Department of Emergency Medicine, ultimately helping to create a fellowship in Administration. Unique to its time, the fellowship curriculum looked beyond the emergency department as a singular entity and instead promoted it as one key point of function in a larger hospital operation. The administration fellowship was the first to incorporate a full MBA into the two-year curriculum. Graduates from this program went on to excel in medical innovation industries and health system leadership.

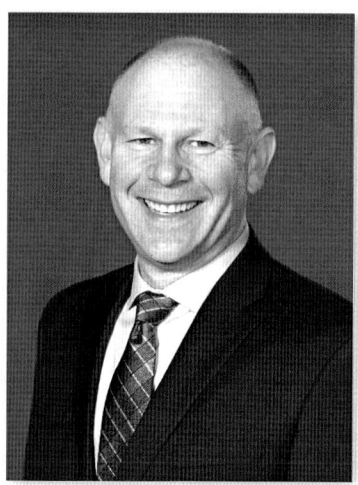

Figure 13: Gary Katz, MD, who, joined the faculty in emergency medicine in 2003, was one of the founders of the administration fellowship at Ohio State.

Katz also promoted emergency medicine as a key point of entry into health system strategy and competed in the Deloitte & Touche business plan competition in 2007, finishing in the top six of all business plan submissions. His proposal, innovative at the time, was to develop the Free-Standing Emergency Department as lower cost, higher service entry point to help patients access the health care system. In the end, the administration, led by Vice President Fred Sanfilippo, MD, PhD, deferred a decision to create such a unit. The thinking offered at the time was that Ohio State was a great academic institution that should concentrate on developing cutting edge treatments for the most serious medical conditions. These capabilities would draw the patients to the medical center regardless of location or convenience.

At the time, however, the medical leadership used the foundation of this plan to develop minute-clinics in cooperation with the Department of Family Medicine and local retail stores. In later years the decision to not create free-standing centers was belatedly recognized and many years later the medical center modified the plan and developed what was called *Advanced Immediate Care*, which was thought to signify a step up in capability from the typical urgent care center but was short of the capabilities of a free-standing emergency department even though the medical staff were emergency physicians.

After leaving full-time work with Ohio State University, Katz continued a close connection with the Department of Emergency Medicine. He facilitated development of a Rural Emergency Medicine elective for residents to learn the important and unique practice aspects of emergency medicine in rural communities. He also maintained considerable national exposure, having served terms as Speaker and Council Officer for the American College of Emergency Physicians (ACEP). During this tenure he represented the council voice of all emergency physicians to the ACEP board. In 2018 he was recognized by his peers with Ohio ACEP's Bill Hall award. Katz also served the greater medical community as a member of the Ohio State Medical Association delegation to the American Medical Association. He is a Lieutenant Colonel in the Ohio Air National Guard and deployed as the State Medical Planner for Ohio and its Adjutant General during the National Guard COVID responses for Operation Steady Resolve.

ERIC ADKINS, MD, MS

Eric J. Adkins, MD, MS, joined the faculty in 2010. He received his undergraduate and MD degrees from West Virginia University in 2001 and completed a five-year residency program at Christiana Care Health System in 2007. He served as Chief Resident in his final year of training. During his years at Christiana, Adkins completed a five-year residency program in both internal medicine and emergency medicine and became board certified in both specialties. He came to Ohio State in 2007 and completed a three-year fellowship in pulmonary and critical care medicine in 2010 and became certified in four medical specialties including emergency medicine, internal medicine and critical care medicine. He also completed a master's degree in medical sciences at Ohio State in 2010. Adkins' extraordinary ability and broad education led to his early appointments to key leadership positions in the department.

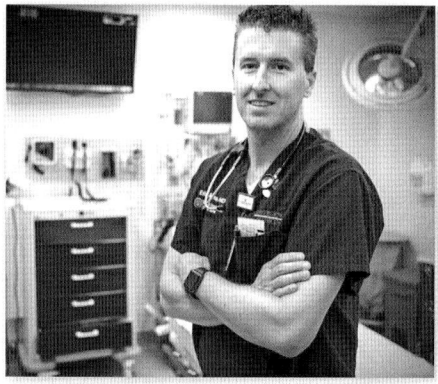

Figure 14: Eric Adkins, MD, residency and fellowship trained in emergency medicine, internal medicine, Critical Care medicine and pulmonary medicine. He is Professor of Emergency Medicine and Critical care Medicine and Vice Chair of Clinical Operations in the Department of Emergency Medicine. He is also the Associate Chief Clinical Information Officer for the medical center.

Adkins was a co-creator of the emergency medicine and internal medicine residency program. He has focused his academic efforts on information technology (IT), patient safety, quality improvement, critical care and ultrasound in the emergency department. He has a joint appointment with the Department of Internal Medicine, Division of Pulmonary & Critical Care Medicine where he practices a portion of his time in the medical intensive care unit. *Columbus Monthly Magazine* has recognized him as a Best Doctor in Emergency Medicine every year since 2013. In 2014 he was presented the "40 Under 40" award by *Columbus Business First*. In 2020, he was recognized by Ohio American College of Emergency Physicians with the Emergency Physician Leadership award.

He is currently is a Professor of Emergency Medicine and Critical Care. He is an Associate Chief Clinical Information Officer for the medical center and the Vice Chair of Clinical Operations in the Department of Emergency Medicine.

In his leadership position he oversees the two Ohio State Emergency Departments and four Ohio State Advanced Immediate Care sites. The EDs account for over 130,000 patient visits each year. Ohio State main campus also features one of the few fully integrated oncology emergency departments. Adkins was also integral in the creation and growth of the Advanced Immediate Care sites. He is the chair of the Integrated Health Information Systems (IHIS) Decision Support and Predictive Analytics Committees for the health system. Adkins is very active in Ohio State's use of Epic and the health system's IT strategy and deployment of new technology.

DANIEL J. "DAN" BACHMANN, MD

Daniel J. "Dan" Bachmann, MD, joined the faculty in 2010. He received his bachelor of arts degree (1997) and his doctor of medicine (2002) degrees from the Case Western Reserve University. He completed a transitional internship at the Naval Medical Center in Portsmouth, Virginia from 2002 to 2003. From 2003 to 2007 he was an officer in the United States Navy; his active-duty time was spent primarily as an Underwater Diving Medical Officer and he received many commendations for his service in the Navy. Bachmann joined the residency program in emergency medicine at Ohio State in 2007 and completed the program as Chief Resident in 2010. As a faculty member, Bachmann was quicky recognized for his expertise in emergency and disaster preparedness by the medical center. In 2014 he was asked to chair the Disaster Preparedness Committee.

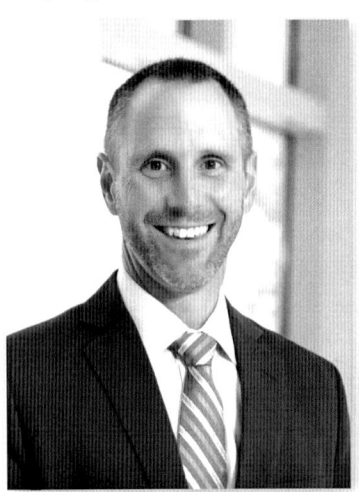

Figure 15: Daniel J. "Dan" Bachmann, MD, a former naval officer, became an expert in disaster relief and medical director of one of the four hospitals comprising the Ohio State Medical Center.

In 2015 he became the medical director of the hyperbaric program, a premier program that offers these comprehensive services: ambulatory and inpatient hyperbaric therapy; on-call hyperbaric physician and nursing team to manage emergent/urgent dives; routine and emergent consultations; capability for treatment of critical care patients; and ability to manage adult and pediatric populations. The program is a major destination for patient referrals throughout the state of Ohio and all adjacent states. During his residency and continuing, he was also the Captain of the Emergency Medicine Team in the *Pelotonia* cycling event benefitting the Arthur G. James Cancer Hospital and Richard J. Solove Research Institute. This is one of the oldest departmental teams in the event.

In 2016 he became the Medical Director for Disaster Preparedness at the medical center. He was recognized in 2019 as the "Ohio Emergency Physician of the Year" by the Ohio Chapter of the American College of Emergency Physicians. Highly regarded as a teacher, Bachmann directs a senior medical student elective the Advanced Competency in Emergency Preparedness & Disaster Response course.

An expert in disaster response, Bachmann has collaborated regionally with several working groups as part of the Central Ohio Trauma System and the Central Ohio Healthcare Coalition. Nationally, he serves as a Medical Team Manager for Ohio Task Force 1, which is a FEMA Urban Search & Rescue Team based in Dayton, Ohio. He has had many deployments to assist in disaster response throughout the country and serves as a member of one of Ohio's Disaster Coalition Advisory Boards.

Bachmann is widely known for his expertise in emergency and disaster medicine and has built an outstanding reputation for academic accomplishments in publishing, speaking and research in these topics. In 2021 he became the Medical Director of Ohio State East Hospital, one of the four major hospital centers that comprise the medical center.

Departmental Anniversary Celebration in 2003

In 2003 the department held a celebration of its 25th anniversary. Although faculty started covering the department as a *hospital* division in 1977, the beginning of the Division of Emergency Medicine *in the College of Medicine* began in July of 1978. The 25th festivity included a banquet and remarks from the founders, including Martin Keller, MD, PhD, who was the highly supportive Chair of the Department of Preventive Medicine when emergency medicine was in its infancy. All residents, former residents and former faculty were invited and the mood was jubilant (Figure 16).

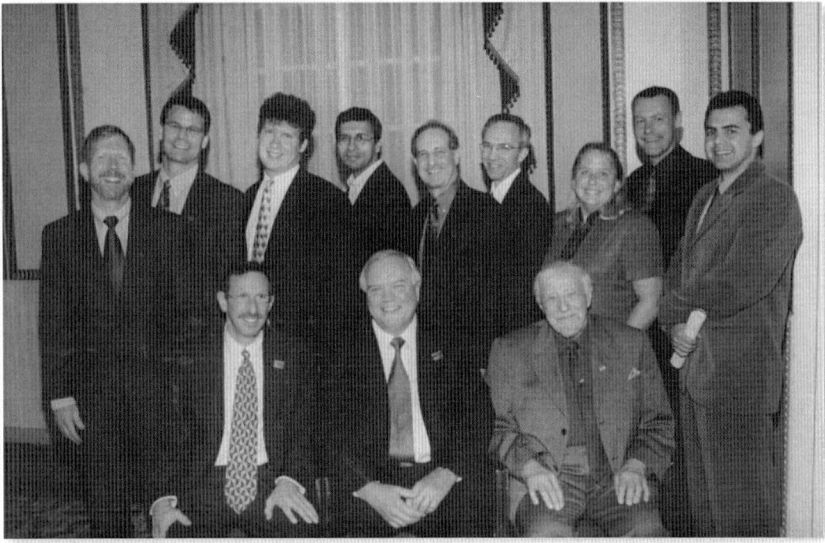

Figure 16: Faculty photo taken at the 25th anniversary celebration at the Athletic Club of Columbus in 2003. Back row from left to right: Michael Dick, MD; Daniel Martin, MD; David Bahner, MD; Sorabh Khandelwal, MD; Richard Nelson, MD; Mark Angelos, MD; Diane Gorgas, MD; Craig Key, MD; and Carlos Torres, MD, PhD. Front row from left: Howard Werman MD; Douglas Rund, MD; and Martin Keller, MD, PhD.

Transition

In 2011 Rund transitioned from Departmental Chair to Professor. One year later, in 2012, he retired from the regular faculty to become Professor Emeritus of Emergency Medicine. By that time, he had served 35 years as the Chief of Emergency Medicine at Ohio State, first as the founder and director of the division of emergency medicine and then as Chair when the department was formed in 1990. At the time of his retirement, he segued into emergency medical services continuing as Medical Director of the Emergency Medical Services program at the Columbus State Community College (CSCC) and Medical Director of the Division of Fire and EMS for the City of Worthington.

During his tenure on the faculty, he had Chaired two other departments on an interim basis: Preventive Medicine and Family Medicine. He chaired the Department of Preventive Medicine from 1988 until 1990, and the Department of Family Medicine from 1994 to 1995 and again from 1997 to 1998. He also served as Associate Dean for the College of Medicine from 2000 to 2011. He served as President of the Ohio State University Physician practice group from its early founding in 1998 to his retirement from the departmental chair in 2011. He had also served as the President of the American Board of Emergency Medicine. Upon his retirement, the College of Medicine commissioned a portrait in recognition of his service in founding emergency medicine at Ohio State (Figure 17).

Upon Rund's retirement, the Dean of the College appointed Mark G. Angelos, MD, as Interim Chair and began the search for a new permanent chair.

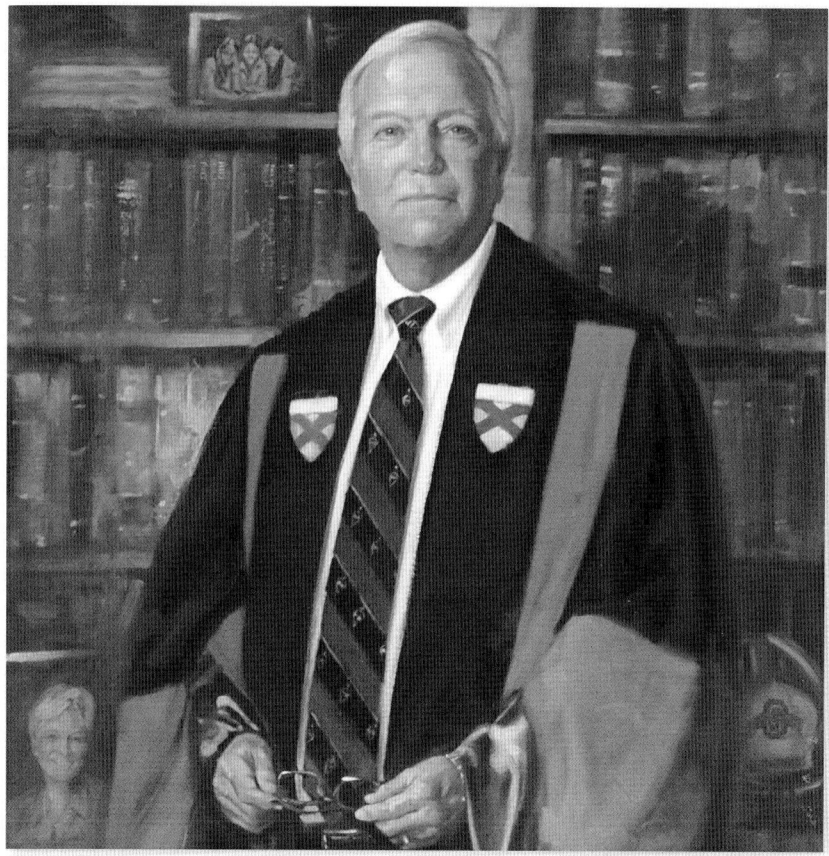

Figure 17: Douglas A. Rund, MD, Founder and Chair Emeritus of the Department of Emergency Medicine at Ohio State, by artist Jamie Lee McMahan. When Rund retired, the College of Medicine, led by Steven Gabbe, MD, Vice President, commissioned a portrait in gratitude for his service.

References

1. Hiestand BC. Personal communication with Douglas Rund. 2022: Columbus, Ohio.

2. Torres CA. Personal communication with Douglas Rund. 2022: Columbus, Ohio.

3. Zelinski DP. Interview with Dan Zelinski by Douglas Rund. 2022: Columbus, Ohio.

4. Bernard AW. Interview with Aaron W. Bernard by Douglas Rund. 2022: Columbus, Ohio.

5. Moseley MG. Interview with Mark G. Moseley by Douglas Rund. 2022: Columbus, Ohio.

Chapter 11
The Terndrup Chair Years: 2013-2015

Douglas A. Rund, MD

THOMAS E. TERNDRUP, MD

Thomas E. Terndrup, MD, was appointed Chair of the Department of Emergency Medicine at Ohio State in July of 2013. Terndrup followed the provisional term of Mark Angelos, MD, who had been appointed Interim Chair in 2011 following the retirement of the original Chair Douglas Rund, MD. Terndrup was the second permanent chair in the department's history (Figure 1).

Terndrup received his undergraduate degree from Juniata College in 1977 and his MD degree from Penn State University in 1981. He completed his residency in emergency medicine at the Atlantic Health System/Morristown Medical Center in New Jersey from 1981 to 1984.

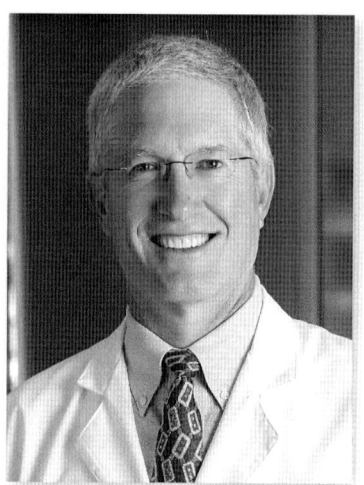

Prior to his appointment at Ohio State, he served as the Chair of Emergency Medicine at the University of Alabama in Birmingham from 1999 to 2006 and the Chair of Emergency Medicine at Penn State University from 2006 to June of 2013. The hospital facility affiliated with Penn State was the Hershey Medical Center in Hershey, Pennsylvania. In 2013 Terndrup accepted the position at Ohio State, and served as Chair until September of 2015. At that time, Mark G. Angelos, MD,

Figure 1: Thomas E. Terndrup, MD, was Chair of the Department of Emergency Medicine at Ohio State from 2013 to 2015.

was appointed permanent Chair of the Department of Emergency Medicine.

The New Emergency Department: 2015

One of Terndrup's early efforts was the planning for the new emergency department. At the time, the objective was to provide over 100 treatment beds, which had been a goal for many years. The hope was that an enlarged facility would help solve the issue of continued overcrowding due in large part to patient "boarding" in the department. Such patients were admitted to the hospital but awaited available beds in the main hospital. In his annual report for 2014, Terndrup reported over 135,000 patient visits at the Ohio State Main and East hospitals, After Hours Clinics and the Clinical Decision Unit.[1]

In his previous experience at Hershey Medical Center, Terndrup developed a facility that minimized prolonged use of the reception area or waiting room by adding additional treatment areas. The staff there also focused on creating treatment efficiencies that allowed patients to be expedited to emergency care rather than have a prolonged wait.

Terndrup carried these concepts to the new Emergency Department at Ohio State with a relatively small waiting area. His vision was to format "our arrival area to be more efficient and reduce our left-without-being-fully-treated population."[1]

The small waiting room was a matter of concern years later when waves of patients with COVID-19 overwhelmed hospitals during the early phases of the pandemic in 2020. The new 2015 emergency department, however, added considerable space to treat patients and included specially designated areas, such as the oncology treatment space. Coincident with the expansion, however, was a shortage of emergency faculty physicians to staff the new and enlarged premises.

In response, a large number of faculty members were recruited. In his 2014 Annual Report, Terndrup listed the following numbers of department employees: 60 faculty, 5 fellows, 48 categorical EM residents and 10 IM-EM residents. Many of the recruited physicians did not stay for the long term. Three who did remain, however, had exceptional careers at Ohio State: Andrew M. King, MD, MEd., Luca R. Delatore, MD, and Ashish R. Panchal, MD, PhD.

ANDREW M. KING, MD, MEd.

Andrew M. King, MD, joined the faculty in July 2013. He was recruited by Angelos but began at the onset of the Terndrup era. King devoted much of his effort toward the education of residents, students and fellows, and started the education fellowship in the department. King was born and raised in Shelby, Ohio, and completed high school there, where he achieved academic and athletic excellence (Figure 2). Years later, he recalled his early mentorship and his first commitment to a career in medicine:

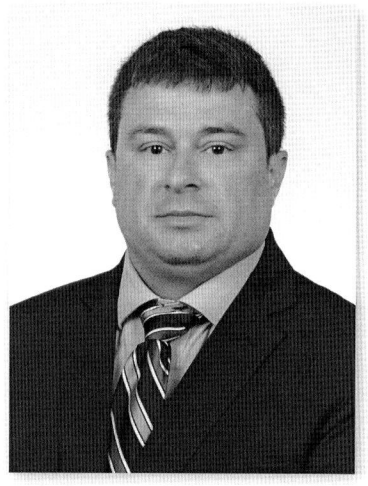

Figure 2: Andrew M. King, MD, MEd, was devoted to education and began the education fellowship in the Department of Emergency Medicine at Ohio State.

> *Without the tireless support of my parents, Clifford and Darlene King, I would not be where I am today. I am the third college graduate in my extended family, and the first to receive an advanced degree and pursue a career in medicine. I committed to a career in medicine at the age of five after witnessing my grandfather's resuscitation and death from MI and associated cardiac arrest; I wanted to prevent other children from experiencing what I experienced.*[2]

King was accepted into an accelerated BS/MD program from high school and went on to complete his undergraduate degree at Youngstown State in three years. He graduated Summa Cum Laude (4.0 GPA) with a degree in combined science in 2005. He was inducted into the Phi Kappa Phi Honor Society and the Clarence Gould Honor Society at Youngstown State. He then matriculated to Northeast Ohio Medical University, where he graduated in 2009 as a member of both Alpha Omega Alpha and the Gold Humanism Honor Society. He served on the student council as a representative for his class for four years and served as secretary, vice president and president. When he began medical school, he expected to pursue orthopedic surgery; however, after a pediatric emergency medicine rotation, he realized that the emergency department was where he belonged.

When King chose Ohio State for his emergency medicine residency, Diane Gorgas, MD, was the program director. Looking back, he was attracted to the program for several reasons:

> *I wanted to stay in Ohio, the program offered a great breadth of training experience, and the opportunity to learn from good people. I really enjoyed my interview day, specifically the program coordinators and program leadership. I also really liked the residents I was able to interact with on the interview day.*[2]

Upon completing residency King accepted a position at Wake Forest University, where he felt could explore all career options. Years later King recalled his thoughts at the time:

> *I was unsure if I wanted to pursue academics or community medicine. I did not have a good understanding of what a career in academics entailed. I thought I would have to perform a lot of research, which did not interest me (although it ultimately was an important part of my contributions). I had mentors that worked in the area, and had the opportunity to work a predominantly community job with a couple of shifts in the academic center. It was in this job that I discovered I had a passion for medical education.*[2]

Recognizing his passion for education and his family ties in Ohio, King accepted a faculty position at Ohio State. In his words he decided to return to Ohio State:

> *to continue my career and give back to the program that helped shape me into the physician that I am today. The medical education component reinvigorated me, and I wanted to have the opportunity to work with learners and to help shape them into excellent emergency physicians and future leaders. Early in my career, I was passionate about establishing a legacy throughout my career, and academics provided an avenue to accomplish all of those goals.*[2]

When King returned to Ohio State, under Terndrup, he found new challenges:

> *It was a time of great transition. Dr. Angelos, who hired me as interim chair, was replaced by Dr. Terndrup. The culture was different. It was a time of accountability and change. The overall culture was challenging for many members of the department. The clinical demands required growth of the faculty as well during this time of transition.*[2]

The emergency department footprint was expanding during Terndrup's leadership but the department was shorthanded. King began working many clinical shifts to make up the shortfall. Despite his heavy clinical load, he was inspired by the thoughts of innovation in education and attended every resident conference he could. During this time, he came under the influence of Sorabh Khandelwal, MD, who became program director in 2015. He appointed King assistant program director. Years later King remembered Khandelwal's mentorship:

> *Everything I have accomplished as an educator I owe to Dr. Sorabh Khandelwal. He took a chance on me as a young, passionate, inexperienced educator, and I spent the subsequent years trying to earn the gift he afforded me. He has been a tremendous mentor.*[2]

King dedicated himself to the challenge of improving education. He developed the education fellowship in 2017 from the ground up. He obtained approval from the university and obtained the endorsement of the Society for Academic Emergency Medicine (SAEM). Fellows in the program included the following physicians: Christopher San Miguel, MD; Krystin Miller, MD; Allison Beaulieu, MD; Kimberly Bambach, MD; and Andrew Kendle, MD. Later King recalled the challenge:

> *I had to advocate that this program should be specific to emergency medicine and not shared with other disciplines. I developed the curriculum, provided all of the education and professional development, and obtained approval from the OSU GME office. I established this program as a national respected program and recruited fellows from across the country. I was also instrumental in the development of a "flipped classroom" based curriculum. The flipped classroom is a pedagogical approach designed to promote higher order learning, and is based on social learning and constructivist learning theories. Learners are expected to learn*

the material independently (traditionally the class lesson) and perform application of material in the classroom (traditionally the homework). We made the decision to transition to this learning approach based on adult learning theory – this is how adults learn and it is proven within the literature.

I also performed a complete overall of our didactic curriculum and produced a curriculum that served as a model for other programs across the country. I became recognized as an expert in curriculum development and represented OSU through scholarship and national presentations. I was instrumental in the development of a resident coaching program, and developed and instituted our longitudinal track program. The longitudinal tracks are designed to help provide professional development to residents interested in the various niche specialties within emergency medicine. The purpose is to help residents develop their curriculum vitae (CV) and learn more about an area of emergency medicine, hopefully spring boarding them to a fellowship.[2]

King was diligent in his scholarly pursuits as well. He published over 40 peer-reviewed papers regarding the accomplishments in education:

As we revamped our entire curriculum, I made sure that each module was written up and published. This helped ensure the promotion of several faculty members due to the number of associated publications.[2]

King received many education research grants and helped create a medical education research collaborative. One publication was featured on the Emergency Medicine Abstracts broadcast and received multiple awards. He currently serves as the chair of the SAEM Education Committee, and has made many national presentations.

King was an outstanding faculty member. During his career he received the following awards: OSU Emergency Medicine Teacher of the Year; Ohio American College of Emergency Physicians Educator of the Year; the Council of Residency Directors (CORD) in Emergency Medicine Faculty Teaching Award; and the CORD Academy for Scholarship Award. He also completed the Master's Degree program in Biomedical Education.

In 2022 King left the faculty to join the OhioHealth Physician Group. In his explanation he mentioned that "over time, my priorities have changed, and the only legacy I want is with my family."

LUCA R. DELATORE, MD

Luca Delatore, MD, joined the faculty in 2014 during the Terndrup administration (Figure 3). Delatore grew up in Steubenville, Ohio, and completed his undergraduate studies at the University of Kentucky. In 2001 he completed medical school at the Medical College of Ohio in Toledo. In medical school he developed his interest in emergency medicine when he was on his trauma surgery month and found that he enjoyed his time with the emergency physicians and several emergency medicine (EM) residents were also working on the trauma service. He then did a student EM rotation at the Mayo Clinic in Minnesota and enjoyed the program. He matched at Mayo for his residency. Following his EM residency, he returned to Toledo and worked in the Flower Hospital where he began to take on administrative responsibilities for the urgent care center. He left Flower Hospital to become a traveling physician or "firefighter" for Emergency Medicine Physicians (EMP), which was ultimately to become US Acute Care Solutions. Years later, looking back on the experience, he reflected:

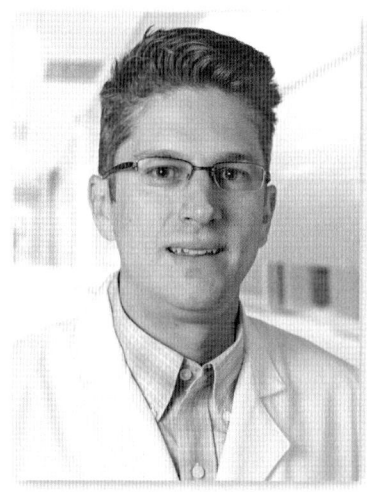

Figure 3: Luca R. Delatore, MD, who pioneered the development of the James Cancer Hospital component of the emergency department and ultimately became Medical Director of the Advanced Immediate Care centers in central Ohio

> *I was a firefighter...I traveled mostly through Ohio. I went to Connecticut, North Carolina and Indiana. If we won a contract bid with a hospital there were about 8-12 of us that would go take over the contract and set it up as we wanted (or as EMP wanted).*[3]

Next, he returned to Flower Hospital where he became the Medical Director of the emergency department for two years. He then transitioned to a strictly clinical role in Hilton Head, South Carolina for six years. Eventually he realized that he wanted to return to Ohio:

> *I looked at jobs [that were] a little bit different and OSU was appealing. Tom [Terndrup] had applications out for faculty but was also interested*

> in me because of my administrative background, and the [new James Cancer Hospital] was getting ready to open. We were getting ready to start the James ED project and Tom brought me in as someone who could be a lead on that project. The whole ED wasn't opened when I started here.[3]

Delatore was appointed Medical Director of a new section of the emergency department dealing exclusively with patients who had cancer or hematologic diseases such as sickle cell. The unit was a cooperative effort between emergency medicine and the James Cancer Hospital ("the James"). The James also provided financial resources which "could be more of a struggle"[3] from the University Hospital. The unit was unique at the time. As Delatore later noted:

> Prior to us opening the James ED, the only other oncology emergency department that had a designated area for cancer patients with designated nursing, protocols for neutropenic fever and all those things was actually in South Korea. People referenced MD Anderson as an emergency department for cancer patients but it was a little bit different. [It has an entire] emergency department for cancer patients only and honestly, it's not staffed by emergency physicians, it is staffed by internists who come down and see patients. So, it is more of a triage unit than it is a true emergency department.[3]

The department chair, Terndrup, also wanted to conduct research in the new unit and publicize its success. Delatore recalled this years later:

> [Dr. Terndrup] knew that opening a new department was going to take a little more focus especially if we wanted to write some of the things we were doing. Running our department, in and of itself, was a lot, so by bringing in someone with a special focus, we were pretty successful in writing up a lot of things about the James ED and presenting it both regionally and nationally. I presented at ACEP. We traveled to Hopkins, we traveled to Mayo, we traveled to MD Anderson. We did a lot of presentations at a lot of sites about what we were doing and why it was successful. So, Tom had the vision to recognize that getting someone with that [exclusive focus] and time allotment was really important.[3]

The cancer specific "James Hospital" emergency department was a great success with patients. Patient satisfaction measures and clinical quality measures were excellent. Specific areas of top performance included providing cutting edge and cancer specific treatments for patients with neutropenic fever and sepsis. Antibiotics and other medications were given at the earliest possible moment. Such efforts vastly improved outcomes. Effective pain management guidelines and care pathways were also greatly appreciated.

> *The benefit of having a cancer specific ED was huge for our patient satisfaction but also for quality. All projects that we took on we presented nationally—the numbers were pretty impressive when we were at our peak.*[3]

The leadership of the department transitioned from Terndrup to Angelos in 2015. Under Angelos some clinical leaders moved on to executive leadership positions in other institutions and others were promoted at Ohio State. During the transitions, Delatore become Medical Director of the entire Main campus Emergency Department, including the James ED. Two years later he again stepped away from his leadership roles to concentrate on being a clinician. In 2020 Angelos retired from the faculty and Jeffrey Caterino, MD, became department chair. At that time the department was developing the concept of Advanced Immediate Care (AIC). Delatore was recruited to become the Medical Director of all the AIC centers connected with Ohio State. The concept was that the centers would provide medical services on demand. Delatore described the range of services:

> *We have a lot of the capabilities of the emergency department. There are no inpatient beds associated with us. We can do most of the testing and medication that you would do at the Main campus. We have IV meds, ultrasound—all the things that you would need in a small ED. I would say our capabilities would match a lot of rural emergency departments, but we are not open 24 hours a day. In that regard it changes kind of what we do. The level of care that we provide is pretty darn high and matches a lot of small communities throughout Ohio.*[3]

The AICs provide needed care to the community and reduce the crowding at the main hospital. The demand for services within the whole system, however, remained high and the need for buy-in by the physicians into the overall goals of the department and the university were described by Delatore:

> *The biggest thing is continuing to get the right culture at Ohio State. It has always been a big thing. I think culture in emergency medicine is*

really, really important and having the right people working with the right mentality is really important as a teaching environment for the residents. If I go in there and I am unhappy during my shift and I am miserable during my shift, the residents learn that is the way they are supposed to be during their shift. That is the wrong method. I think to people I have worked with in the past and still work with—people like Howie Werman who love what they do and continue to work. There are certain people that enjoy what they are doing. I think that is the biggest thing is to try to continue that for the next generation of people who will pass that on knowing that not every job and every shift has to be dismal, and we are lucky to be doing what we are doing. Sam Kiehl is another great example of someone who loved what he did and I hope that I pass that along.[3]

Delatore also noted the major issues facing the emergency department, including crowding, which became worse with the COVID pandemic:

The current state of the department and the hospital is not great. We have lots of boarding and we have lots of issues. Even with the brand-new hospital it is going to be difficult to absorb the growth of Columbus especially when the small communities are becoming less and less capable of caring for simple things. For example, [a community hospital] may send a patient to Columbus [for surgical treatment of appendicitis]. We need to be flexible with the way we grow and be able to adapt. The AICs are important on that because it increases our bandwidth. Yesterday in New Albany, we saw 81 patients over 12 hours. That is close to the record that we've seen there. The good news of that is of those 81 patients I think we only sent three people to the emergency department. If we can decompress the system like that, it is huge. Even if only half of those people would have gone to our emergency department it would have overwhelmed the system. Keeping people out, being flexible, creating new ways of care and access for patients is really important.[3]

ASHISH R. "ASH" PANCHAL, MD, PHD

Ashish R. Panchal, MD, PhD, joined the faculty in 2013. He received his undergraduate degree from Michigan State University in 1996 and received his PhD degree in physiology and biophysics from Case

Western Reserve University in 2001. He completed medical school at Ohio State in 2005 and his residency in emergency medicine in 2008. Following his residency program, he joined the faculty at University of Arizona where he excelled in his academic career with teaching awards and advancing his interests in cardiopulmonary resuscitation (Figure 4).

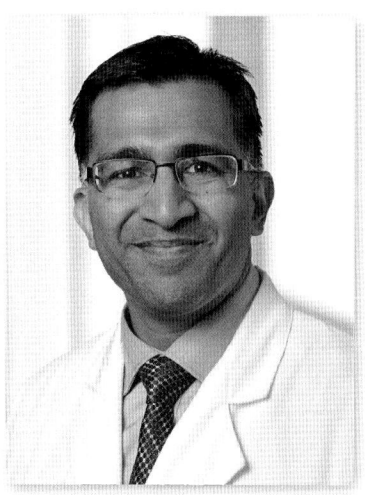

Figure 4: Ashish R. "Ash" Panchal, MD, PhD, Professor, Department of Emergency Medicine, created international reputation for his work in emergency cardiac care and emergency medical services. A highly-funded investigator, Panchal served in influential positions in the American Heart Association, the National Registry of Emergency Medical Technicians and Delaware County EMS.

Panchal was active in the American Heart Association (AHA) in 2013 when he became a member of the Emergency Cardiovascular Care Scientific Subcommittee. At the national meetings, Mark Angelos, MD, and Panchal met often. As Interim Chair of the Department of Emergency Medicine, Angelos frequently tried to recruit Panchal to join the faculty at Ohio State. Panchal recalled years later: "He finally wore me down...I signed and I came in when Dr. Terndrup was put in the chair position."[3] Panchal's family was in Ohio and he was also influenced by Michael Sayre, MD, an Ohio State faculty member who was active in the AHA. Recruited by Angelos and starting under Terndrup, Panchal recalled the early days:

It was a bit of a different situation because being a new chair, people were [not] exactly [sure] what their roles [were] and I was no different because coming in doing a lot of prehospital work and things like that and not having a huge bandwidth in that space, it was a lot of open space for me to find my way around. There was a lot of support to start moving in the direction of enhancing prehospital care. So, it was a very supportive environment to get me started.[4]

Early on Panchal became involved with a study of paramedic airway management that Terndrup had started in Pennsylvania. Panchal's efforts to develop a comprehensive airway management simulation to improve provider skills in using this low-frequency, high-risk procedure ultimately led to the development of a mobile simulation lab. The lab used an airway manikin that required intubation. The paramedics were provided with all equipment needed to intubate or, if unsuccessful, to place an alternate airway. A proctor acted as an assistant and all the paramedic's actions were video recorded. Working with faculty member David Way, Panchal began work on the project. As Panchal recalled years later:

> *We started putting together an analysis pattern using advanced psychometrics to really start thinking about how we can identify competency in EMS professionals to the point that we looked at 131 different items or behaviors in airway techniques. Everything from bag, valve, mask—all the way through to endotracheal intubation. We evaluated all . . . different behaviors to see which ones lead to consistently good outcomes in airway performance in providers. It was a pretty large-scale study when it came to really looking at the nuances of competency-based performance.*[4]

Panchal helped conduct and analyze results obtained not only in Columbus, but also in Terndrup's earlier Pennsylvania studies.[5] In 2022, Panchal authored the Prehospital Airway Management Training and Education: An NAEMSP Position Statement and Resource Document.[6]

In 2016 Panchal became the Research and Fellowship Director at the National Registry of Emergency Medical Technicians (NREMT), located in Columbus a few miles from the Ohio State campus. This was an outstanding opportunity for an academic scholar. Not only did he have access to a vast amount of data, he had the willing assistance of fellows to help him conduct the research.

Years later Panchal recalled the opportunity this provided:

> *The part that was really daunting with this was that my fellows were PhD students in epidemiology. I do have a pretty strong background in epidemiology and was granted a joint appointment in epidemiology, which helped facilitate the relationship that we needed to help the fellows achieve their goals. So now suddenly [this was] part of my job. I was the research director for the registry as well as taking care of these new PhD fellows who I was now training. The fellows were amazing. They*

were street-level paramedics and EMTs who chose to get a master's and then follow up that with a PhD in epidemiology and use their knowledge of prehospital care within their research. That pairing became a very powerful piece. We very quickly were able to publish many papers describing the workforce, the challenges, the occupational risks, and started thinking about how we can improve competency in EMS. So, we evaluated program performance and things like that, all as part of the larger National Registry framework in its EMS mission. That became a big source of my career. Even to this day, I do a lot of research looking at the challenges that are faced by an EMS professional, and at the same time I am still doing my resuscitation work. Then COVID hit and that changed everything for us.[4]*

Panchal began working in areas related to COVID and the workforce in emergency services. He told the story this way:

Some of the early reports from New York were unbelievable about the rate of infection as well as the severity of illness for EMS professionals because they were in the front line. When we started hearing about this one of the things [we noticed was a lot of work being done] trying to understand at risk populations and understand the changes in the serology and virology of people who are exposed to Covid-19. We knew that the vaccine was on the horizon but there was another aspect to this: We needed to know what happens and how does serology change when people are vaccinated, or if they are infected and they are not vaccinated, what is really happening. During this time period we had maybe six weeks to two months to get a grant together for this. It was a large U54 Specialized Center level grant to describe what kind of work we can do to help evaluate with COVID-19 epidemic. It was a grant funded through the National Cancer Institute supported by the National Institute of Allergy and Infectious Diseases (NIAID). Within the six-week period we put together a research group via Zoom, a group from across three or four different Ohio State colleges with something like twenty investigators with four Principal Investigators (PIs). I was one of the PIs and we won the grant—a $10 million U54 grant. We are now two years into the grant, and were refunded for three more years. So, with the full five years, our whole focus is a longitudinal evaluation of prehospital and hospital-based providers and the changes in their serologies when exposed to COVID-19. Part of this is building the longitudinal cohort *and following them over time, and second, doing the serologic and virologic work, including sequencing of the different variants. And last, but not least, it is also about trying to understand how people are feeling throughout the pandemic. One of the studies we are wrapping up right now is looking at the impact and burnout of first responders from before and after the pandemic. My research vision for the future and my bucket list study is to put together the Framingham Study for EMS professionals so we can define their cancer risk, their cardiovascular risk, their occupational risk and these kinds of things have not been done to the extent we follow a population out to really understand this.*[4]

In 2019 Panchal was appointed medical director for Delaware County Emergency Medical Services (EMS). Delaware County is one of the fastest growing counties in Ohio—and in the United States. This agency provides emergency medical services only; there is no fire suppression activity. Panchal quickly applied his previous knowledge in prehospital care to his new agency. Many would say that Panchal has transformed the entire department and added one of the strongest training programs in the country. In September 2022 the Delaware County EMS was awarded the National EMS System of the Year by the National Association of Emergency Medical Technicians and EMS World.

Finally, and just as important, Panchal assumed the leadership of the fellowship program in EMS from Howard Werman, MD. Panchal added considerable academic rigor to the fellowship curriculum and the program grew under his leadership. As Panchal discussed the transition, he recalled this:

The fellowship was always a really core part of the department than when I came in. Howie Werman is an amazing gentleman who really set the stage and really role modeled for a lot of us younger faculty about what a prehospital doc should really look like—for example, our involvement to prehospital care on the national level and what that would look like in the community, and what the impact could be for the community. With that in mind, I started getting more involved in the fellowship work to the point to where he wanted to transition me into the fellowship director role. At that time, we were regularly having a fellow every once in a while. It wasn't as consistent as we would have liked, and some of it was bandwidth issues and some of it was just the fellowship was young.[4]

Panchal accomplished much during his career at Ohio State, becoming: Professor of Emergency Medicine; Clinical Professor, Division of Epidemiology, College of Public Health; Research and Fellowship Director; National Registry of Emergency Medical Technicians Program Director; EMS Fellowship, Medical Director for Delaware County EMS; past Chair of the AHA Emergency Cardiovascular Care Science Subcommittee; and Chair of the 2018, 2019 and 2020 AHA/ECC Guidelines for Cardiopulmonary Resuscitation and Emergency Cardiovascular Care. These AHA guidelines provide the structure for training of over 16 million people per year.

Other Accomplishments in the Terndrup Era

In his 2014 annual report Terndrup noted the continued strength of medical student education. He also noted cost saving measures, such as using Skype for remote interviewing and a hoped-for reduction in overtime pay for faculty. During this time, Diane Gorgas, MD, transitioned from Residency Program Director to the Director of Global Health and Sorabh Khandelwal, MD, took her place. In his report Terndrup also noted that ED admissions generated 41% of University and James Cancer admissions in 2014, stressing the importance of an efficient ED to the overall success of both hospitals.

During Terndrup's term, extramural research funding expanded with an emphasis on funding from the National Institutes of Health (NIH). Grant funding from all sources reached $1,822,206 in 2014. The faculty authored 77 publications in 2013, with two appearing in high impact journals such as *The New England Journal of Medicine*. Rebekah Richards, MD, a 2014 resident graduate, was recruited to be the first clinical research fellow. Research areas within the department included the following:

- Clinical: Geriatrics, neurologic emergencies, acute lung disease, acute coronary syndrome ACS and infectious diseases

- Laboratory: Oxidative stress in cardiovascular disease, cardiac regeneration and use of stem cells

- Educational: Ultrasound training, paramedic airway education

The project addressing paramedic airway education involved extensive videotaping of simulated paramedic intubation exercises, interval education and training followed by reevaluation. Fire departments in central Ohio participated and rated the exercise highly.

Terndrup noted that Emergency Medicine was the third most popular specialty among Ohio State medical students. He listed the following fellowships offered by the department: Ultrasound, Administration, Pediatric Emergency Medicine, Emergency Medical Services, Medical Toxicology and Education.

Terndrup was a successful researcher and had obtained several important grants to support his studies. He remained with the department as a professor until his retirement from Ohio State in 2021.

References

1. Terndrup TE. Annual Report 2014, Ohio State Department of Emergency Medicine, Columbus, Ohio, 2014

2. King AM. Interview with Douglas Rund. 2022: Columbus, Ohio.

3. Delatore LR. Interview with Douglas Rund. 2022: Columbus, Ohio

4. Panchal AR. Interview with Douglas Rund. 2022: Columbus Ohio.

5. Panchal AR, Finnegan G, Way DP, Terndrup T. Assessment of paramedic performance on difficult airway simulation. *Prehosp Emerg Care*. 2020 May-Jun;24(3):411-420. doi: 10.3109/10903127.2015.1102993. Epub 2016 Nov 21. PMID: 27870588.

6. Dorsett M, Panchal AR, Stephens C, Farcas A, Leggio W, Galton C, Tripp R, Grawey T. Prehospital airway management training and education: An NAEMSP position statement and resource document. *Prehosp Emerg Care*. 2022;26(sup1):3-13. doi: 10.1080/10903127.2021.1977877. PMID: 35001822.

Chapter 12

The Angelos Chair Years: 2011-2013, 2015-2020

Mark G. Angelos, MD

Mark G. Angelos, MD, was named Interim Chair of the Department of Emergency Medicine from 2011 to 2013 and permanent Chair from 2015 to 2020. Angelos graduated from the University of Utah Medical School in 1983. He then completed a residency in emergency medicine at Wright State University followed by a critical care fellowship at the University of Pittsburgh. While at the University of Pittsburgh, he worked in the laboratory of Peter Safar, MD, where he was introduced to resuscitation medicine and research. This experience inspired an academic career, which included a laboratory-based research career focused on cardiac resuscitation. Angelos returned to Wright State University in 1987 as a new faculty member.

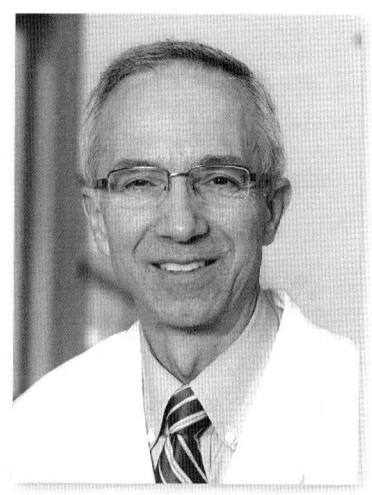

Figure 1: Mark G. Angelos, MD, was Interim Chair of the Department of Emergency Medicine from 2011 to 2013 and permanent Chair from 2015 to 2020.

In 1991 he was recruited to Ohio State as an Assistant Professor, and advanced rapidly on the tenure track. He was promoted to the rank of Associate Professor and awarded tenure in 1995. He was promoted to full Professor in 2000. He served in various roles within the department, including fellowship director, Vice Chair of Research, Vice Chair of Academic Affairs and Chair of the Department Promotion and Tenure Committee.

ANGELOS INTERIM CHAIR YEARS 2011-2013

When Douglas Rund, MD, the Inaugural Chair of the department transitioned to Emeritus status after 21 years in the position of Chair preceded by 13 years as Division Director, the Dean named Angelos as the Interim Chair (Figure 1). He served in this role for the next two years, from 2011 to 2013. This was a time of change and growth within the department. In these two years, Angelos recruited 14 full-time faculty, two part-time faculty and three fellows. During this period all but one faculty member was integrated in to the Faculty Group Practice Plan (OSU Physicians, Inc). Within the department new faculty tracks were developed in alignment with a new college Appointments, Promotion and Tenure (AP&T) document. This growth created a demand for additional administrative space that occasioned a move of the Department Offices from Cramblett Hall to the newly finished seventh floor of the Prior Health Sciences Library in February 2012.

In 2012 a new Department Administrator, Greg Archual, was recruited from University Hospitals of Cleveland (Figure 2). Archual received his Bachelor of Science in Industrial Management from the University of Akron in 1982 and received his MBA from Ashland University in 1987. He also received his Lean/Six Sigma Black Belt certification from Kent State University in 2006 and Academic Emergency Medicine Administration certification in 2018.

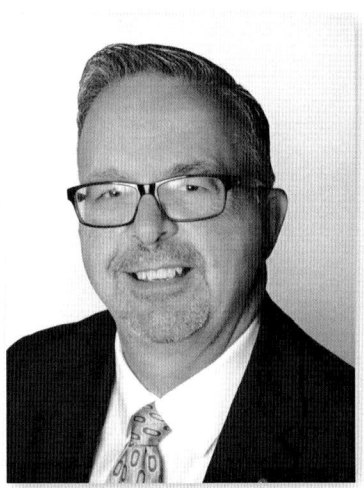

Figure 2: Gregory "Greg" Archual, MBA, became the Chief Operating Officer and Administrator of the Department of Emergency Medicine in 2012.

Archual's work history included both the manufacturing and health care sectors, working 11 years as an industrial/management engineer with a focus on process improvement and systems engineering. His work experience also included 13 years managing an emergency department of a level one trauma center and 14 years of academic emergency medicine practice management. He was hired to be Chief Operating Officer and Administrator of the

Department of Emergency Medicine at Ohio State, where he became responsible for the strategic, financial, and operational success of the department's four missions: clinical, education, research, and faculty development.

Archual became responsible for all operations of the department, which included two emergency departments, three immediate care clinic operations, hyperbaric medicine, a clinical decision unit, and a Physician Advisor Program. He was the Past President of the Academy of Administrators in Academic Emergency Medicine (AAAEM), served on the AAAEM Executive Committee for six years, and was Co-Chair of the AAAEM Benchmark Committee. He helped to facilitate a number of important administrative changes within the department to improve the efficiency and well-being of the faculty. Such changes included design and implementation of a faculty night shift policy and centralization of the clinical shift scheduling process.

Education Mission

During this period, the education mission underwent significant expansion. The residency, considered the jewel of the department, expanded from 12 to 14 residents per year, and the residency curriculum continued to evolve with the implementation of academic tracks for the residents. Growth of other education programs included the establishment of a second residency program: a five-year joint Emergency Medicine and Internal Medicine program. The first resident in this combined program began in 2013. New fellowship curricula were developed for fellowships in Administration, Education and Ultrasound and fellows were successfully recruited. Not all fellowships required accreditation by the Accreditation Council for Graduate Medical Education (ACGME). A fellowship in Emergency Medical Services was developed, which did require ACGME accreditation, however.

Emergency medicine was a popular career choice among Ohio State medical students thanks to excellent faculty role models and extensive faculty involvement in designing the medical school curriculum. Student clinical learning came during the mandatory emergency medicine student rotation. Such activity was responsible for facilitating the successful match of 18 Ohio State students into Emergency Medicine in 2012 and 27 students in 2013, making Emergency Medicine one of the top three specialty choices of all graduating Ohio State medical students.

Research Mission

The department research program also grew in the period from 2011 to 2013. Four new research associates were hired and a new young faculty member, Chun-An "Andy" Chen, PhD, who was successful in obtaining a Pathway to Independence (R00) grant from the National Institutes of Health (NIH), was recruited. This grant, which supported his research for three years, was the second NIH grant received by a faculty member in the department following a NIH K23 grant awarded to Jeff Caterino, MD, in 2010.

Shortly thereafter, the Department of Emergency Medicine partnered with the Department of Neurology and received five years of NIH funding (2012-2017) as the Ohio State site in the Neurologic Treatment Trials Network (NETT) with Michel Torbey (Neurology) as Principal Investigator (PI) and Angelos (Emergency Medicine) as Co-PI. A unique opportunity to showcase the emergency department's research efforts occurred when the department hosted the regional Society of Academic Emergency Medicine (SAEM) Research Conference at Ohio State. For this meeting, Steven Stack, MD, who was on track to become President of the American Medical Association (AMA) in 2015-2016, was the keynote speaker. Stack was an emergency medicine residency graduate from Ohio State.

Clinical Mission

The growth of the clinical mission in the department was a primary driver to expand the faculty. During this time, the medical center made a decision to change to a unified electronic medical record, the Integrated Healthcare Information System (IHIS). This transition, which was hospital wide, occurred on October 15, 2011. As with other institutions that had made this same transition to IHIS, coding difficulties occurred, leading to a dramatic increase in charge lag for the department, resulting in a significant decrease in first-year clinical revenue. However, with the medical center's assistance and due to its strong financial base, the department weathered this decline and made up the deficit the following year.

When the department business unit was a limited liability company (OSU Emergency Medicine, LLC) in the early 2000s, it was part of the medical center practice organization, OSU Physicians. At the time, all departments were urged to maintain a 90-day reserve in case of a financial downturn. Emergency medicine was a leader in meeting this goal.

Other challenges during these years involved the construction of a new James Cancer Hospital, which also included a new Emergency Department. While the Emergency Department never closed, the surrounding construction required the clinical operation and staffing to make innovative adjustments and revampments to accommodate the construction. For example, the 16-bed clinical decision unit (CDU) was relocated to the seventh floor to allow the existing CDU beds in the ED to be re-purposed for acute care. In another innovation, a clinical model was developed to provide after-hours urgent care at the Martha Morehouse Clinic building. The unit opened for business once the clinics closed for the day. This operation was staffed by department faculty from 5 to 11 p.m. weekdays and eight hours on weekend days. During this period, the number of patients seen at Ohio State and Ohio State East Emergency Departments increased to over 120,000 for the year. In order to address this, the department hired the first mid-level providers to work in both East and Main Hospital EDs and in the CDU. At this time, the department reorganized the 24-hour, 7-days-a-week Hyperbaric Service, which emergency medicine had staffed since it first opened in the 1980s. Another department effort was to get all faculty credentialed in bedside ultrasound use and to make this part of the core privileges in emergency medicine. This effort was championed by David Bahner, MD, a faculty member within the department.

ANGELOS CHAIR YEARS 2015-2020

In July of 2015, Dean E. Christopher "Chris" Ellison, MD, appointed

Mark Angelos, MD, as Department Chair with a Chair package aimed at providing resources for the department to support growth in key mission areas. As a new Chair, Angelos reformulated the department's Patterns of Operation to articulate a four-fold mission of the Department of Emergency Medicine at The Ohio State University College of Medicine:

1. *To provide innovative, efficient, safe and compassionate patient care to patients presenting to the Ohio State University Hospital Emergency Departments and After-Hours clinics.*

2. *To be a leader in the education of medical students, residents and fellows in emergency medical care.*

3. *To perform cutting edge research and scholarly investigation to identify the causes, treatments, and prevention of emergency medical conditions.*

4. *To promote faculty development and excellence.*

Over the next four and a half years, the department underwent significant growth and achievement in each of these four areas.

Education Mission

The education mission was led by Daniel M. Martin, MD, Vice-Chair of Education. Martin also served as Residency Director for the EM/IM residency program. Since the initial formation of the residency program in 1981 with four residents per year, the residency grew steadily in size. By 2015, the residency was matching 14 residents into the categorical Emergency Medicine residency and two residents into the EM/IM joint residency per year. Over the next four years, the department was able to secure approval and resources to match 21 residents per year, 19 in the categorical EM residency and two in the EM/IM residency. Two of these resident positions were funded through the department's collaborative arrangement with the Air Force.

To support this growth, additional Assistant and Associate Residency Directors roles were added to support the residency director, Sorabh

Khandelwal, MD. The residency curriculum was improved with the development of a robust wellness component, which included an annual wellness retreat for all residents, establishment of a resident wellness committee, wellness activities throughout the year, including distributing residents into six different wellness families, and monthly wellness dinners sponsored by faculty members. The experience and success of these programs were presented at the annual national Society for Academic Emergency Medicine (SAEM) meeting.

Much of this wellness curriculum was funded through the Samuel J. Kiehl III, MD, endowment established in 2016. Other curriculum changes included a greater involvement of simulation learning into the didactic curriculum. Jennifer Yee, DO, was recruited as an education faculty member and led the simulation component of the residency curriculum, having done a simulation learning fellowship and then served as a simulation medical director prior to coming to Ohio State. The residents received excellent training in bedside ultrasound (US) from the ultrasound faculty, so that they were some of the best US-trained residents in the medical center. Another addition to the curriculum was a state-of-the-art airway course developed and conducted by two faculty members, Colin Kaide, MD, and Ben Ostro, MD. All the residents completed this course.

During this period, there was a new emphasis placed on fellowship training and a number of fellowships were developed within the department. New fellowships included a new revised Emergency Medical Services (EMS) fellowship, requiring approval by the Accreditation Council for Graduate Medical Education (ACGME), an Administrative Fellowship, an Educational Fellowship and a new Oncology/Emergency Medicine Fellowship in conjunction with the James Cancer Hospital. Existing fellowships continued. These were the Ultrasound fellowship and the Research Fellowship. Administratively, a faculty fellowship director was identified for each fellowship and a funding strategy for the fellow and fellowship director was developed. Over these four years, the department was able to attract competitive fellows into each fellowship, although every fellowship was not filled every year. By far, the most popular fellowship was the ultrasound fellowship. A number of fellows were recruited to stay as faculty members in the department. This emphasis on fellowship training proved to influence many of the residents, as each year more graduating residents sought fellowship training within the department and at other institutions. In 2019, seven of the graduating residents went on to fellowship training.

In addition to graduate medical education (GME) and fellowship training, education faculty also developed an impactful presence in undergraduate medical education (UME). A number of department faculty were appointed to named positions within the new medical school curriculum. They worked closely with the large number of medical students interested in emergency medicine each year. They also acquired a reputation for their research and publishing efforts in the medical education literature. This group of emergency faculty consistently ranked first among all Ohio State College of Medicine departments in medical education scholarship. David Way, a medical educator who joined the Department in 2014, very effectively led this group and also helped start a faculty medical education research group within the department.

Research Mission

During the Angelos chair years, focus was placed on growing the department research program to national prominence by developing and supporting a group of laboratory-based researchers and a group of clinical-based researchers. The laboratory researchers were led by Mahmood Khan, PhD, and Mark Angelos, MD, and the clinical investigators were led by Jeffrey Caterino, MD, who also served as the Vice-Chair of Research. The laboratory-based research group was focused on the role of stem cells for treating damaged myocardium. The clinical investigators were focused on industry sponsored clinical trials, large network trials with other emergency medicine centers and Caterino's study of urinary proteins in the elderly presenting to the ED with urinary tract infection (UTI).

In 2016, both groups were successful in landing their first NIH Research Project (R01) grants. Both R01s were 5-year awards and provided significant new resources for each group. At that time, the department was one of the few academic Departments of Emergency Medicine in the nation to have NIH R01 funding for both clinical and basic laboratory research. In 2015, the Department had no NIH funding and did not appear on the Blue Ridge Institute national rankings of NIH funding in academic Emergency Departments. By 2017 the Department achieved a top 10 national ranking (#10) for NIH funding in Emergency Medicine. This same year, seven department faculty members were principal investigators (PIs) or site PIs on funded research programs. The Department's Blue Ridge ranking remained high with a ranking of #15 in 2018 and #14 in 2019.

A travel award program was instituted in the department to support the travel expenses of researchers, including trainees, who were presenting their research at national meetings. A faculty research track was developed in the department to provide some level of protected time for research. In 2019, two additional notable grants were obtained by Department faculty. Lauren Southerland, MD, was the recipient of an NIH Mentored Patient-Oriented Research Career Development Award (K23) grant to study methods for improving care for geriatric ED patients. The duration of the grant was five years. Emily Kauffman, DO, received a $950,000 grant from Franklin County and the Centers for Disease Control and Prevention (CDC) to improve care for opioid dependent patients.

Such successes facilitated the recruitment of additional research personnel, including laboratory technicians, post-doctoral students and graduate students for the laboratory and for the expansion of clinical research support personnel, including student enrollers, research coordinators and faculty researchers. In 2019, the department had its second clinical research fellow, Katie Buck, MD, who was successful in receiving a small grant program (R03) GEMSSTAR award from the NIH to study improving pneumonia diagnosis.

In building the department's research programs for the future, additional young researchers were recruited to the department, including Buck following her fellowship. In 2019, Jason Bishof, MD, was recruited as a clinical investigator from the University of North Carolina (UNC), where he had completed a research fellowship, and where he had received his MD degree in 2014. He completed his residency in emergency medicine at Ohio State and then a fellowship in research at UNC. At Ohio State Bishof was extremely productive in authoring and publishing clinical studies particularly in the area of cancer and emergency medicine. Venkata Srikanth Garikipati, PhD, a cardiovascular basic science researcher, was recruited from Temple University.

National Visiting Professor Series

A national Visiting Professor Series was established, which enabled the Department to bring in nationally renowned Professors of Emergency Medicine for grand rounds presentations and close interactions with faculty and residents each year. It was also an opportunity for the department to showcase itself, which served to enhance the department's reputation.

Douglas A. Rund Emergency Medicine Alumni Society

In 2018 the Douglas A. Rund Emergency Medicine Alumni Society was organized and achieved Scarlet Status, the highest status within the Ohio State Alumni Association in the first year. The Douglas A. Rund Emergency Medicine Alumni Society includes all past and current Ohio State EM residents, EM faculty, past and present and all graduating medical students who matched in EM, either at Ohio State or other EM residency. The department has well over 400 former graduates of the residency program. In conjunction with the Alumni Society, Department dinners are held each year during the Scientific Assembly of the American College of Emergency Physicians (ACEP) in the host city with all alumni and current department members invited. This has been an excellent way to reconnect alumni with current residents, fellows and faculty.

Department Philanthropy

During these years, the department, for the first time, was able to successfully address philanthropy. Due to very generous individuals, a number of endowments were set up within the department.

Samuel J. Kiehl
Endowed Chair in Emergency Medicine

In 2016, Samuel J. Kiehl III, MD, a faculty member in the department made a $1 million donation over five years, which was matched by the department, which enabled the establishment of the first endowed Chair in the department (Figure 3). Initially, the Samuel J. Kiehl Endowed Professorship was established to which Sorabh Khandelwal, MD, was named in 2018. This endowed professorship was transitioned to an endowed Chair in 2020. The purpose of this endowed chair, as stated in the gift agreement, says as follows:

> *The annual distribution shall support program enhancements for resident growth and development...funds shall be directed toward improvement in curriculum, program duration and educational opportunities, critical clinical skills and research training, life and work integration and fellowship awards.*

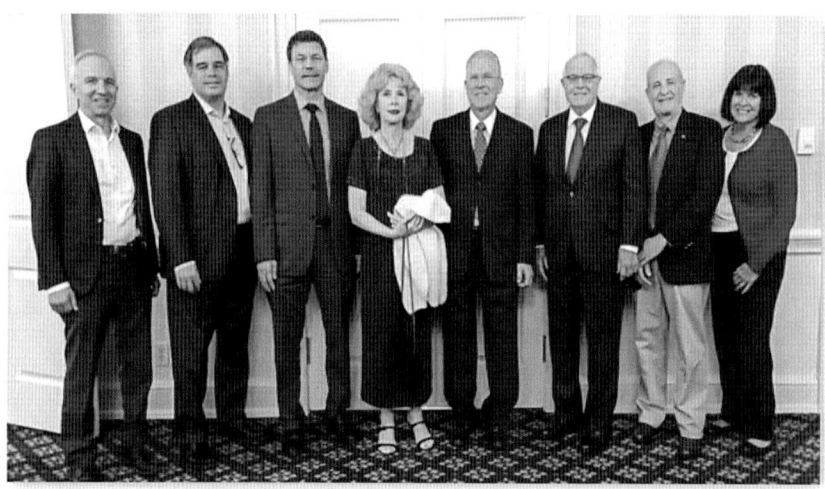

Figure 3: Recognition event at the Scioto Country Club on September 30, 2021, to thank Dr. and Mrs. Samuel Kiehl for their generous gift establishing the first endowed chair in the Department of Emergency Medicine. From left: Mark Angelos, MD; Jeffrey Caterino, MD; Daniel Martin, MD; Terry Kiehl, Samuel Kiehl, III, MD; Douglas Rund, MD; Richard Nelson, MD; and Christine Dailey Shoemaker.

The Ohio State University Endowed Research Chair

A second endowed Chair—the OSU Emergency Medicine Endowed Research Chair—was established in 2018 utilizing funds from the Emergency Medicine LLC. The purpose of this endowed chair is the following:

> *To recruit an established, nationally prominent researcher with a track record of external funding or current funding, including NIH funding, in support of a renowned research program. The faculty member should be a center piece for growing the clinical research program, providing opportunities for research fellow training, mentorship for other faculty members and senior leadership of the department research mission.*

Matt and Melinda Lashutka Endowed Lectureship

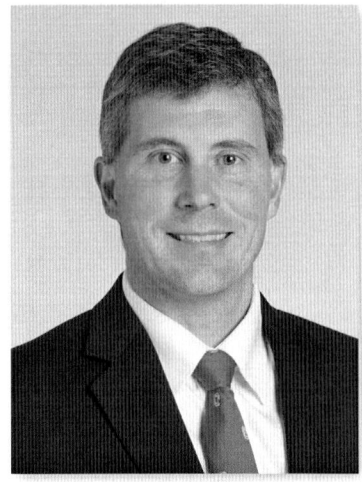

Other endowments include the Matt and Melinda Lashutka Endowed Lectureship which was established in 2017. Matthew K. "Matt" Lashutka, MD, graduated from the Ohio State College of Medicine in 1999 and the residency program in emergency medicine in 2002. (Figure 4) He was chief resident during his senior year. He has practiced in the Cleveland area ever since completing residency. His current position is with Cleveland Clinic where he serves as the medical director for both Lakewood and Lutheran Emergency Departments. This endowed lectureship funds a nationally prominent Emergency Medicine researcher as the keynote speaker for the Department's annual Spring Research Day. Regarding the endowment Lashutka remembered

Figure 4: Matthew Lashutka, MD, finished his emergency medicine residency in 2002. His endowment of the Matt and Melinda Lashutka Endowed Lectureship allows the department to invite a nationally renowned lecturer to present the keynote to Spring Research Day each year.

the intent of the lectureship:

Ohio State means a great deal to me. The medical school and the Department of Emergency Medicine provided me with an excellent education that shaped my career. My wife and I wanted to help OSU continue to provide this same caliber of education for the EM residents of the future, and we were fortunate enough to be able to fund the Endowed Lectureship.[1]

Linda A. Robinson, MD, Scholarship

Finally, the department was able to establish an endowed medical student scholarship through the Linda A. Robinson, MD, scholarship. This scholarship was set up by the Emergency Medicine Alumni Society to honor Linda A. Robinson, MD (Figure 5). Originally from Cleveland, Ohio, Robinson graduated from the Ohio State University College of Medicine in 1986, and went on to join the residency program in emergency medicine, which she completed in 1989. She was the Chief Resident in her final year. After residency, she returned to Cleveland to join the faculty at Case Western Reserve University Hospitals as Senior Instructor and AIRCARE Flight Physician. She returned to the emergency department at Ohio State in 1990 and joined the faculty as an assistant professor and one of the founding hyperbaric physicians.

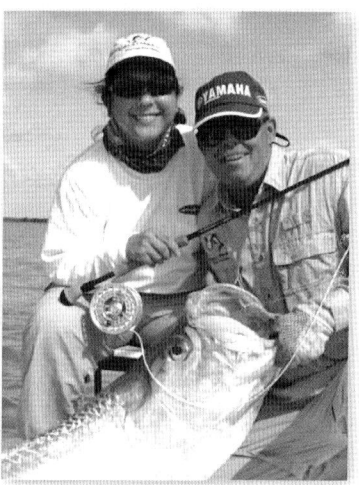

Figure 5: Linda A. Robinson, MD (1958-2017), was an accomplished angler and won many nationwide fishing tournaments. She is shown here with Rick Murphy, a well-known fishing guide and popular host of a television show featuring fishing sports adventures.

Robinson was the first residency-trained woman to become a faculty member in emergency medicine. In 1992 she moved to Miami, Florida, where for the remainder of her career she worked and taught at Jackson Memorial Hospital ED for more than 20 years. During her career at Jackson, she served as Associate Medical Director of the Emergency Care Center and also served with distinction as an ABEM oral examiner.

She was an avid fisherperson, having fished with her father in Ohio and Canada as a child and taking up fly fishing for tarpon when she moved to Florida in 1992. She received a number of accolades in salt water tournaments such as 2002 Grand Champion WWIFC Tarpon Series, 2001 Grand Champion, Golden Fly Tarpon Tournament and 2000 Miami Met Tarpon Master. She lost a tragic battle with cancer and passed away in 2017.

Clinical Mission

The clinical mission grew during the years in both patient encounters and new clinical sites under the direction of Eric Adkins, MD, Vice-Chair of Clinical Affairs. This ongoing growth led to new faculty recruitment. The largest clinical site was the Main Campus ED where over 80,000 patients were cared for each year. The East ED volume and acuity grew year after year, with patient visits increasing to over 50,000 patients per year under the leadership of Mike Dick, MD, Medical Director, and Soni Shellman, MD, Assistant Medical Director. Within the Main hospital ED, Luca Delatore, MD, followed by Mark Conroy, MD, served as Medical Directors.

The department faculty also staffed the Observation Unit, which grew to 20 beds, and the Hyperbaric Medicine Center, in which both chronic and acute conditions were treated by a group of Hyperbaric-trained EM faculty who also provided 24/7 on-call coverage for acute emergencies. Other clinical sites covered by department faculty included two Afterhours Urgent Care sites at the Ohio State Martha Morehouse Clinic and at Care Point Gahanna. In order to provide clinical space for fellows, additional clinical positions for faculty were negotiated in the emergency departments of the following hospitals: Mt Carmel East, Memorial-Marysville, and Licking Memorial Hospital in, Newark, OH. These arrangements allowed the department to expand the number of fellowships.

Geriatric Accreditation of the ED

One of the unique accomplishments of the Main ED was achieving Geriatric ED Accreditation. This was a remarkable effort led by Lauren Southerland, MD. The Geriatric ED Accreditation required the ED to establish protocols, provider training and additional resources, all designed to better facilitate the care of geriatric patients in the ED. The Ohio State University Main Hospital was one of the first EDs in the country to attain this level of certification.

Division of Emergency Ultrasound

The Division of Emergency Ultrasound was created in support of the clinical mission and in response to the leadership of David Bahner, MD, and Creagh Boulger, MD, both national leaders in the use of bedside ultrasound. This was the first Division within the department. The Division was created with eight core faculty members from the Department all with specialized ultrasound training. Between the two Ohio State emergency departments, Main and East, the faculty were performing over 5,000 ultrasound cases per year. Most of these studies were done in conjunction with Emergency Medicine residents, resulting in a high level of competence among residents. The division also provided faculty-training sessions for all department faculty.

Faculty Development

Under the leadership of Diane Gorgas, MD, Vice-Chair of Academic Affairs, the Department instituted a formal faculty mentorship program for all Assistant and Associate Professors in the Department. A plan was developed to assist all mentees to work with a more senior mentor to develop a personal mission statement and develop a three-to-five-year career plan. This mentorship included early discussions and guidance regarding faculty promotion, utilizing members of the Department Promotion and Tenure Committee. Each year, the department had multiple faculty members who were successfully being promoted to Associate Professor and Professor. The number of full

Professors in the Department more than doubled over the five years between 2015-2020.

Faculty Salary Restructuring

In 2018 the Medical Center made a decision to standardize the structure of all physician compensation under a new Medical Center compensation plan. This compensation plan became known as the XYZ plan.

Under the XYZ plan, each department was required to restructure faculty salaries to fit into the new plan. Within the Department these efforts were led by Angelos as the Chair, Archual as the Department Administrator and Caterino, as the Department Finance Committee Chair. Under this plan, faculty compensation encompassed several elements: Academic salary based on university rank (X component); variable portion, based on specialty field, clinical and academic productivity (Y component); and incentive (Z component). This process required approximately two years to develop and implement. Using the plan, the department was able to increase base faculty salaries, excluding incentive, to the 50th percentile using the American Association of Academic Medical Center (AAMC) annual salary benchmarks. This was a significant increase across the board for department faculty.

Gender Equity

During these years, the issue of gender equity within the department was identified, which led to greater awareness and discussion within the department. In 2017, 35% of the faculty were female. This was a very talented group, however, most were at the Assistant Professor level and none were part of the senior leadership group. A Faculty Equity and Parity Taskforce was formed, led by a senior female faculty member and a senior male faculty member to examine gender and equity issues among faculty and make recommendations for improvement.

Over the next few years, a conscious effort was made to develop more female leaders within the department. Part of this effort consisted of providing more specific mentorship in supporting promotion on the various faculty tracks. A review of faculty salaries was made to determine if there was any compensation bias and if inequities were found these were resolved. To improve the culture within the department, all faculty completed implicit bias training. As part of the visiting professor series, a national expert was invited. Esther Choo, MD, from Oregon Health Sciences met with faculty and presented a Grand Rounds Talk, "Gender Bias in the House of Medicine and Why Emergency Medicine is Likely to Crush it."

Department Leadership Development

In order to build the leadership team of the department following a faculty retreat, the senior leadership began meeting monthly to discuss department faculty issues with the guidance of Bob Towner-Larsen, PhD, a well-respected physician coach and Ombudsman at the Ohio State Wexner Medical Center. Towner-Larsen functioned as a facilitator for the group. The group first developed a vision statement for the department, called "Transforming Medicine Through Innovation (TECAR)". This group became the TECAR Group and subsequently worked through five behaviors of a cohesive team: Trust, Engage, Commit, Accountable, and Results. This group included the Vice Chairs, Medical Directors, Department Administrator and the Chair. The group met monthly for two years to learn how to better work as a senior leadership group and how to grapple with department issues. In 2019, a second group of early and future leaders was organized and began to meet monthly with Towner-Larsen to identify and work through key department issues.

The members of the Department all benefitted greatly by an outstanding staff led by Greg Archual, the Department Administrator. Christine Dailey Shoemaker had been with the department since its inception and had a great deal of institutional knowledge that was extremely valuable. While she had worked in many roles, during these years she was primarily responsible for perhaps the two issues of greatest interest to the faculty—the clinical schedule and the payroll. As the department continued to grow, both of these areas grew more complex. Mary Jayne Fortney served as the administrative assistant to the

Chair and facilitated much of the Chair's work. Fortney also had a long history working at the Medical Center; thus, her overall knowledge of the Medical Center and personnel were extremely valuable.

Conclusion

Angelos reported the following to the Dean in 2019:

> *As a department we have been good stewards in partnering with the Ohio State Wexner Medical Center. We exceeded our budget goals, our philanthropic goals, our research goals and our faculty engagement survey alignment score goals.*
>
> *As I retire, serving as Department Chairman has been a singular honor and the capstone of my career. It was a great privilege to serve with outstanding colleagues; students, residents, fellows, staff, and faculty.*
>
> *In my years at Ohio State, I have always appreciated the opportunity to be a part of the discovery, research and education process to improve the care of our patients—something that we are uniquely well-positioned to accomplish as part of a dynamic academic health center.*

In 2019, Dean Craig Kent, MD, offered Angelos a second 4-year term as Department Chair. Instead, Angelos agreed to continue until his planned retirement in 2020 and to work with Dean Kent to facilitate the future department leadership transition. When that time came, Kent announced the appointment of Jeffrey Caterino, MD, as the next Chair.

References

1. Lashutka ML. Personal communication, 2022

Chapter 13

The Caterino Chair Years: 2020-present

Jeffrey M. Caterino, MD, MPH

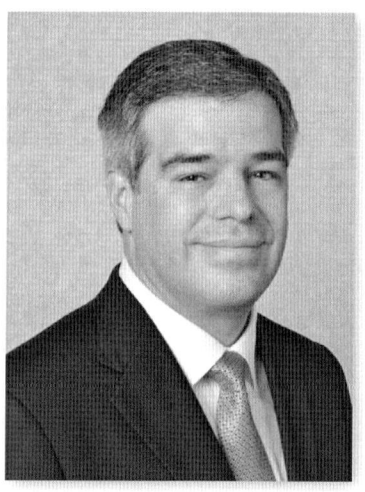

Figure 1: Jeffrey M. Caterino, MD, MPH, was appointed Chair of the Department of Emergency Medicine in 2020. He was highly successful in expanding the research program and leading the faculty in a time of great clinical expansion in the medical center.

Jeffrey M. Caterino, MD, MPH, assumed the role of department Chair on January 15, 2020 (Figure 1). He became the fourth chair of the Department of Emergency Medicine when he was appointed by Dean Craig Kent to fill the position following the retirement of Mark Angelos, MD. He received his undergraduate degree in history from Dartmouth College and his Doctor of Medicine degree from Pennsylvania State University. He then completed a combined emergency medicine/internal medicine residency at Allegheny General Hospital and served as chief resident; he completed his MPH in clinical and translational sciences at Ohio State.

State of the Department, January 2020

With the transition of leadership in January 2020 from Mark Angelos, MD, to Caterino, the department was in a healthy state. Angelos' leadership had done much to move the department forward. Clinical operations had been stable for several years with consistent patient volumes, continued improvement in quality, a steady staffing pattern for the faculty and residents, and clinical operations that were in a comforting rhythm. The research mission continued to grow with new National Institutes of Health (NIH) grants recently funded from Lauren Southerland, MD, and Katherine "Katie" Buck, MD, and the department was in the top 15 nationally for NIH funding. The educators were applying innovative educational techniques across the curricula for both medical students and residents, and the number of residents going into academics was increasing each year.

In short order Caterino's time as Chair was dominated by the COVID-19 pandemic. Despite this enormous challenge, the department continued to move forward with notable successes in its multiple mission areas. Clinical operations eventually adapted to the new reality of a COVID-endemic world. Exciting new clinical opportunities such as the Advanced Immediate Care (AIC) facilities, the first of which opened in August 2021, presented excellent new opportunities for expansion of the clinical mission. The research group grew rapidly under the leadership of Henry Wang, MD, MS, MPH, Vice Chair for Research, to include seven NIH-funded investigators. The education group continued to uphold its national reputation, ranking in the top 30 of emergency medicine residencies nationally. Many faculty members held national leadership positions and were creating innovative programs to advance the science of educating the next generation of EM physicians. The internationally known ultrasound program continued to develop new techniques and expanded to teach point-of-care ultrasound throughout the institution.

The many accomplishments of the faculty served the department well in moving steadily toward the department's vision of *transforming emergency medicine through innovation*. The component goals are outlined in the department's mission statement:

> *To provide innovative, efficient, safe and compassionate patient care to patients presenting to The Ohio State University Wexner Medical Center's Emergency Departments and Afterhours clinics. To be a leader in the education of medical students, residents and fellows in emergency medical care. To perform cutting-edge research and scholarly investigation to identify the causes, treatments and prevention of emergency*

medical conditions and to promote transforming emergency medicine through innovation, faculty development and excellence.[1]

The COVID-19 Pandemic Strikes

Early in 2020 the first months of COVID-19 were among the most challenging ever faced by the department. In January the Hunan Seafood Wholesale Market in Wuhan, China, was closed amid worries of a Severe Acute Respiratory Syndrome Corona Virus outbreak (SARS-CoV-1). Later that month the Centers for Disease Control and Prevention (CDC) instituted the screening of passengers traveling from China to the United States. In February COVID cases began to increase throughout the world and, for the first time, not all were thought to be travel related; some were likely due to community spread of the virus. In March cases were becoming widespread. Many people infected with COVID were dying. Soon schools and businesses were closed throughout the United States. People were advised to stay home and observe social distancing and masking when out for essentials shopping or medical visits.

Hospitals nationwide were on high alert and extensive precautions were taken to prevent the unnecessary spread of the disease within the medical centers. At Ohio State, the Emergency Department had to grapple with the problem and still remain functioning for all patients. In March and April 2020 little was known about the virus itself and questions about its transmissibility, the susceptibility of health care workers to infection, and the potential severity of illness caused great consternation and an urgent need for detailed planning. In March 2020 the Ohio State Wexner Medical Center activated its incident command system, which engaged leaders from all areas of the Medical Center, including clinical operations, supply, nursing, infectious diseases, epidemiology and more. The most immediate concerns and challenges were the identification of patients with COVID in the absence of consistently available testing, protection of the health care workforce, maintenance of adequate supplies of Personal Protective Equipment (PPE) and planning for potential surges of COVID patients.

These initial clinical challenges were characterized by daily changes in knowledge and operations. The department leadership team consisted of Chair Caterino; Vice Chair for Clinical Operations Eric Adkins, MD; medical directors at University Hospital (Mark Conroy, MD) and East Hospital (Michael Dick, MD); and nursing leadership at both hospitals (Erin Farrell, MSN, RN; Ken Gross, RN; Stephanie Sturgis, RN; and Jillian Maitland, MBA, RN). A pattern soon emerged: There would be daily briefings of health system leadership at late afternoon incident command meetings. The ED operations leadership team would then meet to determine what changes needed to be made in the department. These were communicated through a series of daily 7 AM phone calls open to all emergency department faculty, residence, advanced practice practitioners, nurses and staff.

The earliest challenges were those faced by health care systems across the country. Initially, COVID was characterized as a travel-related illness with screening performed only for patients from known hotspots such as China and Italy. Testing was not available locally and required several days to determine positivity. Transmissibility was not yet understood. As a result, the Emergency Department instituted various protocols for testing and isolating patients. One protocol included performing testing only in the limited number of negative airflow rooms as well as outside swabbing.

Although the Ohio State health system always maintained adequate stocks of PPE, uncertainty around its future availability resulted in concerns over PPE shortages. Several community groups and companies donated respirator masks. Others donated food for the clinical staff working on shift. Initial PPE recommendations mirrored those of the CDC and changed frequently. N95 respirator masks were reused throughout each shift and a limited number of reusable respirators were available from the Central Ohio Trauma System (COTS) and private donors. Ohio State partnered with Battelle industries to develop a means of recycling and reusing cleaned N95 masks. A key memory of the early days of the pandemic was the elaborate donning and doffing rituals following each encounter with a patient.

The clinical changes related to COVID spread far beyond the emergency department, complicating previously mundane tasks. New protocols had to be developed for cardiopulmonary resuscitation (CPR), EMS arrivals, patients destined for a catheterization lab, and use of computerized tomography (CT) scans. In just one example, initially stringent CT scanner cleaning protocols led to extended times for obtaining diagnostic studies. Admitted patients with COVID were placed in dedicated COVID units upstairs.

Through all these uncertainties, the clinical operations of the Department of Emergency Medicine continued. There was no ability to work from home or see patients only through tele-visits, although steps were taken to limit clinical staff exposure to COVID. For many patients, only one physician, either a resident or an attending, would see a patient physically in the room and physical exams were limited to avoid close patient contact. Patients with suspected COVID would be given phones so that most communication could be done without health care staff in the room. The faculty used many techniques, some unproven, to decrease exposure. All intubations were initially done by attendings with universal use of video laryngoscopy. Intubation boxes, clear acrylic boxes placed over the patient with holes for the arms of the person doing the intubation, were constructed by Ohio State's College of Engineering based on prototypes tried in China. These were used for months with questionable efficacy in decreasing exposure. This time period was marked by fabulous clinical leadership from the leadership team as well as tremendous collaboration with nurses, respiratory therapy, ED techs, environmental services, and others.

As those working clinically were dealing with the challenges of COVID, emergency department volumes were dropping; and they dropped significantly for an entire year. This was due both to societal fear of going out as well as decreased activity in general. People were advised to remain at home to avoid human contact and possible infection. The ED had an unsettling feel due to low numbers of patients, resulting in significant downtime, but punctuated by high stress periods when taking care of potential COVID patients. This scenario was magnified by the eeriness of coming to and leaving work with no one else on the road, and driving by closed and empty shops and restaurants and the other sequelae of society's response to early COVID. Due to uncertainty around contact spread of the virus, physicians were meticulous in changing clothes and showering immediately when returning home –the last doffing ritual of a shift.

While keeping daily changes in operations at the forefront, the operations leaders also had to plan for many eventualities. Ohio was initially spared large early surges in COVID patients, allowing teams additional time to prepare. In April 2020, however, there was an outbreak in the state prison system. In addition to caring for a large number of patients in the department, emergency department nursing led by Erin Farrell, MSN, RN—and assisted by multiple other nurses—proceeded to conduct surveillance testing of thousands of state prisoners in their institutions, helping to significantly shorten the duration and spread of the outbreak. In addition, due to concerns over potential surges as seen in other areas of the country, the ED operations staff created significant disaster plans to handle a COVID surge. These efforts included setting up outdoor tents at East and University Hospital as well as using space underneath the Ross overhang with a plan for several dozen patient care areas in each of these. Thankfully, a surge requiring their use did not materialize. As testing became available, the ED nursing staff also were critical to manning drive-through swab stations.

Daniel Bachmann, MD, Associate Professor of Emergency Medicine, and an emergency preparedness expert, led much of the institutional response to COVID, including the swab testing stations established throughout Columbus. In 2016 he had become the Medical Director for Disaster Preparedness at the medical center and his expertise in disaster management was essential to the success of Ohio State's preparedness. Later he recalled his efforts during early COVID:

> *My involvement with COVID-19 began before the first case was identified in the U.S. We brought a small group together to discuss the seemingly impossible worst-case scenario of this novel virus becoming a real threat to the health of our country and our world. Unfortunately, as history now knows, that worst-case scenario quickly became a reality and we were engulfed in a global pandemic that was something I never expected to experience firsthand. My focus on the response and preparedness for OSUWMC [Ohio State University Wexner Medical Center] narrowed and I was entirely dedicated to that by March of 2020. For the next 4 months, I didn't work any clinical time in the ED as I was leading the COVID-19 testing operations and serving on our response team. I helped coordinate one of the largest testing sites in central Ohio during that time with additional support to various community members such as the public health department and COTS. When it was clear that*

COVID-19 was not going away quickly, I passed off some of my operational duties to the ambulatory leadership at OSUWMC so that I could get back to emergency medicine. I remained part of the leadership of the response team as we pivoted to other chapters of the pandemic such as creating inpatient capacity and building up a mass vaccination program. I remain connected through my involvement with our Emerging Pathogens committee and we continue to monitor COVID-19 activity as well as the varied threats from other infectious diseases.[2]

Emergency medicine faculty also led in other areas. Howard A. Werman, MD, was one of the early non-occupationally-acquired COVID patients; he was also the first to provide convalescent plasma as an experimental treatment for high-risk patients (Figure 2).

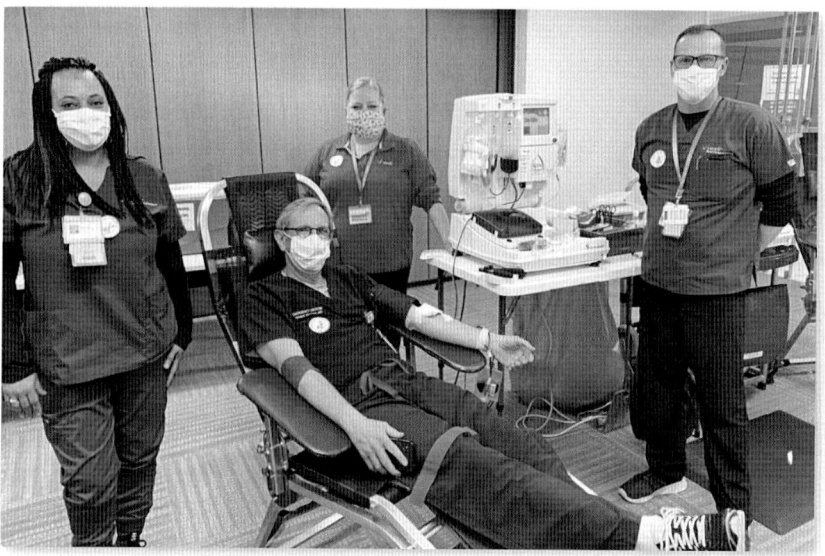

Figure 2: Howard A. Werman, MD, Professor of Emergency Medicine, becomes one of the first COVID-infected patients in Ohio to donate antibody-rich convalescent plasma used to treat patients with severe COVID in 2020.

Covid Vaccines Become Available

Christmas 2020 brought the most welcome gift with availability of the first COVID vaccines. These were approved in early December and by late December they were being administered nationwide to health care workers at highest risk. Supplies were initially limited. However, emergency medicine providers were among the first to receive vaccines. By mid-January, all Ohio State emergency department personnel were vaccinated. This caused a significant change in outlook, approach, and concern among ED personnel. The relative protection offered by the vaccine, particularly from severe illness, resulted in significantly decreased stress levels and concern when caring for patients with COVID. Although the sense that the worst of the pandemic was over would prove illusory, the vaccines collectively allowed emergency department staff to experience decreased stress through the spring and summer of 2021, especially as COVID numbers decreased during this time. The availability of vaccine also allowed students to return to the clinical environment, and clinical research and basic science research resumed.

During this time, emergency department personnel made significant contributions in community health outreach. Many volunteered to staff vaccine stations as vaccines became more available in late winter and spring, helping to vaccinate the population of the state of Ohio. Ohio State had one of the earliest and highest volume vaccine stations statewide and one of the earliest in the country. Dan Bachmann, MD, oversaw many of these efforts.

As part of the faculty's commitment to caring for patients wherever needed, a number of emergency medicine faculty staffed a medical intensive care unit at East Hospital during the winter of 2021. For two months they cared for critically ill ICU patients. This prevented the critical care physicians from being overwhelmed due to the large number of patients with severe illness during the surge, which occurred before widespread vaccination of the population.

Medical Students' and Residents' Efforts During COVID

Emergency medicine residents stood side-by-side with the attendings and other clinical staff throughout the pandemic. The senior residents, with only three months left in training, were critical in the early days of the pandemic to ensuring excellent clinical care both of those with COVID and those without the virus. From the first day, even when there was great uncertainty, the residents continued to put themselves at risk caring for patients. They continued to intubate patients with respiratory illness and perform important clinical duties required to keep the emergency department running.

Due to their inability to meet outside of work, residents lost a lot of the collegiality and support structures that they normally relied on. Throughout the remainder of the pandemic, however, they continued to be tremendous partners in the ongoing care and operations of the department. Residency conference and other learning opportunities switched to virtual for over 18 months. One intervention to meet the need for fellowship outside of work was the implementation of "wellness Thursdays." Simiao Li-Sauerwine, MD, Assistant Program Director, helped organize a series of casual Zoom meetings where various faculty and residents could share their non-medical passions—everything from gardening to learning German to savoring bourbon. Leaders for the week would often assemble goodie bags to be picked up by the participants to use during the meeting.

Medical students were also greatly impacted. As COVID rapidly spread in April 2020, the College of Medicine discontinued clinical rotations for their students and shifted to a completely distance-learning curriculum. Among all of their other duties, Bachmann and Nick Kman, MD, rapidly designed a disaster and pandemic response course for the medical students, with hundreds participating in the course. Once vaccines became available, medical students were gradually reintroduced to the clinical department and resumed their usual roles alongside the residents and attendings.

Research During COVID

As with all other activities, COVID had enormous impacts on the research mission. At the beginning of the pandemic, basic science labs were closed across the university. They remained closed for the better part of a year until staff could be vaccinated and more was understood about the spread of the virus. Although this resulted in a delay of ongoing research activities of these labs, staff and faculty significantly contributed in other ways.

Clinical research was also halted in March 2020. However, the clinical research faculty and staff rapidly identified clinical trials necessary to identify effective treatments for COVID–19. Ohio State Emergency Medicine was among the early leaders in these trials. By late spring, Lauren Southerland, MD, led efforts as part of a multicenter trial to study the effectiveness of hydroxychloroquine prophylaxis on COVID infection rates among health care providers. This study was conducted as part of the Prevention and Early Treatment of Acute Lung Injury (PETAL) network. Likewise, Southerland and Jason Bischof, MD, conducted a study as part of the NIH-funded Strategies to Innovate Emergency Care Clinical Trials (SIREN) network. They led Ohio State's efforts in a clinical trial of convalescent plasma for treatment of ED COVID patients. The department's two research managers, Jennifer Frey and Michael Hill, along with other research staff, successfully managed these trials' completion. Even early in the pandemic these staff members were willing to successfully identify, consent, and administer study interventions to patients with COVID or suspected COVID.

A large number of new techniques to ensure research staff safety when dealing with highly infectious potential subjects were developed – electronic consents, phone interviews, etc. Such contributions were greatly appreciated and recognized. Although the hydroxychloroquine and convalescent plasma studies were negative, they provided important critical information to allow other investigators to focus on other possible treatments for the virus.

As with basic science research, more normal clinical research operations resumed in the spring of 2021. Although continuing to be challenged by concerns over suspected COVID in patients or patients with COVID, and the need for PPE, clinical research operations rapidly returned to their prior level of excellence.

Fall 2021 and Winter 2022 Surges: Delta and Omicron

The summer of 2021 remained relatively quiet with regard to COVID infections. Vaccine stations were closed down with a large proportion of the population having already been vaccinated and large-scale swab stations closed due to decreased community infection rates. By August 2021, however, the Delta variant caused a significant surge in cases. Most patients had minor symptoms but a proportion also had more severe illness. Although more infectious, this variant was less virulent than the initial COVID strain. However, the sheer number of patients infected again threatened to overwhelm the system. Volumes were swollen primarily by mildly ill patients who did not require hospitalization. With tests, vaccines and new treatments available, the real challenge became the increasing volume of patients with COVID symptoms and others with existing and new medical problems which may have been tolerated by patients for a time during the early stay at home period. In addition, monoclonal antibody treatments and an oral agent (Paxlovid) were available for high-risk patients. The volumes in both surges were the highest seen in Ohio and significantly stressed the system simply due to number of patients presenting for testing and possibility of treatment.

Diversity, Equity and Inclusion

In fall 2020, the department formed its first diversity, equity and inclusion committee. This committee was co-led by a faculty member and a resident, with Robert Cooper, MD, as the initial faculty lead. The committee rapidly identified several areas of critical importance for the department: to support the antiracism efforts of the University and the College, and to act in concert with other university and college groups. Initial initiatives included voter registration drives in both emergency departments. Irene Mynatt, DO, from the department and Jackiethia Butsch, Senior Outreach Coordinator for the Office of Community and Civic Engagement at Ohio State, led efforts to increase community collaboration in areas local to Ohio State East. There was a significant educational component as well with residents now receiving additional training in social determinants of health and social emergency medicine. Faculty and resident recruitment was revamped to incorporate holistic principles similar to those used by Ohio State's College of Medicine.

In August 2022, Henry Young, MD, joined the department from the University of Florida as the Vice Chair for Diversity, Equity and Inclusion. He coordinates and spearheads efforts such as those described above to truly apply principles of diversity, equity and inclusion in the care of our patients, our interaction with our community, and in the training of our residents and medical students.

New Clinical Frontiers – Advanced Immediate Care

As part of the Ohio State health system's ambulatory strategy, a series of ambulatory surgery centers with attached multispecialty physician office towers began opening in summer 2021. These facilities include emergency medicine-operated Advanced Immediate Cares (AICs); AIC New Albany opened in August 2021, followed by AIC Dublin in August 2022. The next AIC will be an expansion of the Martha Morehouse Pavilion in 2023, followed by a new site in Powell in 2025. Additional facilities may also be developed.

The advanced immediate care centers are an innovative approach to delivering urgent and emergent same-day health care over the coming decades by providing clinical resources between that of an emergency department and urgent care. Only a few other large health systems in the country have a similar model. Advanced immediate care meets the needs of patients who require more complex diagnostic testing or interventions than delivered in a traditional urgent care, but do not require the services of a full emergency department. Emergency physicians and advanced practice providers staff them and have a suite of laboratory studies, x-ray, CT scan, and both oral and IV medications available. The AICs can care for conditions such as low to moderate risk chest pain, abdominal pain, migraine headache, orthopedic injuries, or potentially serious infections, as well as traditional urgent care conditions. New Albany has been wildly successful with patients, payers and the health system with over 20,000 visits in its first year. Dublin is on pace to meet that in its first year of operation. The AICs deliver cost savings and efficiency to patients; and the health system attracts large numbers of new patients. It is a model that can be successfully replicated in other areas.

In addition, in spring 2022, the department launched a new after-hours clinic located at Ohio State East Hospital, yards away from the East emergency department. This endeavor is supported by Medicaid dollars through the Care Innovation and Community Improvement Program (CICIP) created by the Ohio legislature in 2018. The CICIP is a Quality Improvement program backed by the Ohio Department of Medicaid. The program includes four teaching hospitals throughout the state of Ohio. The new after-hours clinic brings the first urgent care option to the medically underserved residents of East Columbus, with the goal of providing a walk-in option for patients who otherwise might be forced to use the emergency department. The expectation is that the after-hours urgent care clinic will increase rapid access to urgent care services for those who do not need ED services and free up space for more severely ill patients to be seen in the emergency department.

Post-Delta, Post-Omicron and Non-COVID Clinical Operations

With the conclusion of the Omicron surge in winter 2022, COVID transitioned to an endemic disease and low levels of symptomatic patients continued to present through 2022 with periodic spikes in cases. The health system was most limited by overall constraints on capacity driven by an inadequate staffing plight that exists throughout all aspects of the U.S. health care system. Although the prevalence of COVID would wax and wane, small stresses to the system continued to create significant ripple effects. For example, a Respiratory Syncytial Virus (RSV) and influenza surge in the fall of 2022 led to increased boarding, which clogged the emergency departments, creating yet another sensation of crisis. During this time, the AICs also saw large numbers of patients, many of whom were able to avoid visits to the overwhelmed emergency departments because of the availability of the AIC model.

Since 2020, the primary non-COVID challenge facing the Department of Emergency Medicine has been the boarding of inpatients. This is a national trend with constrained inpatient resources exacerbated by various COVID surges, but happens even when those surges are not occurring. The ED has seen record numbers of boarded patients and hours, which has impacted patient throughput and tested physician and staff resiliency. The University Hospital Emergency Department is completely redesigning its patient flow process in order to meet this challenge, with a goal of physicians seeing patients as early as possible in order to expedite evaluation, workup and ensure that beds are appropriately assigned to those who need them.

The department continued to innovate in other areas. One example is the expansion of the medication assisted treatment program (MAT) for opiate dependence. This effort was led by Emily Kauffman, DO, MPH, who secured several million dollars of funding from state and local agencies to improve care of emergency department patients with substance abuse disorder. Both emergency departments now have substance abuse consultation, resources and programs to assist patients in moving immediately from the emergency department to a rehabilitation setting. These resources allow Ohio State to implement best practices in this area as the struggle with substance abuse disorder continues at the local and state level.

Resident and Fellow Education

With the disruption of resident education activities due to COVID returning to normal, the residency program has grown to 63 residents between the categorical emergency medicine and the EM/IM program. The residency also now hosts two Air Force affiliated residents each year. The department continues to recruit high quality residents, with 50% or more of current residents proceeding into fellowship programs or other academic pursuits each year—a goal of the program since its inception. The program is now ranked in the top 30 in the country by Doximity.

Unique educational endeavors include a procedural mastery curriculum developed by Jennifer Yee, DO, and implemented by the core faculty. This innovative program is now being copied throughout the health system. Likewise, the ultrasound division's teaching methodologies—led by Creagh Boulger, MD—are now being adopted systemwide. The goal is to teach point-of-care ultrasound to nearly all specialties.

Fellowship programs continue to recruit future national leaders in their respective areas. The department has from 4 to 7 fellows annually, and offers fellowships in ultrasound, medical education, research, administration, EMS and global health.

Research

Since January 2020, the research mission has accelerated both in clinical and basic sciences. External funding has doubled to over 4 million dollars annually. This amount will continue to grow rapidly as an increasing number of grant applications are submitted and funded.

HENRY E. WANG, MD, MPH, MS

Henry E. Wang MD, MS, MPH, an internationally recognized expert in prehospital resuscitation and airway management as well as sepsis, was recruited as Professor and Vice Chair for Research and joined the faculty in January 2021 (Figure 3). Wang's main research focuses on the design of novel resuscitation clinical trials. He has a long track record of NIH funding and mentoring and he has achieved funding on multiple NIH grants since joining Ohio State. He was a site Principal Investigator (PI) for the NIH Resuscitation Outcomes Consortium, and was lead investigator of the landmark Pragmatic Airway Resuscitation Trial (PART). He is also the founding Editor-in-Chief of the *Journal of the American College of Emergency Physicians Open*.

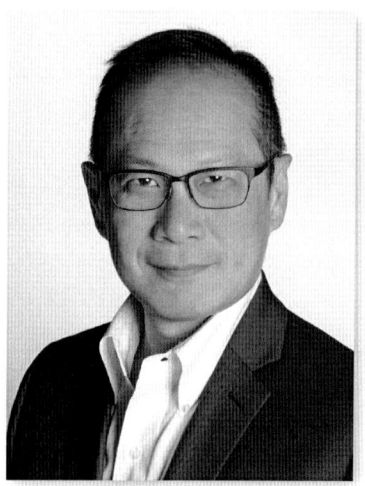

Figure 3: Henry E. Wang, MD, MS, MPH, Professor and Vice Chair for Research in the Department of Emergency Medicine at Ohio State, is an internationally recognized expert in resuscitation and airway management.

EDWARD W. BOYER, MD, PHD

A second senior investigator, Edward W. Boyer, MD, PhD, joined the faculty from Harvard in 2021 (Figure 4). A native of Mississippi, he attended Vanderbilt University before receiving his doctorate in organic chemistry at Columbia University. Boyer completed his medical training at Columbia University College of Physicians and Surgeons in New York City, his residency at the Hospital of the University of Pennsylvania and a medical toxicology fellowship at Boston Children's Hospital. After serving on the faculty at the University of Massachusetts Medical School, he was recruited in 2016 to develop the research

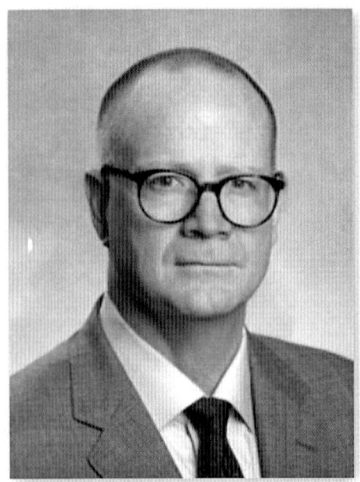

Figure 4: Edward W. Boyer, MD, PhD, is a medical toxicologist and Professor of Emergency Medicine at The Ohio State University.

infrastructure of the Brigham and Women's Hospital Department of Emergency Medicine, where he rose to the rank of Professor at Harvard Medical School.

Boyer's research transcends disciplinary and methodological boundaries. Continuously funded by NIH since 2001, his investigations focus on the intersection of advanced technologies and health care. His studies focus on ingestible biosensors, machine learning-tagged music to decrease pain, mobile interventions to improve antiretroviral adherence, wearable biosensors to detect illicit drug use, digital phenotyping, and delivery of health care interventions via drones. He was the first emergency physician and medical toxicologist to receive a prestigious K24 mentoring award from NIH. In 2018, Boyer was named a Fulbright Scholar to Malaysia, where he used machine learning to study the neurophysiology of kratom use in natural environments. He is, however, most proud of his mentees' accomplishments. Boyer has over 50 mentees in academic practice; most are women and underrepresented minorities and over 70% have received NIH funding in starting exceptional careers of their own.

Other investigators have also had ongoing success. Ashish Panchal, MD, PhD, was one of three principal investigators on a five-year $10 million NIH award to create the Center for Serological Testing to Improve Outcomes from Pandemic COVID 19 (STOP-COVID). This award will study long-term effects of COVID-19 upon first responders, health care workers and members of the general population. Lauren Southerland, MD, is continuing her K23 career development award and is investigating processes of care for older adults in the ED. She is moving on to R01 independent funding awards in the coming years. Katherine Buck, MD, received notice of her K76 career development award also in geriatric EM in Fall 2022. Her work will improve diagnoses among older

ED adults with shortness of breath. Other junior faculty are working towards their first NIH grants while developing their own research programs. Jason Bischof, MD, studies patients with cancer and Michelle Nassal, MD, is a developing resuscitation science researcher.

As a result of these efforts, the department has several nationally recognized areas of clinical research. These include: resuscitation and EMS, geriatric emergency medicine, substance abuse, cancer in emergency medicine, network clinical trials, genomics and cardiovascular disease, medical education research, and ultrasound research. The department is now a sought-after partner in national clinical trials including industry and NIH trial networks (e.g., PETAL and SIREN networks). These and others place the department at the forefront of the most cutting-edge clinical trials in the country.

Ultrasound Division

The internationally recognized ultrasound division adapted to COVID by switching much of their training to virtual learning. David Bahner, MD, has led this division since its inception and is assisted by Associate Ultrasound Director Creagh Boulger, MD, and six other ultrasound faculty. The division is heavily involved in the training of Ohio State medical students who are nationally known to leave the college of medicine with excellent ultrasound skills regardless of their chosen specialty. Likewise, the comprehensive education provided to the emergency medicine residents has generated a reputation for ultrasound excellence among our trainees across the country.

The division remains highly productive academically with multiple published research projects each year led by the research mission leader Michael Prats, MD. The division has expanded the fellowship to train non-emergency medicine physicians in point-of-care ultrasound including family medicine, internal medicine, and pediatric emergency medicine. Starting in 2022, the division will lead the entire institution to train house staff and faculty across disciplines and the use of point-of-care ultrasound to improve patient outcomes. Boulger is the project lead.

Summary

Caterino was initially recruited in 2004 by Douglas Rund, MD, who recognized his exceptional promise for a successful academic career. Years later Rund recalled the following:

> *From the beginning I appreciated Jeff's abilities and great potential for leadership. He completed residency training in both Emergency Medicine and Internal Medicine and was board certified in both. He would be eligible for a dual appointment with Internal Medicine and gain immediate respect in that influential department. His dual qualification would also aid him in joining other investigators in the college to design important studies and ultimately receive federal grants. He was always incredibly perceptive in recognizing areas of need in society and in the department. His focus on the medical problems associated with aging were an example of the former and his ongoing recognition that the finances of the department could be realigned to provide salaries that were more competitive and create incentives was an example of the latter. I knew early on that he had the essential ingredients to be a departmental chair when the time was right.*[3]

Having led the department successfully through the COVID era, Caterino continued to shepherd the department's the progress toward its tripartite mission.

References

1. Mission Statement, Ohio State Department of Emergency Medicine, 2022.
2. Bachmann DJ. Personal communication. 2022: Columbus, Ohio.
3. Rund DA. Personal communication. 2022: Columbus, Ohio.

Chapter 14

Emergency Medical Services

Douglas A. Rund, MD
David P. Keseg, MD

Emergency medical services (EMS) systems provide urgent prehospital treatment and stabilization for illnesses and injuries at the scene of an event and during transport to a hospital. On occasion minor treatment can be provided without transport. Prehospital care has improved dramatically over the past 50 years. In many respects, Ohio State and the Columbus Division of Fire have been a major part of that effort, leading the way in creating modern emergency medical services systems.

The History of EMS and Military Ambulances

Historically, the most significant innovations in trauma care have occurred during wartime, with veterans returning to civilian life to try to implement improvements in ambulance care. In the late 1700s Napoleon's army surgeon, Baron Dominique Jean Larrey, is thought to have developed the first battlefield ambulances. Called "Flying Ambulances," these horse-drawn transport carriages were staffed by junior surgeons and provided early evacuation and treatment for wounded officers. The ambulance structure provided two 16-inch-wide spaces for wounded officers. In his book *American Sirens* Kevin Hazzard describes the initiation of these ambulances in the following way:

> The Napoleonic wars were long and brutal. Bullets, bayonets, grapeshot. Men dropping in columns, left to suffer and die where they fell. No one was there to treat casualties or even decide who should get treatment and in what order so Larrey devised a solution, and in 1797 he brought it to Napoleon: surgeons should be given the same nimble horse drawn

carriages that carried the army's "flying artillery" to use as ambulances. This way, rather than lying in misery...casualties could rapidly be transported to the hospital...Napoleon liked the idea of saving rather that burying soldiers and said yes. In a single brilliant stroke Larrey had invented...the first dedicated ambulance corps.[1]

During the American Civil War, American surgeon Major John Letterman developed the first battlefield ambulance for wounded Union soldiers and a system of medical management of battlefield casualties (Figure 1). The development came gradually during the war. Prior to his reorganization, the military ambulance services were haphazard and shockingly deficient. Henry Bowditch, MD, was an ardent advocate for reform. His perception of the ambulance drivers was that they were "men of the lowest character, evidently taken from the vilest purlieus of Washington."[2] Surgeon General Hammond wrote to the secretary of war about the "frightful state of disorder existing in the arrangement for removing the wounded from the field of battle. The scarcity of ambulances, the want of organization, the drunkenness and incompetency of the drivers, the total absence of ambulance attendants are now working their legitimate results...many [on the battlefield] have died torments which might have been avoided."[2] The medical belief then and today is that injured people treated as rap-

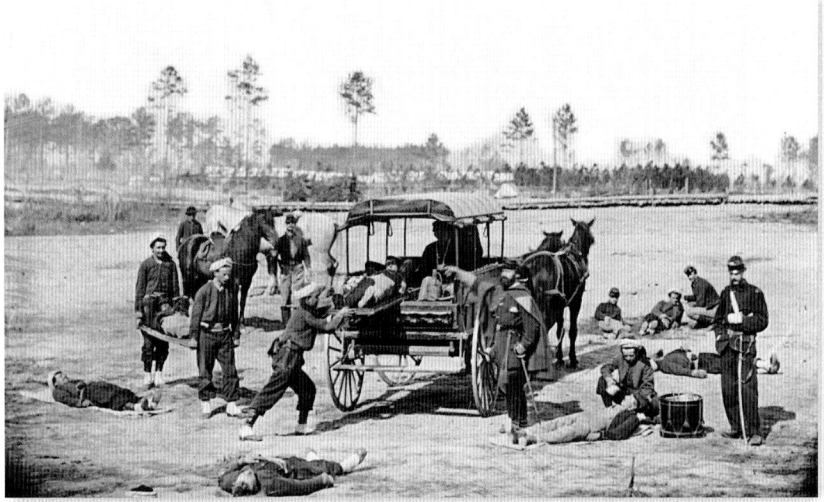

Figure 1: The Civil War horse-drawn ambulance for early evacuation of battlefield casualties was developed by American surgeon Major Jonathan Letterman (Library of Congress).

idly as possible after trauma have better outcomes than those whose treatment is delayed. Toward the end of the war Letterman's reforms improved the ambulance service considerably. Ambulances were redesigned and crews were better trained and better equipped.

During the Civil War, Cincinnati, Ohio, was a center of ambulance manufacture. Hospital-based ambulance services began in Cincinnati in 1865 and in New York in 1868. The ambulances were staffed by a surgical intern or resident. Following the war physicians and others realized the importance of ambulances for managing civilian emergencies.[2]

Ambulances became motorized in World War I (Figure 2). Many were staffed by American volunteers with the American Ambulance Field service, the Red Cross and other organizations. The war saw the beginning of the Triage areas near the front lines where casualties could be rapidly sorted and transferred or provided with treatments as soon as possible.[3]

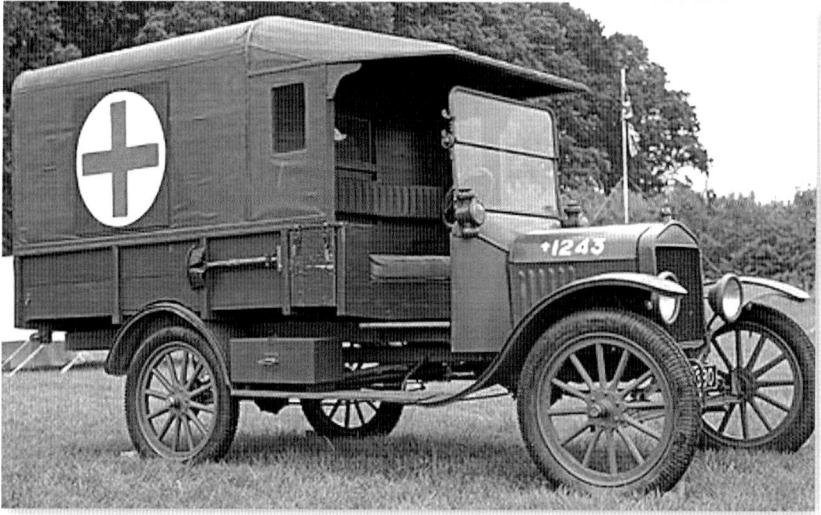

Figure 2: This Ford 1916 Model T Field Ambulance was used extensively by the British and French as well as the American Expeditionary Force in World War I. Its top speed was 45 mph (72 km/h), produced by a 4-cylinder water-cooled engine (Wikipedia, History of the Ambulance).

World War II and Ohio State Future Leaders

World War II ushered in the development of field hospitals, trauma teams and blood transfusions. The war also produced a recognition that the management and evacuation of casualties could be improved. Two Ohio State physician leaders were instrumental in developing evacuation systems for wounded American soldiers during the war: Richard Meiling, MD, and Robert Zollinger, MD. Meiling later became Dean of the Ohio State College of Medicine from 1961 to 1970 and Zollinger became the Chairman of the Department of Surgery, serving from 1947 to 1974.

Born in Ohio, Meiling attended medical school in Germany. He was impressed with systems of airplane evacuation of injured German soldiers during the Spanish Civil War. During World War II he became a high-ranking officer in the U.S. Air Force and pioneered air evacuation for wounded soldiers. Ultimately, he became Assistant Secretary for Defense and Director of U.S. Medical Services. Following the war, he left the military and joined the Ohio State faculty. He specialized in obstetrics and gynecology and became the College of Medicine Dean. Meiling encouraged the development of aerospace medicine within the Department of Preventive Medicine and pioneered the development of a cooperative program for helicopter evacuation of casualties with the Ohio National Guard, which was one of the first in the nation.

Zollinger, famed Chair of the Department of Surgery, was the Chief of Surgery for the Fifth General Hospital in Europe during the war. He developed a system of mobile surgical units and wrote a military medical handbook outlining the steps needed to provide early treatment of the injured soldier. Zollinger was Chair of the Department of Surgery at Ohio State from 1947 to 1974. A strong supporter of the development in helicopter evacuation for injured patients, he lent considerable advice and support to leaders of the new Division of Emergency Medicine at Ohio State.

The Vietnam conflict produced physicians dedicated to immediate trauma casualty care. Such surgeons included Larry C. Carey, MD, the Chair of the Department of Surgery at Ohio State when the Division of

Emergency Medicine was being created. Carey brought tremendous experience and skill to the Department of Surgery based, in part, on his wartime experience. He was an enthusiastic supporter of emergency medicine. Another surgeon who worked with Carey in Vietnam was Charles Cloutier, MD, who joined the emergency medicine faculty in the early 1980s and augmented the department's resources in managing trauma patients.

Civilian Ambulances

In the civilian world before the 1970s, ambulance services were spotty, to say the least. In many cities the police provided transportation (and transportation only) to the hospital. Patients were lucky to arrive at the hospital at all in some of the police ambulances.[1]

Morticians and their hearses were in wide use. The 1966 publication, *Accidental Death and Disability: The Neglected Disease of Modern Society*, describes ambulance services during that era:

> *Very few communities provide sufficient financial support for adequate ambulance services. Where they are provided, they are usually maintained by the fire or police department. Many volunteer, nonprofit rescue squads and local ambulance groups provide commendable service and in many small communities this system would seem to meet basic, but usually only minimal, needs. Approximately 50 percent of the country's ambulance services are provided by 12,000 morticians, mainly because their vehicles can accommodate transportation litters. But in most instances, as is the case of many privately owned*

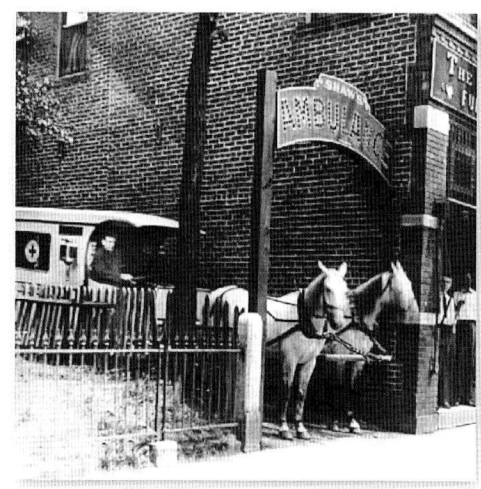

Figure 3: Horse-drawn ambulance operated in Columbus by funeral director H.H Shaw (Courtesy of Shaw Davis Funeral Homes).

ambulances, the vehicles are unsuitable for active care during transportation, equipment and supplies are incomplete, and the attendants are not properly trained.[1]

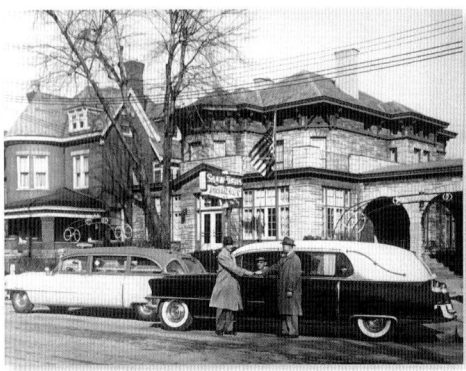

Figure 4: Funeral home hearses doubled as ambulances in the early part of the 20th century. The vehicles were station wagon type hearses too low for the attendants to stand. (Courtesy of Shaw Davis Funeral Homes)

In Columbus, Ohio early horse-drawn ambulances were provided by funeral directors such as Shaw's Ambulance operated by H.H Shaw, a funeral director with an embalming business in the Short North neighborhood of Columbus beginning in 1908 (Figure 3). When motorized vehicles came into use, the motorized hearse continued to double as an ambulance because a person lying down could be transported on a stretcher inside the vehicle; however, ambulance attendants could not stand up and the vehicle carried minimal equipment (Figure 4).

William R. Good was a funeral director at Southwick Good Funeral Chapel located on High Street just north of the Ohio State campus. Years later he recalled his experience as an ambulance operator:

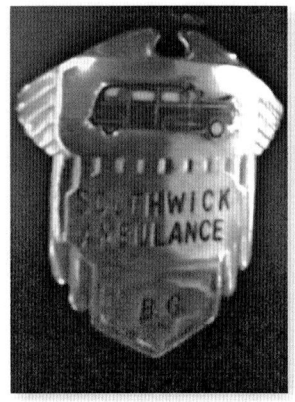

Figure 5: Ambulance operator badge for Southwick Funeral Chapel owner William R. "Bill" Good.

We had a lot of invalid calls, taking people home from the hospital, taking non-emergency cases. Occasionally we would get an emergency case in Columbus. Those of us who were embalmers had a first aid course in embalming school that would prepare us to some extent, but we were very limited. It was a different world back then. Basically, it was: put a person on the cot, haul them to the hospital. In regard to our equipment, we carried an oxygen tank, period. We had a cot, a blanket and a stair chair to get someone from an upper floor.

We also had a back board.

I remember at Christmas time we would always take cartons of cigarettes to the firehouse to thank the firefighters who called us so that they would call us again when they needed a backup or a transport.

I started in the family funeral business in Cincinnati as a teenager. We served a lot of nursing homes that were located in old mansions and there were 50 or more people all through the place and occasionally one of the older folks would break a hip. We would go out there and take them to the emergency room and they would take an x-ray. They would have us stand there and hold these patients without any protection so they wouldn't fall off while they did the x-ray. No consideration of the radiation we received.

In the '50s when a woman had a baby, the funeral home would take her home and give her a baby blanket. That was a common thing. Every woman would go home in an ambulance after having a baby and receive a blanket as a gift.[4]

The History of the Columbus Division of Fire

William T. Hall, a retired firefighter/medic and the Columbus Division of Fire Historian, has chronicled a detailed history of EMS in the Columbus Division of Fire and Ohio State in the *200th Anniversary of the Columbus Fire Department*, published by the Columbus Division of Fire. Hall is the son of William L. Hall, MD, who started the full-time emergency medicine group at Riverside and who became the first full-time physician in the Ohio State Prompt Care fast track area. Hall's history is adapted here with his permission.

In 1933 Fire Chief Ed Welch installed a mechanical respirator (a Pulmotor) in his chief's car to aid in resuscitating firefighters injured or overcome with smoke from a fire. The pulmotor was a gas-powered device that provided cycling breaths, and was particularly effective in resuscitating victims of smoke inhalation or drowning.

One day Welch and two additional firefighters responded with the pulmotor to a call involving a worker who was electrocuted while working on a pole. Hall reports the public's reaction:

> *Their attempts to save the victim were futile, but it happened that a photographer was at the scene and a glowing story and photo of their efforts appeared in the Dispatch newspaper. Thereafter, people began to call the fire department for aid in medical emergencies.*[5]

A year later, a hose wagon was converted into a squad car and the Red Cross donated supplies. A mechanical respirator was placed in the vehicle, which had an open center, and equipment was stored in compartments along the side. There was no possibility of transporting anyone in the vehicle after treatment. Many firefighters were trained in advanced first aid. In 1938 the vehicle was wrecked in a crash and a new hose wagon was converted into a replacement with additional storage and equipment. A new safety package included a siren, a rotating red light (a "Roto Ray" light warning system) and a windshield. Like its predecessor, there was no transport capability. A private ambulance (perhaps a funeral director) had to be called to provide transportation.

In the beginning, 101 men were trained in advanced first aid. This training was voluntary and the men attended classes on their own time. That same year first aid kits were added to all fire apparatus and chiefs' cars as regular equipment. Eighteen first aid demonstrations were given that year and organizations began to request the fire department to staff first aid stations at their activities. As first aid runs increased steadily, a new squad—a 1940 Seagrave Sedan—was purchased and capable of transporting a patient to the hospital.

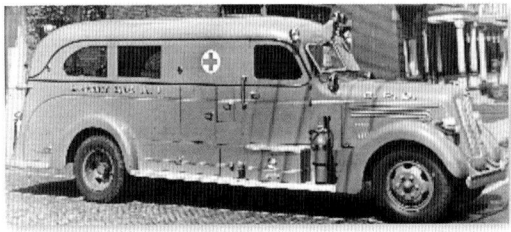

Figure 6: The 1940 Seagrave Sedan had an open back end that had a stretcher and room for attendants to both be seated and covered in the truck.

The vehicle had an open back end to allow a stretcher and attendants to be seated and covered in the back of the truck. The truck also had a small water tank, pump and a one-inch hose line on a reel (Figure 6).

The public readily accepted the new EMS system, and runs increased every year. In 1936, of 2,511 incidents, 52 were for EMS, and in 1937 there were 64. By 1941 EMS calls were up to 1,858 and a second squad—a half-ton Ford V-8 panel truck built by the maintenance shop—was placed in service.

According to Hall, the EMS component of the Columbus Division of Fire increased dramatically as time progressed:

> By 1943 EMS runs hit 5,317 calls for service and a third squad was placed in service. In 1948 the combined runs for all three squads totaled 6,214. In just a short ten years the runs increased from less than 100 to over 6,000. In an effort to help meet the increasing number of calls, the city implemented police ambulances to assist the squads. In 1957 EMS runs exceeded 10,000 calls and a fourth squad was added, with a fifth squad added in 1960. Vehicles of this era were the station wagon, hearse-type large cars like Cadillac, Buick or panel trucks, capable of carrying a patient, attendant, and emergency equipment (Figure 7).

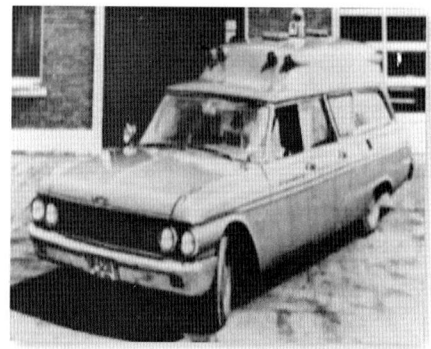

Figure 7: The EMS vehicles of the 1960s tended to be the station wagon, hearse-like cars that accommodated a recumbent patient, but that limited the headroom for rescuers.

In the 1970s new federal guidelines discouraged the use of the station wagon style ambulances. New vehicles were required to have boxlike structures mounted on a truck chassis; rescuers could stand up to treat their patients. This improved design occurred simultaneously with great improvements in patient care, particularly for heart attack victims. The new design requirements for the ambulances and increased expectations for training eventually led to the decline in funeral home transports and the rise in EMS provided by central Ohio fire departments. Ohio State emergency medicine residents experienced their EMS in the new ambulance structures from the beginning of the residency program (Figure 8).

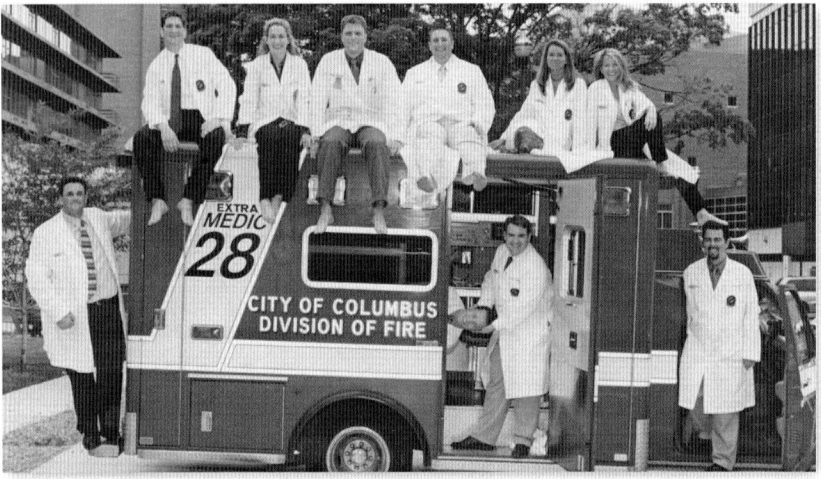

Figure 8: Ambulance requirements in the 1970s called for the larger boxlike structures to be mounted on a truck frame. Emergency Medicine training included participating with crews throughout central Ohio. Pictured above is the class of 2004 on a Columbus Fire medic vehicle. From left are: Robert Paasche, MD; Robert Moskowitz, MD; Anna "Kate" Corbin, MD; Fred Tzystuck, MD; M. Jacob Ott, MD; Matthew Sanders, DO; Amy Ramey, MD; Cynthia Bowers-Lee, MD; and Richard Limperos, MD.

Modern EMS and Ohio State

With the development of advanced treatment methods for heart attack and other emergencies in the 1960s, a new model of care began to emerge: advanced emergency care delivered at the scene of an event by specially trained rescuers. With time the rescuers became known as emergency medical technicians and paramedics. Most historians credit the efforts of faculty leaders at Ohio State as being among the first pioneers in this development. The "Heartmobile" developed at Ohio State and the City of Columbus in 1969 (Chapter 16) initiated the modern system of EMS.

From the initiation of the heartmobile project in 1969 until 1987, Ohio State physicians were medical directors of the Columbus Division of

Fire. The first was Richard Lewis, MD (cardiology), followed by John Stang, MD (cardiology), who served from 1980 to 1984. The third was Douglas Rund, MD (emergency medicine), who served from 1984 to 1987. When Rund was appointed, the Medical Director position was split into two positions: field operations and education and research. Rund was the Director for Education and Research and Richard Esler, DO, was the Director for Field Operations. In 1987 Rund went on sabbatical leave to become a Senior Research Fellow for the North Atlantic Treaty Alliance (NATO) and to study epidemiology at the University of Edinburgh in anticipation of becoming Interim Chair of the Department of Preventive Medicine in 1988 at Ohio State. Upon Rund's departure, the City of Columbus sought independent medical direction and David P. Keseg, MD, replaced Rund as Medical Director for Education and Research. The positions were combined into one in 1991 and Keseg held the position of Medical Director for the Columbus Division of Fire until 2019. Years later he joined the Ohio State faculty and was a key figure in starting the fellowship program in Emergency Medical Services.

Columbus Fire Department Emergency Medical Services, 1991 to 2019

David P. Keseg, MD, became the Medical Director for Education and Research in 1987 (Figure 9). He next took over the medical director for field operations from Richard Esler, DO, who resigned his position in 1991. The medical director position was then consolidated into a single position instead of two. Keseg became Medical Director for the Columbus Division of Fire. He was initially on part time at 20 hours a week. He became full time in 2002 when Ned Pettus became the Fire Chief for the Columbus Fire Department (CFD) and felt that the Division of Fire needed a full-time medical director. Keseg served in this role until his retirement in July 2019.

A Two-Tiered System Changes to a Single System

The Columbus Fire Department Emergency Medical Services (CFD

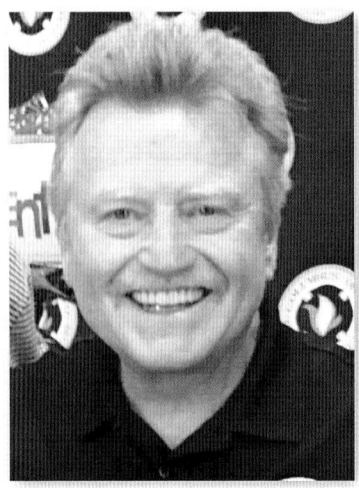

Figure 9: David P. Keseg, MD, was the Medical Director of the Columbus Division of Fire from 1987 to 2019. Later in his career he joined the faculty at Ohio State and helped establish the Fellowship in Emergency Medical Services.

EMS) had started out as a two-tier system that had both Basic Life Support (BLS) and Advanced Life Support (ALS) response components. For many years four of the ALS units were placed strategically throughout the city. The paramedics staffing the ALS units were considered the elite of the EMS providers and typically possessed outstanding lifesaving skills. They tended to perform many procedures including intubations because there were so few to manage so many critical patients. In 1996, in an effort to decrease EMS response time, the department changed to an all-ALS system. A paramedic was required to be on all engines and all medic transport vehicles. This allowed for an ALS capability to be offered on all 911 calls. It also required a larger number of paramedics to be working within the Division of Fire so the training program had to be augmented and new hires had to commit to getting their "medic card" eventually. Training up this number of paramedics was a tremendous accomplishment and required both human and monetary resources.

Innovations

Over time many innovations were initiated with the Division of Fire EMS, including Continuous Positive Airway Pressure (CPAP), intranasal medications, intraosseous lines, Cardiopulmonary Resuscitation (CPR) machines—including the LUCAS chest compression system—and transmission of EKGs to hospital emergency departments. The Division participated in many initiatives with the Central Ohio Trauma System, including trauma care and transport, destination decisions for ST segment elevation myocardial infarction (STEMI) and stroke, and diversion policies. A Comfort Care protocol was developed to address end-of-life situations. The Division was the lead agency to plan for and implement the Stroke Transport Vehicle in collaboration with Columbus' three adult hospital systems.

Infectious disease protocols were developed and implemented and a process for managing exposures was instituted. Protocols to respond to outbreaks of AIDS, SARS, COVID and Ebola were put into place. Infectious disease coordinators were established within the Division of Fire and policies and procedures were established. Keseg successfully championed legislation to allow paramedics to administer influenza vaccinations to their colleagues. Lactate monitors were provided by The Ohio State University Department of Emergency Medicine and utilized in a research project focusing on care of the sepsis patient in the field.

The opiate epidemic impacted the Division of Fire EMS, which administered naloxone (Narcan) to patients throughout the city many times a day. Despite these efforts, mortality rates for opiate overdose increased steadily. The Division, led by Chief James Davis and Matt Parrish, developed the Rapid Response Emergency Addiction and Crisis Team (RREACT) to proactively engage patients who had experienced an opiate overdose in their homes, and try and convince them to seek treatment for their Opiate Use Disorder. This program became a benchmark for many other EMS systems nationally. The Columbus Fire Department also helped to establish the first Addiction Stabilization Center to directly accept from EMS patients who had been successfully revived from an opiate overdose and wanted to seek treatment.

Keseg set up committees within the Division of Fire to focus on EMS equipment, EMS protocols, EMS research, Pediatrics and EMS Week. EMS Week was always an impactful event with each day of the week highlighting CPR education, cardiac arrest survival and other important facets of EMS. The EMS protocol committee met quarterly and updated the protocol to keep it current. The EMS research committee reviewed and vetted many EMS research proposals that involved cardiac arrest, trauma care and pediatrics. Scientific papers were published and the Division of Fire gained recognition in the research community.

Keseg was asked to review and vet the safety of the TASER device for the Columbus Department of Public Safety and the Columbus Police

Department. He testified before Columbus City Council and produced documents attesting to the relative safety of the device. His findings allowed the Columbus Police Department to deploy this device, resulting in improved safety for both the police and the community.

Chief Shawn Koser established the first EMS Quality Management System with Keseg and developed QA/PI policies and procedures to utilize within the Division of Fire. This endeavor allowed the Division to scientifically measure quality of care and match any deficiencies with education to correct them. That area has grown to incorporate more staff members and has increased its capacity.

In 2008 the City of Columbus started to charge Columbus residents for EMS transport, which required the institution of an electronic patient record. Once the electronic patient record was established, the collected data electronically assisted in the Quality Management (QM) process and greatly enhanced EMS leaders' ability to make necessary changes in process and policies. Trends could be followed and planning could anticipate changes in protocols.

Soon thereafter, Keseg joined the Department of Emergency Medicine at Ohio State and became an Adjunct Professor. As a faculty member he helped the Ohio State University Department of Emergency Medicine establish an EMS Fellowship Program. Eric Cortez, MD, was the first fellow to complete the program. Three of the EMS Fellows have elected to stay and work in the central Ohio area.

Early Faculty Commitment to EMS

From the outset, the faculty of the Department of Emergency Medicine realized that EMS was a critically important part of the new specialty. It was one area where the claim of expertise could be substantiated. Cardiologists started the Heartmobile and surgeons pioneered air medical EMS for trauma. But when the Division of Emergency Medicine was formed in 1978, it was soon to be the emergency physician who was expert in the whole gamut of emergency conditions and the first to see the patient upon arrival of the ambulance.

Fire departments and educational institutions were looking for EMS leadership. Richard Nelson, MD, the first residency trained emergency physician in the Division of Emergency Medicine and in all of central Ohio, became the Medical Director of the Westerville Fire Department from 1981 until 1990. He was also the Medical Director of the Grandview Heights Fire Department in the same period. He recruited residents to serve as "assistant" medical directors, which became their residency EMS experience. Among such residents were Howard Werman, MD, Theresa Bridges, MD, and Ronald Pirrallo, MD (Figure 10). Pirrallo established a national reputation for excellence in EMS and eventually became the President of the National Association of EMS Physicians (NAEMSP). Years later he reflected on his experience as a resident:

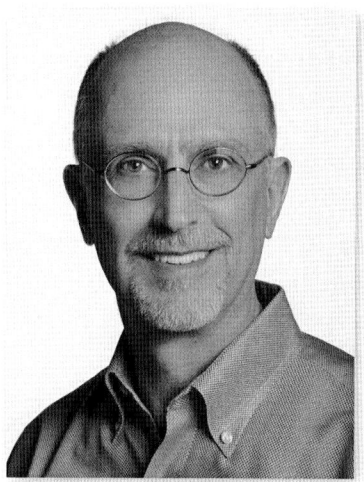

Figure 10: Ronald G. Pirrallo, MD, became a leading national figure in Emergency Medical Services: President of the National Association of EMS Physicians and Vice Chair of the Department of Emergency Medicine at The University of South Carolina School of Medicine. He credits the beginning of his academic career in emergency medical services to the inspiration he received from the Ohio State faculty. Pirrallo finished the residency program in 1990.

My academic career clearly was started in Columbus, Ohio. Howie Werman was my advisor and he introduced me to EMS. My rotation was with the Westerville Fire Department, which led to my embracing emergency medical services, not only in the subspecialty, but as my area of research and innovation. I have photos of me flying in SKYMED. It was my Christmas photo that I sent to family and friends as a senior resident.[6]

Nelson also started the Basic Trauma Life Support program (BTLS) in Ohio around 1985. The program ultimately became the International Trauma Life Support (ITLS) course. He also served on the ITLS Board of Directors and later the editorial board. Nelson and Howard Werman, MD, wrote chapters for the textbooks and Nelson wrote the written exams. Ann Dietrich, MD, Pediatric Emergency Medicine faculty member at Ohio State, started Pediatric BTLS during the same time.

Howard A. Werman, MD, was a resident in one of the first residency classes to graduate in 1984. He was asked by Nelson to serve in one of the "assistant" medical director roles in Westerville. Nelson fostered Werman's love for prehospital medicine and was an inspiring role model as well. Werman had an outstanding career in EMS. Werman gradually became the EMS expert in the department. He was the medical director for the university's own Ohio State EMS and Fire Prevention service in the 1980s. He soon became the Medical Director for the university's initial helicopter program, SKYMED, in 1988. When the helicopter program reconfigured in 1995 and became MedFlight, he became the Medical Director and remained in that position for most of his career.

During his tenure Werman held important leadership positions in EMS. He served as Chair of the Board of Directors of the National Registry of Emergency Medical Technicians (NREMT). He also served on the national American College of Emergency Physicians (ACEP) and Ohio ACEP EMS Committees, the State EMS Board and Trauma Subcommittee and was a liaison representative to NREMT from the National Association of EMS Physicians. He also served as Medical Director for Grandview Heights and Mifflin Township Fire and EMS. Additionally, he served as a member of the Governor's Advisory Council on EMS.

Columbus State Community College

The EMS Technology program at Columbus State Community College began in the late 1970s when the college was still named the Columbus Technical Institute. The program provided fire science instruction and education to qualify for an EMT Certificate and a Paramedic certificate. The program also always offered a two-year Associate Degree in EMS. In 1981 Douglas Rund, MD, FAEMS, was asked to become the medical director of the program. He remained in that position for the next 40 years (Figure 11).

The Columbus State link with Ohio State has always been strong. Over the years there have been efforts to link a Bachelor's degree offered at Ohio State to the associate degree from Columbus State to complete a 4-year degree program in EMS. The effort was never completed. The

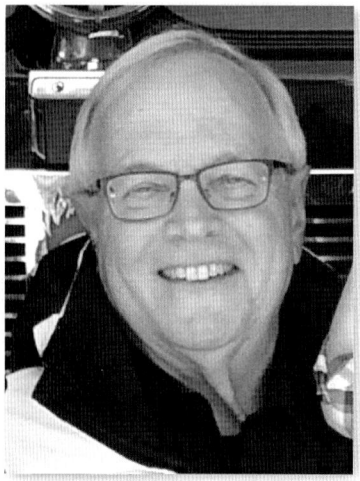

Figure 11: Douglas A Rund, MD, FAEMS, was the Medical Director of the Columbus State Community College EMS Technology Program, serving from 1981 to 2021. He served as the Medical Director for Education and Research for the Columbus Division of Fire from 1984 to 1987 and Medical Director of the City of Worthington Division of Fire and EMS from 2003 to 2024.

program has had associate and co-directors over the years. Following Rund's retirement from the Director position in 2021, Creagh Boulger, MD, and Brooke Moungey, MD, became the medical directors.

Boulger was an exceptional resident in emergency medicine finishing the program in 2011. Working almost constantly, she became a critical contributor to the ultrasound program where she established a nationwide reputation for excellence. She also became a departmental leader in the trauma program. An outstanding physician, Boulger was a perfect choice to help direct the EMS program at Columbus State in 2011. She was selected Professor of the Year by the College of Medicine graduating class of 2017. In many respects, her election for this prestigious award fulfilled one of the early dreams of the founders: to be recognized for excellence in the education of the medical students. She made the rapid ascent to the rank of full Professor in 2022 (Figure 12).

Brooke M. Moungey, MD, completed her medical training at the University of Wisconsin School of Medicine and Public Health, followed by residency training in Emergency Medicine at the University of Wisconsin Hospital and Clinics. During that time, she served as a Flight Physician for the University of Wisconsin's Medflight program and subsequently completed Fellowship training in Medical Education. Moungey joined the core faculty at Ohio State in 2018 as an Assistant Professor. Since that time, she has applied her expertise in curriculum design and implementation to the education of medical students, residents and EMS providers. She became the EMS Course Director for the EM and EM/IM residency programs as well as the faculty lead for the EMS Longitudinal Track,

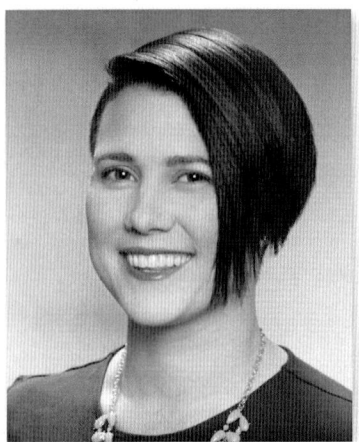 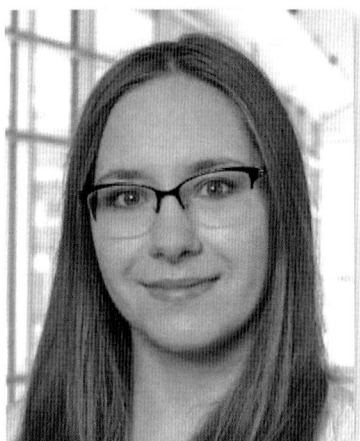

Figure 12: Creagh Boulger, MD, is the Medical Director of the EMS Technology program at Columbus State Community College and Professor of Emergency Medicine at Ohio State. She is expert in emergency medical services, trauma and ultrasound. She was elected Professor of the Year by the College of Medicine graduating class in 2017.

Figure 13: Brooke M. Moungey, MD, is the Associate Medical Director of the EMS Technology Program at Columbus State Community College. She is expert in teaching and educational methods.

which is designed to give resident physicians opportunities to prepare for Fellowship training in EMS.

She also continued her passion for EMS outside the hospital, and became an Associate Medical Director for Delaware County EMS and Columbus State Community College's EMS programs. In addition, she now serves as Medical Director for a number of Union County EMS agencies, including Allen Township Fire Department, Leesburg Township Fire Department, Marysville Division of Fire, Northern Union County Joint Fire and EMS District, Southeast Hardin Northwest Union Joint Fire District, Union Township Fire Department, and the Union County Sheriff's Office (Figure 13).

The Ohio State Center for Emergency Medical Services

The Ohio State University operated its own Emergency Medical Services (EMS) service within the Division of Public Safety until the early 1990s. The service had excellent paramedics and Howard Werman, MD, was the Medical Director. When Ohio State discontinued this service in 1991, the university had to rely on the City of Columbus to provide emergency medical services on campus, which provided an excellent opportunity to try something new. The university had just added its entire student body and staff to the potential workload to the Division of Fire. At the same time, the Division was looking for additional educational resources to train its paramedics. The result: the creation of the Ohio State Center for EMS. The initial concept was to model itself after the Center for EMS in Pittsburgh, which was supported by all of the health care systems in the city and housed at University of Pittsburgh Medical Center (UPMC). To show its initial support for the concept, the Ohio State College of Medicine arranged transport for key medical and administrative leaders and high-ranking officers and influential paramedics within the Columbus Division of Fire to travel together to Pittsburgh for a visit to the center.

Highlights of the Center for EMS at UPMC included an *education center* for its paramedic training program and emergency medicine residency, an *active research program*, the Department of Emergency Medicine offices, offices for their air medical transport program (partially staffed by EM residents) and a communication center where active medical direction was provided to the City of Pittsburgh EMS, a third-service within the city structure.

Following the visit by leaders from Ohio State and Columbus Fire, a proposal was drawn up to create such a Center on the Ohio State campus with the concomitant location of the Division of Fire working EMS station and education center on the Medical Center campus. The guiding visions for the proposed Center were innovation in emergency medical services, regional paramedic education and a robust effort to study and publish the center's accomplishments. Such efforts would enhance out-of-hospital care for all in central Ohio and help re-establish its national reputation for excellence in EMS. A budget was prepared, which included city and university cost sharing. Unfortunately, the University decided not to support the proposal and the project was shelved. An opportunity was lost.

In 2000 Craig Key, MD, joined the faculty. Key had been an assistant EMS medical director for the City of Houston under Paul Pepe, MD. One of his first assignments was to revisit the original planning document for the Center for EMS (CEMS). He pulled the original document "off the shelf," reworked it and reestablished the Center for EMS in 2004. Through his leadership the Center advanced its academic mission for innovation, education and research. One of the accomplishments of the Center under Key was the development of unique medical conferences such as a leadership conference co-led by the Department of Emergency Medicine and the Fisher College of Business at Ohio State.

In 2017 Ashley Larrimore, MD, became the medical director of the Center for EMS. Under her leadership the span of activity increased. In her words:

> *We expanded a lot of the education we were doing. We were doing conferences; we were doing a lot more outreach. During the time I was there we had the Cardiac Arrest Registry to Enhance Survival (CARES) underneath the Center for EMS for a bit. We expanded the people who were working with us. We had a data person and more senior outreach people so we were able to spend more time at our departments which was great. We were focusing a little bit more on our EMS provider wellness. So, we were partnering with the James mobile kitchen to do meals, talk to them about healthy eating; sometimes we would bring an athletic trainer out to talk a little about keeping themselves healthy on the job in terms of lifting. I think the focus has now shifted somewhat from doing some of the bigger external programs to focusing on individual agencies and partnering in terms of medical direction.[7]*

Over time the center has had many leaders and reporting relationships. One of the center's current areas of emphasis regards the recognition, on scene management and transport of patients with time critical diseases such as stroke, myocardial infarction, sepsis and major trauma. The current mission statement for the center reflects the significance of this focus:

The Center for Emergency Medical Services (CEMS) at the Ohio State University Wexner Medical Center serves as an expert resource for all prehospital activity by conducting targeted outreach, providing expansive and comprehensive education, and finding innovative ways to improve quality in partnership with our emergency department, time critical disease clinical teams and local EMS.[8]

Following Larrimore, Michael Dick, MD, became the center director. He was also the Medical Director of Ohio State East Emergency Department and the Upper Arlington Fire Department. Following Dick's untimely death in 2023, Travis Sharkey, MD, PhD, who is a graduate of the EMS fellowship and is Associate Medical Director of the City of Worthington Division of Fire and EMS, became the center director.

The Center works on new innovations such as improving feedback for EMS agencies that transport patients to Ohio State. New data platforms streamline record sharing between the Emergency Department and other medical center sites. As a result, hospitals can now automatically and securely share clinical outcome data with EMS so care teams can review and improve protocols to support better patient outcomes.

The CEMS also helps provide comprehensive EMS medical direction, quality improvement and systems design services for local EMS agencies and the communities they serve. This vital role helps to improve the quality of care that patients receive in the prehospital setting.

The EMS medical directors in the center are board certified emergency physicians with extensive training and EMS experience. Each has completed the requirements set forth by the State of Ohio for the position of medical director and has knowledge and training in the following areas:

- Medical aspects of care consistent with the mission profile of both ground and air ambulance services;

- Aspects of ground service EMS units, including pertinent regulatory and safety issues, vehicle capabilities, and equipment requirements and performance;

- Operational aspects of communications equipment and dispatch procedures;

- Training in prehospital and interhospital transport issues and laws;
- Medical control and medical command issues, such as protocols, standing orders, triage and the capabilities of care providers; and
- Quality improvement theories and applications.

Table 1 lists the central Ohio EMS Medical Directors who are faculty members of the Department of Emergency Medicine at Ohio State.

Table 1. Central Ohio EMS Medical Directors*

AGENCY	MEDICAL DIRECTOR
Clinton Township	Nicole McAllister, DO, MA
Columbus State EMS Program	Creagh Boulger, MD Brooke Moungey, MD
Delaware County EMS	Ashish Panchal, MD, PhD, FAEMS Brooke Moungey, MD Nicole McAllister, DO, MA
Medflight	Ashley Larrimore, MD, FAEMS
Muirfield Memorial Tournament	Travis Sharkey, MD, PhD
National Trail Raceway	Craig Key, MD
Newark Fire Department	Ashley Larrimore, MD, FAEMS
Thorn Township Fire Department	Ashley Larrimore, MD, FAEMS
Union County Agencies	Brooke Moungey, MD
Upper Arlington Fire Department	Michael Dick, MD, *until 2023*
Whitehall Fire Department	Ashley Larrimore, MD, FAEMS
Worthington Fire and EMS	Douglas Rund, MD, FAEMS Travis Sharkey, MD, PhD

* All are also faculty members of the Department of Emergency Medicine at Ohio State.

References

1. Hazzard K. *American Sirens*. New York: Hachette Books; 2022:48.

2. Bell RC. *The Ambulance*. Jefferson, NC, and London: McFarland and Company; 2009.

3. Rund DA and Rausch TS. *Triage*. St. Louis, MO: Mosby; 1981.

4. Good WR. Interview with Douglas Rund. 2022: Columbus, Ohio.

5. Hall WT. *200 Year Anniversary. Columbus Division of Fire*. Sikeston, MO: Acclaim Press; 2023.

6. Pirrallo RG. Interview with Douglas Rund. 2022: Columbus, Ohio.

7. Larrimore AD. Interview with Ashley Larrimore, MD, by Douglas Rund. 2023: Columbus, Ohio.

8. https://wexnermedical.osu.edu/healthcare-professionals/center-for-ems.

Chapter 15
Air Medical Transport

Howard A. Werman, MD
Steven Steinberg, MD

History of Air Medical Transport

The first known use of air transport was reported to have occurred during the Franco-Prussian War during the Siege of Paris. Hot air balloons were reportedly used to evacuate wounded soldiers from the battlefield. Whether this transport actually occurred is a matter of some controversy.[1] What is known is that fixed wing aircraft were used to evacuate wounded soldiers during WWI. This first use of aircraft under these conditions was attributed to the British who used biplane aircraft to retrieve a wounded soldier from Turkey in 1917.[2] Both the French and British used airplanes to evacuate wounded soldiers during the colonial wars in Northern Africa and the Middle East during the 1920s.

In the United States, wounded soldiers were evacuated by helicopter from the jungles of Burma during World War II.[3] The dedicated use of rotary winged aircraft was first observed during the Korean conflict, as depicted in the television show *M.A.S.H.* However, it was during the Vietnam War when helicopters became instrumental in the retrieval of wounded soldiers from the battlefield during Operation Dustoff.[4] Trauma surgeons returning from Vietnam recognized the value of moving injured soldiers from the battlefront to a field trauma hospital; it wasn't long before the same model was adopted for the civilian trauma population.

The first civilian use of aircraft for medical evacuations was probably found in scarcely populated areas of Canada, Australia and Scandinavia. The first known civilian aircraft used for medical evaluations was credited to Walter Schaefer in Los Angeles in 1947. The concept of dedicated helicopters for medical transport was credited to several government and civilian entities who were early adopters of this new paradigm, including Superior Ambulance, the Maryland State Police and St. Anthony's Flight for Life, which is generally recognized as the first hospital-based air medical transport program in the United States.[5] In 1980, a year before The Ohio State University Medical Center started its residency, 32 programs operated 39 helicopters and flew about 17,000 patient missions each year.

The development of trauma systems in the United States coincided with the increase in popularity of the air transport programs, which were bolstered by civilian air medical transport's role in reducing trauma mortality. Baxt and Moody published their findings in *JAMA* in 1983, demonstrating that compared with patients transported by ground, patients transported by air transport had a 52% reduction in mortality.[6] Further work published in 1985 calculated the expected mortality in a group of patients based on their trauma severity scores. There was a 21% reduction in expected mortality among these patients treated and transported by air. The study was conducted using data from seven air transport programs throughout the United States.[7]

As a result, many trauma centers saw air medical transport as an integral part of expanding their service to rural and suburban communities, which led to a significant expansion in both the number of programs and air transport resources throughout the United States. According to the Atlas & Database of Air Medical Services (ADAMS) Database, in 2017 nearly 300 air transport programs operated over 900 fixed and rotary winged aircraft, completing over 500,000 patient transports annually.

Early Development of an Air Transport Program at Ohio State

The development of an air transport program at Ohio State University Hospital started within the Department of Surgery, thanks to Robert Zollinger, MD, Chair of the Department of Surgery. Zollinger, who had an impressive background in combat trauma from his service in WW II, recruited Stuart Roberts MD, to Ohio State in 1967. Roberts was familiar with Operation Dustoff used during the Vietnam conflict and felt that helicopters could be used to transport injured and critically ill patients to Ohio State (Figure 1).

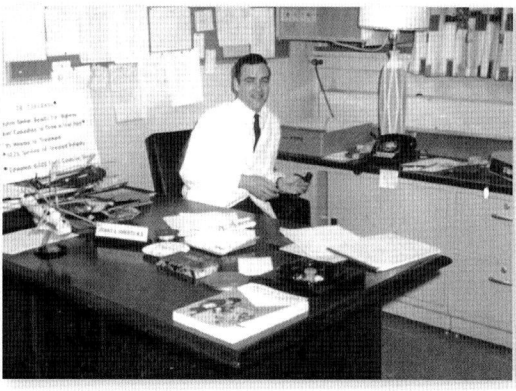

Figure 1: Stuart Roberts, MD, in his office at Ohio State *(photo courtesy of Cynthia Roberts)*.

The first opportunity came in November 1967 when Roberts mobilized the Army National Guard to transport a patient with a dissecting thoracic aorta to Ohio State. Following this first successful transport, Roberts worked with the Governor's office, Army National Guard and State Highway Patrol to establish the first air transport program using a dedicated aircraft. The helicopter was equipped with two stretchers, medical equipment, and communications capabilities. His goal was to "test the feasibility of the use of helicopters equipped with appropriate communication devices to (1) move critically ill patients from community hospitals to the medical center (University Hospital), and (2) move physicians and medical equipment directly to the accident site on major highways to evacuate victims to the medical center."[8]

The Medicopter program was staffed by residents, attending physicians and nurses. During the first 50 transports, 25 were transported directly from the accident scene, of which 94% survived. Roberts eventually recognized the need to train paramedics to assist in staffing the program, which led him

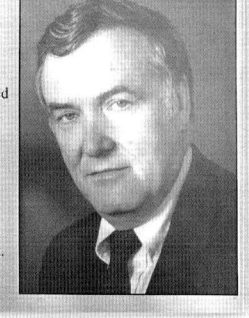

Figure 2: This plaque on the Ohio State Helipad honors the contributions of Stuart Roberts, MD *(photo courtesy of Cynthia Roberts)*.

to develop a manual to train these individuals in the early stabilization and care of trauma patients. Roberts left Ohio State in 1972 and the program was ultimately not sustained. A plaque on the current helipad honors Roberts and his many contributions to Ohio State (Figure 2).

Development of an Air Transport Program at Ohio State

Roberts' departure left a void in air transport resources in central Ohio until 1982, when Grant Medical Center established the LifeFlight program, thanks to the advocacy of Robert Falcone, MD. LifeFlight was based on Grant Medical Center's rooftop helipad. The program provided access to trauma patients in central and southeastern Ohio and allowed rural hospitals the ability to transport complex medical patients to Columbus. This air transport resource was often used by Ohio State Emergency Medicine residents such as Michael Kelley, MD, Robert Behrendt, MD, Mark Smith, MD, Ken Kidwell MD, and Howard Werman, MD, who were able to 'moonlight' in smaller rural hospitals in southeast Ohio.

Eventually, the administrative leadership of the Medical Center recognized the value of the 'flying billboard' in expanding referrals to the institution and reached out to Grant Medical Center to explore the potential to participate in the LifeFlight program. When these talks failed, the Ohio State Medical Center CEO Michael Covert reached out to two other area hospitals (Mount Carmel East Hospital and St. Anthony's Hospital) and decided to form a consortium with the purpose of establishing a competing air transport program. The new program was called SKYMED and the program operated a Sikorsky S-76 aircraft with a nurse and paramedic crew. David Kerins was hired as the new program's executive director and Olga Chavez, RN, was the program's chief flight nurse. The program was based at Lane Aviation at Port Columbus Airport. For a time both SKYMED and LifeFlight operated concurrently (Figure 3).

The SKYMED program began operations in November 1987, with John Drstvensek, MD ("Dr. D"), serving as the program's first medical director. A medical advisory committee was established and includ-

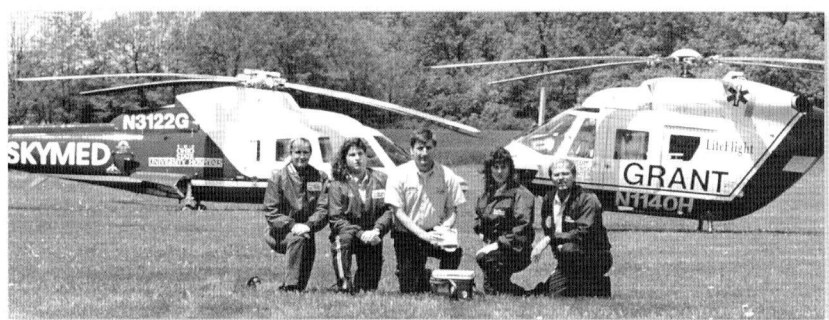

Figure 3: Columbus SKYMED and Grant LifeFlight prior to the programs' merger in 1995 (photo courtesy of Woody Schubert, EMT-P).

ed Drstvensek, Richard Schlanger, MD, and Howard Werman, MD. Operating costs for an air transport program are quite expensive and within months, the two other hospitals in the SKYMED consortium realized that they failed to generate the referrals to justify supporting this costly endeavor. By March 1988, Mount Carmel East Hospital and St. Anthony's Hospital withdrew from the consortium and Werman assumed the role as program medical director. At the time, Werman was serving as the medical director for three ground Emergency Medical Services (EMS): Ohio State University EMS and Fire Prevention, Grandview Heights Fire and EMS, and Mifflin Township Fire and EMS. Additionally, he was serving as a member of the Governor's Advisory Council on EMS under Richard Celeste.

The program grew in popularity based on the strong referral patterns to the medical center. In addition, Columbus Children's Hospital (as it was known at that time) joined the consortium in order to support its strong neonatal and pediatric transport programs. In fact, in order to maximize the availability of the helicopter resource, a unique program was established whereby neonatal teams were delivered to the referral hospitals by helicopter and were retrieved by ground resources.[9]

Eventually, the SKYMED program added an additional aircraft that operated 12 hours daily. This came at a time when the LifeFlight program announced the addition of a third base in Coshocton, Ohio. This escalation in competition between the two programs drew the attention of business leaders in town who were alarmed by rising health care costs and were concerned about safety issues in the medical transport industry. They exerted pressure on Grant Medical Center and the Ohio

State University Medical Center to merge the two programs and in mid-1993, talks began.

The formal merger took place on April 18, 1995, and the MedFlight program was created. At the time of the merger, the program operated four BK-117 aircraft: two at Columbus at Don Scott Airport; one in Wellston, Ohio; and one in Coshocton, Ohio. Rodney Crane was the program's President and CEO and Cathy Jaynes, RN, was the chief flight nurse. Medical direction was provided jointly by Robert Falcone, MD, and Werman. Approximately one year later, Grant Medical Center and Riverside Methodist Hospital joined forces to become OhioHealth. Riverside Methodist Hospital operated a ground critical care service, which was incorporated into the program. In addition, MedFlight operated a fixed-wing aircraft from 1997-2007. Finally, in 2010, the MedCare ground basic life support and advanced life support transport services were added to the program (Figure 4).

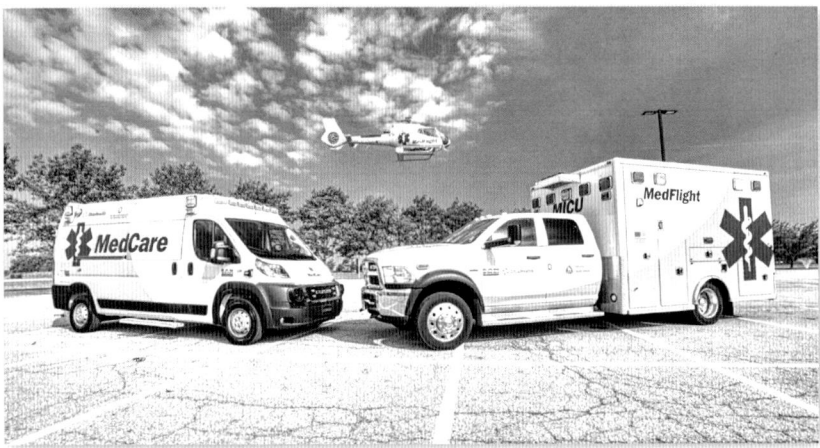

Figure 4: MedFlight Air and Mobile ICU alongside a MedCare Ambulance *(Photo courtesy of Todd Bailey).*

Currently, the program supports nine air transport bases as well as six ground critical care bases throughout the state. The ALS/BLS program completed almost 50,000 transports in 2021 throughout central and southeast Ohio and is rapidly expanding.

Medical Direction

Ashley Larrimore, MD, FAEMS (current Ohio State Emergency Medicine faculty member), and Bradley Raetzke, MD (Ohio State residency graduate), serve as the program's co-medical directors. Larrimore received her Doctor of Medicine degree from George Washington University School of Medicine in 2011. She completed her residency at the University of Massachusetts in Worcester in 2014 and her fellowship in emergency medical services at the University of Cincinnati Medical Center in 2015. She then joined the Department of Emergency Medicine at Ohio State as the first fellowship trained EMS physician in the department. Air medical care and transport has been her passion from the outset. In 2021 she took over the MedFlight directorship from Howard Werman, MD. In the past she had served as the medical director of the Center for EMS from 2016 to 2021 (Figure 5).

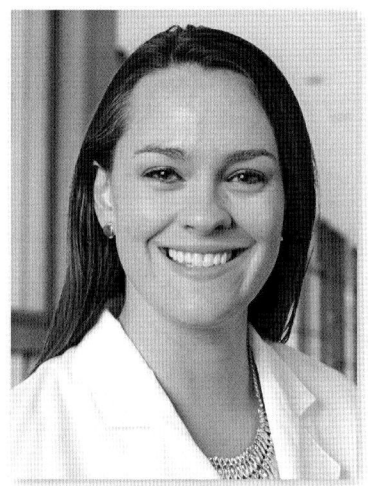

Figure 5: Ashley Larrimore, MD, FAEMS is the current co-medical director of MedFlight

Larrimore was honored as the medical director of the year in 2022 at the Annual Ohio Emergency Medical Services Star of Life Awards ceremony presented by the Ohio Department of Public Safety's Division of EMS, the State Board of Medical Fire and Transportation Services (EMFTS) and the Ohio Chapter of the American College of Emergency Physicians. She is also the Medical Director of the Newark Division of Fire and EMS, and the Whitehall Division of Fire and the Thorn township Fire Department.

In looking at the achievements of MedFlight, especially during the COVID epidemic, Larrimore recalled the following:

> We have actually been having a few really exciting years at MedFlight. When MedFlight purchased MedCare it allowed us to do everything from BLS all the way up to critical care or medical care transport. We

also changed the way our MICU division is running; we are constantly focusing on our training. With each incremental change we are able to do a little bit more. We are partnering with Ohio State to be able to transport ECMO patients which has been very exciting. We have really been focusing with our education team and with our leadership in trying to do more, just knowing the types of patients that we are caring for. Although we had already been seeing increasing numbers of very sick patients for a while, when COVID hit one of the things we recognized is that suddenly we were seeing more and more life-threatening respiratory illnesses. We were having to learn to deal expertly with very challenging ventilator management and it really pushed our crews to be able to do more and better.

We have also been able to expand the types of equipment that we have, we are working to make sure that every person in the company is really brought up to a higher level of critical care thinking. My favorite part of emergency medicine is those really sick patients that we get. We figure out what's wrong with them, we get them stabilized and they go on and survive and do well. Emergency physicians should get full credit for that. These are the patients that we have the biggest impact on. Then to be able to be doing that and maybe indirectly impacting thousands of those patients a year through MedFlight and our people is so rewarding. It's incredible to hear about the types of cases that our EMS clinicians are handling in the field and if you look back to the birth of EMS, you go from ambulance drivers to professionals who must manage increasingly complex cases and figure out how to manage the patient with more and more sophisticated knowledge of pathophysiology. It is so fulfilling to see how far we have come.[10]

Ohio State Emergency Medicine attending physicians and residents provide on-line medical support to the MedFlight nurses and paramedics. The Emergency Medicine residents ride as observers as part of the program, participate in quality improvement activities, conduct chart reviews and take part in the program's annual Core Competency training activities. In addition, the Ohio State Wexner Medical Center's EMS fellows participate in these activities at MedFlight as well.

Innovations/National Recognition

The MedFlight program has achieved several important recognitions for its innovation and safety. Each year medical support team members speak at the national Air Medical Transport Conference about their clinical, quality assurance, operations, educational and administrative innovations for which MedFlight has been known as an industry leader.

The primary achievement of this program has been the outstanding growth in the program from four aircraft performing almost 2,500 missions to a full EMS service from basic life support ambulance to air critical care transport. In fiscal year 2021, the aircraft completed 4,315 transports and ground critical care completed 2,764 missions.

There have been individual accolades for the program as well. In 2006, Werman was awarded the Barbara A. Hess Award, which recognizes an individual who has significantly contributed to the enhancement, development and promotion of the emergency medical industry through their research or educational efforts.

In 2012, MedFlight received the American Eurocopter Vision Zero Safety Award for its safe operations as well as the program's safety initiatives, which served as a model for other programs in the industry. And finally in 2014, MedFlight was recognized as the Association of Air Medical Service's Program of the Year. The recognition honors an emergency medical transport service (national or international) that has demonstrated a superior level of patient care, management prowess, high-quality leadership through visionary and innovative approaches, customer service, safety consciousness, marketing ingenuity, community service, and a commitment to the medical transport community as a whole.

Howard A. Werman, MD, was also honored at the Ohio Star of Life ceremony in 2021 when he received the Jack B. Liberator Lifetime Achievement Award. Werman was honored for dedicating over 40 years to emergency medical care. The award noted that he had built incredible collaborations with leaders in the field of EMS and contributed numerous publications to the areas of resuscitation, patient transport, trauma and EMS practices. The text of the award also noted that "his charisma and passion have had a positive impact on EMS through his lifetime of leadership." [11]

Finally, a number of peer-reviewed publications by faculty, residents and medical students have been generated as part of the program, as indicated in the list below:

Werman HA, Falcone RE, et al. Helicopter transport of patients to tertiary care centers after cardiac arrest. *Am J Emerg Med*. 1999;17:130-134.

Falcone RE, Herron H, Dean B, Werman H. Emergency scene endotracheal intubation before and after the introduction of a rapid sequence induction protocol. *Air Med J*. 1996;15(4):163-7.

Herron H, Falcone R, Dean B, Werman H. 8.5 French peripheral intravenous access during air medical transport of the injured patient. *Air Med J*. 1997;16(1):7-10.

Stanhope K, Falcone RE, Werman HA. Helicopter dispatch: a time study. *Air Med J*. 1997;16(3):70-2.

Falcone RE, Herron H, Werman HA, Bonta M. Air medical transport of the injured patient: scene versus referring hospital. *Air Med J*. 1998;17(4):161-165.

Jaynes CL, Blevins G, Werman HA. Evaluating interfacility ground and air transport of the critical cardiac patient. *Air Med J*. 2022;21(2):37-41.

Larsen JT, Dietrich AM, Abdessalam SF, Werman HA. Effective use of air ambulance for pediatric trauma. *J Trauma*. 2004;56:89-93.

Werman HA, Schwegman D, Gerard J. The effect of etomidate on airway management practices of an air medical transport service. *Prehospital Emerg Care*. 2004;8:185-190.

Werman HA, Jaynes C, Blevins G. Impact of a triage tool on air versus ground transport of cardiac patients to a tertiary center. *Air Med J*. 2004;23(3):40-5.

Werman HA, Herron H, Deppe S, Betz S, et al. Clinical clearance of spinal immobilization in the air medical environment. *J Trauma*. 2008;64:1539-42.

Sinclair TD, Werman HA. Transfer of patients dependent on an intra-aortic balloon pump. *Air Med J*. 2009; 28:40-46.

Thomas H, Judge T, Lowell MJ, MacDonald RD, Madden J, Pickett K, Werman HA, et al. Airway management success and hypoxemia rates in air and ground critical care transport: a prospective multicenter study. *Prehosp Emerg Care*. 2010;4:283-293.

Hiestand B, Thomson D, Cudnik M, Werman HA. Succinylcholine versus roccuronium in prehospital air medical transport. *Prehosp Emerg Care*. 2011;15:457-463.

Cudnik MT, Werman HA, White LJ, Opalek JM. Prehospital factors associated with mortality in injured air medical patients. *Prehosp Emerg Care*. 2012;16:121-127.

Jaynes CL, Werman HA, White LJ. A blueprint for critical care transport research. *Air Med J*. 2013; 32(1):30-35.

Jaynes CL, Cook P, Farmer R, Werman HA, White L: Assessing satisfaction and quality in the EMS/HEMS working relationship. *Air Med J*. 2013;32(6):338-342.

Garey ML, Greenberger S, Werman HA. Ruptured splenic artery aneurysm in pregnancy: a case series. *Air Med J*. 2014; 33(5):214-7.

Krebs MG, Fletcher EN, Werman HA, McKenzie LB: Characteristics of nontrauma scene flights for air medical transport. *Air Med J*. 2014;33(6):320-5.

Jaynes C, Valdez A, Hamilton M, Haugen K, Henry C, Jones P, Werman HA, White LJ. Survivors perceptions of recovery following air medical transport accidents. *Prehosp Emerg Care*. 2015;19(1):44-52.

Werman HA, Zielinski A, Raetzke BD, Nappi JF. Limb reimplantation in air-transported patients: a 4-year review. *Air Med J*. 2016;35(4):239-241.

Pathan SA, Soulek J, Qureshi I, Werman HA, et al. Helicopter EMS and rapid transport for ST-elevation myocardial infarction. *J Emerg Med Trauma Acute Care*. https://doi.org/10.5339/jemtac.2017.8.

Krebs W, Higgins T, Buckley M, Augustine JJ, Raetzke BD, Werman HA. Botulism outbreak in a regional community hospital: lessons learned in transfer and transport considerations. *Prehosp Emerg Care*. 2019;31(1):49-57.

Billups K, Larrimore A, Li J, Werman H, Shirk MB. Impact of paralytic agent on post-intubation sedation. *Air Med J*. 2019;38(1):38-44.

Patterson PD, Moore CG, Guyette FX, Doman JM, Weaver MD, Sequeira DJ, Werman HA, et al. Real time fatigue mitigation with air-medical personnel: the SleepTrack TXT2 randomized trial. *Prehosp Emerg Care*. 2018:Oct 29;1-14.

Miyagi H, Evans D, Werman HA. Are there field triage criteria that can predict low-yield air medical transports? *Prehosp Disaster Med*. 2019;34(6):596–603.

Gilliam C, Evans DC, Spalding C, Burton J, Werman HA. Characteristics of scene trauma patients discharged within 24-hours of air medical transport. *Int J Crit Illn Inj Sci*. 2020;10(1):25-31.

References

1. Lam DM. To pop a balloon: aeromedical evacuation in the 1870 siege of Paris. *Aviat Space Environ Med*. 1988;59(10):988-991.

2. http://fly.historicwings.com/2013/02/first-aero-medical-evacuation/ accessed 12/23/2022.

3. Wartenberg S. Rescue in Burma. *Vertiflite*. 1987;33:36-39.

4. Dorland P, Nanney J: Dustoff: *Army Aeromedical Evacuation in Vietnam*. Washington, DC: Center of Military History, US Army; 2008.

5. Thomas F. The development of the nation's oldest operating civilian hospital-sponsored aeromedical helicopter service. *Avait Space Environ Med.* 1988;59(6):567-570.

6. Baxt WG, Moody P: The impact of a rotorcraft aeromedical emergency care service on trauma mortality. *JAMA.* 1983;249:3047-3051.

7. Baxt WG, Moody P, Cleveland HC, et al. Hospital-based rotorcraft aeromedical emergency care services and trauma mortality: a multicenter study. *Ann Emerg Med.* 1985;14:859-864.

8. McClung F. "Aerial Ambulance; A helicopter with medical personnel aboard speeds accident victims to the hospital in an Ohio experiment." *Bee-Hive.* United Aircraft. Summer 1968; 9-13.

9. Werman HA, Neely BN. One-way neonatal transports: A new approach to increase effective utilization of air medical resources. *Air Med J.* 1996;15(1):13-17.

10. Larrimore AD. Interview with Ashley Larrimore, MD, by Douglas Rund. 2023: Columbus, Ohio.

11. https://content.govdelivery.com/accounts/OHEMS/bulletins/3180074

Chapter 16

The Columbus Heartmobile: History and Influence

Craig B. Key, MD
Douglas A. Rund, MD

In the late 1960s as America was fascinated by manned space flight and the race to the moon, another innovation was quietly being developed in prehospital care. Following the lead of a cardiologist, Frank Pantridge, MD, of Belfast, Northern Ireland, a small group of physicians in the United States began to provide advanced prehospital care as never done before.[1,2]

Five cities, including Columbus (Ohio), Los Angeles, Miami, New York and Seattle, each developed the first metropolitan advanced out-of-hospital care systems in the United States. Among the physicians who led this innovation were Drs. James V. Warren, Michael Criley, Eugene L. Nagel, William J. Grace and Leonard A. Cobb. Each of these physicians was interested in treating cardiac problems such as "possible heart attacks" and cardiac arrest, which was termed "sudden death." These programs developed largely independent of each other.

Miami

Eugene Nagel, MD, was perhaps the first physician to provide advanced training to firefighters. As early as 1964 he began training firefighters in closed-chest massage, now known as CPR. By 1969 Nagel had trained firefighters to resuscitate patients from cardiac arrest. In June that year, Miami had its first hospital discharge of a cardiac arrest patient.[3]

New York

At St. Vincent's Hospital in Manhattan, William Grace, MD, began what was the United States' first mobile coronary care unit in 1968. Grace used ambulances based at St. Vincent's to transport physicians to the scene of cardiac emergencies. Like most early advanced prehospital medical programs, Grace targeted only cardiac patients.[3]

Columbus

Mobile coronary care in Columbus began with the Heartmobile program in April 1969. James Warren, MD, and team formulated the first vehicle specifically designed as a mobile coronary care unit, the Heartmobile, based on a recreational vehicle platform (Figure 1).[1] As in Manhattan, physicians were dispatched to assist with the care of cardiac patients. Unlike Manhattan, the Columbus program engaged firefighters to work alongside the physicians. Designed to transport the care and facilities of the Coronary Care Unit directly to the patient, the Heartmobile in Columbus facilitated patient treatment while en route to the hospital. In contrast, ambulances in New York were small and did not allow significant patient care during transportation.[4]

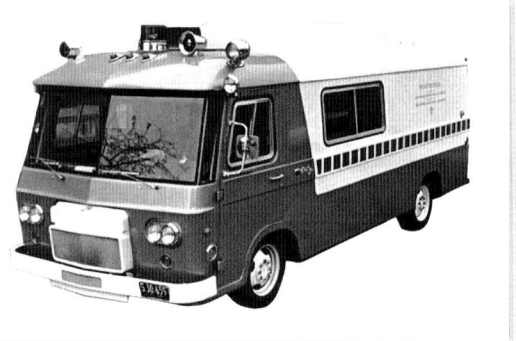

Figure 1: The Heartmobile, introduced in 1969 by Ohio State and the Columbus Division of Fire, was the starting point for subsequent EMS development in Columbus.

Los Angeles

December 1969 marked the beginning of mobile coronary care in Los Angeles, where Squad 59, an old forestry service station wagon, was housed at a small fire station on the grounds of Harbor General Hospital. It was there that Michael Criley, MD, trained the firefighters who responded with a nurse from Harbor General.[3]

Seattle

Using a system very similar to the Columbus Heartmobile program, Seattle established the Medic One program in March of 1970. Firefighters were trained at Harborview Medical Center and responded with physicians in a large recreational vehicle officially called Medic One. Firefighters affectionately referred to Medic One as "Moby Pig" (Figure 2).[4,5]

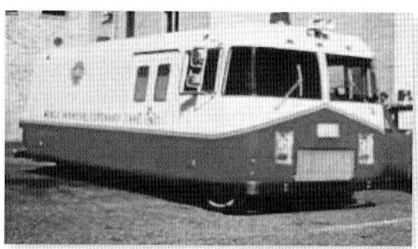

Figure 2: Seattle firefighter/medics nicknamed the initial Medic One emergency vehicle "Moby Pig."

The vehicle was a renovated Winnebago that "looked like an inverted bathtub." It was awkward to drive and usually overloaded with equipment.[6]

Background

In 1962 Bernard Lown, MD, published a report about the successful result of externally applied direct current (DC) electricity to treat and restore the heartbeat of a patient with a fibrillating heart.[7] Ventricular fibrillation was a leading cause of cardiac arrest and death in patients with heart attack, but treatments were limited and death was the usual outcome for untreated fibrillation. An effective intervention in this process would thus save many lives. The early apparatus needed to defibrillate was large and heavy. Hospital Coronary Care Units were developed to be able to treat patients with myocardial infarction and intervene in lethal arrhythmias with electricity and medication such as lidocaine. The Ohio State University Hospitals opened the first Coronary Care Unit in Columbus in 1964.

In time, defibrillator equipment became smaller in size but still not easily portable in those early years. Nevertheless, Frank Pantridge,

MD, a cardiologist in Northern Ireland, developed a mobile coronary care vehicle with a "relatively portable" defibrillator weighing over 150 pounds.[8] Pantridge and his colleagues began working on smaller instruments. By 1969 his work and that of others had resulted in much smaller defibrillation units. James Warren, MD, a cardiologist and the influential Chairman of the Department of Medicine at Ohio State, was known to travel extensively and met Pantridge in the United Kingdom. Pantridge had begun operating his "flying squads" in 1966 to respond to out-of-hospital patients with myocardial infarction and sudden death in Belfast.[9]

Warren adopted Pantridge's ideas and began discussions about mobile coronary care with the Columbus Division of Fire given their increasing commitments to out-of-hospital medical care. With the help of Dave Ellies, a local industrialist, the Advanced Coronary Treatment Foundation, the central Ohio chapter of the American Heart Association and the Regional Medical Program, a coalition was formed.[1,9,10] By April 1969, the Heartmobile program had been grafted into the existing Columbus Division of Fire's emergency medical care system and operated as a joint effort between the Columbus Division of Fire and the Ohio State University Medical Center.[1]

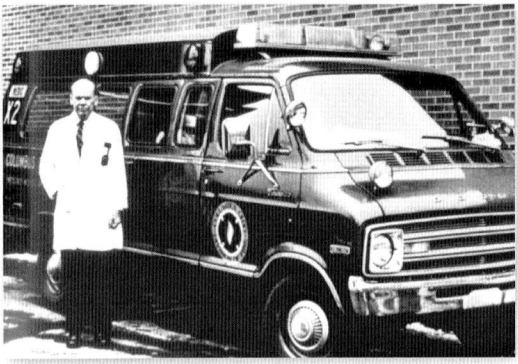

Figure 3: James V. Warren, MD, Chair of The Ohio State University Department of Medicine, was the originator of the Heartmobile in Columbus.

Warren served as Chair of the Department of Medicine from 1961 to 1979 (Figure 3) and had also been President of the American Heart Association. Building on the work of Pantridge, he and fellow cardiologist Richard Lewis, MD, not only created one of the first mobile coronary care units in the United States, they were among the first to initiate the concept of the Emergency Medical Services (EMS) as we know them today. Warren was a steadfast and strong supporter of emergency medicine in the early days given his dedication to improving cardiac care in the prehospital setting. He was also curious about faculty longevity; he once opined to Rund, "I thought emergency medicine was a 'young man's game'."

Columbus firefighters were trained at the Ohio State Medical Center and were taught lifesaving skills such as endotracheal intubation, cardiac defibrillation, insertion of intravenous lines and administration of medications effective in treatment of cardiac arrest. The first instructors were cardiologists and anesthesiologists.

Throughout this process, Ohio State faculty members involved in this project studied and published their experiences in highly regarded medical journals; their studies are now regarded among the landmark articles of EMS history. In fact, some of the first reports of tracheal intubation by firefighter medics taught by Ohio State anesthesiologists ushered in EMS procedures for airway management throughout the country. Innovations in prehospital clinical care, education and research characterized these pioneering accomplishments.

One of the pieces of the puzzle that brought the rapid entrance of emergency medicine into the Department of Preventive Medicine in 1978 was the early involvement of the preventive medicine faculty in the Heartmobile and Columbus EMS. Department Chair Martin Keller, MD, PhD, warmly welcomed emergency medicine. He and his colleagues were studying and writing extensively about myocardial infarction and the impact of mobile coronary care units.[12,13] His wife, Geraldine, another faculty member, was studying EMS dispatch. Emergency services were therefore one of the Kellers' primary research efforts. At meetings and other venues, they met the leaders of other early EMS systems such as Nagel and Grace. Keller and colleagues from cardiology studied the impact of advanced EMS units extensively and shared the effectiveness of mobile coronary care unit in treating and transporting the sickest of the patient with acute myocardial infarction.[13]

In 1971 it became clear to the Heartmobile program leaders that the firefighters could manage patients on their own without the doctor, and the Heartmobile was replaced with four "medic" units throughout the community. The firefighters staffing these units had advanced training and skills and became "paramedics."

Among the first reports about training paramedics to perform endotracheal intubation was the work done by Bernard C. "Bernie" DeLeo, MD. DeLeo was an Ohio State anesthesiologist who devoted a great deal of time and effort to teaching endotracheal intubation skills to the new Columbus paramedics. He is considered a pioneer and a legend in Ohio State history for his ground breaking work in training paramedics to intubate.

The paramedic training included lectures by anesthesiologists and supervised practice with the Laerdal intubation manikin. Squad personnel were required to place the tube successfully in 15 seconds. Even though most of the teaching was done on a manikin intubation head, DeLeo also taught the firefighter paramedics to intubate in the operating room. The new trainees would be distributed throughout the city in such a way that "there would be one experienced man for each medic at all times."[14]

In one study, DeLeo compared the effectiveness of intubation by paramedics working on their own "under standby orders" after the termination of the Heartmobile project in 1971 to the performance of intubation by the physicians who staffed the vehicle from 1969 to 1971. In the summary of his study, he reported the following:

> *For the years 1972 through 1974, fire rescue squad personnel, working without direct medical supervision in Columbus, Ohio, successfully completed 91 percent of the endotracheal intubations they attempted. Under similar circumstances, physicians completed only 8 percent. Complications of vomiting and aspiration as a result of intubation and resuscitation have been reduced from 30 percent with a physician-staffed vehicle to 3 percent with fire rescue-staffed vehicles. No significant complications were encountered by either group. Endotracheal intubation is a physical skill which can be readily mastered by rescue squad personnel and, therefore, should be a part of any mobile emergency care system.[14]*

DeLeo also noted that the "medic squad personnel in Columbus have successfully placed endotracheal tubes in victims found in bathtubs, ditches and even in an electrocuted lineman when he was still on the ladder."[14]

The "Heart Shack"

Initially, the Heartmobile was located in a small temporary building that was erected on the campus of Ohio State directly adjacent to the Emergency Department. This building later became known as the "Heart Shack." According to Lewis, the dean of the College of Medicine did not want the Heartmobile housed on the medical center campus. Warren had had the building constructed nearly overnight without the dean's knowledge. When the dean found out, he was upset, but allowed the structure to stand (Figure 4).[11]

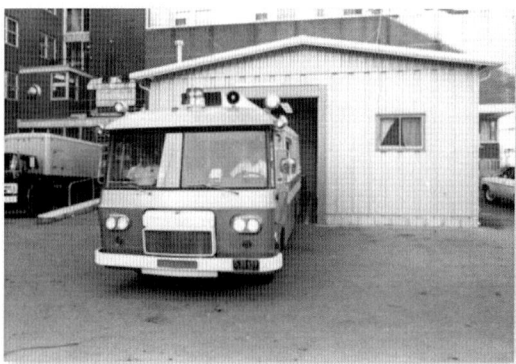

Figure 4: The "Heart Shack" was a temporary building near the emergency department and located in the parking lot which initially housed the Heartmobile. Shown here is the Heartmobile exiting the "Shack," which eventually became a classroom where Columbus firefighters were trained in electrocardiography, intravenous lines, intubation and cardiac medication. The EMS skills taught there were transformative and were eventually copied by all other fire departments in the country.

The Heart Shack had sleeping quarters for the firefighters who were off their regular shift. They were paid but volunteered for the extra duty. When a call for assistance was thought to be cardiac in nature, a resident or cardiology fellow was paged and responded from the 11th floor Coronary Care Unit. Three firefighters and a physician would then respond to the call. Average response times were 12 minutes, with most of the delay being related to the physician responding to the Heartmobile. It was difficult sometimes to get the doctor on board quickly. As their experience grew, the firefighters learned the required skills so that, over time, they would be able to function independently by following a set of standing orders. The standing orders were the forerunners of modern EMS protocols and the firefighters were among the first of a new type of ambulance staff: the paramedic.

Medical Leadership in the Columbus Fire Department

In July 1969, Richard P. Lewis, MD, joined the faculty at Ohio State as an Associate Professor of Medicine in the Division of Cardiology. A 1957 graduate of Yale College, Lewis received his MD from the University of Oregon in 1961. He became a resident at the Peter Bent Brigham Hospital affiliated with Harvard in Boston and completed his residency in 1964. He then served as a fellow in cardiology at the University of Oregon from 1964 to 1966. Following his fellowship, he was commissioned as a Captain in the United States military corps and completed a two-year tour of duty as Associate Chief of Cardiology at the Madigan Army Hospital in Tacoma, Washington. He then became an instructor in the Department of Medicine at Stanford in 1968. At Stanford he taught student Douglas Rund, MD, who would later establish the emergency medicine program at Ohio State.

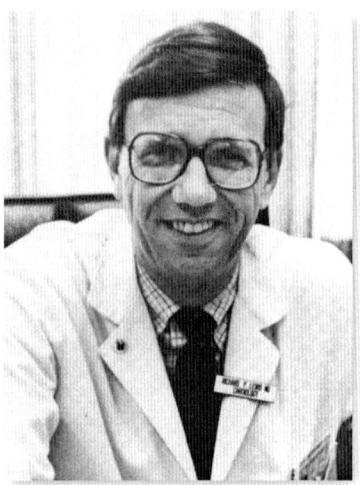

Soon after his arrival at Ohio State, Warren approached Lewis and asked him if he had any interest in the Heartmobile program. As Lewis put it: "Well, I had never given it any thought at all. But you don't turn down things for your new Chairman."[9,10] Lewis supervised the Heartmobile project from July 1969 and collected data on every Heartmobile run to judge the effectiveness of the program. He went on to become Medical Director of the Columbus Division of Fire Emergency Medical Services (EMS) program from 1971 to 1981 (Figure 5).[2]

Figure 5: Richard P. Lewis, MD, supervised the Heartmobile project and worked to evaluate its effectiveness and publicize the revolutionary innovation he helped create.

During the early days of the Heartmobile program, there were regular meetings between Lewis and the coronary care directors from around the city. Emergency Department nurses were quickly included in those meetings. The cooperation of the nurses and coronary care units was crucial to the Heartmobile program's acceptance within the medical community.

Early in the Heartmobile program, Warren and Lewis recognized a problem with a lack of physicians interested in responding with the Heartmobile. Further, fellows and residents from Ohio State who responded with the Heartmobile were a significant source of delay while the firefighters waited for them to appear in the parking lot to take the run. In addition, mandatory telemetry was causing additional delay. The wait for a physician to read the ECG from the hospital and issue orders could seem like an eternity in the setting of a life-threatening cardiac emergency.

On December 6, 1969, a conference was presented at Ohio State entitled "A Workshop: On the Operation of a Mobile Coronary Care Unit". This workshop was conducted in cooperation with the Ohio State Regional Medical Program and the Central Ohio Heart Association. Present along with Warren and Lewis were Pantridge from Belfast, Grace from New York and Hirschman (one of Nagel's colleagues) from Miami. Other representatives came from across the nation, including Houston, Los Angeles, Maryland, Seattle and others. Considerable discussion centered on who should provide advanced coronary care in the future, e.g., physicians, firefighters, nurses, etc.[4]

Experience indicated that the immediate interpretation of the electrocardiogram (ECG) sent by telemetry to the physician in the hospital was disappointing and unreliable. However, by 1971 it was apparent to Warren and Lewis that properly trained firefighters and paramedics could read the ECGs as well as resident physicians. James J. Hughes, Jr., Columbus Director of Public Safety, who was involved in the Heartmobile program from the start, agreed with Warren and Lewis and approved the firefighter-only operation.

On July 1, 1971, the Columbus Division of Fire took over Heartmobile operations. Firefighters began treating patients at emergency scenes without direct physician supervision.[1,2] Medics were established at stations 2, 10, 15 and 16, and were supplemented with basic life support squads at stations 1, 6, 7, 8, 14, 17 and 21, along with rescue squads at stations 2, 16, 17 and 23.[2] Liability for the paramedics' actions, initially a worrisome issue, was assumed by the City of Columbus. Each of the other cities mentioned earlier that initially responded with sending physicians to the scene ultimately abandoned physician care in favor of the paramedics—firefighters or ambulance personnel who were trained to provide advanced medical care.

The Columbus medic system rapidly spread to the local suburbs, where smaller departments cooperated with the Columbus Division of Fire to jointly provide emergency care to the central Ohio community.[15] Among the first of these departments was the Sharon Township Division of Fire, today known as the Worthington Division of Fire and EMS.

In July of 1971 when firefighters began to respond to medical emergencies without physicians in Columbus, the Heartmobile was moved to a Columbus Fire Station. Meanwhile, the Heartmobile's previous building on the medical center campus, the "Heart Shack," was converted to a classroom. A 96-hour paramedic course was developed and taught by Kathryn (Katy) Sampson, a Coronary Care Unit nurse, and a team that included Drs. Richard Lewis, Stephen Schaal, Phillip Fulkerson and later, John Stang. Stang, a cardiologist and renowned educator, served as medical director of Columbus Fire from 1981 to 1984. Firefighters from Columbus, Franklin County and other surrounding counties, including Delaware, received their paramedic training from the Ohio State team. Sampson and the Ohio State team influenced most of the early paramedics in central Ohio.[1,15]

Heartmobile Influence on Modern EMS

While the programs in each of the cities discussed above grew largely independent of each other, the Columbus Heartmobile program did influence EMS in Ohio and nationally. Within the central Ohio area, fire department-based EMS is clearly the dominant model. This predominantly fire-based EMS resulted from the influence of the Columbus Division of Fire model for prehospital care that developed out of the Heartmobile program. The Heartmobile is also credited with being the first program of its type to provide advanced treatment to patients with non-heart related medical problems.[9]

According to Lewis, Cobb from Seattle visited the Heartmobile program during its infancy, and about a year later, the Seattle Medic One program, which closely resembled the Heartmobile project, was launched.[11] Both programs were based at a university medical center and operated as cooperative efforts between the fire department and the medical centers. Both programs initially responded with physicians and firefighters together, later replacing the physician with firefighter paramedics. The Medic One vehicle (Moby Pig) and the Heartmobile were both large recreational vehicles converted to bring the resources of the Coronary Care Unit to the patient. Cobb also used Regional Medical Program funding—part of Lyndon B. Johnson's Great Society Policy—just as Warren had done in Columbus.

Although the Heartmobile preceded the Medic One program by about a year, Cobb removed the physician from Medic One before Warren and Lewis converted the Heartmobile to firefighter-only in July 1971. Both programs flourished in the 1970s. Along with the Los Angeles paramedic program, Columbus and Seattle had the best survival rates for cardiac arrest patients. Early survival rates for ventricular fibrillation/tachycardia cardiac arrest in these three cities ranged from 25% to 33%.[12, 15, 16, 17] A study of the impact of the Columbus paramedic program also demonstrated a reduction in the mortality rates for heart attack patients.[12] Furthermore, the study showed that a knowledgeable population could appropriately activate the Advanced Life Support System.

Today Seattle has perhaps the finest EMS system in the country. The city conducts significant research on resuscitation, and survival rates for cardiac arrest are the best of the 50 largest cities in the United States.[18] Along with Cobb, Michael Copass was also instrumental in the development of the Seattle Medic One System and directed the system for many years. In 2014 Michael Sayre, MD, of Ohio State moved to Seattle became the medical director of Medic One. He was only the third person to serve in this role since the beginning of the program in 1969.

The Heartmobile Today

The Heartmobile is a 1967 Clark Cortez recreational vehicle powered by a 6-cylinder engine and front wheel drive system. Custom Coach Corporation of Columbus, Ohio, customized the interior following the design of Dave Ellies Industrial Design Company also of Columbus. Armco Steel Corporation of Middletown, Ohio, built the patient table and the B. Coburn Company of Buffalo, New York, manufactured the patient monitoring system.[19]

After the Heartmobile was retired from service as an emergency response vehicle, the Columbus Division of Fire used it for several purposes, including as a mobile recruitment vehicle for the department. When the Columbus Division of Fire retired the vehicle, they planned to sell it at auction. Fortunately, William Hall, a paramedic/firefighter with Columbus and director of the Central Ohio Fire Museum, had the foresight to requisition the vehicle for the Museum. He removed it from the Fire Department storage lot and hid it until he could convince the city to donate it to the Central Ohio Fire Museum.[20] The exterior of the vehicle was in rough shape but the engine and transmission were repaired and serviced and became operational. Today, the Heartmobile has been completely restored to its 1969 configuration and is located in the Central Ohio Fire Museum, 260 North Fourth Street, Columbus Ohio, 43215-2511.

References

1. Warren JV, Hill FM, Faehnle L. *The Columbus Story of Mobile Emergency Care*. Department of Medicine, The Ohio State University College of Medicine; 1976.

2. Stang JM, Keller MD, Lewis RP. Mobile pre-hospital coronary care – Columbus, Ohio. In Adgey AAJ (ed). *Acute Phase of Ischemic Heart Disease and Myocardial Infarction*. Boston, MA: Martinus.

3. Page JO. *The Paramedics*. Backdraft Publications; 1979.

4. Proceedings of: *A Workshop: Mobile Coronary Care Unit*. Department of Medicine, The Ohio State University College of Medicine. Dec. 6, 1969.

5. HistoryLink.org: historylink.org/essays/output.cfm?file_id=2330

6. Gilmore S. Rusty motor home part of Medic One's history. *The Seattle Times*, November 28, 2011.

7. Lown, B, et al. New method for terminating cardiac arrhythmias: use of synchronized capacitor discharge. *JAMA*. 1962;182:548-595.

8. https://en.wikipedia.org/wiki/Frank_Pantridge

9. Eisenberg ME. *Life in the Balance: Emergency Medicine and the Quest to Reverse Sudden Death*. New York, NY: Oxford;1997: 240-2.

10. Transcript of Mickey Eisenberg's interview of Richard Lewis, MD. April 28, 1992.

11. Personal communication with Richard Lewis, MD. May 2005.

12. Lewis RP, Lanese RR, Stang JM, Chirikos TN, Keller MD, Warren JV. Reduction of mortality from prehospital myocardial infarction by prudent patient activation of mobile coronary care system. *Am Heart J*. 1982;103:123-30.

13. Keller, MD, et al. A study of the impact of mobile coronary care units. Report to the Department of Health, Education and Welfare (C1RO HS 02078). 1978.

14. DeLeo BC. Endotracheal intubation by rescue squad personnel. *Heart Lung.* 1977; 6(5): 851-854.

15. Lewis RP, Fulkerson PK, Stang JM, Sampson KL, Dutko HG. The Columbus emergency medical service system. *Ohio State Med J.* 1979;75:39.

16. Eisenberg MS, Horwood BT, Cummins RO, Reynolds-Haertle R, Hearne TR. Cardiac arrest and resuscitation: a tale of 29 cities. *Ann Emerg Med.* 1990;19:179-86.

17. Stratton S, Niemann JT. Outcome from out-of-hospital cardiac arrest caused by nonventricular arrhythmias: contribution of successful resuscitation to overall survivorship supports the current practice of initiating out-of-hospital ACLS. *Ann Emerg Med.* 1998; 32:448-53.

18. Merrill, L. EMS experts, journalists praise 2003 USA TODAY series that changed the industry. Accessed July 25, 2023. https://www.ems1.com/cardiac-care/articles/ems-experts-journalists-praise-2003-usa-today-series-that-changed-the-industry-XV4y1xYumr1e-J8zn/

19. *Design in Action.* Dave Ellies Industrial Design, Inc. Columbus, Ohio (no publication date).

20. Personal communication with William Hall. May 2005.

Chapter 17

The Emergency Department

Richard N. Nelson, MD
Douglas A. Rund, MD

Ohio State's original emergency room was on the ground floor of Starling-Loving University Hospital. Operational in 1924, it was named in honor of Lyne Starling (1784-1848), a founder of Columbus and benefactor of Starling Medical College and Starling Loving, MD (1827-1911), an early dean of Starling Medical College, which was a predecessor of the Ohio State College of Medicine.

Operating rooms and delivery rooms were on the top floor, with huge windows to illuminate the surgical fields (Figure 1). By contrast, the emergency room was on the ground level so that patients could access the hospital protected from the elements through the covered doorway

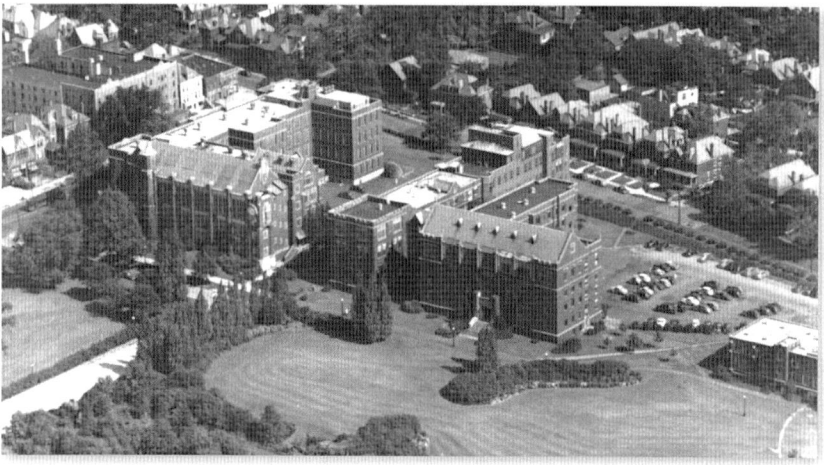

Figure 1: The Starling-Loving University Hospital (center) was constructed in 1924. Large top-floor windows served as sources of lighting and ventilation for the operating rooms and delivery suites. The emergency room entrance was in the rear of the building, alongside parking.

(Figure 2). In 1934 the hospital consisted of 276 beds. The emergency room was basically a single room. Emergency transport services of that era were comparatively primitive, with many transports made by funeral directors in their hearses.

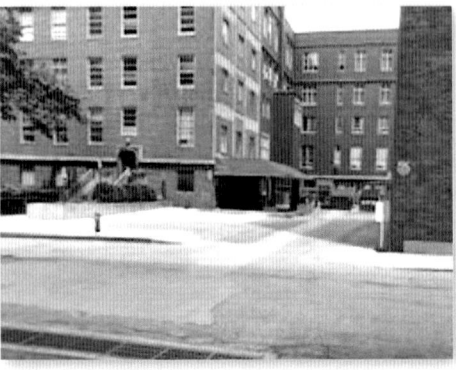

The emergency room was a small 720 square-foot space. The original floor plan shows a single "emergency and dressing" room and an attached "examination room"

Figure 2: The original 1924 ground-level emergency room entrance to what was then the Starling-Loving University Hospital later became a loading dock in the rear of the building, renamed Starling-Loving Hall in 1951.

(Figure 3). Treatment areas such as this in many hospitals of that era resulted in the term *emergency room*, which is still used by some today. Adjoining the emergency room was a room for the "house doctor," an original term for the current term "house staff" (interns and resi-

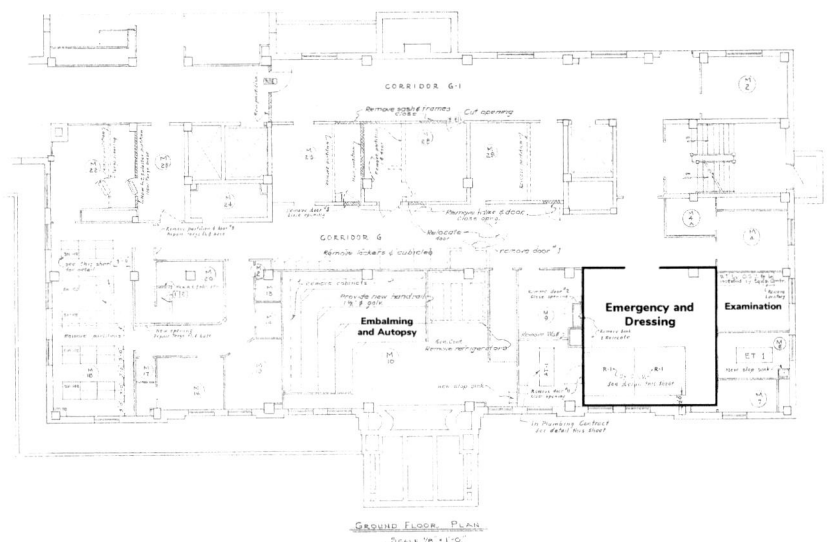

Figure 3: Original floor plans of the ground floor of Starling-Loving Hospital shows the emergency room (ER) that operated from 1924 to 1951. The morgue, with body storage, embalming and autopsy procedures, was adjacent to the ER.

dents). Alongside the emergency room was the "embalming and autopsy" room. The scale drawing shows theater seating in the adjacent postmortem room where students could view the necropsy.

Students could be watching the postmortem dissection while, next door, the house doctor was attending to emergency patients. This layout next to the morgue was probably not terribly reassuring to a trepidatious emergency patient. The emergency room was also near other ground floor services: radiology, fluoroscopy, cystoscopy, pharmacy, kitchen, dining room and the dietician.

Many years later the renowned Ohio State cardiologist Mary Beth Fontana, MD, remembered being seen in the emergency room as a child:

> *My visit to the ER when in the basement of Starling-Loving occurred in the late 40s. My younger brother hit me on the top of my head with a hammer. I remember entering the doors at the back of Starling-Loving and sitting on an exam table while they attended to the large lump on the top of my head. I don't remember getting x-rays or anything else. There was no waiting.*[1]

The organization and patient composition of the early emergency room is somewhat unclear, but it was most likely staffed by the "house doctor" and nurses. Patients included those of the few private physicians on staff, Ohio State students and other patients.[2] In 1938 the Ohio State *outpatient department* moved to Starling-Loving from the State Street Dispensary. A report from 1939 gives a hint as to what might have been the makeup of these "clinic" patients:

> *Our greatest problem has been to turn away large numbers of people who obviously can go to private physicians. The type of patient has changed greatly since we have moved [to Starling-Loving]. The vagrants in the vicinity of 6th and State Streets are not so much in evidence. Also, more people are being sent by doctors from out of the city.*[3]

University Hospital

In 1951 the new university hospital containing the new emergency room was constructed (Figure 4). A 12-story facility, the hospital was considered ultramodern and state-of-the-art when it first opened and was the primary teaching hospital for the College of Medicine. An underground tunnel connected it to Starling-Loving Hall.

The "emergency room" was located on the ground floor on the far west side in what would later become a loading dock area. The 12-bed facility included: two 4-bed wards (separated by curtains), a trauma room, a cast room, an ENT/dental room, an Ob/Gyn treatment area and an x-ray room (Figure 5).

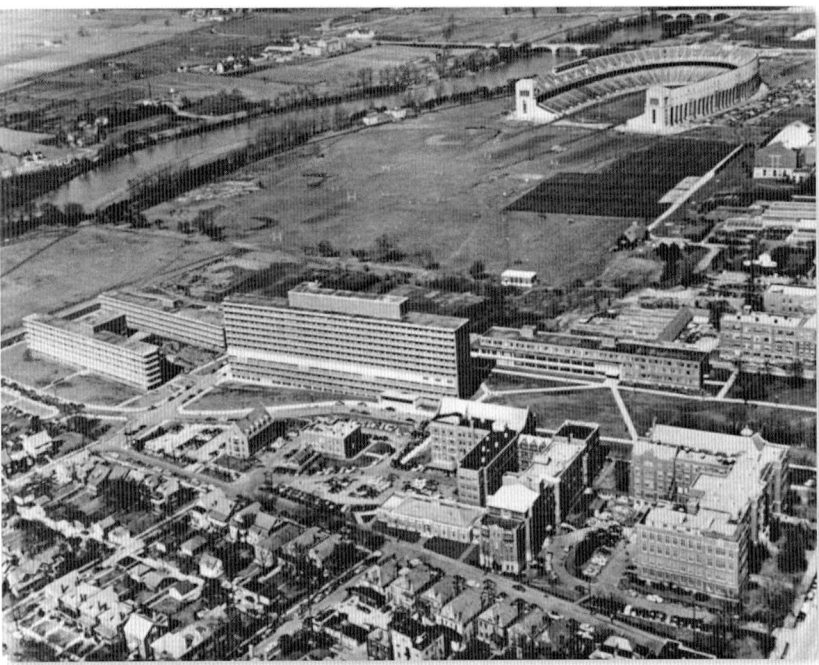

Figure 4: The "new" university hospital (center) was constructed in 1951. The emergency room entrance was in the rear of the main hospital. Means Hall (front left center) was the old tuberculosis hospital and Upham Hall (behind Means) was a psychiatric hospital. Both halls served as the Department of Emergency Medicine administrative offices over the years as the department grew. The famous Ohio State "Horseshoe" football stadium is in the background.

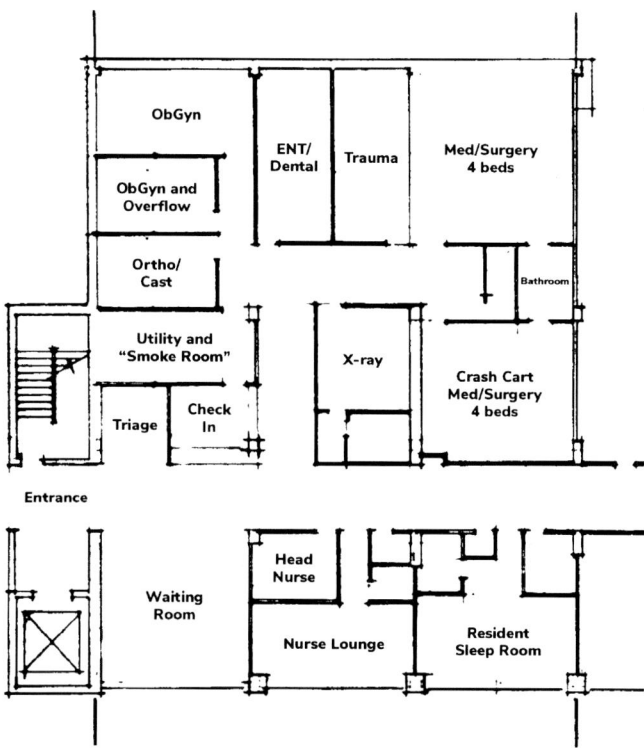

Figure 5: This was the emergency room layout at Ohio State from 1951 to 1979. In 1977, 28,000 patients were seen in this facility.

The emergency room (ER) entrance also served as the hospital's ambulance entrance. The patient mix was similar for years: students, out-of-town referrals, private patients of the faculty, and patients who used hospital teaching clinics for regular care. Until 1977, interns fresh out of medical school primarily staffed the unit. In 1983 the Board of Trustees renamed University Hospital Doan Hall in recognition of former College of Medicine Dean Charles A Doan, MD.

In 1977, with 28,000 patients being seen in the emergency room, the facility was sometimes crowded. On the rare occasion that it was overflowing, the interns would call more experienced residents to "come down" from their inpatient duties to help. There were quiet periods as well. Overnight residents could sleep in the bedroom across the hall.

Years later Kate Bullock, RN, recollected the quiet periods from the early 1970s (Figure 6):

> At nights it got a little quiet. The place was empty every now and then. We would put out a page "Dr. Needa Fourth" because we wanted to play cards in the trauma room. We wanted to play bridge and we needed a fourth player. The operator would go along with it. But we figured if someone rolled in the place that they would land in either Room 1 or 2, places for heart patients and overdoses, but we thought if there were any traumas that would come in, we would be right here.[4]

Periods of relative quiet were sometimes interrupted by pandemonium in those early days. On April 29, 1970, Ohio State students protesting the Vietnam War along with other issues, including demands to add Women's and Black Studies to the university courses, clashed with highway patrolmen in riot gear in front of Hamilton Hall just yards from the hospital. Many of the resulting multiple injuries were treated in the ER.[5]

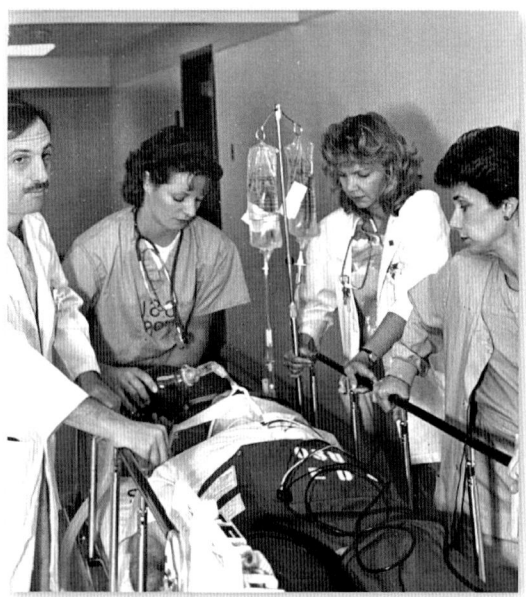

Figure 6: Richard Nelson, MD (far left), works alongside (center to right) Sara O'Neilly, RN, Marla (Unterzuber) Milstead, RN, and Kathleen "Kate" Bullock, RN.

The trauma room and x-ray rooms were small and advances in communication were slow. Mary Jane Fellers, RN, worked in the emergency room starting in 1976. Years later she recalled this method of transmitting laboratory results to the emergency department:

> There were no computers or printers in the ER in the 1970s, and results of lab tests ordered on ER patients had to either be called directly to

> the unit clerk or else hand-delivered on paper. At some point in time, someone came up with the idea of equipping the lab with a closed-circuit TV camera linked to a TV monitor in the ER. The staff would have blood and UA results on a lab requisition and shoved under a screen so we could see their handwritten results. Of course, if the lab sheets weren't positioned perfectly under the camera lens, some results could be cut off, prompting a phone call from the ER requesting to "move the report half an inch to the left" or "up a quarter inch" such that all results were visible.[6]

Although it is hardly conceivable by later standards, the interns and junior residents were seeing, treating and discharging patients without any faculty supervision, a standard occurrence at university hospitals before emergency medicine became a specialty. Interns and residents of that era learned in a trial by fire. The faculty had also been unsupervised as house staff; therefore, recognition of the deficiency was slow to develop in university hospitals. During Rund's own medical residency at the University of California in San Francisco in 1971, interns were treating patients on their own with the aid of a medical manual for house staff. No attending physicians were ever present. During the day an advanced resident was present. At night the resident slept. The half joking whispering among interns was that having to waken the resident from sleep was a "sign of weakness."

At Ohio State, Bullock later remembered these times with no staff:

> [The physician director] would come along every once in a while, especially when JCAHO was about to happen. He was tall and there were emergency cords on the wall right outside the rooms, and he would come along with a white glove and get after us for not cleaning way up there. There were times that we should have called in a lot more staff. [There were a couple times when] there were 50 students or people participating in riots that required care and it was awful. We had one doc running around. I don't know why we didn't call in somebody else to help in that small little place.[4]

Emergency medicine faculty were just being recruited in 1978. Douglas Rund, MD—and David Roberts, MD, in the final year of his cardiology fellowship—were beginning to staff the ED intermittently, working from 10 AM to 10 PM, but the emergency room was still basically staffed by one or two interns working 16-hour shifts and a surgical resident on duty for 24 consecutive hours as it had been for years. The days of full-time attending coverage had to wait until the move to the new emergency department in 1979 when 24-hour coverage by attendings finally started.

Nursing

In the early days of faculty coverage, the medical staff and the nursing staff were an extremely close-knit group. Faculty physicians were few and optimal patient care required close cooperation and intense mutual respect for each other. The nurses had far more experience than the interns and residents and could handle many of the clinical situations quite well by themselves. They were especially expert in the first phases of patient contact and getting the appropriate work up started. Patients with suspected cardiac chest pain typically needed an electrocardiogram, blood work, intravenous line and possibly a chest x-ray. Bullock recalled those early days:

> *We just did what we could, as best we could to stabilize the patient. I thought, I know how to draw ABGs, I've seen it a thousand times. Nurses were allowed to do that. We didn't have pulse oximeters. I drew the ABGs and sent them off to the lab and did everything we could to stabilize the patient and then woke the resident. We took some liberties. We just had to do what we had to do.*[4]

In the early days of attendings, coverage reliance on the experienced nursing staff was especially important considering the potential for an attending stretched thin with too many patients. Nearly every doctor had a story of a nurse "saving the day" by rendering indispensable assistance in managing their patients. In many ways, the relationship was like a family. There was also good-natured humor and enjoyment in each other's company (Figure 7).

The nurses also appreciated the new attending emergency physicians. Years later Fellers recalled:

> *... we couldn't believe it when we got docs who wanted to work the ER "full time" .... what a difference in level of decision making! Before that*

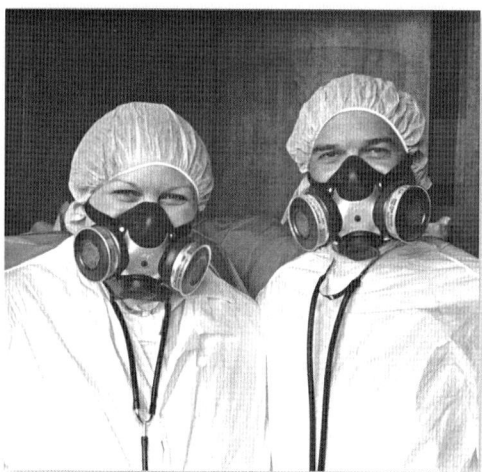

Figure 7: Head nurse Tondra "Toni" Rausch, RN, and Douglas Rund, MD, pictured here in the isolation gear of the 1980s, co-authored *Triage*, describing "state-of-the art" methods for determining urgency and priority needs. The relationship between physician and nurse was close in the department's early days.

it was always the residents or interns asking us what they should do next (that's if they were smart enough to know they should do that).[6]

Patients who presented to the ER on their own would start out at the front desk where they were met by a registrar. The need for a system of triage, the sorting of patients according to their injury severity, became apparent as the volume of patients kept increasing. Years later Fellers recalled:

Actually, I don't think we even used the word "triage" until Doug [Rund] came. The ward clerks staffed the front counter/did registration and would physically walk back to let us know there was a patient to see out front. When we were busy, they might come back and say, "there are 5 patients in the box," meaning that they had registered 5 patients and put their 4 carbon ER sheet in the stacking tray for us to get when we could. They would let us know if there was someone who they "felt" we should see right away. Squads always just came right back through the double doors so we would at least lay eyes on those patients right away. As crazy as the system was, I don't recall the ward clerks ever missing a really sick patient that we should have brought back sooner.

Actual triage started, I think, in 1977. We cordoned off a small part of that front area with a screen, two chairs—one for the patient, one for us—and a small desk that held the thermometers. The clerk would let us know there was a patient and we would then come out and triage them at the front before taking them back. There were only two nurses and two attendants on night shift...so it's not like there were a lot of extra staff to sit in triage waiting for a patient.[6]

By the time the Division of Emergency Medicine was established in 1978, the volume of patients continued to grow, signaling a need for a larger emergency department.

The New Department of 1979 in Rhodes Hall

In the summer of 1979, the Emergency Department relocated to its vastly expanded new space on the ground floor of the new Rhodes Hall (Figure 8). The new emergency department encompassed 28 separate rooms in 17,000 square feet of space. Ambulances and patients were protected under a covered entryway when arriving and unloading. A significant new feature was the separation into a "medicine" and a "surgery" side. The attending physician ran from side to side seeing patients. The 7-bed "medicine" room included the gynecology treatment area. The 4-bed "surgery" area was used for minor wounds and minor trauma with the beds separated by curtains. When the department was packed, patients could be placed in any available bed regardless of complaint.

Two large rooms, Trauma 1 and Trauma 2, were in the center. Each room held two beds that were used for critical medical and surgical/trauma patients respectively. These rooms were large and accommodated the equipment used for resuscitations. Additional rooms included an orthopedic (cast) room, psychiatric seclusion room, two x-ray suites, isolation room (E6), and a radiation and chemical decontamination room. A prison inmate unit was on what was then called the "east corridor." While the unit was designed for prison inmates, it pre-dated Ohio State's longstanding relationship with the Ohio Department of Rehabilitation and Corrections by a number of years and was only occasionally used for prisoners. Other east corridor rooms included an ENT room complete with slit-lamp for eye examinations, and a dental room mainly staffed in the evenings by oral surgery residents.

Another east corridor room contained a small laboratory, a holdover of academic medicine practices of the '60s and '70s. Clinicians would perform dipstick and microscopic urinalyses with the aid of a centrifuge and microscope. Nurses would routinely "spin down" the urines

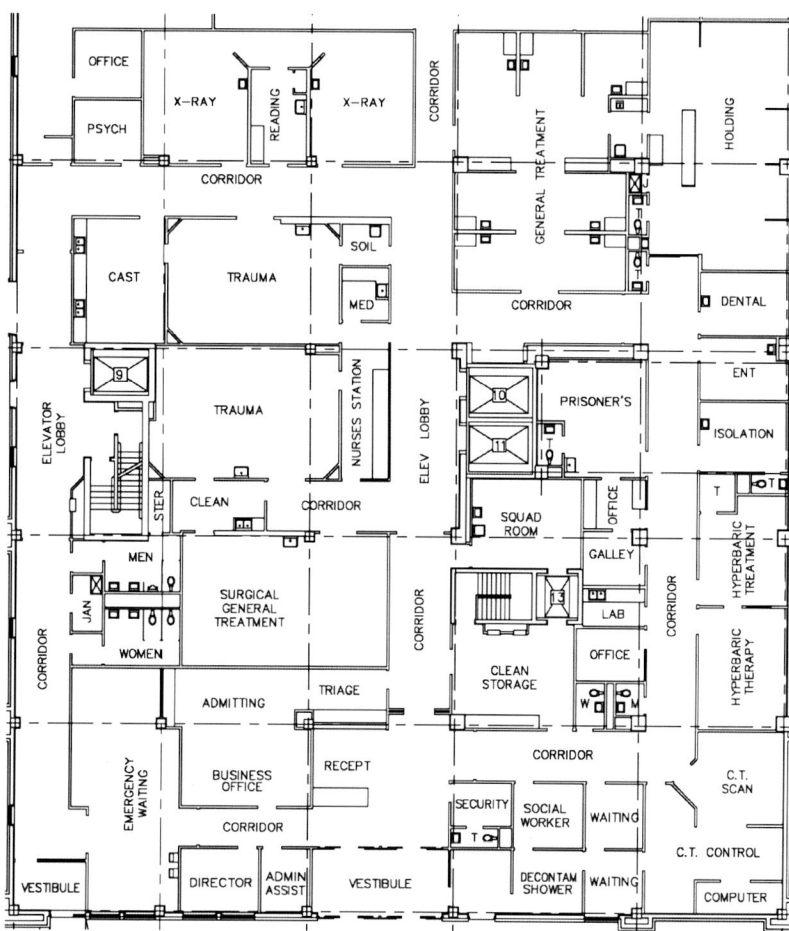

Figure 8: The new ED went through several iterations after it was constructed in 1979. While the "holding" area was one of the concepts developed later, the major features remained the same: the "medical-general treatment" side, the "surgical" side, and the trauma/resuscitation rooms (center).

and the sediment was examined under a microscope by the resident or the attending. The practice ended in 1988 when the federal Clinical Laboratory Improvements Amendments (CLIA) essentially prohibited such testing outside of an "official" lab.

An alcohol lamp and reagents were also available for gram stains, often used to examine sputum samples for pneumococci, spinal fluids for bacterial meningitis, and urethral discharges for gonococci. Finally, stool guaiac testing, using the three required reagents in separate bottles complete with eyedroppers, could be used to rule out GI bleeds in this pre-hemoccult-card era. Other common tests included vaginal wet prep, stool microscopic exams and urine pregnancy tests.

The new unit provided far greater capability than the old unit and served the division well until the next major revision in 1995. Pauline "Polly" Hansplant, RN, who worked in the emergency department from 1979 until her retirement in 2014, recalled she could not understand why the utility room between the surgery room and Trauma 1 contained an autoclave, a steam sterilizing unit common in operating rooms. Such a unit was rarely if ever found in typical emergency departments. The mystery was solved when Charles "Charlie" Cloutier, MD, a general surgeon who had served in a field hospital in Vietnam with surgery chair Larry Carey, MD, began working part-time as an emergency attending. Cloutier, who would later start Ohio State's trauma program, explained that he immediately recognized the surgery side of the ER as a common military field hospital design in which the 4-bed surgery room would serve as a triage area and the trauma room would function as an operating room. The incongruous autoclave between the two rooms confirmed his design assessment.

This side room was also affectionately known as "Pete's office" in honor of Cecil "Pete" Martin, a longtime ED tech who would take his cigarette smoking breaks there. Martin had been imprisoned early in his life but rehabilitated completely and worked so effectively and compassionately in the prison infirmary that his release was strongly advocated by Ohio State physicians working there. Smoking by staff was allowed in the two utility rooms.

The decontamination chamber, another unique feature of the new department, was located in the front of the department near the covered entryway and was designed to treat patients contaminated by radioactive materials or toxic chemicals. The department became the de facto destination for contaminated patients from anywhere in central Ohio and beyond. The "room" consisted of a robust water supply along with stocks of personal protective equipment. One or two staff drills were held each year. In later years, a formal agreement was reached with Battelle Research Institute to provide secondary decontamination services to its employees who were involved in workplace accidents involving toxic substances. In return, Battelle physicians and staff would provide Ohio State emergency physicians, nurses and residents with educational presentations on chemical, biologic and radiation decontamination.

By the time the new department opened in 1979, the clinical laboratory was no longer using the closed-circuit TV system to report results. According to Fellers:

> *The "new system" we used with the new ER was a "VT terminal" ... one of those early PC monitors. There was a dot matrix printer attached next to it, so we could print the lab results if we wanted to. It was sooo hi tech.*[6]

Studies were typically limited to the basics: complete blood count electrolytes, blood urea nitrogen creatinine, glucose, amylase, coagulation studies, arterial blood gases, cultures, and urinalysis. The tests usually took one to two hours to complete. It was not unusual for a lab test to be inadvertently omitted from the requisition form, thus requiring it to be re-ordered and sometimes re-drawn, resulting in another one- or two-hour delay. X-rays were also basic.

The medical center had a computerized tomography (CT) scanner; however, it was an early generation model and only used for head studies. Abdominal and chest CTs would only become available later in the '80s. Any CT had to be approved by the radiology resident of the day (the "Rad OD"). Plain films were done in one of two x-ray rooms in the back of the department near Trauma 2 and were read by the emergency physicians followed by an over-read by the radiologists later in the day or the following day. Emergency physicians filled out a card describing their interpretations so that the department could be notified, usually the next day, if the initial interpretation was erroneous. Otherwise, the final radiology report usually appeared in the physician's mailbox a few days later. General consults were similarly challenging.

The paper charts, with carbon paper, consisted of a "front sheet" and "nursing notes" sheet. Charts would start off in a hard gray folder and be placed on the counter in the medicine or surgery sides. Colored plastic tags attached to the hard folders would alert the clinician to the patient's status: green for patients to be seen, yellow for labs/x-ray/meds/consults ordered, red for ready for admission or discharge.

Large white boards the walls of the larger rooms listed the patients, their complaints and status, along with occasional and sometimes questionable editorial remarks.

Most emergency departments used a similar "tracking" system. Such systems were not terribly protective of patient confidentiality, but were also not yet illegal— this was almost 20 years before HIPAA. Histories and physician examinations were handwritten on the front sheet. Nursing notes were similarly recorded. Orders were also placed on the same front page as the history and physical examination, and all consult requests, including those for x-rays, had to be manually stamped and filled out by the physician caring for the patient.

Consultants, always residents, had to be paged, and their response to the page was not necessarily timely and often depended on inpatient rounding or commitments in the operating room. Consultants had to see the emergency patients and make a determination as to whether or not they required admission. Most internal medicine patients, regardless of subspecialty, had to be seen by the Medical Admitting Resident (MA) on call, who ultimately determined dispositions.

Often in the evenings it was not unusual for the MA to be consulted on 10 or more patients, who were usually seen in order of when the consult was received. Not surprisingly, this meant even patients who were ultimately admitted to the hospital had to wait a long time before an admission/discharge decision was made. Medical records were available upon request from the medical records department on the first floor of the hospital. Records had to be manually located by clerks and then sent down by cart. Patients who had multiple prior hospital admissions often had multiple volumes of paperwork sometimes appearing in overflowing stacks and piles on carts from medical records.

"Starter packs" were another ED aspect during this time. Patients would often be discharged from the ED after most pharmacies had closed and many did not have insurance coverage and could not afford their prescribed medications, often essential antibiotics. To mitigate these problems, the ED and pharmacy put together starter packs of medications, which usually consisted of a few days' supply of prescribed drugs in a brown paper bag. Drugs of abuse were generally not included in the approved list of starter pack medications. This system worked reasonably well until 1996, when the practice was discontinued due to more stringent regulation of prescription medication dispensing.

The Emergency Team Working Together

In the new emergency department, the relationships between all staff remained close and some could say "like a family." Working in a high-stress environment such as the ED inevitably resulted in parties and other opportunities to "let off steam." The earliest of the Christmas parties featured Santa Claus who arrived in an off-duty Columbus emergency squad. Staff gathered in private homes, laughing, having fun and enjoying each other's company.

Summertime meant parties at homes in backyards or around pools. Songs were created such as the not quite famous "No Beds at Riverside." The song, sung to the old-time tune "Down by the Riverside," was originally created because the Riverside emergency department had a high patient volume and had to divert occasionally and the closest hospital was University Hospital, "just 3 miles south" as the song lyrics went. Douglas Rund, amiable singer and bluegrass guitarist, would sing and accompany the songs along with his close friend Gary Smith on the washtub bass.

The Silver Saddle Award, presented at the annual Christmas party, went to the staff member who was responsible for what was considered the greatest "happening" while on duty during the year. The "trophy" itself was a chrome bedpan and included a roll of toilet paper on which was recorded previous winners and descriptions of their supposedly brainless deeds, written on the "scroll of honor." Nurses typically selected other nurses the winners, however, in 1984, Richard Nelson, MD, received the award because a patient under his care had stolen an empty ambulance from the emergency parking area. The patient had been turned down for admission by the psychiatric consultant. Upon discharge from the ER, the patient went out the front doors and found an empty prison ambulance–motor running–which had just brought a patient with a broken jaw. The patient jumped in the ambulance and drove it about 20 miles before being apprehended by the police. The patient ultimately got their wish and was readmitted.

Other popular diversions included night shift picnics on the helipad, cookouts on the Means Hall lawn and champagne breakfast parties thrown at someone's house by the nurses immediately after a night shift.

Perhaps part of the closeness that developed was due to the incredibly serious patient cases the doctors and nurses needed to address. There was also tremendous compassion for the patients. Julie Mitchell, RN, recalled a beautiful story of that era years later (Figure 9):

> We had a patient who was seriously ill. He needed infusion therapy for his illness and pain medication. He came in often and we knew him well. He was always soft spoken and complimentary to staff. Unfortunately, his repeated infusions caused a severe infection. He came to the ED on a Sunday, accompanied by his brother, and was put in one of the rooms back on the old east corridor. I went in to do an assessment, and to draw labs. I can remember being quite taken back when I saw him, as he had become quite emaciated, pale and weak.

> Making some small talk, I asked if they had had a hard time getting to the ED with all of the increased traffic in the area due to it being the last day of the state fair. His eyes widened, and he said, "Today's the last day?" I said yes. He looked at his brother, and said sadly, "I never got my candy apples."

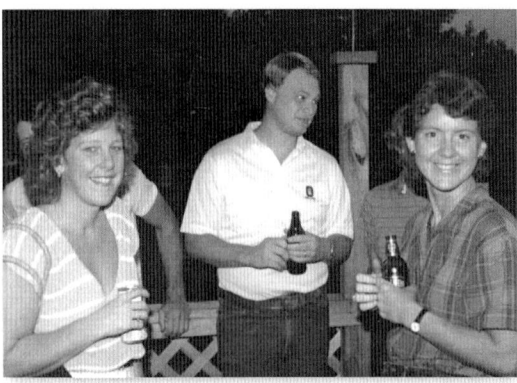

Figure 9: Truly working as a team and getting together off duty are (from left to right) Julie Mitchell, RN, Glen Lundgren, RN, and Delores "Dee" Tschirner Goodwin, RT, (R)(M) socializing with colleagues.

> While I was sending his labs, I saw the hospital coordinator, and relayed this story to him. About an hour later, he came back to me and asked me if I could get someone to cover for me for about 20 minutes or so. I said yes. He had called the state patrol and asked if they could dispatch an officer to

come and pick me up and get me over to the fairgrounds.

The officer took me, LIGHTS AND SIRENS, over to an access gate at the fair, escorted me to where the food vendors were, where I bought 6 candy apples. I'll never forget the look on our patient's face when we went back to his room and handed him that white bag. He opened it and when he looked at those apples he just cried. So did his brother...so did I. He passed away a few weeks later.[7]

Delores "Dee" Tschirner Goodwin, RT, was an outstanding radiologic technologist who worked exclusively in the emergency department (Figure 8). She was a perfect example of an interdisciplinary team member so integrally important to the team and its mission. Years later she recalled some of her experiences:

I started my dream job back in 1976, that being a radiologic technologist at OSU Medical Center as it was called back then. I remained employed there for 30 more years spending 15 in the ED exclusively. I remember those years as the best of my 45-year career. As the "X-ray gal" (as we were referred to back then) I have some great memories from this time. Great experiences![8]

She remembered being on her way to work one day listening to her car radio and hearing about a nearby shooting and "hitting the gas" to get to the ED in time. She also remembered assisting getting a woman out of a car and finding a baby being birthed right then and there. She always worked professionally with patients and had an outstanding sense of humor. She had a true dedication to the emergency department and always helped the team in any way she could.

Anyone who ever worked in the Ohio State Emergency Department between 1979 and 2014 also knew Paulina "Polly" Hansplant, RN (Figure 10). She was the quintessential ER nurse: a smart, funny, take-charge type of professional physicians loved to see on during their shifts. There was no ambiguity with Hansplant: She would tell you exactly what she thought and she was almost always right. Born in Philadelphia, raised in Chillicothe, and graduating high school in 1969, she immediately entered nursing school at Mount Carmel in downtown Columbus. She lived with the other students in the school's dormitory. Before the end of her first year, in her own words:

I was kicked out because I just was not nurse material. My grades were fine; it was just my moral character. We would sneak out at night and go over to Josie's Bar. We would get pizza and low alcohol beer and go up to Lazarus department store at least two nights a week; it was open until 9 and only two blocks from the school. Four of my besties all were excused (they didn't call it expelled) because we were way too rowdy.[9]

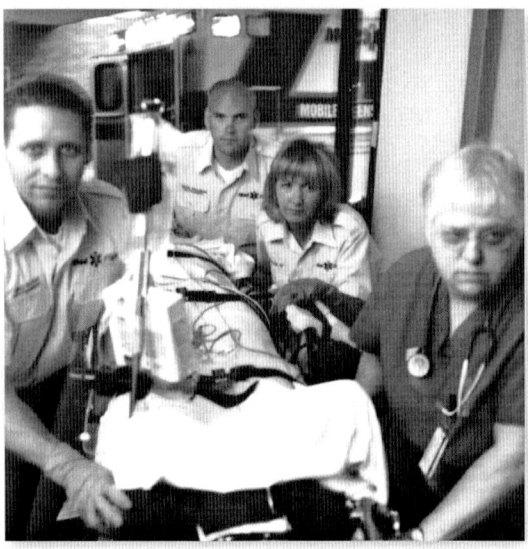

Figure 10: Paulina "Polly" Hansplant, RN (far right), was one of the most experienced nurses in the emergency department. She also worked as a flight nurse. Here she is bringing in a patient from the Medflight ground vehicle along with (from left) Mike Isham, Mark Willison, and Gina Marcum.

After her excusal, she worked as a student nurse assistant and took some classes at Ohio University. She completed the nursing program at Capitol University, where student nurses wore highly distinct and vivid uniforms, thus becoming "one of the purple people." In addition to her work in ED, she had a long and successful career with Medflight as a flight nurse, taking care of critical patients on countless hospital transfers and scene runs.

The Ohio State Emergency Department in the 1980s

The first application to start a residency program was submitted to the Liaison Residency Endorsement Committee (LREC) on August 6, 1980. The program officially started on July 1, 1981, with four first-year and two second-year residents. Richard Nelson, MD, joined the faculty in July, 1981 after completing a residency in emergency medicine at Akron City Hospital. As the first faculty member to have completed a residency in emergency medicine, he developed and led the program.

When the residency started in 1981, attendings worked single coverage in two shifts: 8 AM to 6 PM, and 6 PM to 8 AM. The 14-hour night shifts could be brutal or could be relatively quiet. Towards the beginning of the academic year, attendings were allowed to go home at night when department activities "settled down" usually around 2 AM. By the middle of the year, however, there was a general agreement that the faculty would stay in the department until their shifts officially ended at 8 AM. There still was a sleep room available for the attendings when the department was sufficiently slow. Patient volume in 1980 was 36,000 per year.

In the beginning, EM residents were shared with residency co-sponsor Riverside Methodist Hospital. First-year residents spent most of their months on rotations outside the department. Emergency medicine attendings supervised mostly first-year internal medicine and surgery interns and a smattering from ob-gyn, family medicine and anesthesiology residents. Many of these rotating interns were quite good. They seemed to enjoy the wide variety of patients they saw, especially patients with conditions they did not normally see on their regular rotations.

Although the new department was divided into "medical" and "surgical" sides, there was no attempt to assign rotating interns to a particular side. Medical interns would routinely see trauma patients and patients with abdominal pain. Surgery interns would routinely see patients with chest pain and shortness of breath. During the 1980s oral surgery residents did two-month rotations and were extremely popular among the attendings. Although most had DDS and not MD degrees, they were highly motivated, hard-working, and very fast learners. They did not shy away from complicated medical patients, and were excellent with procedures. The shift with an EM resident, though rare, was most welcomed in those early days.

Gradually through the 1980s, the residency grew from four to eight residents per year. By the end of the decade, their presence in the department became more noticeable and more consistent. At the same time, residents from other departments became fewer as some programs decided to curtail their residents' emergency rotations in favor of the ever-expanding specialty services. By the mid-1980s, there were no required emergency medicine rotations for surgery residents, who were needed on the transplant, cardiac and oncology services. Similarly, internal medicine interns were cut back from 2-month to 1-month rotations.

Common Life-Threatening Conditions in the 1980s

The ED was always been the prime destination for patients with acute, life-threatening conditions. Certainly, in the 1980s, myocardial infarctions, strokes, chronic obstructive pulmonary disease exacerbations and drug overdoses were commonplace. Treatments for such conditions were primarily supportive. Thrombolytics and stents for patients with myocardial infarction were not yet available. In fact, treatment of that era for acute myocardial infarction was limited to oxygen, morphine, nitroglycerine, cardiac monitoring, treatment of arrhythmias, and rest. Even aspirin had yet to be determined to be efficacious.

Common overdoses at the time included narcotics, alcohol and PCP (phencyclidine, or "Angel Dust"), a dissociative hallucinogen often mixed with marijuana that usually won the user an all-night stay in the department treated with a dubiously effective forced acid diuresis using intravenous ascorbic acid along with the probably more effective benzodiazepines. One of the most feared overdoses involved tricyclic antidepressants, particularly amitriptyline (Elavil). It was not unusual for a totally alert and normal-appearing patient to walk into the ED seeking help following their ingestion, and within an hour or two end up on a ventilator or dead from refractory ventricular arrhythmias and shock despite gastric lavage and bicarbonate drip, the mainstays of tricyclic overdose management at the time.

The symptoms of HIV infection were first described in 1981, though the infection was undoubtedly present for a number of years prior. At first, no one knew what was causing this strange illness that occurred predominantly in homosexual males and resulted in severe immunodeficiency resulting in the host contracting rare opportunistic infections such as Pneumocystis carinii (now Pneumocystis jirovecii) pneumonia (PCP) and Kaposi's sarcoma. For a while, the disease was known as GRID (Gay-Related Immune Deficiency). Until an actual viral etiology was discovered, speculation in the medical community and general public was that the cause was possibly related to hepatitis B virus, as those who contracted GRID often tested positive for hepatitis B. There was even an idea that the disease was related to the inhalation of nitrous oxide gas via "Whippets," which was also common among those with the disease.

By 1982, when it became apparent that this new disease was not limited to gay men, the name was changed to Acquired Immune Deficiency Syndrome (AIDS). The true viral etiology was discovered in 1983, and by 1986, the name was changed to HIV. For several years after its discovery in 1981, there was not much known about this new disease or even how serious it was. Once accurate testing was established in the mid to late 1980s, rates of progression to full-blown AIDS and subsequent mortality rates could be determined.

At first, mortality rates were thought to be fairly low, as most newly infected patients would be asymptomatic for a number of years. Even when testing was available, few patients were tested or knew their HIV status. It was not unusual to see a patient in the emergency department with fulminant "PCP pneumonia" as their first manifestation of any, let alone advanced, HIV infection. Within a few years, it was determined that almost all patients eventually progressed to full-blown AIDS, making the true mortality rate close to 100%. This fact had a tremendous effect on the medical community, particularly among surgeons and emergency physicians who were in constant exposure to blood and body fluids, the most likely mechanism for transmission. Simple needle sticks, which used to be commonplace, were suddenly a cause for great consternation among medical workers. Even splashes by urine, saliva or other body fluids carried unknown consequence, with the worst-case scenario being conversion to HIV positivity and almost certain premature death, not just to the medical worker, but also to their intimate partner.

The medical device industry came up with new products that made needle sticks from phlebotomy and IV insertions less likely. The "shirt-and-tie-to-work" era for emergency physicians ended abruptly.

Most clinicians were encouraged to wear clean scrubs to work, with a special hospital storeroom available to sign out clean scrub suits and return used ones. Employee Health was involved with following up on all significant exposures, usually for six to 12 months, though it would be several years before post-exposure prophylactic medications were available. With the HIV epidemic, for one of the first times, medical workers now feared their patients, causing them to question their profession and creating a barrier between them and their patients when providing care in the ED. History would repeat itself in 2020 with the onset of the COVID-19 pandemic.

Another relatively common illness from the 1980s that has since almost disappeared was Toxic Shock Syndrome (TSS). First described in 1978, TSS was eventually linked to high absorbent tampons in addition to skin infections, abscesses and strep infections caused by toxins produced by Staph aureus or Strep pyogenes. University Hospital physicians saw many cases owing to its proximity to the huge Ohio State student population. Patients typically presented with sudden onset nausea, vomiting and diarrhea associated with hypotension, an erythematous rash that would desquamate in a week or so, elevated creatinine and liver functions, and low platelet counts and coagulopathy in severe cases. Most patients ended up in the intensive care unit. Emergency physicians learned to include the questions, "Are you on your period? Do you use tampons?" whenever a female with vomiting or diarrhea presented.

Emergency Department Administration

The emergency department had always been a department *within the hospital structure*. In 1978 when the Division of Emergency Medicine was formed within the Department of Preventive Medicine, academic faculty were actively recruited and hired, but it was not until 1990 that an academic Department of Emergency Medicine was formed. Although many in the hospital called the emergency unit the *Emergency Room*, the term *Emergency Department* was favored by the leaders of emergency medicine striving so hard to become a full academic department. After 1978 the physicians were faculty members employed by the Ohio State University. By the end of the practice plan lawsuit in

1979, however, physicians were also simultaneously employed by their practice corporation, Emergency Care Associates, Inc., which had its own administrator responsible for corporate billing and finance. The emergency physicians, like the other physicians in the hospital had two employers: the university and the practice corporation.

For the hospital emergency department itself, ED administration was led by head nurse Toni Rausch, RN, until 1987. Rausch reported to the director of outpatient and clinic nursing for the hospital whose office was far from the ED. Rausch was considered the ED administrative director for all intents and purposes. This changed in 1987 when the hospital hired Tim McQuone as administrative director to whom Rausch and all other ED staff would report.

A non-clinician with a Master of Science Degree in Healthcare Administration from Gannon University, McQuone had previously been Trauma Coordinator at Hamot Medical Center (now University of Pittsburgh Medical Center Hamot) in Erie, Pennsylvania. His official title was Director of Emergency Department and Trauma Services and he reported directly to Kamilla "Kam" Sigafoos, the hospital's chief operating officer. His appointment reflected the growing consensus by hospital administration that the "ER" of old was maturing into a department that would play a substantial role in the growth of the hospital.

The other factor in McQuone's appointment was the hospital's interest in becoming a level 1 Trauma Center, made possible by several factors: recent state legislation establishing designated trauma centers and Ohio State's SKYMED medical helicopter service. The Department of Surgery also named Charles Cloutier, MD, the director of the trauma service. Michael Townsend, MD, later replaced Cloutier as director of the new Division of Trauma Surgery. Years later, McQuone remembered his arrival in 1987:

> *My first impression of the ER (not ED yet) was that it had fantastic physician and nursing individuals. Yet the ER with great history was utilizing most of its energy fighting the same battles each day. We had nursing issues, we had physician issues, and not department issues. This was a service that had a history of being told "no," and (to me) forgot how to fight. Each day was a battle to survive with little to no development of a strategic plan to build a better system.*[10]

Interestingly, in subsequent years external consultants would question this two-track method of organization: the physicians reporting to the department chair and the nurses and staff reporting to the hospital administrator. One of the consulting reports recommended that all emergency medicine staff report to the Chair of Emergency Medicine, thus unifying efforts to reach desired goals with a single reporting relationship for all employees in the emergency department. The recommendation was never implemented.

Mass Events and Referrals

With the Ohio State football games ensuring crowds of over 100,000 on campus on fall Saturdays, the excitement of the game could be too much for some fans with sometimes as many as three patients with myocardial infarction being admitted. Another challenge for Ohio State and emergency medicine involved the sports program and the treatment of Ohio State athletes. Ohio State had a superb sports medicine program under Robert "Dr. Bob" Murphy. Prior to 1978, however, the emergency department at Ohio State was staffed by interns and residents. By contrast, Murphy and his orthopedic colleagues were on staff at Riverside would see injured athletes themselves and questioned the ability of the interns to deal with athletic injuries. If an athlete required knee surgery, therefore, it was generally performed at Riverside Methodist Hospital.

Similarly, the Ohio State Student Health Center was staffed by a private group of physicians not affiliated with Ohio State, and up until 1991 students with suspected appendicitis or other surgical emergencies would be referred to Mt. Carmel Hospital ED for consultation and admission. Over time, however, the emergency department and Ohio State physicians became the preferred providers for all students, including athletes.

One memorable event in the ED's history occurred on May 28th, 1988, when Ohio Stadium hosted Pink Floyd as its first ever rock concert. As part of their "A Momentary Lapse of Reason" world tour, the band played to 64,000 enthusiastic and often inebriated fans, making it the largest concert ever in Columbus up until that time.[11] Administrator

McQuone recalls at least 10 to 15 ticketed fans never made it to the stadium and instead detoured to the ED to be treated for mostly conditions involving various intoxicants but also some traumatic injuries. Indeed, those working in the ED during the concert recall very busy evening and night shifts. That was the first of many concerts to be held at the stadium. By the time Pink Floyd returned six years later on May 29th, 1994, the medical center and especially emergency physicians had a seat at the table in formulating specific plans for such large-scale events.

With the annual Ohio State Fair held less than a mile from the medical center, the emergency department received plenty of business from fair workers and patrons. Many of the conditions were so unusual and sometimes so bizarre that an informal log sheet was hung up in the department where nurses and physicians could add their cases to the list. The title of the log sheet was "It's State Fair Time." Richard Nelson, MD, recalled seeing three patients with alligator bites on the same day after an alligator wrestling side show. Another event, the "Globe of Death," which involved two or three motorcyclists riding close-quartered on the inside of a wire-mesh globe, resulted in fortunately minor head injuries. Common entries on the list included "EtOH enthusiasm," "food poisoning," and "severe vertigo from Tilt-a-Whirl."

Rehabilitation and Corrections

In the late 1980s, University Hospitals became the main referral hospital for the Ohio Department of Rehabilitations and Corrections (ODRC). Many Ohio State medical faculty members were opposed to the decision, citing security issues and low reimbursement as well as lack of input into Ohio State's selection as the "prison hospital." This new designation meant that most prisoners within the state correctional system would eventually end up at Ohio State, often being transferred many miles via EMS or prison transport. A notorious transport service run by the state was based at Orient Correctional Institution in the town of Orient in Pickaway County, about 20 miles from the medical center. Physicians and nurses in the ED referred to this basic ambulance service as the "Orient Express."

Overall, working with inmates and correctional officers in the ED went smoothly. Most ED transfers were entirely appropriate and the admission rate was fairly high. The Lucasville riot of 1993 caused concern but only a few inmates were ever transferred.[12] Emergency physicians also enjoyed a good relationship with Larry Mendel, DO, the medical director of the prison system and a part-time emergency physician. He would often come to faculty meetings and spend time in the ED to better familiarize himself with department processes and procedures. He developed an early version of telemedicine services based at Ohio State for remote evaluation of inmates and for a short time, included a telemedicine station in the ED.

While the hospital administration supported the ODRC relationship, they were concerned with public perceptions. Inmates could not always be segregated in specific parts of the ED or hospital if they were too sick for those designated areas. Indeed, it was not unusual for a "VIP" patient to find themselves in an ICU bed next to an ODRC patient. The ED did make some concessions to appearances by having inmate transports arrive through the backdoor entrance to the ED, away from most other patients and families. Serious incidents occurred only rarely (see Inmate Incident).

Early Marketing Efforts and Ask-a-Nurse

Promoting health services was a relatively new phenomenon in the 1980s, but U.S. medical center marketing efforts continued to grow, as competition among hospital systems and physicians for patients and market share characterized the modern American health care system. Consequently, substantial marketing and advertising efforts by both institutions and physicians began in ernest.[13] Indeed, the American Medical Association's (AMA) code of ethics in 1847 considered advertising by physicians to be *"derogatory to the dignity of the profession."* This was reaffirmed and expanded in 1957 when the code determined *"Solicitation of patients, directly or indirectly, by a physician, by groups of physicians, or by institutions or organizations is unethical."*

This concept of advertising as beneath the lofty goals of health services began to unravel in 1975 when the Federal Trade Commission

> **Inmate Incident**   *By Jeffrey M. Caterino, MD, MPH*
>
> I was the sole attending in the department when we had a stat level I trauma alert. At that time, there was an outpatient MRI building adjacent to the emergency department. Apparently, a prisoner had his shackles removed for MRI. He then pulled out a spork (plastic spoon and fork combo) which had been sharpened at one end, stabbed his guard in the neck, and ran out the door. The guard was immediately brought to our trauma bay. At that point there was no warning and the trauma team was not present. We immediately began our protocols and were attempting to determine the seriousness of this penetrating neck injury. Within a minute the second level I trauma was called overhead. The fleeing prisoner had been shot and captured.
>
> Still without response from the trauma team who had not yet arrived, we split our teams. I remember turning to one of the guards who had a radio: "Where did they shoot the prisoner?" I asked. "Just outside of Means Hall," he said. I stared at him for a second then repeated with different emphasis "*WHERE did they shoot the prisoner?*" "Oh...in the head." So, we now prepped for a possible gunshot to the head in addition to our penetrating neck injury. As the prisoner was wheeled into the trauma bay, the trauma team began arriving. The guard's injury after imaging turned out to be superficial. Likewise, the prisoner had a minor graze wound of the scalp. He had wisely fallen to the ground after being shot. He was returned to prison.

determined that entities that prevented advertising, engaging in price competition and other competitive practices by health care providers actually violated antitrust laws. Ironically, the AMA was among the defendants when this went to court. In 1982, the U.S. Supreme Court confirmed the ruling, but not before the American Hospital Association had already adopted guidelines on advertising, which were quite conservative in scope and focused primarily on patient education.

One of Ohio State's first ventures by into this new competitive environment occurred in the early 1980s. At the time, the consensus among hospitals and even many emergency physicians was that the emergency department care was the most expensive of all medical care. Of course, the vast majority of this expense resulted from facility charges set by the hospital. The professional fee submitted by the emergency physician was relatively small by comparison. The perception of high costs, along with rising ED patient volumes led to the notion that everything should be done to keep patients out of the emergency department lest the health care system became insolvent. This concept was later debunked, although the perception still exists in some minds to this day.

One idea that emerged was to keep patients out of the emergency department and provide an opportunity for them to speak by phone with a trained nurse and perhaps avoid an unnecessary and expensive visit. Ultimately, the goal was to increase hospital and physician referrals while directing patients to the appropriate level of care. This program was started and marketed by Los-Angeles-based Adventist Health System and purchased by Ohio State in 1983. The program was initially under the emergency department, however later was moved to the hospital's Marketing and Communications department. Mary Jane Fellers, RN, an assistant head nurse in the ER, was selected to head the program. The hospital medical director, Hagop Mekhjian, MD, with input from emergency physicians, reviewed and signed off on the protocols.

Patients would call the well-publicized 24-hour hotline and speak to a registered nurse trained in phone triage. Patients would then be given several options: Follow suggestions by the phone nurse, within the limits of their protocols, follow up with their physicians in a specified timeframe, or go to the ED for evaluation and treatment. Over the years of its existence, the program was probably responsible for a net gain of patients presenting to Ohio State's emergency department. Fellers later recalled the following:

> *Eventually the program just became too expensive for the hospital to support. We started with 4.8 RN FTEs and we peaked at somewhere around the low 20s. Over time it became apparent that the actual payer for a program like this should have been a health care plan and not the hospital, because the opportunity for actual savings was to keep patients out of the hospital rather than drive them in. The program ultimately ended in July 1998.*[6]

Another New Emergency Department, 1995

By the early 1990s, Emergency Medicine had become a full academic department within the College of Medicine and the faculty and the residency program had grown substantially. By 1993 there were eight residents in the department each year in addition to the fellowship programs in research. Not only were there more EM residents, but with the decision to centralize the program in 1990, most resident rotations were in the emergency department at Ohio State.

The old concept of dividing the ED into "medicine" and "surgery" sides, established with the 1979 expansion, no longer made sense. EM attendings covered the entirety of the department, and EM residents vastly outnumbered rotating residents from medical and surgical specialties who never really benefited from a divided ED anyway. Also, the old design did not permit any discretionary space to establish popular modern ED programs, such as the observation unit and fast track, and simply involved too much walking back and forth with no ability to keep the majority of patients within visual site of the physicians.

A new ED expansion and remodeling in 1995 would address such issues. The project's leads were nurse manager Patti Finerty and James "Jim" Hoekstra, MD. Clinicians and administrators, met regularly and contributed to the project. The medical center hired a young architect, Arden Freeman, to design the new department. Because the new ED would include portions of the old department, the construction would take place in phases and over two or three years, with periodic partial ED shutdowns. The effort was a logistical challenge, but proper planning and cooperation by staff fortunately kept disruptions to a minimum. The entire project was finally completed in 1998: ED beds increased from approximately 28 to 45 beds.

The "new" emergency department was a substantial improvement over the old one. One important design feature was a large main room with approximately 24 patient rooms around its periphery. Physicians and nursing staff work stations were in the center as was the glassed-in "control center" in which unit clerical staff and the EMS radio were stationed. Physicians and nurses could now have direct visualization of most of the ED patients without having to walk between the old "medicine and "surgery sides."

The rooms were fairly small and the only rooms with doors were the negative airflow room and the psychiatric room. For all other rooms curtains sufficed for privacy. Other areas of the new ED included the two trauma rooms which remained in their original places, a 6-bed observation unit in what was previously the "medicine side", and a Fast Track area located in the east corridor. The area for prisoners was now moved to the north side of the ED. Radiology rooms, CT scan and the two-chamber hyperbaric unit remained in the same spots.

Prompt Care and Fast Track

Prompt Care began in 1988 to provide urgent care services and perhaps decompress the emergency department. Initially housed on the ground floor of the university hospital clinic building, the center offered walk-in care from 10 AM to 6 PM on weekdays. William "Bill" Hall, MD, was hired to cover Prompt Care four out of five days with the remaining weekdays covered by family physicians Stephanie Cook, DO, Robert Guthrie, MD, and various EM faculty members. Hall was one of the founders of the Riverside Methodist Hospital emergency physicians' group and was one of the first group of presidents of the Ohio Chapter of the American College of Emergency Physicians from 1974-75. The Bill Hall Award was named in his honor and is awarded annually to a past or present member of the Ohio ACEP Board of Directors to recognize their contributions in advancing emergency medicine and patient care.

By 1992 there was considerable interest to decompress the busy ED by triaging appropriate lower acuity patients directly to Prompt Care. These efforts were only partially successful due to several factors. First, the recently enacted Emergency Medical Treatment and Active Labor Act would have required a physician to perform a medical screening exam verifying that the patient did not have an emergency medical condition prior to sending them across the street to Prompt Care. A medical screening exam in a low acuity patient represents most of the entire medical interaction. The physician could complete the visit with a prescription and instructions in less time than in sending the patient across the street. Patients would also have to cross the street or travel by tunnel with an ED guide. Upon arriving at Prompt Care, if they should require an x-ray, they would have had to be sent back across the street again. Consequently, this triage of ED patients never occurred.

Prompt Care was eventually moved to the ED. With growing patient volume there was interest in expediting care for low-acuity patients. Under the old system such patients might have to wait hours for what would ultimately be a brief visit. There were attempts to establish a "Fast Track" area of the ED beginning in March, 1996, with Prompt Care continuing to run concurrently across the street during weekday hours. This area was located on the old east corridor of the ED. By February, 1998, Prompt Care was moved to the Fast Track area of the ED and the hours expanded to 11 AM to 11 PM on weekdays and 2 PM to 10 PM on weekends. Eventually only emergency medicine faculty worked in the Prompt Care area, which was now called Fast Track to avoid confusing patients who were used to the old Prompt Care across the street.

Fast Track soon became very busy. Despite only being open less than half the time, Fast Track saw almost 25 percent of total ED patient volume. This was also a popular area for medical student clinical education, who were able to have more patient contacts, perform more procedures, such as suturing and incision and drainage of abscesses, and receive more individual instruction from the faculty. Eventually, nurse practitioners and physicians' assistants were hired to staff Fast Track alongside the attending emergency physician, who often concurrently staffed the Clinical Decision Unit. Physicians working in the Fast Track area had to see patients quickly but be thorough enough to not miss an unsuspected emergency—a hidden "land mine."

Wound Care

Many hyperbaric programs across the country sought new sources of revenue through wound healing. In November 1998, faculty members Richard Boggs, MD, Sorabh Khandelwal, MD, and later Colin Kaide, MD, began to spearhead efforts to establish a wound care center affiliated with the hyperbaric oxygen (HBO) unit. The Ohio State Wound Care Center was soon established, with most of the wound services being performed in the small treatment rooms adjacent to the ED hyperbaric chambers. As the center grew, a company called National Wound Healing took over management of the center and in 2006 moved it to a larger space at the Camera Center (now Martha Morehouse) on Kenny Rd.

The center was multidisciplinary, emergency physicians working alongside podiatrists, plastic surgeons and general surgeons. The center also added its own hyperbaric unit at the Camera Center while maintaining the two in the ED. National Wound Healing held national HBO courses in Columbus, which drew physicians nationwide. Eventually, the Wound Care Center grew into The Ohio State University Comprehensive Wound Center under the Department of Surgery.

The Ohio State Emergency Department in the 2000s

September 11, 2001

One memorable event for all Americans at that time were the hijackings and subsequent attacks on New York City and Washington, DC. By the time the second airliner crashed into the south tower of the World Trade Center at 9:03 AM on that Tuesday morning, it was obvious the U.S. was under attack. Regularly scheduled Tuesday morning residency conferences were taking place when ED Medical Director Rick Nelson, MD, interrupted the 9 AM speaker, Doug Rund, MD, to announce the unfolding shocking events. The projection system in the conference room was re-tuned to TV news broadcast so that residents and faculty could witness what was going on.

Hagop Mekhjian, MD, hospital medical director, called an emergency meeting of hospital leadership. Nelson attended the meeting representing the emergency departments and recalls the immediate concerns on everyone's minds: What is happening? Who is responsible? Will there be more attacks? How will this affect us and what can we do? This last question was crucial in that everyone in the room understood that Ohio State was not only a level 1 trauma center but also central Ohio's only adult burn center. Continued attacks and mounting casualties would surely overwhelm medical resources on the east coast, making it likely that patients would ultimately need to be transferred to other areas of the country for care. Burn injuries would potentially make Ohio State an institution in high demand. Years later Kamilla "Kam" Sigafoos, Chief Operating Officer of the medical center at the time, recalled that day and that meeting:

> *I remember driving into work that morning, I had the radio on, and they talked about the first tower being hit. I thought we're at war but we don't know who with. When I got to the hospital and the second tower had been hit, it was interesting; everybody wanted to go home. The secretaries, the different staff, even some of the nursing folks, they wanted to go home. And I'm like, "You can't go home right now. We need you guys here." And then Hagop called a big meeting, and whether it was right or wrong, we shut down anything that looked elective. At the time, Hagop and others thought that we might get a lot of burn patients and we did not end up getting any burn patients. And we caught a lot of grief for that, because people said well, Riverside is still seeing surgical patients. We're closing down our OR but Riverside and Mt. Carmel aren't. And then of course it didn't end up impacting us directly.*[14]

One of the few positive things to come out of the 9/11 event was the impromptu role the Central Ohio Trauma Systems (COTS) played that day. Until then, there was very little real-time communication between area hospitals regarding events that might impact other hospitals' operations. The Columbus Medical Association and Foundation had established COTS a few years earlier to improve coordination of hospitals with regards to trauma patients. COTS staff quickly realized there was a significant amount of telephone traffic between hospital emergency departments asking for information as to what was occurring and how that might impact Columbus area hospitals.

They set up a clearinghouse to provide up-to-date information that hospitals and emergency departments could access with one call rather than having to call multiple hospitals. Questions included whether hospitals were shutting down elective surgeries and routine hospital transfers, and about needed equipment should the hospitals be overwhelmed by transfers from New York. COTS ultimately formalized this plan as a 24/7 Healthcare Incident Liaison service. The service would play an important role in years to come with Hurricane Katrina in 2005, the H1N1 pandemic of 2009, the COVID-19 pandemic of 2020, and numerous smaller more local events that impacted hospital and ED function.

Another event that occurred shortly after September 11th that ultimately proved even more disruptive to emergency department operations were the anthrax mail attacks. Starting on September 18th and lasting approximately five weeks, weaponized anthrax spores were sent through the U.S. mail, ultimately infecting 22 people and killing five. The attacks were initially thought to be related to the same group of terrorists behind the 9/11 attacks, however the source of the anthrax spores was eventually determined to be from the government's biodefense labs at Fort Detrick in Maryland with the perpetrator being a scientist working there.

Although no one in Columbus up to that point had been exposed or infected with anthrax, the local emergency departments, particularly Ohio State, responded to large numbers of patients wanting to be checked for anthrax due to exposure to strange powders in various locations. Occasionally a patient would present to triage with the actual powder they were exposed to, wanting it to be analyzed but not realizing that should it have actually been weaponized anthrax spores, everyone in the near vicinity of the triage area would have been exposed to potentially lethal amounts of anthrax. Also, the ED area itself would have been contaminated and would have been required to undergo extensive decontamination procedures. A protocol was soon established for both the handling of potentially dangerous substances and the diagnosis and treatment of exposed patients and staff. After a few months, anthrax cases across the country ended, media coverage died down, and patients stopped presenting to the ED for possible anthrax exposure.

Advances in Information Technology

By the late 1990s it had become apparent to all that handwritten charts, even with physician dictation for histories, physical exams, and clinical course, was inadequate. An early tracking system called Clinicomp, which had been used on Labor and Delivery and earmarked for the ED was never implemented. Emergency patients at Ohio State were becoming more complex; rapid access to medical information was critical. Also, tracking patients using a white erase board visible to staff, patients, and visitors essentially violated the 1996 HIPAA law.

Another significant deficiency in handwritten charts was the work needed to carry out simple orders. Orders for laboratory tests, x-rays, medications and consults were written on the chart with unit clerks filling out the paperwork, sending the blood collection tubes and forms through the pneumatic tube system, and paging the appropriate people. If one omission was made in this complex process, it could be one to two hours before that error was noticed and another one to two hours to correct the error. Probably the most significant deficiency of the paper record was the inability of doctors, nurses, unit clerks, techs and consultants to have simultaneous access to the chart. Physicians and nurses would waste a tremendous amount of time merely searching for the chart they needed to review, write on and implement orders.

By the early 2000s the hospital had committed to a mostly paperless information technology system in the emergency department. The goal: Install a common hospital-wide and accessible system utilized by all departments. However, a commercial system that was suitable for the medical center did not yet exist even though some hospitals had developed their own "home-grown" systems. With a great deal of support from the hospital Information Technology (IT) department, emergency department leaders started a quest for a Clinical Information System (CIS) that would include patient tracking/tracking, documentation, order entry and discharge instructions.

Patti Finerty, RN, former ED nurse manager and current Patient Care Resource Manager and Rick Nelson, MD, ED Medical Director, led the efforts to find such a system. After approximately one year of meetings, site visits, demonstrations and user evaluations, the hospital selected a product called IBEX (Healthdata Systems, Inc), a subsidiary of Picis, Inc. The hospital and ED pursued an aggressive implementation schedule and phase 1 of IBEX began operation on November 4, 2004, with tracking and triage. A few months later Phase 2 (physician documentation) was added, and Phase 3 (order entry) was added much later in early 2007, though a hybrid system of order entry was employed beginning in 2005. The discharge instruction component was a separate program called Discharge 1-2-3, which was largely developed by Ohio State EM faculty member Colin Kaide in association with Callibra, Inc.

The IBEX CIS was a huge success. The ED became the first department in the medical center to essentially go paperless. Although there was initial staff and physician trepidation about going to such a new system, particularly the concern that documentation would require much more time than handwriting or dictating, it became quickly apparent that the advantages far outweighed any disadvantages.

Allowing multiple workers simultaneous access to charts was a tremendous advance and spared clinicians much wasted time searching for charts. Physician documentation was quick and easy as well.

IBEX used a system that allowed physicians and nurses to generate what appeared to be a clinical narrative by clicking on certain key words on a screen. More complicated information could be added using either the keyboard or a Dragon voice-activated dictation, which was integrated into the system. As an added bonus, physicians did not have to review and sign their charts days later as they did when the carts were dictated. The charts were usually completed once the patient left the department. When the order entry module went on-line, physicians were amazed at a dramatic decrease in lab and medication errors compared to the old paper system.

Finally, IBEX tracked levels of service based on documentation, giving physicians immediate feedback as to missing documentation that would prevent a higher level of billing from being generated. This combination or rapid turnaround of charting and immediate feedback on levels of service resulted in a substantial improvement in physician revenue for the department. Once fully functional in 2007, IBEX remained the main IT platform for the emergency department for five years before it was ultimately replaced by a systemwide platform, Integrated Healthcare Information System, with Epic at its core, in 2012.

Emergency Department Clinical Pharmacist Program

In the beginning, like most emergency departments across the country, neither of the Ohio State emergency departments had on-site pharmacists. In fact, it wasn't until the 1990s that most EDs, including Ohio State, transitioned from a "cabinet with paper log documentation" to an automated dispensing cabinet. Ohio State went with the Pyxis product. The subject of pharmaceuticals was broached briefly during a September 6, 2005, faculty meeting regarding how emergency physicians should respond to questions likely to be asked by surveyors during an upcoming JCAHO (currently The Joint Commission) visit. The minutes read as follows:

> *Joint Commission will be visiting OSU Medical Center in early October. One of the issues has been pharmaceuticals in the emergency department. According to Joint Commission standards, a pharmacist must be involved in the dispensing of hospital medications except in an emergency situation. Currently there is no pharmacist in the emergency department. Thus, the physicians must perform the role of checking for appropriateness of medications, assuming it does not go through the pharmacist. If residents or attendings are asked by the Joint Commission surveyor how they ensure that medications given in the emergency department are appropriate, the proper response should be that they check for allergies as well as medication interactions prior to ordering specific medications.*

As it turned out, that Joint Commission visit presaged things to come. Mary Beth Shirk, PharmD, who would later be the first clinical pharmacist in the ED, worked in the ICU and Pain Service at the time of the 2005 Joint Commission visit. Years later she recalled the following:

> *During the site visit, they opened a drawer in one of the unlocked trauma bay airway carts and found unsecured controlled substances, either morphine or hydromorphone. Back in 2005 the mindset in the ER was: "that's not a problem."*

This event, along with the realization that more patients were on many different types of medications with higher potential for drug interactions and side effects, prompted nursing and physicians to see a role for pharmacists in the ED. Nursing and physician staff soon began identifying other potential functions of pharmacists in the ED and advocated for their presence like that in other hospital units such as the ICUs. Rund was one of those who pushed for pharmacists in the ED.

Another impetus for having pharmacists in the ED related to a new set of Joint Commission standards proposed in 2006. One of the standards required prospective review by a pharmacist of first dose administration of medications. This would have created a difficult situation in EDs, particularly those without pharmacists, when it came to administering emergency drugs in a timely fashion. Another new standard required medication reconciliation on all ED patients, much the same as that required for hospital inpatients. These Joint Commission rules were eventually softened after letters were written by a coalition of EM organizations, including American College of Emergency Physicians, American Academy of Emergency Medicine, and Emergency Nurses Association.

The medical center eventually provided funding and Shirk began working in the ED in January 2007. She recalled her priorities for this newly established position: *We first focused on needed operational improvements, then moved to establishing and expanding clinical services, and finally extending our teaching reach to include disciplines beyond just our own.*

The EM pharmacist impact was felt immediately. In the first two years of the program, these procedures and efforts were put into place: The State Pharmacy Board's new Ohio Automated Rx Reporting System was introduced; the medications stored in the ED Pyxis® were adjusted to meet urgent needs with consideration given to frequency of use and safety; a determination was made whether ED's embossing system would be compliant for Medicaid patients whose tamper proof scripts were mandated; physicians were surveyed about the most common home going medications and then developed home going medication instructions and labeling for these products; rapid sequence intubation kits were created; and prebuilt orders for ED management of blood-body fluid exposure, take home medications, and HIV medication kits were developed.

Mary Beth Shirk, PharmD, received her Doctor of Pharmacy degree from Ohio State followed by a two-year fellowship in Drug Information. In 2007 she took on a newly created position in the medical center as Specialty Practice Pharmacist in Emergency Medicine. She conducted high quality research, initiated and monitored pharmacotherapy, led quality improvement activities, provided coverage for arrest, stroke and trauma, and provided high quality education for pharmacy, nursing and medical staff.

She retired in 2020 and received numerous prestigious awards during her career. Erin Reichert, PharmD, became the second pharmacist in the ED in August 2009, and covered the evening shifts. With two full-time pharmacists in the ED, coverage was provided for just less than 50% of the hours each week and none yet on weekends or holidays. A later incident of trauma during pregnancy resulted in recognition of the need for a pharmacist in cases regarding mothers and newborns. Shirk later noted, "OB actually met with the ED and pharmacy folks with the result that there would be a pharmacist at all level 1 traumas 24/7." Trained central operations pharmacists would provide coverage in Shirk and Reichert's absence.

An EM pharmacy residency program was established in 2011 with Shirk as director. A two-year post-graduate program with the second year focusing on Emergency Medicine, this was the 12th such program in the United States. In 2012, the program received its accreditation by the American Society of Health-System Pharmacists. Ohio State's program began with one resident per year and expanded to two per year in 2014. By 2022 there would be almost 100 programs across the country.

By 2017 the EM pharmacist program had expanded to seven pharmacists in the ED in addition to the two residents, and further expanded to Ohio State East in 2018. The EM pharmacy team has a robust research program whose faculty and residents are well represented at the Department of Emergency Medicine's Spring Research Day each year as well as at national and regional meetings. Their research has not only been published in the pharmacy literature but also in the emergency medicine, EMS, toxicology and trauma literature.

The 315 Exit Ramp to Medical Center Drive

Having grown up in Columbus, Douglas Rund, MD, was puzzled by the absence of a state Route 315 exit ramp to the Ohio State Medical Center. His concern developed soon after he was recruited by the university to start an emergency medicine program in 1977. Rund soon sought out physician and historian George Paulson, MD, who explained the history. When state Route 315 was built in the 1960s and 70s, the freeway had to be rerouted on its way north from downtown to avoid crossing Union Cemetery just south of Riverside Methodist Hospital. According to Paulson, Riverside Hospital agreed to provide the needed land for the freeway reroute in exchange for two freeway exits to the hospital. This was done and the freeway proceeded northward.

The absence of at least one similar exit to the Ohio State University Hospital baffled Rund in many ways: The hospital, after all, provided tertiary care for serious acute events of all sorts, including patients with life-threatening cardiac disease and accident victims with major trauma who clearly needed the resources provided by the medical center and needed them quickly. In addition, this was a state hospital so why had the state Department of Transportation not provided an exit when the freeway was initially constructed? Rund's initial quest for answers led him to the office of Richard Jackson, Vice President of Business and Finance in the 1980s. An article in *Business First* published in 2002 described the meeting:

> It has been more than 20 years since Dr. Douglas Rund got his first glimpse of plans for new Route 315 ramps that would steer traffic to and from Ohio State University Medical center. "I'll never forget that day when Dick Jackson unrolled those blueprints for the ramps," Rund said. "That was especially impressive to a young faculty member like me." But the high hopes of Rund and others at Ohio State were to be dashed for two decades when the project didn't climb to the top of the state's funding list. That meant emergency vehicles, patients, and visitors from the south and east had to follow a convoluted route over city streets and university roadways to reach the medical center. That trip should become faster and easier by the end of 2004 when construction on two new ramps is completed, according to Ohio Department of Transportation (ODOT) officials. With funding finally in place for the $9.6 million project, they say two years of construction should begin this fall.[17]

To Rund, the construction of the ramps made obvious sense. Existing traffic patterns at that time required that northbound vehicles on 315 had to exit at Lane Avenue and double back to the hospital. The proposed ramps were estimated to shave 12 precious minutes off the trip.

Years passed and the university made no progress in convincing the state to add the freeway ramp, which also led to a distrust of the agency itself. The Director of Health Services Facilities Planning at the medical center, Ralph Hudson, soon joined Rund in the seemingly fruitless quest to create a freeway exit to the hospital. Hudson was quick to point out the benefits for all patients who would be the real beneficiaries. Frustrated by years of inaction, Rund and Hudson approached Manuel Tzagournis, MD, Vice President for Health Sciences, who contacted U.S. Congresswoman Deborah Price (Columbus) who also supported the exit and who then secured federal support. The eventual funding included contributions from the university and the federal government.

The medical center could finally be accessed from the south by the exit to Medical Center Drive. It literally "took an Act of Congress" to get it done. The advocacy for an exit for vehicles heading south from Worthington and points north of the campus was never successful. The Department of Transportation apparently felt that such a ramp would require an enormously high structure towering over the Lennox Town Center and the proposal was never approved.

Further ED Expansion and Clinical Decision Unit (CDU)

Despite a large increase in ED beds that came with the 1998-completed ED expansion, there was still limited capacity to observe patients over longer periods of time than typical for ED visits. The old seven-bed "medicine side" of the 1979 ED had been converted into a 6-bed Extended Emergency Unit, but patients eligible for placement there initially were limited to three specific diagnoses: chest pain, stable congestive heart failure and asthma. The hospital and the ED wanted to establish a much larger observation unit of up to 20 beds. One of the metrics the hospital-wide Clinical Quality Management Committee tracked on an ongoing basis were the numbers of admitted patients discharged within 48 hours. It was believed that many of these patients could be managed by emergency physicians in an ED Observation unit and thus reduce the numbers of "unnecessary" hospital admissions.

The Institute of Medicine's June 14, 2006, report, *The Future of Emergency Care in the United States Health System,* presented the severe problems facing the nation's emergency care system and offered recommendations for improvement. One recommendation cited clinical decision units (CDUs) as a way to improve hospital efficiency and reduce ED overcrowding.[15] Within a month after the report's release of the report, a delegation from Ohio State's Emergency Department—Assistant ED Medical Director Mark Moseley, MD, Chair Doug Rund, and practice manager Rich Sobieray—traveled to Rochester, New York, to tour the CDU at Strong Memorial Hospital to learn about some of the best practices. Moseley was eventually asked to lead the Clinical Decision Unit. Years later he remembered his thoughts at the time:

> *I was an emergency physician. I hadn't done a lot of observation medicine because it just wasn't a thing in the emergency medicine circles other than at a few select sites. But again, being very curious and supported, I attended a training course at Emory. I got very involved in ACEP and SAEM observation medicine section. In 2009 we opened our CDU. That was very instrumental in my career and something that made a big impact in the department, and something to this day I remember as being a seminal event for me, realizing that with appropriate planning and the right support from leadership, you can do something truly extraordinary. We had people coming from all over the country to see what we did. We went from that small little CDU of six beds that we had to a beautiful 20-bed CDU. At one point we were putting almost 6,000 patients a year in that unit. We totally positively impacted length of stay in the ED and [reduced the number of patients who] left without being seen.[16]*

Advanced Practice Practitioners (APPs)

In 2009 Advanced Practice Practitioners (APPs) began work in the main campus Emergency Department with the opening of the Observation Unit. Mark Moseley, MD was the first collaborating physician. The APPs have been key players in managing the conditions of admitted patients ever since, with the number of APPs having grown from less than 10 to almost 20. Today there are two main 12-hour shifts for the Observation APPs, 7 AM and 7 PM, 7 days a week.

Moreover, 38 patient care protocols have been developed, with the department experiencing great success in rapidly managing patients with transient ischemic attacks, chest pain and heart failure exacerbation and those in need of GI consultation, and others with more complex issues such as frailty and hospice placements.

Over time, the APPs broadened their skill set beyond the Observation Unit to expand to the ambulatory sites at AfterHours Care at Martha Morehouse, the Advanced Immediate Care Clinics at New Albany and Dublin, and in the oncology pod in the new ED. The concentration of patients with cancer in this pod made a partnership with the James Cancer Hospital attractive. With some James funding, a group of APPs was hired to solely provide care in this pod in conjunction with the ED attending physicians. The APPs came from different areas, including inpatient oncology services, intensive care units and the ED. By working solely in this pod, this group of APPs has developed expertise in acute oncology and has a successful collaboration with emergency medicine attendings.

The new advanced immediate care centers have also provided an opportunity for innovative physician–APP collaboration. Each center is staffed by an emergency physician along with an APP, a model that now accommodates over 20,000 patients per center each year. For many years Daniel Christopher "Chris" Fulks, CNP, MS, MPA, has been the lead physician for the Main campus and the Immediate Care sites in Dublin and New Albany. Mark Conroy, MD is the current collaborating physician.

The CDU became the Observation Unit

During the COVID-19 pandemic the CDU's name was changed to the ED Observation Unit (EDOU). Farhad Aziz, MD, named director in 2019, was an Ohio State undergraduate alumnus and received his medical degree from the University of Toledo. He completed his EM residency and fellowship in medical education at the University of Kentucky. Looking back, he recalled the accomplishments of the observation unit:

Shortly after I took over, we had to adjust our hours and functionality due to COVID-19. During the timeframe of COVID-19 we were able to expand to occupy the Post Anesthesia Care Unit (PACU) to accommodate for an expanding protocol list and increasing numbers. Unfortunately, the PACU was not a sustainable venture at the time as COVID-19 led to a decrease in patient volume throughout the hospital. We expanded our protocol list to accommodate approximately 30 different protocols, ranging from general chest pain protocols all the way to working up and managing transient ischemic attacks (TIAs) and cerebrovascular accidents (CVAs). In July 2022 we expanded to include the 12-bed medex unit on the 11th floor into our observation unit. This was staffed by our advanced practice practitioners (APPs) and our faculty. In March 2023 we expanded from 24-hour APP coverage to include 12 hours of APP cross coverage to manage volumes. On average we are accommodating 17 patients in our EDOU and hope to expand to 30 patients. It is truly remarkable how well our APPs manage the unit and turn over approximately 15-25 beds every day. It truly is a service to our department and to the hospital.

Quality Improvement

The 1990s saw an interest by emergency physicians nationwide to not only provide excellent patient care, but to make efforts to improve that care over time. Ohio State had a large and robust Clinical Quality Management Committee, which looked at patient care issues. This committee was multidisciplinary, including all specialties and non-medical members who represented the public. One such member was Charles Y. Lazarus, Chairman Emeritus of Federated Department Stores and past chair and board member of the Ohio State University Hospital board of trustees.

Lazarus took an active role in the committee's activities and was known for focusing the committee's attention on patients rather than processes, particularly when discussions got "too deep in the weeds" and risked losing perspective on the most important things. The Department of Emergency Medicine had its own Clinical Quality Management Committee that reported to and was represented on the hospital committee. The department committee included physicians, nurses, administrators and quality improvement specialists.

Several improvements in quality focused on cardiac care. The treatment of patients with ST segment elevation myocardial infarction improved markedly in the early 2000s due to improved collaboration between cardiology and the emergency department including pre-hospital emergency medical services (EMS). Patients with chest pain seen by EMS were quickly evaluated on the scene with a 12-lead electrocardiogram (ECG). The tracing was transferred to Ohio State wirelessly and interpreted by the emergency medical staff almost simultaneously. Based on the ECG and the report of the EMS crew, patients were taken quickly from the ED to the catheterization laboratory for coronary artery opening and revascularization of the myocardium. Eventually the crews could bypass the ED and take patients directly to the catheterization suite. Under the guidance of emergency physicians Brian Hiestand, MD, and Craig Key, MD, and cardiology faculty members, including Ernest Mazzaferri, Jr., MD, the performance improved dramatically: In 2006 the time between patient arrival and opening the artery (door to balloon) was 176 minutes; in 2009 the time was 53 minutes.

The scope of services and quality of patient care expanded in several areas in the early 2000s and two areas were highly impactful: ultrasound and advanced techniques in airway management. Ultrasound became a routine diagnostic procedure for many procedures, including placement of central lines and drainage of cutaneous abscesses; and many faculty became credentialed in three areas: the focused abdominal scan in trauma (FAST), detection of presence or absence of intrauterine pregnancy in women with abdominal pain and a positive pregnancy test and detection of cardiac motion in cardiac arrest.

There were also significant advances in difficult airway management. The EM physicians, even then, were considered the experts in acute airway management. In order to provide the most-cutting edge care, the department avidly adopted new devices that became approved for airway management during this time period. These included a number of airway adjuncts and indirect laryngoscopy solutions such as the use of the GlideScope, the fiberoptic intubation device, the AirTraq device and ongoing training in their uses in difficult airway scenarios. Other advances included continued ongoing education in the use of various airway adjunct devices such as tracheal introducer, laryngeal mask airway (LMA), fastrack LMA, and the lighted stylet, and yearly difficult airway labs, which included the use of all airway devices and practice in the techniques of open and percutaneous cricothyrotomy. Education also included small group sessions on an algorithmic approach to the difficult airway.

A New Hospital and a New Emergency Department

In 2010, construction began on the new James Cancer Hospital and Solove Research Institute, named for its founder Ohio State cancer surgeon Arthur James, MD, who desired a comprehensive cancer hospital to Columbus. The original hospital was opened in 1990 on the east side of the medical center, but its success ultimately created the need for a larger facility. In 2010 ground was broken for "The New James" on the west side of the medical center. This was to be a 21-story building costing $1.1 billion, the largest construction project in Ohio State's history and the third largest cancer hospital in the country. An important part of this construction project was an ED expansion westward and occupying the east side of the ground floor of the James.

Planning for the ED expansion went on for at least two years. Tammy Moore, RN, nurse manager of the ED from 2008 to 2012 recalls: "I believe the initial discussions began in 2010 and were initiated due to the growing demand for ED services and our limited beds. We were seeing high 'left-without-being-seen' metrics, and wait times were on the rise with inability to clear our waiting rooms in appropriate times. All of this was impacting patient care and patient experience."

Like the 1995 expansion, the new design required input from virtually all categories of personnel who worked in the ED, including physicians, nurses, administrators, security, facilities, Transfer Center, contractors, EMS, lab, imaging, and Ohio Department of Corrections. Mark Moseley, MD, ED medical director at the time, played a particularly critical role. Physicians from other departments were also involved, with Steven Steinberg, MD, founding director of the Division of Trauma, Critical Care and Burn, playing an important role in the design of the new trauma rooms.

The new ED expansion opened in January, 2014, preceding the James Hospital's completion, which opened in December, 2014. The completed ED, including the expansion, consisted of 94 total beds, with most of the rooms having sliding glass doors. The front entrance on 10th Ave. offered valet services for ambulatory patients and a rear entrance on 12th Ave. for EMS and corrections arrivals. Specialty areas within the ED include a Hyperbaric Oxygen unit with three monoplace chambers, three large trauma rooms, six critical care rooms, a 20-bed ED Observation Unit, 15-bed James Oncology unit, 16 psychiatric beds, eye room with slit lamp and retinal camera, decontamination room, and rooms in the Arrival Zone of the ED where physicians and APPs can examine, order labs and imaging, and often disposition patients.

Areas outside the ED that are covered by emergency physicians and APPs include the 12-room Medical Express unit on 11 West Rhodes Hall for observation patients and the James Immediate Care Clinic, located on the 5th floor of the James and staffed with James APPs. Specialized designations include Level 1 Trauma Center, Regional Burn Center, and Level 1 Stroke Center. Ohio State ED was also the first in the Midwest to achieve Level 1 Geriatric Emergency Department Accreditation by the American College of Emergency Physicians.

Growth of Patient Care Space in the Past 100 Years

The emergency room of 1924 through 1951 consisted of a single emergency and dressing room with a side examination room. The total area was 720 square feet. The emergency department 100 years later occupied 58,197 square feet and included well over 100 beds in the department itself with 28 additional beds on other floors. The growth in space proceeded in stepwise fashion with new construction in 1951, 1979, 1995 and 2014. Increasing patient demand created an insistent need for additional space over the years. Figure 11 shows the growth of the emergency department patient care space over the past 100 years.

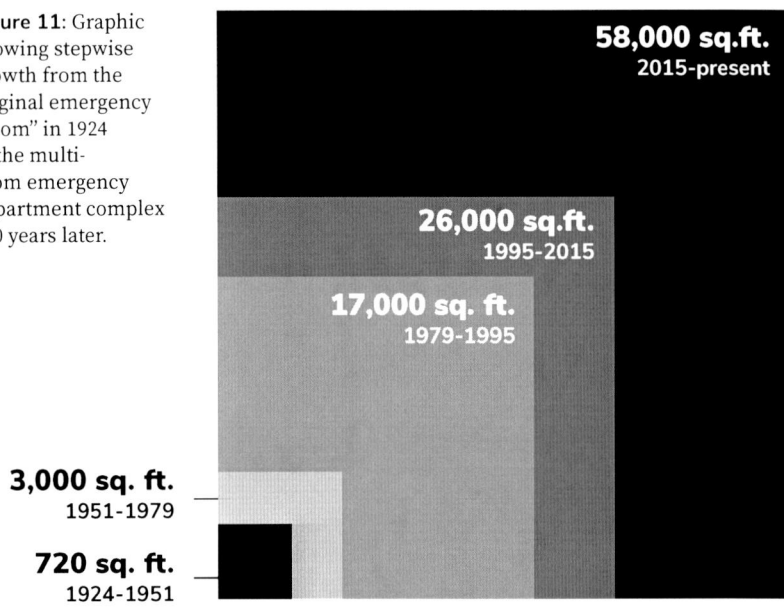

Figure 11: Graphic showing stepwise growth from the original emergency "room" in 1924 to the multi-room emergency department complex 100 years later.

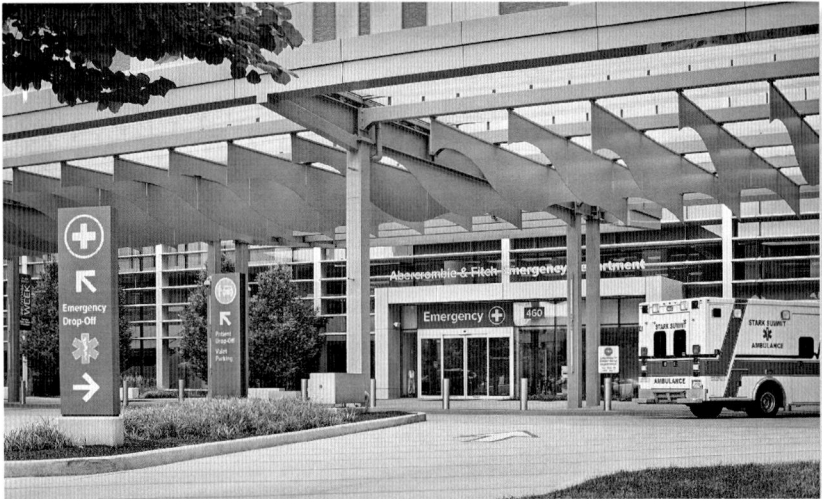

Figure 12: Entrance to the emergency department in 2023

References

1. Fontana ME. Personal communication. 2022.

2. Williams JH. Personal communication. 1978.

3. Hudson PW. Ed. Letter from Director of Dispensaries, Elijah J. Gordon to John Upham, Dean of the College of Medicine, dated June 20, 1939. The Ohio State University College of Medicine 1934-1958. The Ohio State University. 1981: 271.

4. Bullock K. Interview with Kathleen "Kate" Bullock, RN, by Douglas Rund. 2021: Columbus, Ohio.

5. Ferenchik, M. OSU turmoil of 1969-1970 remembered. *Columbus Dispatch*, Oct. 5, 2017.

6. Fellers MJ. Interview with Mary Jane Fellers, RN, by Richard Nelson. 2022: Columbus, Ohio.

7. Mitchell J. Personal communication. 2022.

8. Goodwin D. Personal communication. 2023.

9. Hansplant P. Interview with Paulina Hansplant by Richard Nelson. 2022: Columbus, Ohio.

10. McQuone T. Interview of Timothy McQuone by Richard Nelson. 2022: Columbus, Ohio.

11. Deitch L. In 1988, Pink Floyd rocks the 'Shoe in stadium's first-ever concert. *Columbus Dispatch*. May 8, 2022.

12. Newberry PG. Lucasville: What happened at the 1993 prison riot that was Ohio's longest and deadliest. *Cincinnati Enquirer*. June 28, 2022.

13. Oxman D. Hospital advertising. *The Hospitalist*. Jan. 2, 2007.

14. Sigafoos K. Interview of Kamilla "Kam" Sigafoos by Richard Nelson. 2023: Columbus, Ohio.

15. IOM Report: The future of emergency care in the United States Health System. Institute of Medicine. *Acad Emerg Med.* October 2006;(13)10.

16. Moseley MG. Interview with Douglas Rund. 2022: Columbus, Ohio.

17. Bell J. Med center ramps up. *Columbus Business First.* January 28, 2002.

Chapter 18
Ohio State East Hospital

Michael R. Dick, MD
Richard N. Nelson, MD
Douglas A. Rund, MD

Ohio State East Hospital was originally St. Anthony Hospital, founded in 1890 by The Sisters of the Poor of St. Francis (later the Franciscan Sisters of the Poor) and dedicated on November 22, 1891. The hospital accepted its first patients the following month. Located on the east side of Columbus at Hawthorne Street and Taylor Avenue in what is now the King-Lincoln Bronzeville area, St. Anthony Hospital could accommodate over 200 long-term patients. In 1904 an additional floor was added, and in 1939 a three-story wing increased bed capacity to 270 (Figure 1).

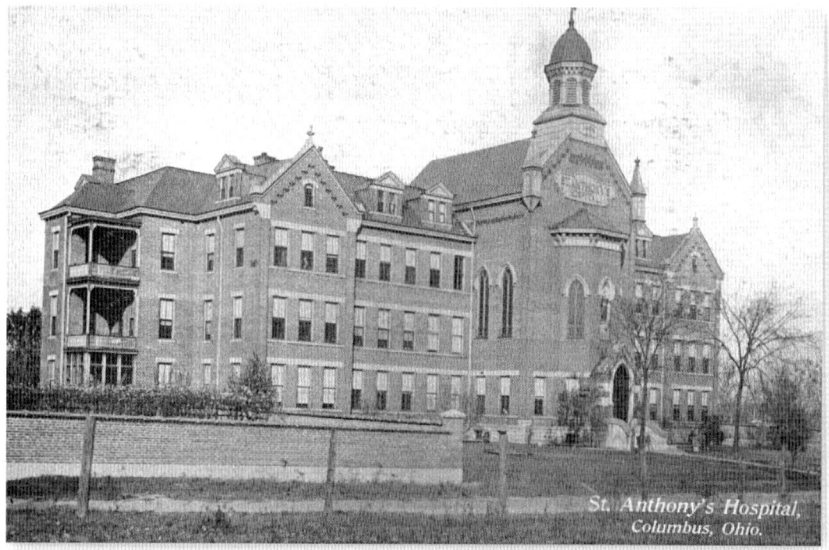

Figure 1: St. Anthony Hospital (the precursor to Ohio State East Hospital) was founded in 1890 by the Sisters of the Poor of St. Anthony.

St. Anthony was initially set up to care for older patients with chronic conditions in order to free up patient beds at St. Francis Hospital, the first hospital established by the Sisters in 1847 in downtown Columbus. St. Francis Hospital was the first to combine patient care and clinical teaching in the same facility in the United States.[1] Ohio medical students received their training at St. Francis up to the mid-20th century. The hospital used two-thirds of the building; Starling Medical College was housed in the remainder.

Starling Medical College, the predecessor of the Ohio State College of Medicine, existed until 1907. In 1929 the Franciscan Sisters of the Poor organized a School of Nursing, which moved to St. Anthony Hospital when St. Francis closed in 1955. St Francis was razed in 1957 and the site was occupied by Grant Hospital thereafter.

In 1969 St. Anthony's original red brick gothic building was demolished and replaced with the iconic cylindrically shaped 16-story tower (Figure 2). Designed by Leon A. Ransom, a prominent Columbus African American architect, the new St. Anthony Hospital continued to serve the people of Columbus, particularly those living on the east side.

The new facility's emergency department (ED) was located on the tower's ground floor. Because of the tower's cylindrical shape, the ED was small and oddly shaped, with one curved hallway reflecting the building's circular design. John Sigafoos, RN, who worked there at various times and was assistant nurse manager in 1999, recalled years later:

> *Beds were on the outside of the curve and the nursing station and radiology were on the inside of the curve. It was like a quarter of a racetrack. We had four beds on one side and six on the other with a significant amount of distance from one end to the other. We used to run back and forth like crazy.*[2]

Emergency Medical Associates, Inc. (EMAI), one of the earliest emergency physician groups in Central Ohio and founded by T. William Evans, MD, in 1971, provided physician staffing for the hospital's emergency department until the late 1970s. One of the emergency physicians who worked for EMAI at St. Anthony ER was Douglas Rund, MD, who had just moved back to his hometown of Columbus after completing an EM fellowship at Stanford University.

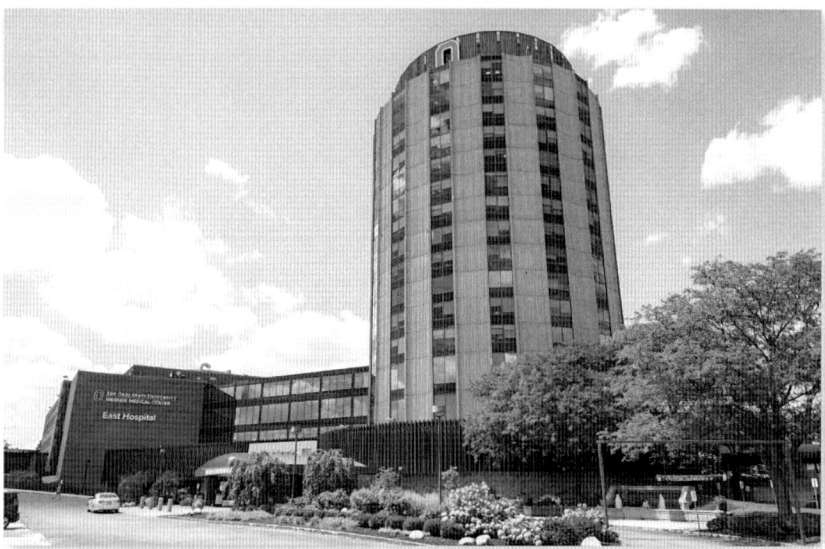

Figure 2: The original emergency department at OSU East Hospital Tower was on the tower's ground floor. Today, the department is on the ground floor of the brick structure to its left. The original round tower's shape made it difficult to use the rooms.

By the 1980s, St. Anthony, like many small community hospitals, was struggling financially. Managed care and limited Medicare and Medicaid reimbursement reduced the not-for-profit hospital's ability to achieve financial success. Larger hospitals could garner higher revenue through specialty surgery services not offered at St. Anthony. Trauma patients were often brought to St. Anthony due to its proximity to the inner city, though trauma patients, like many of St. Anthony's other patients, were uninsured and therefore did not contribute to the bottom line. Later, Ohio designations of trauma centers further limited St. Anthony's draw.

During that era the drop in the number of women entering religious life eventually led the Franciscan Sisters of the Poor to divest their hospitals nationwide. After years of financial difficulty, St. Anthony was sold in 1991 to Tennessee-based for-profit Quorum Health, which renamed the hospital Park Medical Center. Changing to a for-profit entity did little to improve revenues and actually further limited its patient base. The ED saw a decrease in patient volume, dropping to as low as 1,000 patients per month. Most of the emergency physicians who worked there were neither residency trained nor board certified in emergency medicine. In the 1990s the three major hospital systems in Columbus were expanding by actively acquiring other hospitals to increase their market share.[3]

Ohio State leaders were concerned that being left out of these rapidly growing multihospital systems would result in stiffer competition. Rather than acquire other hospitals, Ohio State settled for negotiating transfer agreements, primarily for trauma patients, and providing limited specialty physician presence at a few outlying smaller hospitals. Similarly, while emergency medicine physician groups in other settings were acquiring contracts to staff departments in other hospitals both near and far, Ohio State's Department of Emergency Medicine faculty members concentrated on academic rather than business pursuits.

Douglas Rund, MD, and Richard Nelson, MD, the department's Chair and Vice Chair, respectively, in the 1990s, were routinely approached by small hospital administrators about staffing their EDs. None of these discussions led to any agreements and the Ohio State faculty limited their practice to University Hospital.

When EMAI stopped staffing the St. Anthony Hospital emergency department, the contract was taken over by a local independent group led by Nino Diiullo, MD, a family physician. This was a common occurrence in the early days of the specialty of emergency medicine. Diiullo was joined by his business partner, Will Coppel, MD, another Ohio State graduate who left a surgery residency at Ohio State to work in the emergency room.

After St. Anthony was sold to Quorum in 1992, Diiullo and Coppel became less involved with emergency medicine and more focused on developing urgent care centers. Park hospital administrators then approached Rund about having Ohio State emergency physicians staff the hospital emergency department (ED). At the May 5, 1992, faculty meeting, however, there was little enthusiasm for the concept. Eventually the emergency departments at both St. Anthony and Columbus Community Hospital (formerly Mercy Hospital) were staffed by an emergency medicine contract management group out of Warren, Ohio, called 4M Emergency Systems. At the time, both Park Medical Center and Columbus Community, a physician-owned hospital were in decline and ED volumes at Park were less than 15,000 patients per year. EMS was reluctant to take patients to Park.

By 1998, quiet negotiations began between Ohio State and Quorum for the sale of Park. University Hospital was often full, resulting in typically long delays for admitted emergency patients going to their inpatient rooms. In addition, Ohio State had a well-deserved reputation as a hospital focused on research and education. This did not always completely resonate with many in the general public, some of whom seemed to value easy hospital access and customer amenities over cutting-edge medicine. The hospital also had always been a large teaching hospital so prospective patients may have felt that they were under the care of students and residents. Also, the fact that Ohio State medical center physicians were capable of providing state-of-the-art care for all conditions, including rarer more complex medical conditions, may have led some to believe that more routine conditions did not require the services of an academic medical center.

Park Medical Center was located in an area which had started to decline in the 1960s. Some attributed part of the decline to the construction of the local freeways that divided the traditional neighborhoods. By 1998 the hospital had a poor payer mix. When the sale of Park was finalized in early 1999, Ohio State made the decision that the newly acquired hospital would focus on two services: Family Medicine and Orthopedics. Family Medicine had long struggled to find a niche competing against the large highly specialized academic departments at Ohio State. Its residency program in particular had difficulties finding suitable inpatient rotations in which the residents would be considered full members of the team and not "just rotators." Being based at what would soon be called Ohio State East, Family Medicine would be an important player in both inpatient and outpatient services for the hospital.

Orthopedic Surgery at Ohio State had been a division under the Department of Surgery, however, with the Park acquisition, it became a department in 1999. Thomas Mallory, MD, a Grant Hospital orthopedic surgeon and pioneer in joint replacement surgery, performed the first total hip replacement surgery in Columbus in 1971. He was hired by the university to chair this new department. Having orthopedic services at Ohio State East would guarantee a reliable flow of insured patients not only from the east side of Columbus but also from the entire central Ohio area.

Other services that would continue included Talbot Hall, which provided inpatient and outpatient drug and alcohol addiction rehabilitation services, and the emergency department. Discussions were held on whether an emergency room should even be continued owing to low patient volumes and poor reputation. One idea involved housing one of the University Hospital's MedFirst urgent care/primary care centers at East in lieu of an emergency department. In the end it was decided that Ohio State East would be a mostly full-service hospital (excluding obstetrics) that included an emergency department. Services at the hospital would feature orthopedics and family medicine. Moreover, the Department of Emergency Medicine at Ohio State would provide physician staffing for the emergency department.

Seeking Opportunity
By Douglas A. Rund, MD

In 1998 leaders at Ohio State were mulling the acquisition of an additional hospital to increase clinical capacity and help maintain its market share by competing with the other hospital systems in Columbus: OhioHealth and Mount Carmel. My next-door neighbor was the Chairman of the Osteopathic Heritage Foundation Board. I knew that the foundation was planning to sell its hospitals, Doctors North and Doctors West.

Seeing a great opportunity for Ohio State, I arranged a meeting to discuss this with Bernadine Healy, MD, the College of Medicine Dean, Manuel Tzagournis, MD, Vice President, and the Osteopathic Heritage Board leadership. We met at Doctors West Hospital and toured the facility. We knew that Park Medical Center was about to be placed on the market. From my standpoint, we had a choice to acquire either Doctors or Park. The former included the facility on Dennison Avenue in the Short North district and Doctors West on West Broad Street.

Healy envisioned offering specialized surgical services at Park, such as orthopedic surgery, and Tzagournis noted the increase in hospital capacity that Park offered the university. The university ultimately purchased Park and asked the Department of Emergency Medicine to provide physician staffing for its emergency department. Ohio State finally bought Park Medical Center for $12.7 million. The Doctors facilities were well over 10 times as much. The complexion of hospital services in Columbus would certainly have changed if the university had instead acquired the Doctors locations.

Ohio State Emergency Medicine Provides Physician Staffing

The Department of Emergency Medicine (EM) saw providing physicians to staff Ohio State East ED as a huge challenge. Patient volume at Ohio State Main ED, as it became known to distinguish it from East, had increased substantially since the newly renovated ED was completed in 1995, and the hiring of new faculty members was not keeping up with needed added coverage shifts. By 1999, volume at Ohio State had reached 54,000 patients per year. Many of the EM faculty members were not enthusiastic about working in a new practice environment, presumably without residents or even medical students to teach, which was the reason many chose to work at Ohio State in the first place.

Finally, and perhaps most important, the Department of Emergency Medicine, like other academic departments in the College of Medicine, was largely self-supporting and highly dependent on patient care revenue. Ohio State East had a high percentage of uninsured and Medicaid covered patients. Medicaid reimbursement in the 1990s did not come close to covering physician salaries and other department expenses, such as secretarial and administrative staff as well as medical liability insurance and billing costs. Emergency Care Associates Incorporated (ECAI), the department's practice corporation, determined that the hospital would have to heavily subsidize the department's practice income for things to work out financially. This was something that the hospital had never done before with emergency medicine. By the spring of 1999, after the sale of Park Medical Center was finalized, Park officially became Ohio State East (or simply, East). The Department had to recruit truly excellent physicians in a short time. Fortunately, department leaders recruited several outstanding and highly qualified emergency physicians to take over ED staffing.

MICHAEL R. DICK, MSc, MD

In 1999, Michael R. Dick, MD, MSc, was asked to serve as the Medical Director of the Ohio State East ED in 1999 (Figure 3). The son of a railroad worker, Dick, who grew up in Shelby, Ohio, knew the value of hard work. Dick became a paramedic in Colorado in 1977, completed his undergraduate degree at the University of Colorado in 1978 and continued to practice as a paramedic after moving to Columbus in 1978. He completed his Master of Science degree at Ohio State in the Department of Pathology in 1980 and continued in graduate school before enrolling in medical school at Ohio State. From 1982 until 1989 he also worked as a flight Paramedic for Lifeflight Emergency Medical Transport and as a paramedic in the emergency department at the Columbus Childrens Hospital from 1980 to 1989.

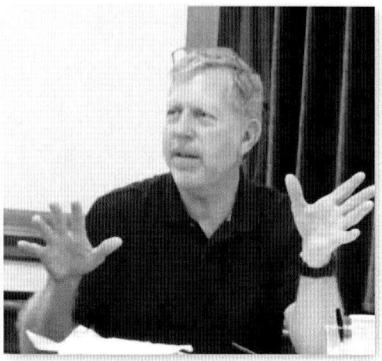

Figure 3: Michael R. Dick, MD, leads a discussion in 2015.

He was inducted into the Alpha Omega Alpha Honor Medical Society in 1988 and in 1989 received his MD. He went on to complete his residency in Emergency Medicine at Ohio State in 1992 and then a fellowship in Critical Care Medicine in the Departments of Anesthesiology and Surgery in 1993. Following his fellowship, he joined the faculty in the Department of Emergency Medicine.

Dick was obviously an accomplished physician with far-ranging skills when he joined the faculty, and in 1999 the Department of Emergency Medicine asked him to lead the new department at Ohio State East. It was imperative, however, that he recruit a staff of similarly superior physicians. The reputation of the previous hospital staff was so low it was felt that the new staff had to be exceptional. First and foremost, the physicians needed to be superb clinicians and provide the best possible patient care in order to improve the hospital's reputation. Dick rapidly recruited the best physicians available and provided the leadership and role modeling needed for his new physician staff. His expertise in critical care was a bonus for his patients and supported his vision for the future of his department: to provide the best care possible to all who came for care.

Years later, in an interview with an Ohio State reporter regarding his career, Dick shared the following recollections:

> *I am grateful that Ohio State invested in East Hospital. It's a special*

> *place to work. I have been so fortunate to work with such a wonderful group of physicians, nurses, staff and administrators. In some ways it has become a stepping stone for many of our top medical center leaders. I do hope they never forget where they came from. I've always felt that every person, whether they're a CEO or someone on Medicaid, deserves the same quality of care. And because of where we're located, we have the opportunity to provide that care for people who are really, really in need.[4]*

He also shared some of the emergency department's successes under his leadership:

> *The East Hospital ED, with support from other departments, has developed a program for the care of patients with acute heart attacks and strokes. We are now a Level III Trauma Center. Our ED leads the central Ohio region in providing state-of-the-art care to patients with drug addiction. I see the East ED as the unusual blend of public health and outreach, while treating minor problems one minute and cardiac arrests and gunshot wounds the next. All these programs have been established and maintained independent of the full complement of resources available at University Hospital.[4]*

During his career Dick became Chairman of the Medical Services Advisory Board in Upper Arlington and later Medical Director of the Center for Emergency Medical Services (EMS) at Ohio State. He was recognized in 2022 for his service to EMS, receiving the highest honor for an EMS clinician and leader during the Star of Life Program: the Jack B. Liberator Lifetime Achievement Award. Presented by the Ohio Department of Public Safety's Division of EMS, The State Board of Emergency Medical, Fire, and Transportation Services and the Ohio Chapter of the American College of Emergency Physicians, the award noted the following:

> *Dr. Dick has dedicated over 40 years to emergency medical care. He joined the OSU faculty in 1993, where he's made an outstanding impact on the clinical practices in the community of EMS giving lectures to broad EMS audiences. He has championed many EMS programs such as stroke, trauma, and cardiac protocols and Project DAWN (Deaths Avoided With Naloxone) that prevents deaths using naloxone (also known as Narcan). Naloxone is a medication that can reverse an overdose caused by an opioid drug (heroin, fentanyl, or prescription pain medications).*

He started the first emergency department naloxone distribution program in Franklin County in 2015 that is now considered a standard of care. He is revered as an expert clinician and still serves as an outstanding resource for the medical community.[5]

Dick began recruiting emergency physicians to staff Ohio State East in 1999. Two of the first physicians hired were Ann Haynes and Kurt Neltner.

ANN M. HAYNES, MD

Ann M. Haynes, MD, received her Doctor of Medicine degree in 1992 from Northeastern Ohio Universities College of Medicine (Figure 4). Her undergraduate degree was from Youngstown State University. She graduated summa cum laude from college and was elected a member of the Alpha Omega Alpha Honor Medical Society in medical school. Following medical school, she completed the emergency medicine residency program at Ohio State. She then worked in several community hospitals, including Good Samaritan in Zanesville and Grady Memorial in Delaware.

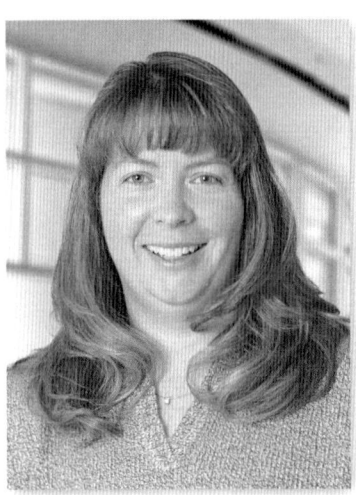

Figure 4: Ann M. Haynes, MD, was one of the first attending physicians at the newly acquired Ohio State East Hospital.

In 1999 she joined the Ohio State faculty to become one of the original East faculty members staffing the emergency department. Haynes grew up in the Buckeye Lake area and made it her home since. Over her career she served on the Door to Balloon committee at the startup of the East ST Elevation Myocardial Infarction (STEMI) program. Along with cardiology she worked on the STEMI protocols and procedures. The program turned out to be quite successful.

She also spent several years focused on improving the timeliness and care of sepsis patients and improving compliance with the CMS sepsis core measures. At the time, no EM residents were assigned there and faculty worked single coverage 12-hour shifts. Years later she recalled the changes that had occurred at East over her career, including huge growth in the patient population, development of programs for stroke, addiction and sexually transmitted diseases. Over the years the faculty coverage expanded to two to three attendings at a time with additional advanced practice provider (APP) and resident coverage. She also recalled the following:

> *We had a sleeping room. With a bed. That we actually had time to sleep in some nights. [The facility was] a round tower [that was] a dysfunctional design for an ED. Curved walls and curtains separating tiny treatment spaces led to a lot of bumping into each other. That first year, we delivered a lot of babies in the ED. The community saw the OSU sign and assumed we had the same services as the Main campus. One of my most memorable patients was an elderly veteran who was part of the D Day invasion. He talked about how scared he was that he would drown. He didn't know how to swim and got dumped off in chest high water and in chaos.*[6]

KURT A. NELTNER, MD

Kurt A. Neltner, MD, joined the faculty in 1999 as part of the new core staff at Ohio State East (Figure 5). Neltner graduated from Thomas More College with his bachelor's degree in biology in 1991 and completed medical school at the University of Kentucky College of Medicine. He completed his residency in emergency medicine at the University of Illinois at Peoria and worked for one year at Proctor Hospital, also in Peoria.

Tom Gavin, MD, an existing faculty member who had graduated from the residency program in 1993, agreed to work most if not all his shifts at East.

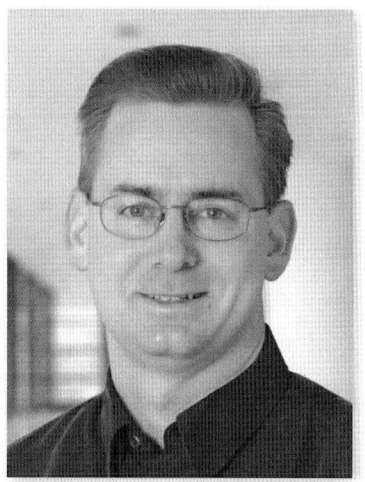

Figure 5: Kurt Neltner, MD, joined the emergency medicine faculty in 1999 to become one of the first members to staff the emergency department at Ohio State East Hospital.

These four emergency physicians—Dick, Haynes, Neltner, and Gavin—worked full time at East. They could not, however, completely staff the emergency department. Several faculty members from Main also agreed to work some of their shifts at East. In addition, a few of the physicians who had worked for 4M Emergency Systems, the previous staffing group, stayed on temporarily in a limited capacity. The Department of Emergency Medicine officially took over staffing at OSU East on July 1, 1999. Soon additional faculty members were recruited.

SONDRA "SONI" SHELLMAN, MD

Sondra "Soni" Shellman, MD, joined the faculty at East in March 2000 (Figure 6). She completed her BS in Human Nutrition at Ohio State University in 1990, and graduated from Ohio State with her MD degree in 1994. She completed residency training in emergency medicine at North Carolina Baptist Hospital/Wake Forest University in 1997. Her first position out of residency was working in the community at Licking Memorial Hospital in Newark, Ohio.

Shellman missed the breadth of services a system such as Ohio State could give her patients and when staffing at Ohio State East expanded, she came aboard. In the beginning, she aided administratively with tracking quality data such as 72-hour returns. In 2007, Ohio State East ED hired its first two Advanced Practice Providers and the APP program began. Shellman became the East APP collaborating physician in 2008 and today still holds this position, advocating for this provider group. For her efforts, she was awarded the APP Champion Physician Award in 2014.

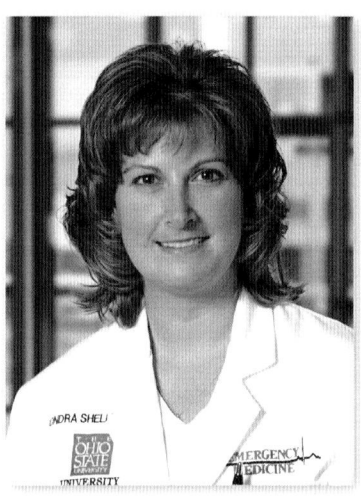

Figure 6: Sondra "Soni" Shellman, MD, joined the faculty in 2000 and worked exclusively at Ohio State East during her career at Ohio State.

In 2012, Shellman helped nursing develop the SANE (Sexual Assault Nurse Examiner) program at Ohio State

East and became the Assistant Medical Director that year as well. As part of her administrative duties, she also began coordinating emergency medicine, family medicine and podiatry residents' rotations through the East ED. In 2016, Shellman was promoted to Associate Professor and continues her role as one of two assistant medical directors at East. Thinking back on the development of the East Emergency Department, Shellman recalled:

> *I remember the very first East faculty meeting I attended, which was the night before my first shift at East. Mike Dick, the medical director, talked about the facility itself and how he was working on a number of things to improve the physician's job so that we could focus on being excellent patient providers; hot water and modern equipment were a premium in those days! I was struck by how impassioned he was to make East a premier emergency department. From the beginning, everyone working at East including physicians, nurses, and staff had the same common goal: to not only make East Hospital successful, but to have East Hospital provide care to people who truly had nowhere else to go. We started with the basic principles of emergency medicine and have been able to branch out to include services at East that previously we had to transfer patients away from East to obtain. All this growth was the vision of Mike Dick. Working at East has been and still is truly a family environment; we have shared so much over the 20-plus years I have been there.*[7]

MARK L. DEBARD, MD

Mark L. DeBard, MD, joined the faculty in 2001 (Figure 7). Born in Des Moines, Iowa, and growing up in Centerville, Ohio, DeBard graduated from the University of Dayton in 1972 and earned his MD from Ohio State in 1975. He joined the attending staff at St. Elizabeth Hospital in Dayton in 1976 and became board certified in family practice from 1978 to 1985 and board certified in emergency medicine from 1981 to 2019.

DeBard was the recipient of the 2007 Excellence in Teaching Award from the Ohio State Department of Emergency Medicine, and received the 2011 Distinguished Educator Award from The Ohio State University College of Medicine. He became active in the American College of

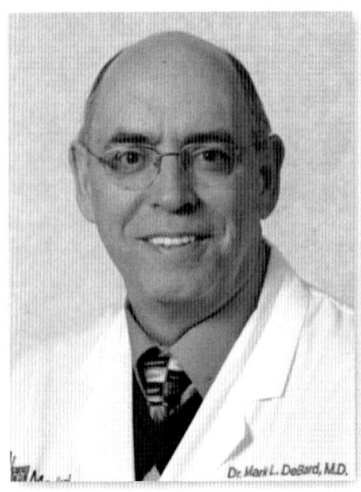

Figure 7: Mark L. DeBard, MD, practiced at Ohio State East from 2001 until his retirement in 2016.

Emergency Physicians (ACEP) and held numerous leadership positions in the state and national organization. He became speaker of the national ACEP Council from 2003-2005, and received their highest honor, the John G. Wiegenstein Award in 2013. DeBard's research and expertise encompassed food and waterborne illness, medical marriages, the sexual assault examination, and excited delirium syndrome.

He prompted the ACEP Council to pass a resolution to study patients with agitated delirium with unexpected deaths. The subsequent expert panel task force, which he chaired, identified Excited Delirium Syndrome as a clinical entity which the ACEP Council and Board subsequently endorsed as a medical diagnosis in 2009. Along with Richard Nelson, MD, in 1992 he also helped Ohio ACEP establish a statewide protocol for examination of the sexual assault patient. He then convinced national ACEP to establish a national task force to establish standards for the examination of sexual assault patients throughout the country.

DeBard retired in 2016 and became Professor Emeritus (Figure 7). Years later, DeBard recalled his experiences as a faculty member at Ohio State East:

> *I was a practicing clinician and Attending Physician from 1976 until my retirement 40 years later in 2016 at the age of 65. I chose Family Practice for my residency upon Ohio State Medical School graduation in 1975 as I liked everything but had never heard of emergency medicine, nor had I set foot in the emergency room during my 3 years as a medical student. But as an intern I loved the ER and moonlighted heavily. Uniquely, I staffed and ran my inner-city, 40,000 patients/year training center ER by myself as an accredited attending while I was a second-year resident, replacing two psychiatrists. Trial by fire with on-the-job training. I*

became a board-certified emergency physician in 1982 with the third EM board exam ever given.

I came to OSU East in 2001 because it reminded me of my old closed inner-city hospital in Dayton and offered an academic teaching environment like we had at Wright State Medical School. At that time, we worked in the small old emergency department, single physician-only coverage, with 18,000 visits/year. When I retired in 2016, we had a modern and growing ED seeing 50,000 patients/year with double physician coverage, multiple midlevel providers, residents, and medical students, along with the best practical nurses with whom I had ever worked. These nurses were a very stable and hugely motivated and talented group that all felt like family and had each other's backs—and mine. In 2001 until the new ED was built the docs could even grab a few hours of sleep in a back room at night.

I loved our annual Christmas parties in an informal setting, seeing the loving-life side and families of all those who worked with us. And towards the end of my career, I think we provided a model of how midlevel providers can become health care partners with nurses and emergency physicians in a cooperative effort to provide the best and most efficient care for patients.

MELISSA FENNER, MD

Melissa Fenner, MD, grew up in the Cleveland area (Figure 8). She graduated from Smith College in 1995 and returned to Ohio, later graduating with her MD degree from the University of Cincinnati College of Medicine in 1999. She completed her EM residency at Ohio State in 2002. She moonlighted at Ohio State East during her PGY3 year—before the residency had a presence at the hospital. After she completed medical school, Fenner joined the Ohio State faculty and practiced primarily at East. She stayed on as an Assistant Professor for 12 years. During her tenure she participated in the medical student education mission giving lectures, mentoring, and serving on various committees such as the admission committee. For many years she wrote a column in *The Columbus Dispatch* about emergency medicine.

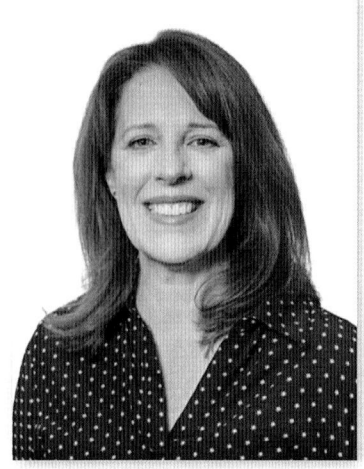

Figure 8: Melissa Fenner, MD, completed her residency in 2002 and joined the core faculty group staffing the Ohio State East emergency department.

Fenner's family moved south in 2014 and she left academic medicine. She began working in a large community hospital, a level 3 trauma center, in the Charlotte, North Carolina area. Soon after starting in her new hospital, she became Medical Control for a hospital-owned EMS agency. In that role she began supervising over 125 paramedics, five first responder agencies within York County South Carolina, and serves as Medical Control for the county emergency management agencies as well. Fenner has been the Assistant Facility Medical Director for Emergency Medicine at Piedmont Medical Center in Rock Hill, South Carolina, since 2015 with several stints as the Interim Director over the years. She is currently serving as Secretary/Treasurer at Piedmont Medical Center through 2025.

BRANDY L. (HELMINIAK) ZIMMER, MD

Brandy (Helminiak) Zimmer, MD, received her MD degree from the University of Buffalo School of Medicine in 1999 (Figure 9). She received her undergraduate degree in biology from SUNY Genesco and completed the emergency medicine residency program at Ohio State in 2002. She began moonlighting at East soon after the department was staffed with Ohio State physicians. After graduation she continued to work at East as a faculty member.

Years later, recalling her experiences during this part of her career Zimmer remembered the following:

> [Eventually all my time] was devoted to working alongside some of the most amazing physicians, nurses, and staff in the brand-new Ohio State East emergency department. My 13-year career was the basis of solid friendships that formed into a sisterhood and ultimately the best work

family a physician could ask for. Four of the initial full-time physicians at East were women. This was influential in building a stronger workforce for women in medicine. I have fond memories. Dr. Dick, our medical director, encouraged everyone's participation in our monthly meetings. I remember pushing a stroller with a new baby to our meetings and all the other physicians' children playing in the back of the meeting room. Dr. Dick welcomed all our children with opened arms (and doughnuts and pastries for them). It was a wonderful way to reiterate that our work families and our home families would be forever entwined.[8]

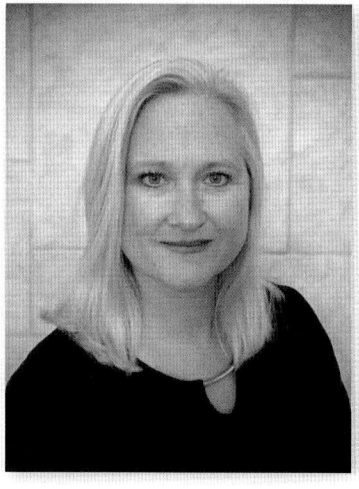

Figure 9: Brandy (Helminiak) Zimmer, MD, completed her residency in 2002 and joined the core faculty group staffing the Ohio State East emergency department.

Zimmer eventually entered practice in a community hospital south of Columbus.

The Turnaround in Emergency Services

The emergency medicine business corporation, Emergency Care Associates, billed patients and payors for physician services at Ohio State East through Ohio State University Physicians Inc., as it did for patients at the Main campus. In addition, however, the hospital agreed to provide a calculated monthly subsidy to make up for shortfalls in collections. This subsidy became critical since the collection rate for self-paying patients—almost 20 percent of the EM practice—was extremely low at under 3 percent. This subsidy allowed the Department of Emergency Medicine to maintain its financial health while making an essential contribution to Ohio State East's future success under the Ohio State umbrella.

Ohio State East Hospital quickly showed an amazingly rapid turnaround from where it had been as Park Medical Center under Quorum

Health. The Department of Orthopedics did most of its surgeries at East, thus keeping the operating rooms and inpatient beds occupied. The Department of Family Medicine, and later, General Internal Medicine, admitted many of their patients to East, where Richard Schlanger, MD, a graduate of the Ohio State surgery residency program, led a small but busy general surgery service.

Talbot Hall continued with its addiction and alcohol rehabilitation services, one of the few such private ventures in the region. The emergency department, under Dick's leadership, saw a substantial increase in patient volume and EMS traffic in just a few months. In fact, Dick reported just two months after the Ohio State purchase, that volume had increased from 1,200 to 1,800 patients per month with up to 35% of patients arriving via EMS. He believed they would soon need double coverage of physicians in addition to resident coverage. It was also anticipated that a new emergency department would also soon be required.

By 2003, Ohio State East emergency department continued to show considerable growth in patient volume and outgrowing the ED, which was also outdated. Physicians, nurses and administrators met regularly to draw up plans for a new, state-of-the-art emergency department, and held a ground breaking ceremony March 31, 2004.

The new emergency department would occupy renovated space on the south side of the hospital. It would expand from 7,000 square feet to

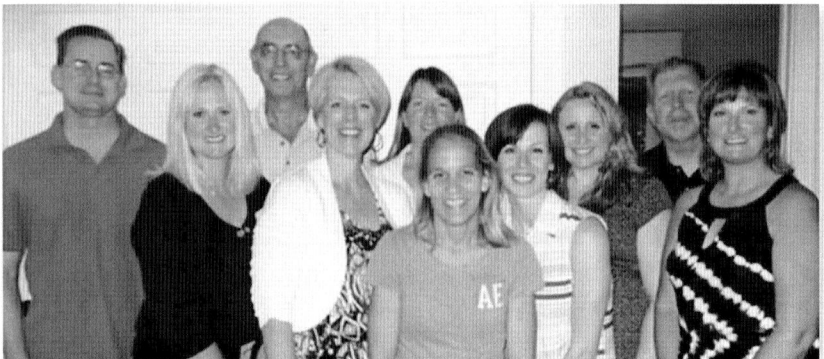

Figure 10: Ohio State East faculty and staff in 2014, left to right: Kurt Neltner, MD; Brandy Helminiak Zimmer, MD; Mark DeBard, MD; Melissa Fenner, MD; Ann Haynes, MD; Heather Matejovich, CNP; Carol Petke, RN, CNP; Sommer Lindsey, MD; Michael Dick, MD; and Sondra "Soni" Shellman, MD.

15,000 square feet of space, and feature 26 private rooms, a larger waiting room, and two specialized suites for patients with breathing disorders.

By the time the emergency department moved to the south building in 2005, patient volume continued to dramatically increase. All physicians working in the emergency department were Ohio State faculty members and were board eligible or board certified in emergency medicine. Many of the shifts were now double covered and EM residents and Ohio State medical students would do rotations in the ED. There were discussions about adding nurse practitioners and physician assistants to the provider staff. Several physicians practiced exclusively at East and in 2007 advanced practice practitioners became an integral part of the team (Figure 10).

Advanced Practice Practitioners (APPs)

In April 2007 the Department of Emergency Medicine launched the Advanced Practice Provider (APP) program to address rapidly increased patient volume at Ohio State East. Envisioned by Gary Katz, MD, the program involved mid-level providers, such as physician assistants and nurse practitioners to evaluate lower acuity patients. Heather Matejovich, CNP, who had previously been an emergency nurse in the Ohio State East ED, was hired to administer the program at the start. The next year Soni Shellman, MD, took over the administrative duties of the APP Program at East, including scheduling, hiring, and becoming the main collaborating physician and advocate for this group of providers.

Originally the APPs covered one shift only and worked daily 4 PM to 2 AM. In 2018 Adalyn Harrah, CNP, the lead APP, was appointed to assist with the group's increasing administrative duties. Today, not only do these highly qualified individuals evaluate lower acuity diseases and injuries, but they are comfortable managing complex disease processes alongside supervising physicians. Matejovich continues to work as an APP at East and her colleagues are an extremely close-knit group.

DARALEE R. HUGHES, MD

Daralee R. Hughes, MD, completed her undergraduate training in biology at the University of Notre Dame and received her MD degree from Ohio State in 2011. Following medical school in 2011 she entered her Emergency Medicine Residency at Ohio State where she participated in the residency Academic Track in Focused Ultrasound. She developed a digital portfolio for ultrasound images and created a vertically-integrated medical student ultrasound curriculum.

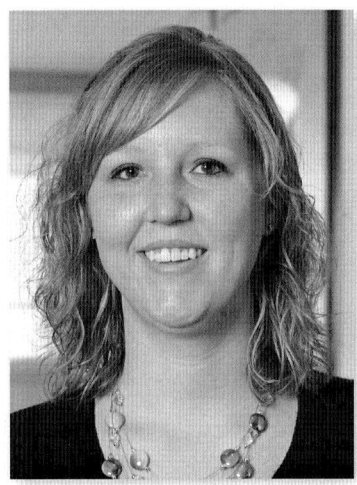

Figure 11: Daralee R. Hughes, MD, joined the East faculty in 2014 and pioneered the advancement of ultrasound there.

She went on to participate in national conferences, with poster and oral presentations at the American Institute of Ultrasound in Medicine (AIUM) annual convention as well as the World Congress for Ultrasound in Medical Education conference. While a resident she assisted with revision of the residency ultrasound curriculum as well as the quality assurance process. She co-authored five publications as a resident, the most notable being "I-AIM: A Model for Teaching and Performing Focused Sonography".

After graduating from residency in 2014, Hughes became an assistant professor in Emergency Medicine at Ohio State East Emergency Department (Figure 11). She instituted a clinical ultrasound program for the ED, which gave the department the ability to save, review and bill for the ultrasounds performed. She also helped the department understand more of the nuances with ultrasound billing and coding, which led to improved reimbursement for ultrasounds. This effort led to another poster presentation and publication, "Billing I-AIM: A Novel Framework for Ultrasound Billing."

SOMMER E. LINDSEY, MD

Sommer E. Lindsey, MD, joined Ohio State as a member of the core East faculty in September 2013. Her areas of interest included underserved populations, early detection of HIV and syphilis, and prevention of sexually communicable diseases. She completed her undergraduate degree in psychology at The University of Chicago, post-baccalaureate work at Drexel University in Philadelphia, and earned her medical degree from University of Cincinnati College of Medicine. She completed her residency at UCSF in Fresno, serving as Chief Resident in her final year.

EMILY B. KAUFFMAN, DO, MPH

Emily B. Kauffman, DO, MPH, completed her dual residency training in emergency medicine and internal medicine at Louisiana State University-New Orleans and received her master's in public health from Ohio State (Figure 12). She started her Ohio State career in 2012, dividing her clinical time between hospital medicine and emergency medicine. In 2013, Kauffman became Assistant Program Director for the newly formed Emergency Medicine and Internal Medicine residency program and served in this role until 2020.

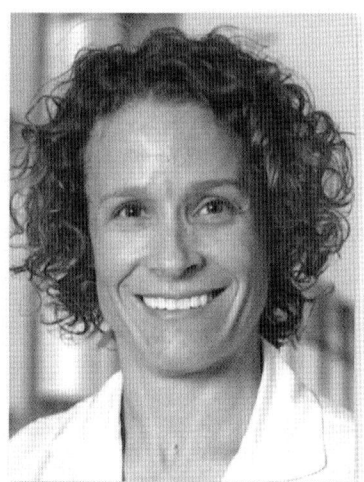

In 2017, she pivoted toward addressing the opioid epidemic in Ohio and was appointed as a co-investigator on an internal ED grant to start buprenorphine administration as evidence-based care for patients with opioid use disorder. This initial grant led to a $1 million award from the Ohio Department of Health to pilot and expand this project from the East ED. The department was the first ED in Franklin County to offer take-home naloxone, buprenorphine dosing, peer support and fentanyl test strips. This

Figure 12: Emily B. Kauffman, DO, MPH, created ground-breaking practices at Ohio State East emergency department in the management of opioid addiction disorders.

program continues to be funded by state and federal grants and has expanded to include an addiction consult team on the main campus ED staffed by a dedicated nurse practitioner, social worker and peer recovery supporter.

Board certified in addiction medicine, Kauffman now manages all addiction programming through the Emergency Department and continues to integrate with departments across Ohio State to ensure that addiction care is mainstream and expected as a part of the patient experience. Since 2019, she also has served as co-investigator on the NIH HEALing Communities Study as an Emergency Department Intervention Design Team lead implementing evidence-based programming to select high-risk emergency departments in 16 counties throughout the state. This includes naloxone dispensing, improved linkage for patients with opioid use disorder (or any type of substance use disorder) and buprenorphine dosing.

Kauffman served as a principal investigator on several federal and statewide funded grants implementing evidence-based treatment for addiction in the ED with Ohio State East as the pilot site for Franklin County. Due to her ground-breaking work, she was awarded the 2020 Emergency Physician of the Year by the Ohio Chapter of the American College of Emergency Physicians. She is an associate professor with additional interests in infectious diseases and community health.

ANDREW T. GATHOF, MD

Andrew T. Gathof, MD, graduated from the University of Notre Dame in 2008, completed medical school at the University of Louisville in 2012 and Emergency Medicine residency training at Ohio State in 2015 (Figure 13). He then joined the Ohio State faculty and has worked almost exclusively at Ohio State East Hospital ever since. Drawn to East Hospital because of its unique combination of community an academic medicine, Gathof enjoyed the smaller environment, close professional relationships, medical education opportunities, and underserved patient population that working at East Hospital afforded. He joined the administrative leadership team at Dick's urging a few years after completing residency, and began taking extra coursework,

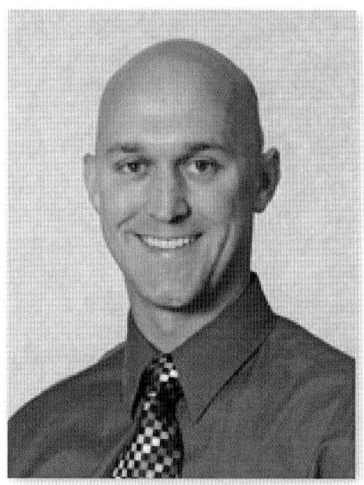

Figure 13: Andrew Gathof, MD, is one of two Assistant Medical Directors at Ohio State East.

including the Ohio State Faculty Leadership Institute and the ACEP ED Director's Academy.

Gathof is currently serving as one of two Assistant Medical Directors for the East Hospital Emergency Department. He and the rest of the East Hospital ED faculty take great pride in providing high quality medical care in a geographic part of Columbus that is a relatively underserved. In discussing his career at East Gathof noted the following:

I have been fortunate and immensely grateful to have the mentorship of Dr. Michael Dick, who has been the Medical Director there since the hospital was initially acquired by Ohio State and Dr. Sondra Shellman, the other Assistant Medical Director at East.[10]

Emergency Medicine Leads the Way Forward

In 2023 Daniel J. Bachmann, MD, Associate Professor of Emergency Medicine became the medical director of Ohio State East Hospital. He outlined the hospital's capabilities:

East is a level 3 trauma center. We have a catheterization lab staffed 24/7 for cardiovascular emergencies including STEMI. We are a certified stroke center. We have an ICU stepdown unit and multiple operating rooms including 2 robotic systems. We have an endoscopy unit and dialysis unit. We have approximately 220 beds in the hospital.[11]

Bachman's leadership exemplifies the progress of emergency medicine at Ohio State since its emergence in 1978. Moving into leadership positions system-wide, emergency physicians are highly prized for their breadth of vision, administrative skill and expert guidance of complex medical systems.

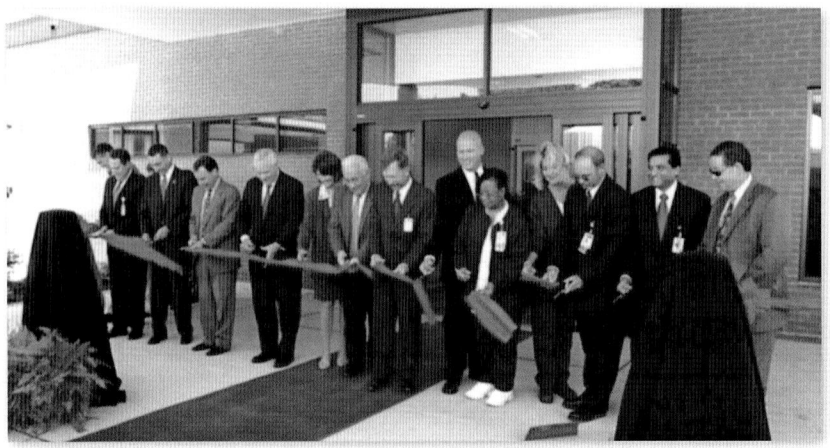

Figure 14: Michael Dick, MD (center of photo) cuts the ribbon to celebrate the opening of the new Ohio State East Emergency Department in 2004.

Encapsulating the story of the Ohio State East Hospital emergency department, Michael Dick summarized a remarkable 25-year history:

In 1999, due to Medical Center leadership, including Drs. Rund and Nelson, Park Medical Center was purchased. Originally St. Anthony Hospital, Park had a storied history as one of the first hospitals in Columbus, as a religious institution, as a trauma center, and ultimately as a facility in rapid decline with a terrible reputation. This decline had an untoward impact on the poorer population on the near east side of Columbus. With the continued support of Ohio State, the Department of Emergency Medicine, and ultimately with the support of my colleagues – nurses, physicians and APPs – we have been able to provide services that were not and are not part of mainstream emergency medicine. These include the best SANE program in Columbus, the first ED to dispense Narcan, comprehensive STI testing with referral to our ID colleagues for treatment. In addition, we are now starting treatment with buprenorphine when the patient is in the ED. We provide immunizations. Patients are referred to a variety of locations to continue their treatment. None of this could have been done without the support of my colleagues as noted above. It truly has been a team effort. I could not have asked for a better career.[12]

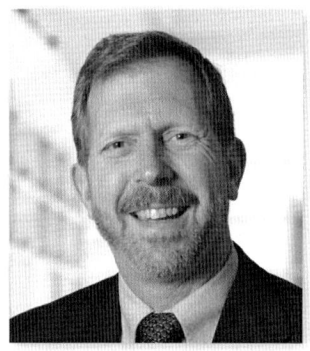

~ *In Remembrance* ~

Mike Dick passed away peacefully surrounded by family at his home in Powell, Ohio, on the afternoon of May 3, 2023. He was only 67 years old and had been courageously battling cancer for the previous two years. Despite the challenges brought by his illness and aggressive medical management, he continued to serve as OSU East Emergency Department Medical Director until the very end. He even worked clinically in the ED well into January 2023, and also found time and energy to author this book chapter. Just prior to his death, Mike was notified of his induction into the 2023 cohort of the Mazzaferri-Ellison Society of Master Clinicians, only the second OSU emergency physician to be so honored.

It is difficult to express what Mike's loss will mean to our department. He was not just a leader, but also a friend and trusted colleague. His legacy will continue to live on through his many accomplishments, contributions, innovations, and our memories of him. Perhaps the most fitting tribute was expressed by Mark DeBard, MD, Professor Emeritus, who worked with Mike at OSU East Emergency Department from 2001 until his retirement in 2016.

> *Lastly, a word about our Medical Director, Mike Dick. What a fabulous leader! He embodied competency, vision, and hard work like no ED Director I have ever seen. His vision brought us from a disrespected shabby inner-city failure to a modern, academic, community-driven modern ED. It was his vision that made us a stroke, MI and trauma center. It was he who pushed us to upgrade our skills and lead in educating residents and medical students. It was he who provided the protective*

external interface to attendings and administration. And all this while being the best and most competent practicing clinician I have ever seen, a model for all we physicians, every one of whom I would have gladly let care for my family. OSU East is what it is today because of this man.[9]

References

1. Rodgers K. St. Anthony's Hospital. Historical Reflections: The Medical Heritage Center blog. The Ohio State University. October 15, 2012. https://library.osu.edu/site/mhcb/2012/10/15/st-anthonys-hospital-2/

2. Sigafoos J. Interview of John Sigafoos by Richard Nelson. 2023: Columbus, Ohio.

3. Galvin B. Area hospital restructures. *The Lantern*. April 23, 2001.

4. Thompson J. https:// wexnermedical.osu.edu/blog/doctor-dick-won't-let-anything-stop-him-from-working. May 11, 2021.

5. Star of Life Awards 2022. https//ems.ohio.gov

6. Haynes EM. Personal communication. 2023.

7. Shellman S. Personal communication. 2023.

8. Zimmer BL. Personal communication. 2023.

9. DeBard ML. Personal communication. 2022.

10. Gathof AT. Personal communication. 2023.

11. Bachmann DJ. Personal communication. 2023.

12. Dick MR. Personal communication. 2023.

Chapter 19

The Fundamentals: Medical Student Education

David P. Bahner, MD
Nicholas E. Kman, MD
David Way, MEd

In the early 20th century proprietary medical schools folded into universities partially due to the Flexner report of 1910, which criticized the inconsistent quality of the medical education offered by for-profit schools and emphasized the need for scientific research and appropriate laboratory facilities in medical schools. Thus, in 1914, the Ohio State College of Medicine was founded by the merger of several private medical schools.

Respect for academic medicine during the 20th century had to be earned, however. For Ohio State medical students' clinical education, the early departments had to rely on part-time faculty and community practitioners while gradually developing a full-time faculty with the capacity for scientific research and therapeutic advances.

By the latter half of the century, starting in the 1970s, the new specialty of emergency medicine began to take shape. The people propelling the specialty forward in these early days carried a significant burden. They paved the paths, fought the fights, and handled the friction that occurs when something new comes along in a large academic medical center. Gradually, leaders like Douglas Rund, MD, Richard Nelson, MD, Howard Werman, MD, and Chuck Brown, MD, garnered increasing respect for the budding specialty of emergency medicine both at Ohio State and nationally. They were key figures with the leadership skills to carry that load.

Rund's people skills allowed him to recruit the faculty needed to manage both the academic and clinical burdens of operating a 24/7/365 department. These skills also enabled him to navigate the growing pains of the new specialty of emergency medicine, which has evolved in the United States throughout the last half century and continues to do so. Throughout his own medical education, which included fellowship years at Stanford University, Rund recognized the importance of excellent educational programs. He experimented with new models to streamline medical student education.[1]

The leaders at that time recognized that, in essence, the raison d'être of a medical school was student education. If they could focus on that aspect of the College of Medicine, they could establish a relatively non-controversial way to establish the identity of emergency medicine as a true specialty. This was also the approach David Bahner, MD, took in establishing ultrasound as a subspecialty. Prior to 1978 there were no student rotations in the emergency room at Ohio State because there were no faculty there to teach them. Only after the establishment of a Division of Emergency Medicine with the addition of a full-time faculty could there be student education.

The earliest course was the clerkship in emergency medicine for fourth-year students. The earliest didactic teaching in emergency medicine had a distinct flavor of preventive medicine. Lecture topics included ones such as "broad overviews of the EMS system" and "how EMS was integrated into the overall health delivery system." The student experience included riding as observers with the emergency units of the Columbus Division of Fire and spending time at the Fire and EMS Dispatch Center. Emergency medicine was staking out exclusive claim to emergency medical services as part of the untiring effort to create a distinctive new specialty. To provide clinical experiences for medical students, the department relied heavily on student rotations in all of Columbus's major hospitals. These experiences, combined with the lecture series, continued throughout most of the 1980s, and comprised the emergency medicine educational format for Ohio State medical students.

Emergency medicine faculty were eager to participate in College of Medicine student programs. The curriculum varied over the years as different educational structures were developed. From the beginning lectures delivered by experts were the standard method for teaching the foundational sciences such as anatomy and pathology. This was eventually referred to as the lecture/discussion (LD) format. In the early 1970s, a group of other academics developed alternative pathways: the Independent Study Program (ISP) and the Problem-Based Learning (PBL) pathway.

Independent Study Program (1970-2012)

The two-year Independent Study Program (ISP) was established in 1970 as a research project funded by the Department of Health, Education and Welfare through the Health Services Manpower Program, and led by principal investigator Lloyd Evans, MD, Assistant Dean at the Ohio State College of Medicine. Originally called the Pilot Medical School, the program had several goals: stimulate students to be self-directed learners, emphasize proficiency in a flexible time frame and use the computer as an instruction and evaluation tool. The computer was the hospital's IBM System digital computer under DOS with magnetic disc and tape drives and 8 IBM computer terminals. Computer use in instruction was quite innovative at the time. Students would log onto the computers to take practice tests, and used the computer's feedback to assess their knowledge and identify areas requiring more study before taking the post test.

The ISP curriculum was divided into modules exploring the normal human (year one) and pathophysiology (year two). Each of the modules was organized predominantly by organ system and contained specific learning objectives and learning resources, which were usually textbooks. Instead of delivering lectures, faculty members constructed each module and could supplement them with additional learning resources to facilitate student learning such as clinical correlation sessions or computer-based instructional programs. There were suggested completion dates for taking posttests and maximum times by which they must be completed. The program was also portable and available to other institutions.

Years later Mary Beth Fontana, MD, described some of the program's benefits:

The flexibility of the program allowed students to pursue research, to progress more quickly in areas where they were already proficient, and to study certain areas in more depth. Progress could be fast enough to complete medical school in three years or elect the five-year option, allowing for family issues or work outside of medical school if needed. About 10% to 35% of the incoming class selected ISP, some of whom came to the Ohio State University College of Medicine because ISP was an option. Students with advanced degrees or who were pursuing a concurrent advanced degree were particularly attracted to the program. Good time management skills, self-discipline and motivation were necessary to be successful. The students had their own library, study carrels and computer terminals.[2]

The Independent Study Program also provided opportunities for new educational initiatives. A new anatomy course integrating clinical imaging techniques and computer-assisted instruction was first used in ISP and then expanded to the entire class. Components of the Physical Examination course and the Medical Humanities and Behavioral Science course were piloted with ISP students before being integrated into the course for all students. The requirement of passage of National Board of Medical Examiners shelf exams to progress through the curriculum was unique to the program along with a higher passing standard for successful program completion. Both became requirements of subsequent curricula. Many students who later became emergency medicine residents or fellows studied in the ISP program. Many aspects of the program were easily transitioned into the Lead. Serve. Inspire. (LSI) curriculum, which became the only preclinical curriculum in 2012.

Problem-Based Learning Pathway and Emergency Medicine

The Problem-Based Learning Pathway (PBLP) was initiated during the 1991-1992 academic year. PBLP was offered as an alternative pathway for medical students to complete their foundational science requirements during the first two years of medical school, and like ISP, became an attractive feature to prospective medical students.

The Problem-Based Learning Pathway was founded on the principles of Social Learning Theory. To be successful, students not only were required to develop self-directed learning skills like in ISP, but were also required to learn group process skills. Initially, the program could accommodate 24 students per class. This was eventually expanded to 35 students. Students were divided into small groups of seven or eight and met three times a week during the first year and two times a week during the second year. A physician and a behaviorist facilitated each group. Students received actual patient cases on paper and would work through the cases one page at a time to identify learning issues that they agreed to study in between group sessions.

Emergency medicine physicians Howard "Howie" Werman, MD, and James "Jim" Hoekstra, MD, became enthusiastic PBL champions and both facilitated second-year PBL groups. The first class had 24 first-year students. David Way, MEd, a College of Medicine program evaluator, conducted personal interviews with the first class. His first interview was with Sorabh Khandelwal, MD, the future EM faculty member and residency program director. During the interview, Khandelwal expressed dismay at the fact that the new program was not quite ready for implementation.[3] The students had outpaced the faculty's ability to deliver the paper cases needed for student learning. The program director ultimately confessed that the proposed program had been controversial with the college faculty and administration. Had it not rolled out when it did, it would have never been implemented.

During the following academic year, Way was assigned to the PBL program as a facilitator. During the history of the PBL Pathway, which was offered from academic years 1991-1992 through 2003-2004, it produced 22 medical students who went on to become emergency physicians, including Timothy Reeder, MD; Brian Gelb, MD; Lesley Perez, MD; Sorabh Khandelwal, MD; and Ashish Panchal, MD, PhD.

DAVID P. BAHNER, MD, AND EVIDENCE-BASED LEARNING (EBL)

David P. Bahner, MD, joined the faculty at the conclusion of his residency in 1998. Within his first year, following the lead of the original leaders to gain acceptance by focusing on undergraduate medical education, he introduced an extracurricular elective called Evidence-Based Learning (EBL). Within this elective, Bahner introduced medical students to the specialty of emergency medicine. With the help of his sister Diana Bahner, a program coordinator, the course became an efficiently run, multiday seminar for medical students to explore and experience what a career in academic medicine was like. One unique feature of the program involved medical students contributing to actual emergency medicine cases by conducting searches of key literature on a mobile computer at the patient's bedside. The literature was used as evidence for selecting the appropriate diagnosis and the appropriate treatment, thus the practice of applying evidence to the medical care provided.

JAMES W. "JIM" HOEKSTRA, MD

In many ways, the story of the rise of educational leadership at Ohio State should start with James "Jim" Hoekstra, MD (Figure 1). He was recruited in 1988, a time when the Division of Emergency Medicine was first applying to become a full academic department. The prevailing wisdom in 1989 was that the faculty had to demonstrate to the university that the division was worthy of elevation to departmental status. The faculty had to teach a variety of student courses. The leadership, including Hoekstra, had to "create" new courses on the spot: "seminars in emergency medicine," "individual studies" and "research electives."

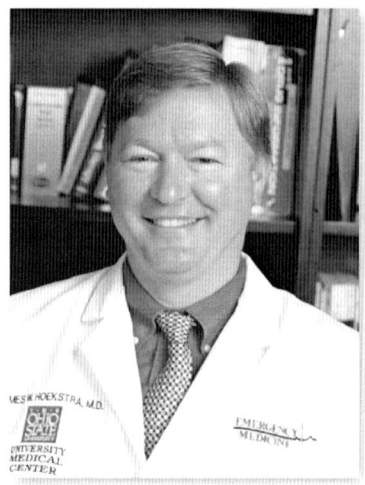

Figure 1: James W. Hoekstra, MD, made a lasting impact on Ohio State medical student education.

Hoekstra became famous for his teaching at the bedside in the emergency department. His "hands-on" teaching included instruction about skills like splinting, suturing, or performing cardiopulmonary resuscitation. A highly regarded clinician and effective educator, he connected with learners and many would come away smiling and smarter from Hoekstra's wisdom and pragmatism. He made learning fun and learners became confident in their skills after spending time with him.

After listening to Hoekstra explain and show how to throw a corner stitch or put on a thumb spica splint, learners could practice and become proficient. He made sure to highlight the common pitfalls to avoid and the "must remember" key points for each procedure, styling an effective teaching method for teaching others. He was dedicated to service leadership and helping others help themselves.

When Hoekstra left Ohio State to become the chair of emergency medicine at Wake Forest University, he left behind his legacy as a star within the ED. His research addressing cardiovascular emergency care highlighted his academic career, yet it was his educational prowess that had such a lasting impact on the many who were lucky to learn from him. Hoekstra showed it could be done and how to do it. The rest was up to those who knew him and learned from his academic model: Show up, work hard, work with others, strive for excellence, lead, and serve.

The Differentiation of Care (DOC) Program (1993-2006)

In 1993 the Associate Dean of Medical Education, Seth Kantor, MD, called for a revision of the fourth-year curriculum. His proposed change, called "taking back the fourth year" was intended to provide more structure to a program that had been comprised mostly of elective rotations. In 1993 Hoekstra was appointed to the fourth-year curriculum committee called the Differentiation of Care (DOC) Subcommittee. Their charge: to develop a curriculum to provide students with standard experiences in different patient care settings. The DOCs included four "selective" rotations in which students could select the site of their clinical work but would meet one day a week for didactic education.

DOC 1 covered care for the "undifferentiated patient." Classically speaking, this was treatment delivered in the emergency department. DOC 2 covered care that would be delivered in the ambulatory setting.

DOC 3 was about chronic care and the care of special needs populations. And finally, the DOC 4 was a sub-internship. Eventually, the DOC 4 was redefined as a sub-internship in medicine or subspecialty of medicine. A DOC 5 was later added, which became a sub-internship in a surgical or perioperative subspecialty.

Hoekstra became the department's Director of Medical Student Education in 1991 and the first DOC 1 director in 1994. In preparation for the DOC 1, he recruited clinical sites for student clinical experiences, developed a written examination covering the course objectives, and recruited David Way in the Office of Academic Services to develop grading guidelines, clinical performance evaluations, and a system for evaluating the clinical sites and didactic programs.

The DOC curriculum was rolled out during the 1995-1996 academic year. DOC 1 students could select to do their clinical rotations from an initial list of 11 sites, most of which occurred in the emergency department: Berger Hospital in Circleville, Columbus Children's Hospital (eventually Nationwide), Children's Outpatient Clinic, Grant Hospital, Marysville Hospital, an Ohio State Urgent Care Center (MedOhio), selected rural hospitals, Mt. Carmel Medical Center, Riverside Methodist Hospital, the Ohio State Student Health Center and the Ohio State University Hospital.

During the DOC 1, medical learners were evaluated on their history taking and physical examination skills, case presentations, diagnostic skills, general medical knowledge, professional demeanor, ability to perform routine clinical procedures, clinical judgement, problem solving skills, clinical documentation, and interpersonal communication skills with other members of the team and patients. Students learned basic procedures like suturing and splinting in a lab setting. Students also had to pass an in-house multiple choice knowledge examination covering content related to patient pathologies commonly seen in an emergency department.

Early program evaluation results reflected medical student enthusiasm for the DOC 1. When asked whether they would recommend this experience to fellow students, over three quarters of the students responded with "definitely." Nearly 50% of the students thought that the DOC 1 didactic sessions in emergency medicine were better than most of the didactic sessions they had experienced across the entire four-year curriculum.

Hoekstra was named the Assistant Dean for Clinical Education in 1998 and Associate Dean for Clinical Education and Community Outreach in 1999. In this new role he led the development of an ambitious program called the 2006 Curriculum, a modern curriculum designed for medical students who would start clinical practice in 2006. One of the biggest challenges Hoekstra faced in leading the development of the 2006 Curriculum was to get the individual clinical departments to give up some of their clerkship time and to partner with other departments to deliver clinical education.

Over the years, emergency medicine faculty members followed in Hoekstra's footsteps to become involved with undergraduate medical student education: Sorabh Khandelwal, MD; Nicholas Kman, MD; Laura Thompson, MD; Cynthia Leung, MD; Michael Barrie, MD; Lauren Branditz, MD; Christopher San Miguel MD; and Matthew Malone, MD. Each brought personalities, skills, interests and experiences to foster relationships with medical students and to build upon Hoekstra's reputation and work ethic.

SORABH KHANDELWAL, MD

In 1999, Hoekstra entrusted the DOC 1 Clerkship to Khandelwal, who became the DOC 1 director. With the help of Sharon Pfeil, department administrator, Khandelwal enhanced the DOC 1 curriculum over time. Years later Khandelwal reflected on the DOC 1 clerkship and its evolution under his leadership:

> *A year after I came back to Ohio State after residency, Dr. Hoekstra was moving up to higher levels of responsibility in the college, so he offered me the position of DOC 1 clerkship director, which was called Differentiation of Care. It was a required clerkship for all fourth-year medical students, but interestingly it could be done in any undifferentiated care setting. So, that could be the emergency department, urgent care centers [or other sites]. At that point, emergency medicine didn't have a strong foothold in the College of Medicine and was considered one of multiple undifferentiated sites that a student could rotate through. I saw the op-*

portunity to push emergency medicine a little bit in the College of Medicine as I thought it really should have been a required rotation instead of a part of the undifferentiated care elective. So, numerous conversations and much politicking eventually got emergency medicine put into the fourth-year rotation as a required clerkship. Students could no longer do their rotations at urgent care centers and other places that were undifferentiated and I think that played a role in the growth of emergency medicine within the medical center. Once it became a required fourth-year clerkship, I think you could see the impact of that over the next multiple years in terms of what we accomplished.[4]

As the medical school curriculum evolved and the needs of students for emergency medicine education expanded, Khandelwal began to develop a new program called the Advanced Topics in Emergency Medicine (ATEM). This curriculum was designed specifically for senior medical students who had interest in a career in emergency medicine.

Khandelwal reflected on this period of growth:

We expanded emergency medicine's presence in the undergraduate medical student curriculum by also adding a third-year EM elective. We really had much more of a foothold in the college, maybe that's not the right word, but more of a presence at the early stages when students are choosing a specialty. I think it is easy to see the popularity of EM in our medical school. The interest in EM and the department's offerings have slowly become greater and greater as we grew our faculty, and our faculty became more invested in the College of Medicine. Students then started seeing the benefits of emergency medicine. Now, I think we are a top specialty of choice.[4]

Advanced Topics in Emergency Medicine (ATEM)

Advanced Topics in Emergency Medicine (ATEM) was established in 2007. The ATEM course curriculum included: journal club presentations, specialty-specific didactics, certification in advanced trauma life support and pediatric advanced life support, high acuity code pager response, operating room experiences for tube thoracostomy and intubation, small group clinical lectures with skills lab scenarios, ultrasound, EMS lectures, grand rounds presentations, and teaching shifts with senior residents.

To align with the American Council on Graduate Medical Education (ACGME) assessment standards, the ATEM curriculum was revised to be based on educational milestones for incoming interns in emergency medicine. A required "boot camp" component was added to the course as a capstone assessment in order to provide future residency program directors with additional information about the graduate's abilities.

By 2015 ATEM was folded into a series of courses that became the EM Clinical Track, a recommended schedule for any student committing to the specialty of emergency medicine as a career. This competency-based curriculum offered medical students the opportunity to achieve and demonstrate proficiency in all 23 of the Level 1 EM milestones, which was the expected level of performance for incoming interns in emergency medicine. The EM Clinical Track Curriculum was published in an article entitled "Promoting Achievement of Level 1 Milestones for Medical Students Going into Emergency Medicine."[5,6]

NICHOLAS E. "NICK" KMAN, MD

Nick Kman, MD, completed medical school at Ohio State and EM residency at Wake Forest University (Figure 2). Hoekstra had left Ohio State in 2003 to assume the Chair of Emergency Medicine at Wake Forest and worked closely with Kman, who had become chief resident at Wake in 2006 but was then recruited back to Ohio State in 2007. Years later he described the student education leadership in the department as he saw it at the time: "I started to work with Sorabh and I realized that he was really kind of a one-man show when it came to medical student education."[7]

Kman took over directorship of the ATEM course, and began transitioning it into a college-approved, longitudinal elective that medical students would complete throughout their fourth year. He saw it as a "bootcamp" or intern preparation course for students in their final year. Over time he became an expert in preparing fourth-year students

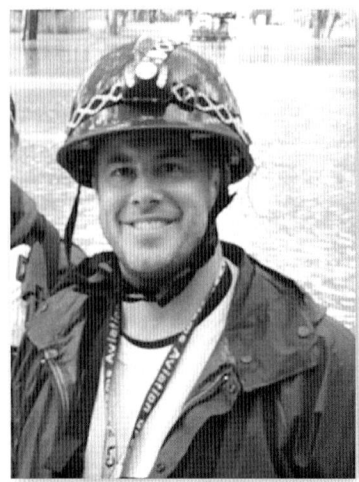

Figure 2: Nicholas "Nick" Kman, MD, became an expert in disaster response during his career at Ohio State. Working with Daniel Bachmann, MD, he developed a longitudinal course in Emergency Preparedness and Disaster Medicine in 2015. He is shown here responding to hurricane Harvey in Houston in 2017.

for residency, which made him a perfect candidate to become the director for Part 3 of the new Lead. Serve. and Inspire. (LSI) curriculum, which was rolled out in 2012. To quote Kman's description of that period:

In 2010 the College of Medicine decided it was time to move away from the traditional 2+2 medical school curriculum which had been 2 years of foundational sciences, a traditional clinical year of required clerkships, and a traditional senior year of clinical electives. They moved to a three-phase or three-part curriculum that they would call the LSI – Lead. Serve. and Inspire. curriculum. The LSI curriculum was rolled out in the fall of 2012. At that point, with just one class in the pipeline, the College really focused on Part 1 or the foundational sciences. It wasn't until the first class of LSI students were entering Part 3 (Med 3 and 4) in December of 2014, that I applied and was hired as the Part 3 Director. My job was to develop and create a new fourth-year curriculum that would have a continued EM component and bootcamp for all students but would also provide clinical tracks related to the medical student's chosen specialty for all the medical students going into all specialties. One of the things that was a little interesting about the transition from the old curriculum to the new curriculum resulted from a change in the academic calendar. As a result, in May, 2014, there was a period when the students needed a series of electives to cover a gap of time created by the transition.

Dan Bachmann and I submitted a proposal for an elective course in Disaster Medicine, which was ultimately approved. We ran the course in May 2014 as an elective, but it eventually became an Advanced Competency elective that students could choose as part of their EM Clinical Track. The Disaster Medicine Course continues to this day and has become very popular among students planning careers in emergency medicine.[7]

Kman's involvement with the College of Medicine resulted in his becoming an integral part of the new LSI three-part curriculum completed over four years. The LSI Part 1 replaced the first two preclinical years with 18 months of instruction in the foundational sciences supplemented with clinical experiences. The LSI Part 2 was a conversion of the third year required clinical clerkships in the seven original clinical departments to three phases called "rings." Each ring covered a general area of medicine: specialized medical care; surgical and reproductive care; and caring for patients within special populations.

The LSI Part 3 replaced the traditional fourth year, which had included both elective and "selective" clinical rotations. One of Kman's visions was that Part 3 could be focused on helping students complete the advanced competencies (or Level 1 milestones) for their chosen specialty. Part 3, therefore, became a series of coordinated experiences to learn advanced clinical management and clinical competencies all customized to enable the student to achieve level 1 milestones in their specialty of interest. Students selected rotations to meet fourth-year requirements, but also had some flexibility to explore content that would be relevant to them in their future chosen specialty. Kman would ultimately lead Part 3 of the Ohio State LSI curriculum and would mentor residency graduate Christopher San Miguel, MD, to take over the third-year EM elective and eventually the EM Longitudinal Clerkship. Cindy Leung, MD, and Lauren Branditz, MD, would eventually lead the ATEM course, one of the electives within the EM Longitudinal Clerkship.

The Disaster Medicine Elective and the Pandemic Course

In 2014 Kman and Bachmann moved a set of activities in Disaster Medicine from an informal Emergency Medicine Interest Group Curriculum (EMIG) into a full four-year elective course. This course would become a popular Advanced Competency Course in Emergency Preparedness and Disaster Response. Students would participate in FEMA certifications and complete a comprehensive disaster scenario active shooter simulation that required the skill of mass casualty triage.

They attended lectures on Personal Preparedness, Community Resources for Disaster Response, Infectious Agents of Bioterrorism, Response to Natural Disasters, Review of Ebola Viral Disease, Radiological Emergencies, Biosecurity & Outbreak Response, Toxic Antidotes, and Pandemic Influenza. Additionally, they had the opportunity to participate in a regional full-scale disaster exercise, tour a research facility with BSL-3 level pathogens, and assist with on-scene care for a mass gathering event of greater than 10,000 people.[8]

COVID-19 brought an interesting adaptation to the Disaster Medicine Elective. On March 7, 2020, students were removed from the clinical setting due to concerns of the novel coronavirus. Kman was asked to adapt the disaster medicine program into a course that could teach all students about COVID-19. On May 4, 2020, the course began for 212 Med 3 and 4 students. When it concluded on June 1, learners returned to the clinical setting. This course was integral in getting the learners ready to return to the clinical setting. They received lectures, participated in tabletop exercises, and reviewed pandemic plans that were being implemented by various physicians and leaders statewide. Finally, the students learned new medical campus policies due to COVID-19, were taught basic levels of competence in Personal Protective Equipment and learned about environmental safeguards, including social distancing requirements.

SHARON E. PFEIL

Sharon Pfeil, who joined the department in 2003, provided critically important administrative support for the student education program. Prior to her recruitment, she had worked as assistant to the Dean of the College of Medicine for 18 years (Figure 3). Upon joining the department, she became the coordinator for the emergency medicine fourth-year clerkship. She was also administrative assistant to Douglas Rund,

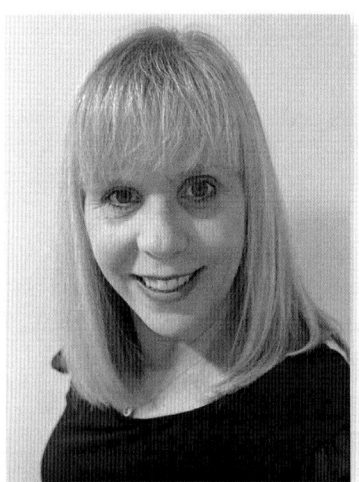

Figure 3: Sharon Pfeil joined the department in 2003 and became responsible for all administrative tasks in student education. She was vitally important in the establishment of many of the department's innovative new courses.

Professor and Chair.

During Pfeil's tenure, the new EM education programs increased substantially through the addition of elective and selective courses, including the 10-month longitudinal courses of Honors Ultrasound, Advanced Topics in Emergency Medicine, Emergency Preparedness and Disaster Management, a two-week third year Emergency Medicine elective and an ultrasound immersion elective. She was instrumental in helping to develop and implement these courses over the span of her career.

Third-Year Elective in Emergency Medicine

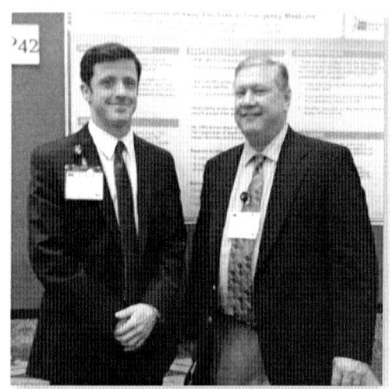

Figure 4: Aaron Bernard, MD, and David Way, MEd, present their poster on innovations introduced in the third-year emergency medicine elective at the Southern Group on Educational Affairs conference in Lexington, Kentucky, 2011.

The third-year, two-week elective in emergency medicine was started by Aaron Bernard, MD, in 2010. Bernard created the course, in part, to give students an early glimpse of emergency medicine so that they had ample time to consider EM as their future specialty and prepare their residency applications. Students attended EM conferences and worked shifts in the main ED, the wound care area and the fast track area. They also participated in MedFlight medical transports and had some experiences with hyperbaric oxygen (HBO). Bernard, with the help of Pfeil and Way, studied the effects of medical student's access to emergency medicine education during the third year (Figure 4).[7]

Advanced Management in Hospital-Based Care- Emergency Medicine (AMHBC-EM)

In 2015 DOC 1 transitioned to Advanced Management in Hospital

Based Care-Emergency Medicine (AMHBC-EM). The AMHBC course involved experience in both the intensive care unit and the emergency department, supplemented with a didactic component. The course also featured comprehensive assessments and has incorporated virtual reality into both teaching and evaluation. Pfeil remembers that the college piloted the program with Internal Medicine (AMHBC-Mini I) for two months in 2014 before the eventual rollout to the entire LSI class. Each rotation within the course is one month in length. All fourth-year students must complete the requirement. Kman offered additional information about the fourth-year curriculum:

Part 3 is the fourth year. When I took the course as a fourth-year student it started in July. One thing that is different now is that the course starts in May. Back then the fourth year was kind of a hodge podge of electives, and frankly it was pretty light by comparison. It was also very hard to know what you wanted to do and get all the things you wanted to do done prior to residency match time. Now, students have more advanced time to decide and then to prepare for residency. The preparation is a lot more rigorous. They still do electives, but they also do bootcamp courses and four required courses.

There are a lot more assessments in the Part 3 Curriculum. For example, emergency medicine now has an NBME content exam that all the students must take and pass, and we have a simulation that the students are graded on. We use virtual reality for both training and assessment; we have different observed standardized clinical evaluations—we call those Objective Structured Clinical Examinations (OSCEs). The assessment in Part 3 is much more robust than when I was a medical student.[7]

Honors Ultrasound

Honors ultrasound (HUS) started in 2005 with the help of Bahner, Rich Limperos, MD, and the work of two students – Burke Hatch and Spencer Proctor. The first offering of the course enrolled 14 students. There have been some years with upwards of 40 students, and some years with as few as 20-25 fourth-year students. In 2012, the HUS course transitioned into an advanced competency within the new LSI curriculum. This HUS course was described in an article in *Academic*

Medicine and served as a model for the longitudinal advanced competencies offered in the Lead. Serve. and Inspire. Curriculum in the third and final part of the 3-part medical student curriculum. Focusing on point-of-care ultrasound modules, expert lectures, hands on experience, journal club presentations, and an honors project linked to the student's career goals, the Honors Ultrasound Course achieved significant success. As the course was founded with Bahner and Limperos as the early faculty, new faculty members including Creagh Boulger, MD, Michael Prats, MD and Jessica Everett, MD, were added and continued to lecture and mentor the fourth-year students as they engaged in mastery of point-of-care ultrasound. In 2023-2024, 38 students were enrolled in HUS, including students who plan to enter residencies in EM, IM, general surgery, anesthesiology, ENT, Radiology, Obstetrics and Family Medicine. The course requires a minimum of 150 hours of ultrasound scanning time, which is designed to be sufficient for them to attain basic and advanced competencies in diagnostic ultrasound and competencies in using ultrasound to guide procedures. Due to its rigorous requirements, the HUS course prepares students to be future leaders in ultrasonography and ultrasound education.

Birth of Simulation and The Clinical Skills Education and Assessment Center

While the adage "see one, do one, teach one" described much of clinical teaching for decades, it sorely needed an update for the 21st century. Ethical concerns based on learners with limited experience conducting procedures on live patients for learning purposes continued to be questioned on into the 1970s. The use of simulations, a practice used for training in the airline industry, became a promising alternative to the "do one" tradition of learning through performing procedures on patients. Performance assessment and the use of standardized patients for teaching and assessing medical communication skills had been evolving since the 1970s. The development of task trainer simulations for learning procedures, and the creation of simulated clinical environments for training with patient actors, however, were resource intense alternatives to the traditional apprenticeship method of medical education. Subsequently, due to the costs involved, it took a confluence of events to become widely adopted by medical education.

In the mid-late 1990s, the National Board of Medical Examiners announced a clinical performance examination to assess communication skills. Around the same time, the Accreditation Council for Graduate Medical Education (ACGME) announced that it would require residents in all specialties to demonstrate competence in performing all common clinical procedures. In response to these changes, the clinical curriculum reform initiated in 2000 called for defining and delineating ways to teach and assess over seven pages of clinical skills that had not uniformly been covered in the existing curriculum. The curriculum documents suggested that these were skills that needed to be mastered by all medical students before graduation. These new requirements and other external pressures would become the catalyst for building a new simulation center.

Hoekstra led an educational committee to plan, fund, build and staff a simulation center that could serve the entire medical community at Ohio State, including the College of Medicine and Public Health, College of Nursing, College of Dentistry, University Hospitals, and the School of Allied Medical Professions. With letters of support from the Deans of Dentistry, Nursing and from Surgery Chair Christopher Ellison, MD, who would become the future interim dean, the skills center proposal was approved and funding was secured. By the end of 2002, the Clinical Skills Educational and Assessment Center (CSEAC) began to take shape.

The CSEAC opened in 2004, and its initial location was the basement of Prior Hall, which coincidentally had been the academic and administrative office of the Department of Emergency Medicine until it outgrew the space. The CSEAC consisted of 14 patient examination rooms outfitted with one-way mirrors and digital video recording equipment, a classroom outfitted with task-trainers for teaching procedures, and a space with a high-fidelity patient simulator. This portion of the CSEAC was eventually named the Ann Crowe Essig Patient Simulation Learning Laboratory as a memorial for the mother of a former medical school graduate and faculty member Leroy Essig II, MD.

In 2010, two floors were added to the five-story Prior Hall with the sixth floor entirely dedicated to the expansion of the CSEAC, allowing

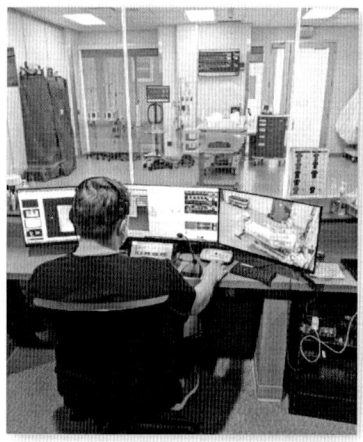

Figure 5: A simulation technician sits in the control room looking through a two-way mirror at a mock patient care room with a high-fidelity patient simulator on a gurney.

it to become a site for multidisciplinary health science education. The addition provided 18,000 square feet of dedicated space for ultrasound and procedures training, a seminar room and four simulated operating theaters. Badly needed space for storing and building simulations and task trainers was also added. The current CSEAC configuration is the product of the vision Hoekstra put into motion when he administratively navigated the logistics of creating one of the first simulation centers in Central Ohio. It is perhaps a coincidence, but fitting that the academic and administrative office of the Department occupies the space on the seventh floor of Prior Hall because the Department of Emergency Medicine has become the leading user of the CSEAC.

The Center's importance to simulation innovation and research is perhaps understated, particularly now that simulation has become such a critical component of medical training. The CSEAC and the educa-

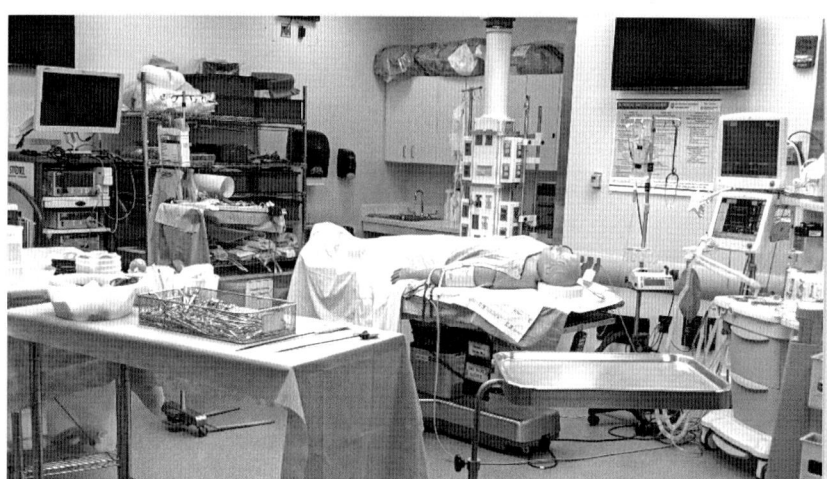

Figure 6: A mock operating room with a high-fidelity simulator in the Ohio State CSEAC contains all the elements for elevated learning.

tion that goes on within, represents a major paradigm shift in medical training, facilitating the move from the "see one, do one" model on real patients to training learners to master a procedure through simulation before they are permitted to participate in procedures on live patients. Hoekstra's leadership through this transition for Ohio State helped to forge a long-lasting symbiotic relationship between the College of Medicine and the Department of Emergency Medicine. The CSEAC that he helped create continues to be a source of inspiration and a resource for emergency medicine educators to develop a pipeline of future EM physicians (Figures 5 and 6).

Virtual Reality: A New Chapter of Simulation Begins

Entrustable Professional Activities (EPAs), were introduced into the medical school curriculum during the early 2010s. These were integrated foundational competencies required of all practicing physicians. One specific EPA, #10, was specific to the acute care environment. This EPA required a physician to recognize an unstable patient and initiate evaluation and management. In 2015 the simulations in AMHBC EM began to focus on EPA-10. During their Emergency Medicine Clerkship, medical students participated in an assessment in which they were required to successfully manage one of six emergent patient (EPA-10) cases in high fidelity simulation. In 2021, the clerkship added a formative virtual reality (VR) simulation for teaching EPA-10.[10]

The advantages of VR-based simulation education are extensive. VR simulators are already being used to educate and assess emergency medicine specialists, surgeons and other health care subspecialists in complex procedures that are too dangerous to practice on live patients. VR advocates have noted that virtual standardized patient simulations can reduce cost, faculty time and resources needed to assist students in developing their clinical skills. Two cases were converted into virtual reality simulations using a commercial VR simulation platform and incorporated into the clerkship. Medical students have become very enthused about using this modality to train for their summative assessment.

JENNIFER YEE, DO

Jennifer Yee, DO, completed a simulation fellowship at Summa Akron City Hospital in 2017 after she completed her residency training there. She joined the faculty at Ohio State shortly thereafter and began to direct simulation for the emergency medicine residency program (Figure 7). She recalled her goals and challenges:

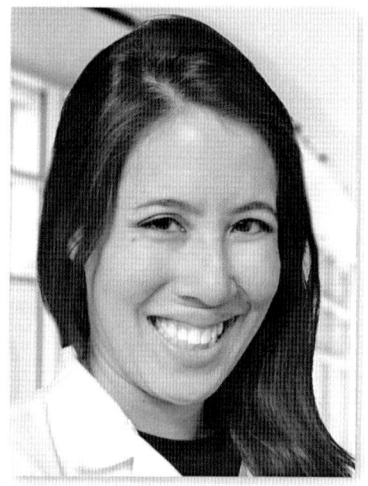

Figure 7: Jennifer Yee, DO, joined the faculty in 2017, specializing in medical simulation. She heads the medical simulation program for the Department of Emergency Medicine.

As a medical student, I was told to avoid the word "exciting" when explaining my interest in emergency medicine–however, it was a fitting way to describe our simulation cases. I was fascinated at the ability to translate textbook knowledge and suddenly see it come to life in front of me. I was able to practice rendering care to sick "patients" without worrying about harming real people, receive immediate individualized feedback, and slowly build my autonomy and confidence while pushing the boundaries of my medical knowledge.

Once I arrived at Ohio State, I continued developing curricula for our weekly resident conferences while branching out to projects involving tying milestone assessments to simulation and best practice methodology for teaching procedures. Over time, one thing I noticed was a lack of translation of closed loop communication practices from the simulation laboratory to the clinical setting. When discussing this with the program director, I told him that I wished I had a real-time auditory stimulus to "buzz" the residents whenever they would yell an order out into the air without directing it to any one individual. This snowballed into what is now known as the "alarm study," where aspects of human factors are being studied in the simulation lab to determine ways to reinforce communication practices during medical resuscitation cases.

While working on this project, out of necessity, a new question arose: How do we demonstrate procedural competence for our emergency medicine residents? We have been evolving away from the "see one, do one, teach one" model, and it had been assumed that with time and experience, our residents would demonstrate competence–but this was not rigorously demonstrated in a standardized fashion. The department funded my attendance for a workshop on simulation-based competency assessments. Upon my return, I worked with Dr. Panchal to develop a competency-based procedural curriculum during orientation so residents would be able to demonstrate competence in the simulation lab before they ever touched a physical patient. The OSUWMC Graduate Medical Office eventually supported the roll out of our curriculum, called Simulation-Based Mastery Learning (SBML) to all incoming PGY-1 residents who will be expected to place central venous catheters during residency. Residents from IM, Surgery, OB-GYN, and other programs now undergo the SBML curriculum as part of their orientation.

The Department continues to support and encourage my professional growth so that I may continue with my passions of teaching and pursuing educational research projects, including partnerships with interdisciplinary teams. Helping our residents to explore their interests to find what excites them professionally continues to drive me. Additionally, I am motivated by advancing their skills and knowledge in the simulation lab and in the department. As medicine moves towards a competency-based structure, I anticipate the need for simulation to grow exponentially over the future.[11]

Educational Research and Scholarship

Since 1999, the Department of Emergency Medicine has maintained a tradition of scholarly productivity through national presentations and published articles. This tradition started with Hoekstra's involvement with key parts of the Ohio State medical student experience, which paved the way for productive career paths of others who have become key figures on the medical education stage. By 2008, the department's surge in educational publications quickly surpassed other departments throughout the medical center. Growing and innovating while working with others in the college and collaborating with other educators across the nation became a successful model for producing educational scholarship.

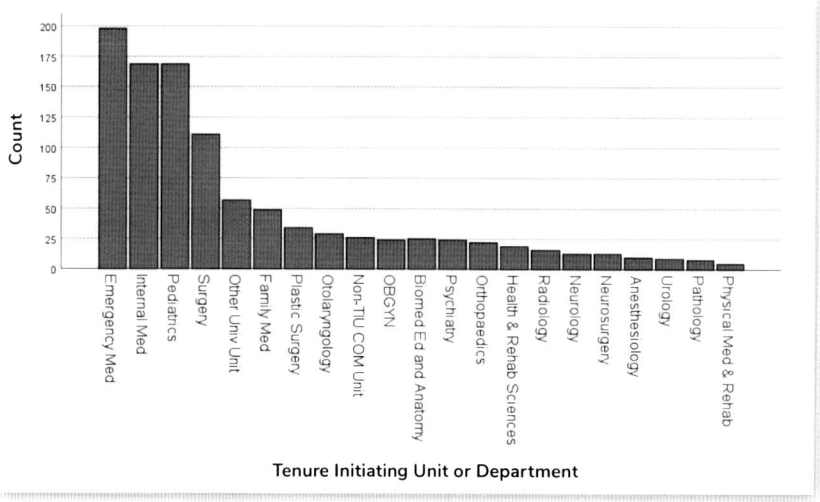

Figure 8: Number of Ohio State authorships in medical education related peer-reviewed publications from 1999-2000 through 2021-2022 by academic unit (TIU) as of October 4, 2021. (Note: Published abstracts and book chapters are not included).

DAVID P. WAY, MEd

Throughout David Way's 30-year tenure with the Ohio State University College of Medicine, first as a specialist in evaluation and assessment, then as a contributor to faculty development, he has been integrally linked to the Department of Emergency Medicine. In 2007 he was assigned by then Vice Dean of Education, Catherine Lucey, MD, to become a founding member of the Center for Education and Scholarship (CES).

The CES rolled out the Faculty Teaching Scholars Program (FTSP), an 18-month certificate program for training faculty in the skills they needed to become successful in their academic careers. One of the primary goals of FTSP was to increase the scholarly productivity of those most involved with medical education. A number of faculty members from Emergency Medicine completed this rigorous program in teaching and learning skills, educational research and program leadership, including Sorabh Khandelwal, MD; Aaron Bernard, MD; Nicholas Kman, MD; Jillian McGrath, MD; Diane Gorgas, MD; and Ashish Panchal, MD. As the program was being phased out in 2014, Thomas Terndrup, MD, the new Chair of Emergency Medicine, offered

Way a full-time staff position with the department.

Once in the department, Way's focus continued to be on increasing the scholarly productivity of the emergency medicine educators. He began resuscitating a backlog of rejected and incomplete manuscripts, seeing them through to publication. He continued to work on the projects the FTSP graduates initiated during their program, helping guide them to publication. Eventually he turned his attention to providing research mentorship to junior faculty and guiding them on their path to promotion. Along the way, the Department of Emergency Medicine became the leading producer within the medical center of publications in medical education research and innovation, producing more publications than departments two or three times its size (Figure 8).

Moreover, by 2020, emergency medicine faculty and staff were 11 of the top 25 education research authors in the medical center. These included Way, himself, along with Khandelwal, Bahner, King, Kman, Panchal, Mitzman, Barrie, Bernard, Greenberger, and McGrath.

Way also contributed to the funded research that Terndrup brought with him to the department, an Agency for Healthcare Research and Quality grant to train and assess emergency medical service (EMS) professionals in comprehensive airway management. His work on this project resulted in the publication of a standard performance assessment instrument for validly assessing comprehensive airway management.[12] More recently, he has been working with Kman, Panchal, McGrath and Sharkey on development of a virtual reality simulator for training and assessing first responders to triage and treat mass casualty incidents (Figure 9). The program, called First Responders, has attracted the attention of the local, regional, and national media.[13] Furthermore, the program, even while still in its infancy, has been highly requested by EMS agencies across Central

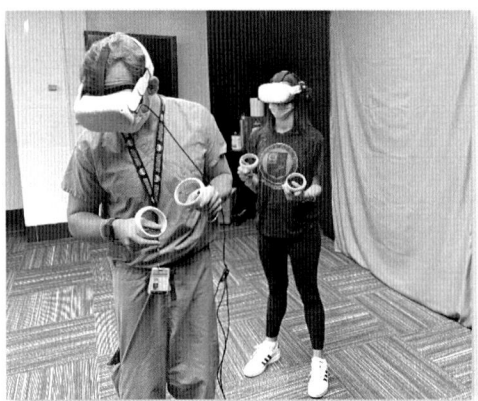

Figure 9: Medical students use the first responder mass casualty incident virtual reality simulator.

Ohio. Way remembered his relationship with emergency medicine:

> *I always had a special affinity for the Department of Emergency Medicine, even before becoming part of the department. Jim Hoekstra's and Howie Werman's enthusiasm and interest in medical education was infectious early on in my career. I cherished the opportunities to work with them as part of the PBL program and in contributing to the development of the DOC 1 program. Meeting Sorabh Khandelwal as a student and eventually getting to work with him in the FTSP program and as residency program director has been a special highlight of my career. I always seem to get a laugh out of him by bringing up stories from the past.*
>
> *Another longtime associate, David Bahner, has also been fun to follow in his career, all the way from his struggles to get ultrasound recognized as a viable clinical skill to his current success as a national leader in ultrasonography.*
>
> *I am very thankful to have been a part of the professional lives of those EM physicians who participated in the FTSP program: Sorabh Khandelwal, Nick Kman, Diane Gorgas, Aaron Bernard, Jillian McGrath, and Ash Panchal, all of whom became incredible leaders in the field. Finally, working arm-in-arm with Andy King, Jennifer Mitzman, and Jennifer Yee along with the PEM faculty, Maya Iyer and Delia Gold to produce scholarship that has received national recognition has been another great career highlight of mine.*[14]

Course Offerings in Emergency Medicine

The medical student educational program and mentorship has resonated with Ohio State students. For many years from 8% to 10% of the graduating medical school class has chosen emergency medicine for their residency training. The educational contributions of emergency medicine faculty created an overall culture of education within the department. As new faculty members brought energy to build on established curricula, existing faculty helped mentor and allowed them to make changes and evolve the educational service lines.

This structured mentorship and innovative education became a hallmark for the Ohio State Department of Emergency Medicine. Courses in emergency medicine have continued to be popular with Ohio State medical students. Table 1 lists the student enrollment for courses offered by the Department of Emergency Medicine in the 2020-2021 academic year. The number of courses has expanded over the years and the Department of Emergency Medicine continues to extend its influence at Ohio State.

Table 1.
Student enrollment in courses offered by the Department of Emergency Medicine 2021-2022 academic year

Course	Enrollment
AMHBC – didactic Emergency Medicine	**163**
Honors Ultrasound Emergency Medicine	**22**
ATEM Emergency Medicine	**21**
MS3 Elective Emergency Medicine bedside teaching	**39**
Pandemic and Disaster Preparedness and Response Emergency Medicine	**225** *MS3 (190) and MS4 (35)*
Ultrasound Immersion Emergency Medicine	**6**

References

1. Rund DA, et al. Clinical learning without prerequisites: students as clinical teachers. *J Med Educ.* Jun 1977;52(6):520-2.

2. Fontana ME. Personal communication. 2023.

3. Way D. Personal communication. 2023.

4. Khandelwal S. Interview with Sorabh Khandelwal by Douglas Rund. 2023: Columbus, Ohio.

5. Kman NE, et al. Advanced topics in emergency medicine: curriculum development and initial evaluation. *West J Emerg Med.* November 2011;12(4):543-50.

6. Leung CG, Thompson LR, Way DP, Kman NE. Promoting achievement of Level 1 milestones for medical students going into emergency medicine. *West J Emerg Med.* 2017;18(1):20-25.

7. Kman NE. Interview with Nicholas Kman, by Douglas Rund. 2023: Columbus, Ohio.

8. Pollard KA, Bachmann DJ, Greer M, Way DP, Kman NE. Development of a disaster preparedness curriculum for medical students: a pilot study of incorporating local events into training opportunities. *Am J Disaster Med.* 2015;10(1):51-59.

9. Bahner DP, Adkins E, Patel N, Donley C, Nagel R, Kman NE. How we use social media to supplement a novel curriculum in medical education. *Med Teach.* Jun 1, 2012;34(6):439-44.

10. Thompson LR, Leung CG, Green B, Lipps J, Schaffernocker T, Ledford C, Davis J, Way DP, Kman NE. Development of an assessment for Entrustable Professional Activity (EPA) 10: Emergent patient management. *West J Emerg Med.* 2017;18(1):35-42.

11. Yee J. Personal communication. 2022.

12. Way DP, Panchal AR, Finnegan GI, Terndrup TE. Airway management proficiency checklist for assessing paramedic performance. *Prehosp Emerg Care.* 2017;21(3):354-61.

13. Kman NE, Price A, Berezina-Blackburn V, Patterson J, Maicher K, Way DP, McGrath J, Panchal AR, Luu K, Oliszewski A, Swearingen S, Danforth D. First responder: virtual reality simulator to train and assess emergency personnel for mass casualty response. *JACEP Open*. Feb 2023;4(1):e12903.

14. Way DP. Personal communication. 2023.

Other UME Articles

Leung CG, Malone M, Way DP, Barrie MG, Kman NE, San Miguel C. Preparing students for residency interviews in the age of COVID: lessons learned from a standardized video interview preparation program. *AEM Edu Train*. July 2021;5(3):e10583.

Walrod B, Conroy M, Boucher LC, McCamey KL, Hartz CA, Way DP, Jonesco MA, Albrechta S, Bockbrader M, Bahner DP. Beyond bones: Ultrasound-enhanced instruction of soft-tissue musculoskeletal structures for first-year medical students. *J Med Ultrasound*. July 2019;38:2047-2055.

Walrod B, Schroeder A, Conroy MJ, Boucher L, Bockbrader M, Way DP, Bahner DP. Does ultrasound-enhanced instruction of musculoskeletal anatomy improve physical examination skills of first-year medical students? *J Med Ultrasound*. 2018;37:225-232.

Thompson L, Exline M, Leung CG, Way DP, Clinchot D, Bahner DP, Khandelwal S. A clinical procedures curriculum for undergraduate medical students: the eight-year history of a third-year immersive experience. *Med Educ Online*. 2016;21:29486.

McGrath JL, Bischof JJ, Greenberger S, Bachmann DJ, Way DP, Gorgas DL, Kman NE. 'Speed-Advising' for medical students applying to residency programs: An efficient supplement to traditional advising. *Med Educ Online*. 2016;21:31336.

Prats MI, Royall NA, Panchal AR, Way DP, Bahner DP. Outcomes of an advanced ultrasound course: Preparing medical students for residency and practice *J Med Ultrasound*. 2016;35(5):975-82.

Bernard AW, Martin DR, Moseley MG, Kman NE, Khandelwal S, Carpenter D, Way DP, Caterino JM. The impact of medical student participation in emergency medicine patient care on departmental Press Ganey Scores. *West J Emerg Med*. 2015;16(6):830-838.

Khandelwal S, Way DP, Wald DA, Fisher J, Ander DS, Thibodeau L, Manthey DE. State of undergraduate education in emergency medicine: A national survey of clerkship directors. *Adv J Emerg*. 2014;21(1):92-95.

Bahner DP, Goldman E, Way DP, Royall NA, Liu TY. The state of ultrasound education in U.S. Medical schools: Results of a national survey. *Acad. Med*. 2014;89(12):1681-1686.

Chapter 20

A Tradition of Excellence: The Residency Program in Emergency Medicine

Douglas A. Rund, MD
Diane L. Gorgas, MD

The creation of an excellent residency program in emergency medicine was always one of the highest priorities of the emergency medicine faculty from the beginning. A focus on this goal guided many of the early decisions as the department grew.

When the first application for approval was submitted in 1980, there were no emergency physicians in the country who were certified by the newly created American Board of Emergency Medicine (ABEM) because the first examination was just being given in 1980. Douglas Rund, MD, Ohio State's first emergency medicine program director, and Samuel Kiehl, MD at Riverside, passed the examination and thus became among the very first board certified emergency physicians; only 248 individuals in the nation were certified after this first exam.

Leadership

When Richard Nelson, MD, joined the department he was the first residency trained emergency physician in central Ohio. Rund immediately asked Nelson for help with setting up the program and over time Nelson became the de facto program director even though Rund retained the program director title until 1990. Technically, Nelson was the director of the program at Ohio State and Marian Schuda, MD, was the director at Riverside Hospital.

This was a challenging time in the history of Emergency Medicine, as the total number of training programs nationally was around 30. The house of medicine was still settling into the idea that emergency medicine was a bona fide specialty that focused on the care of any patient with any condition at any time, all unified by their need for immediate diagnosis and treatment. Ohio State's early leaders in residency education stood firm in the need for a training program and assured the longevity of the program in future years.

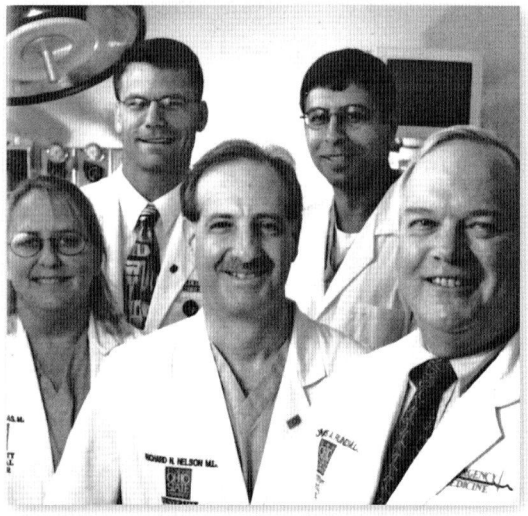

Figure 1: The program directors of the residency in emergency medicine at Ohio State through the years. From left to right: Diane Gorgas, MD (2010-2015), Daniel Martin, MD (1990-2010), Richard Nelson, MD (1981-1990), Sorabh Khandelwal, MD (2015-present) and Douglas Rund, MD (1981-1990).

Throughout the entire history of the program there were only five residency directors: Douglas Rund, MD (1981-1990); Richard Nelson, (MD 1981-1990); Daniel Martin, MD (1990-2010); Diane Gorgas, MD (2010-2015); and Sorabh Khandelwal, MD (2015-present) (Figure 1).

DANIEL M. MARTIN, MD, MBA

Daniel M. Martin, MD, MBA, was the Ohio State Emergency Medicine residency program director in 1990, a time when the program underwent the most restructuring (Figure 2). Martin received his medical degree from the Indiana University School of Medicine, did an internal medicine residency at the University of Iowa Hospitals and Clinics and completed his emergency medicine residency at the Medical College of Wisconsin, serving as Chief Resident during his final year. He joined the Ohio State Department of Emergency Medicine as an Assistant Professor in 1988.

Being residency trained and boarded in both specialties, Martin worked to improve ties with the Department Internal Medicine in order to develop Emergency Medicine training. Despite the reduction in support from Riverside, the program expanded in 1988 to include six residents per year. The following year the department entered into an agreement with the U.S. Navy to offer training to one officer per year. The arrangement with the Navy ended in 1994 but in future years agreements were made with other branches of the service.

Martin oversaw several key changes during his directorship: The program expanded to 12 residents per year; the medical center began paying the residents stipends (which initially came from faculty practice income); the trauma rotation transitioned from the early experience at Maryland Shock Trauma Center in Baltimore to Columbus (Ohio State and Grant Medical Center); and a unified and cohesive community medicine rotation at Ohio State East was launched.

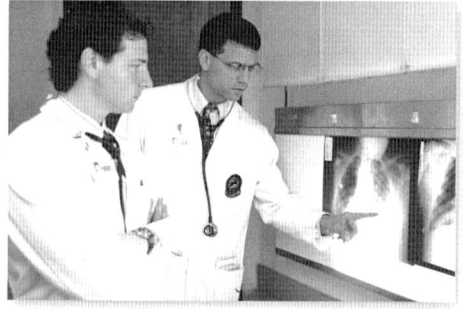

Figure 2: Daniel M. Martin, MD (right) became director of the residency program in 1990. He is shown here in 1995 with resident Phillip Bielecki, MD (left), reviewing x ray films that were in use at that time before the era of digital images.

DIANE L. GORGAS, MD

In 1994 Diane L. Gorgas, MD, joined the faculty as an Assistant Program Director, focusing on learners' extra-clinical educational needs (Figure 3). She revised the conference curriculum and off-service rotations and instituted a flipped-classroom model for resident education, moving away from the "sage on the stage" to more of a "guide on the side" philosophy. Her work significantly influenced resident education, with didactic presentations ebbing and small group conference sessions with faculty leaders increasing.

When Gorgas took over program directorship in 2010, her leadership style focused on collaborative, grass roots engagement. She increased

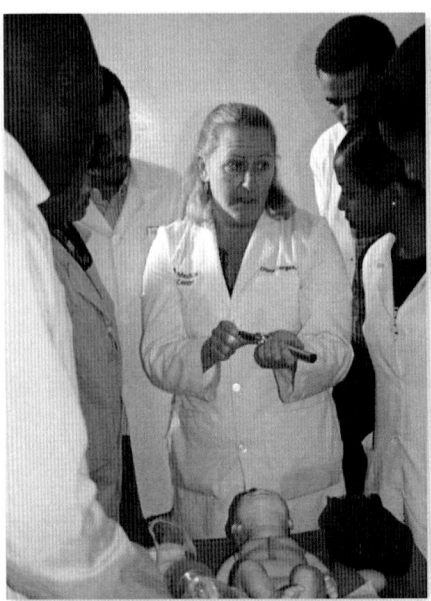

Figure 3: Diane L. Gorgas, MD, served as Program Director from 2010 until 2015. Here she is teaching neonatal resuscitation to pediatric residents at Black Lion Hospital in Addis Ababa, Ethiopia.

the number and ownership of Assistant and Associate Program Directors as she grew the training program from 8 to 14 residents per year. Her driving vision: "If you want to go fast, go alone. If you want to go far, go together."

The other tenet she held fast to was recruiting for contribution, not fit. Gorgas changed the rubric and traditional value system, which rewarded sameness and "fit" in applicants, and instead created an environment that valued potential program contribution, an endeavor that led to more diversity among resident ethnicity, race, gender and geographic location. Her recruitment strategy was lauded by the university (Shining Star Award) and nationally by SAEM's Academy for Diversity and Inclusion in Emergency Medicine.

Gorgas' leadership was recognized nationally and she was elected to the Accreditation Council for Graduate Medical Education's Review Committee for Emergency Medicine (RRC-EM) where the values and vision of Ohio State's EM training program influenced national standards in program requirements and the value of EM education.

In 2015 she left the program directorship to become Executive Director of the Health Sciences Center for Global Health, but continued to serve in resident education, and currently leads the American Board of Emergency Medicine's Becoming Certified Initiative, which focuses on revolutionizing the initial certification of residency graduates.

SORABH KHANDELWAL, MD

In 2015 Sorabh Khandelwal, MD, took over leadership of the training program as the number of Accreditation Council for Graduate Medical Education (ACGME) accredited residencies was rapidly increasing (Figure 4). At the time, the pressures on every program to continue to match talented students to their ranks was felt more acutely than ever. Increased requirements for graduation coupled with decreased mandated protected educational time for core faculty meant pushing colleagues and peers to spend more uncompensated time in direct learner contact.

During Khandelwal's leadership, the faculty split into much more well-defined tracks given the designation of Clinical Research, Clinical Excellence and Clinical Educator Pathways in the promotion system. The core educator group (on the Clinical Educator Pathway) fell under the umbrella leadership of Martin as Vice Chair of Education, but the GME core educators had to be engaged and increasingly contributory under Khandelwal's leadership.

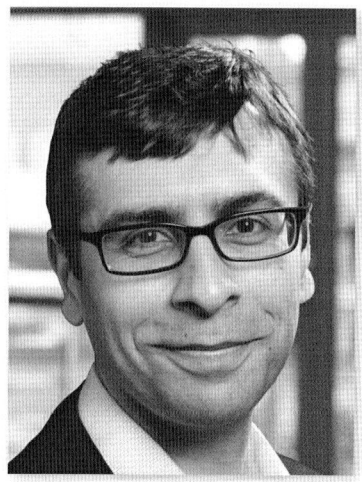

Figure 4: Sorabh Khandelwal, MD, became the Program Director in 2015 and serves to the present. His four guiding principles are innovation, wellness, academics and diversity.

Among the accomplishments achieved during Khandelwal's leadership were the securing of a $2 million endowment focused on resident wellness and the establishment of the Samuel J. Kiehl III, MD, Professorship in Emergency Medicine. Khandelwal was the first occupant of this named chair. He also partnered with the United States Air Force to become the civilian site for its Operational Emergency Medicine program. He improved diversity within the program and helped change the culture to a more academic focus with almost 50% of residency graduates opting to enter fellowship training in one of Emergency Medicine's subspecialties.

One of Khandelwal's earliest goals for the program was to be more focused on the preparation of academic physicians:

> *I think the challenge was putting a vision in place. I really wanted an academic culture... I told faculty members that we were switching to a very learner directed model with small group sessions, etc., and that I really wanted an academic culture. [My] goal was [that] 40%...of our residents...go into academics. I remember friends of mine in the program who came up to me and said, "I don't think this is going to work, I think this is crazy. We are going to recruit the wrong type of people." [We are now] recruiting from a tremendous geographic region from [excellent] schools. Ultimately the program is the gem here.[1]*

Khandelwal's vision was to construct the program on four pillars: innovation, wellness, academics and diversity. His continuing goal is to recruit the best candidates possible.

Associate Program Directors in Later Years

GEREMIHA G. EMERSON, MD

Geremiha G. Emerson, MD, graduated from the University of Cincinnati College of Medicine in 2012 (Figure 5). He did his residency training at Vanderbilt University Medical Center in Nashville Tennessee. After serving an additional year as Chief Resident, he left Vanderbilt to join the faculty at Ohio State in 2016. In 2017, he joined the residency leadership team, serving as Assistant and subsequently Associate Residency Program Director. Within this role, Geremiha focuses on resident remediation and curriculum development. His passion: teaching clinical reasoning and interpretation of electrocardiograms.

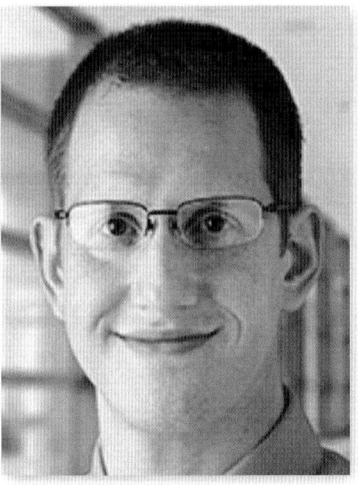

Figure 5: Geremiha G. Emerson, MD, is an Associate Director of the Residency Program in Emergency Medicine. He focuses on curriculum development and resident remediation.

SIMIAO LI-SAUERWINE, MD

Simiao Li-Sauerwine, MD, completed her undergraduate studies at Pomona College and medical school at the University of Pittsburgh, where she earned a combined MD and Master of Science in Clinical Research as a Doris Duke Clinical Research Fellow (Figure 6). She completed her residency training in Emergency Medicine at Northwestern University McGaw Medical Center, where she was awarded multiple Outstanding Teacher Awards and elected to the Best Resident Role Model award by her peers.

She worked initially as Assistant Program Director at Ohio State and then became Associate Program Director. A medical education researcher and a nationally recognized speaker on—and with interests in—physician well-being and equity in academic medicine, Li-Sauerwine is the Chair-elect of the Council of Residency Directors in Emergency Medicine Well-being Committee.

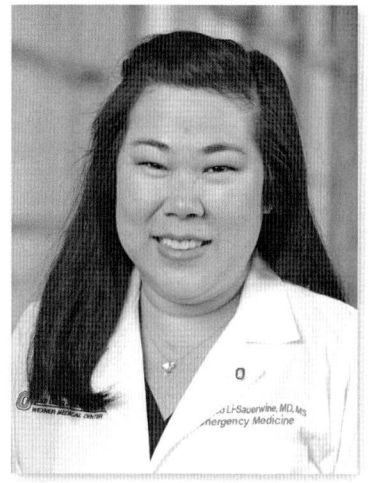

Figure 6: Simiao Li-Sauerwine, MD, is an Associate Program Director for the emergency medicine residency at Ohio State. Her interests include physician well-being and equity in academic medicine. She directs the Sam Kiehl III Emergency Medicine Resident Wellness Endowment.

She also directs the Sam Kiehl III Emergency Medicine Resident Wellness Endowment and is founder and faculty lead for the Residents and Faculty Female Tribe (RAFFT), a longitudinal professional development curriculum and mentorship group for women in academic emergency medicine. Recognitions for her achievements include The Ohio State University College of Medicine Clotilde D. Bowen MD Women of Excellence Faculty Award.

Emergency Medicine/Internal Medicine Residency Program

In 2013 Daniel R. Martin, MD, MBA, Professor and Vice Chair of Education, started the Emergency Medicine Internal Medicine Residency Program. The program was built from two collaborative and intertwined departments, internal medicine and emergency medicine, each of which had already independently housed competitive and academically productive residencies. Many ties between EM and IM existed prior to the creation of the joint training program, both clinically and academically, and the merging of the two into a joint training pathway was a natural consequence.

Years later Martin recalled the impetus for starting the program and its successes:

> *We were often asked by medical students and residents to develop a combined EM IM program because our parent categorical programs had required rotations together and both programs were highly regarded. Although starting a new program can be challenging, in this case Dave Wininger (IM PD) and Mike Grever (IM Chair) were very excited and supportive. Our program differed from many in that it was based at a university hospital and residents could interface with many practice sites. We also offered many research and mentorship opportunities afforded by two departments highly ranked in scholarship. Finally, we offered a unique 3 block opportunity in the 4th year called "mini-fellowships" in which residents could investigate areas or research, clinical or other passions. To date, residents have travelled abroad during this time to experience medicine in other countries and others have delved deeper into scholarship, education, and administrative leadership.*
>
> *Our 4th and 5th year residents are some of the best clinicians in our medical center. The expertise they gained from caring for the sickest of the sick often made them the "go-to" person when encountering a critically sick or injured patient. Residents would start with a combined 6 weeks of orientation then flip back and forth between both departments every 3 months spending 50% of their clinical time in each department. In 2022 the award for best clinical resident in EM went to two PGY5 EM IM residents (Scott Cardone and Serena Hua) and Scott Cardone was also recognized for best clinical MICU resident. Their combination of clinical and procedural expertise with servant leadership and humanism also has resulted in frequent recognition for excellence in educating a variety of learners.[2]*

The program has two residents per year in a five-year curriculum.

Most EM/IM residents have chosen academic pathways after completion of the residency, with 8 of the first 12 graduates entering critical care fellowships and 2 others entering pain and palliative fellowships. Martin stressed the important lessons learned from the combined residency: humanism and dedication to the health of all patients in need, collegiality, and the ability to function equally well on a ward or in the emergency department. Martin added:

> *Although workforce concerns have led to slight decrease in EM residency applicants of late, EM IM programs have become more competitive. Most EM IM graduates are able to combine practices either as an EM physician and hospitalist or as an EM physician and critical care specialist. Some have also included observation medicine in their practices and often these graduates are active educators of residents and medical students. Currently discussions are beginning about expanding the program.*[2]

Assistant/Associate Program Directors (APD)

Emily Kauffman was the first APD in EM/IM and served as a hospitalist at Ohio State East in addition to maintaining a robust practice in EM. Her passion for advocacy and program development in substance use disorders has seen her time and talents in these areas grow beyond the capacity to maintain program leadership. Other leaders who followed her in the APD role include Jennah Morgan, MD, Greg Eisinger, MD, Sarah Greenberger, MD, Travis Eastin, MD, and Andrew King, MD. From 2011 to 2015 Jillian McGrath, MD, was Associate Program Director.

The Residents

The first full class of four residents began in 1981, with the initial program including three main clinical sites: Ohio State University Hospital, Riverside Methodist Hospital and Columbus Children's Hospital. Clinical experience in the emergency department was divided equally between Riverside and Ohio State. In 1990 the program changed when the Ohio State Residency Review Committee for Emergency Medicine

(RRC-EM) required that most of the clinical practice must take place in the primary academic institution. Their reasoning was that resident training was so divided among the institutions that it was difficult if not impossible to create an impactful presence at one hospital.

With more of the residents' rotations occurring at Ohio State, residents would become a more constant and consistent presence at the "mothership" (according to one reviewer), and would allow for a schedule that encouraged resident-to-resident teaching and graded responsibility as the resident progressed through the program.

In 1990, in response, Riverside applied for approval to begin its own emergency medicine residency program. There was good justification for starting a program. The patient population was the largest in the area and the physicians were superb clinicians and teachers. Ultimately, a competing program in Columbus was not accredited at the time, so Ohio State remained the sole training program in the city.[3]

This transition was difficult for many reasons. To start, Riverside had come to Ohio State's rescue in 1980 when the program had to increase the resident compliment from one to four per year. In addition, the clinical experience for residents was different at each institution. Years later, Mark Smith, MD, who was a member of the second class of residents in 1985, remembered this about the differences in the practices:

> *We enjoyed the off-service rotations but we all really looked forward to getting back in the ER, because that is what we did. And we spent again, half our time at OSU ER and the other half at Riverside ER. You got different patient populations. I don't know that I saw more than half a dozen acute MIs at OSU ER during my whole time there. You would see that many in a day or two at Riverside. It was just that patient population. On the other hand, you really didn't see complex cases. There were the bread-and-butter cases at Riverside and complex medical cases at OSU. So, you got the experience both ways. Then of course the pediatric training at the Children's Hospital was superb.*[4]

The Early Years Before 1990

Unfortunately, images of the early classes are not available because the group photos were not taken until 1992. The class of 1985 included three physicians who finished the program: Eric Davis, MD, Mark Smith MD, and Gregory Decker, MD. Davis completed his residency in emergency medicine and a research fellowship at Ohio State and enjoyed a productive academic career. He ultimately became Professor of Emergency Medicine at the University of Rochester. Decker continued to teach at the university on a part-time basis. He developed and taught the popular and always oversubscribed first responder course for first year medical students.

Students knew well that, *since they were in medical school—even in year one*—they were expected by their peers to know what to do in emergencies even though their course work consisted of the basic sciences. The first responder course taught such things as cardiopulmonary resuscitation, stabilization of the trauma patient in the field and emergency childbirth. Decker worked in the OhioHealth system throughout his career as part of the Mid-Ohio Emergency Services (MOES). Many Ohio State residency program graduates began practicing with the MOES group, including other early residents Warren Yamarick, MD (1987), and Steve Eskin, MD (1988) (Figure 7).

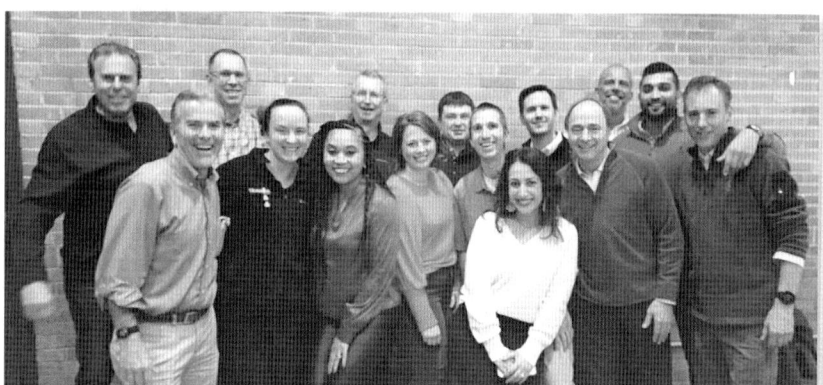

Figure 7: Mid-Ohio Emergency Services physicians who were graduates of the Ohio State residency program and their year of graduation. From left: Steve Eskin, MD ('88); Warren Yamarick, MD ('87); Andy Jenkins, MD ('07); Erica Kube, MD ('09); Laura Espy-Bell, MD ('14); Tom Gavin, MD ('93); Sarah Sisbarro, MD ('12); Andy King, MD ('12) ; James Falk, MD ('15) ; Tamara Halaweh, MD ('15); Brad Raetzke, MD ('11); Greg Decker, MD ('85); Brian Seifferth, MD ('97), Imran Shaikh, MD ('16); and Buck Marshall, MD ('06).

Class of 1985

Mark Smith, MD, joined the Mount Carmel medical group after graduation. Years later Smith remembered this about his residency experience:

> I remember one particular case where the oral surgery residents rotated through the ER. The emergency medicine residents were definitely the senior residents when they were rotating through because the oral surgeons needed back up. I remember one where the oral surgery resident came to me with a case. I think it was a chest pain, and he was pretty unconcerned about it, and I went and talked to the patient and sure enough they had a dissected thoracic aneurysm.
>
> I do remember that my favorite night shifts were shifts where the attending would say "It's yours" and go to sleep. Those were my favorite shifts because how else would you learn responsibility other than taking it.
>
> I was an intern and at that time we had the medical areas and the surgical area. From the medical area you could see a couple of beds in the surgical area, and they had the typical curtains across the doorways. I could see this patient rocking back and forth behind the curtain. All I could see was his feet and ankles. Tom [Bullock] said, "that guy's got a kidney stone." From 50 feet all he could see was his feet and ankles and Tom made a diagnosis. I said, "how do you know?" and he said, "nobody paces like that unless they have a kidney stone." I remember thinking he was a wizard.
>
> Another patient was walking on the football field and got some indigestion. I went and talked to him and thought, yes, it was indigestion and then you [Rund] came in and said, "I think we are going to look into this a little further." He ended up with four bypasses. That's another one. You taught me on that one.[3]

Class 1986

The class of 1986 included Howard Bernstein, MD, Frank Birinyi, MD, Cheryl Lee, MD, and Ronald Taylor, MD. Years later Birinyi remembered this about his residency experience:

I remember the program as being small. We just had two other interns. It was just me, Cheryl Lee and Ron Taylor. It was the third class so the other classes were similarly small so when we had conference on Tuesday it was a small crowd. If you were off-service at OSU and, let's, say Internal Medicine, you were definitely a guest. Back in that era internal medicine ruled the hospital. One illustration is that I did two months of "hem-onc" [hematology-oncology]. That's where internal medicine needed bodies so that is where they put us. It didn't necessarily correlate with the training that was necessary. At Riverside I was treated well. I think that having the two hospitals exposed you to a wider group of teachers and I think gave you a good training. When you train at Ohio State and then you applied for a job in Ohio there were no further questions. When people asked you about your background, how competent are you? You say, I trained at Ohio State. They move on to the next subject.[5]

Cheryl Lee, MD, was the first woman in the program. Lee graduated from Northwestern University Medical School in 1983, before it became the Feinberg School of Medicine. She was attracted to emergency medicine (EM) because of the EM/IM residents at Northwestern, who she recognized as extremely talented. She quickly learned that it was the EM aspect of the dual program that interested her. After graduating from the Ohio State University EM Residency in 1986, Lee joined the faculty at the University of Buffalo. She was not only the sole woman on the faculty, but also the only EM boarded attending in the department where she supervised residents from internal medicine and surgery.

Class of 1987

The class of 1987 included only three residents: Warren Yamarick, MD, Teresa Bridges, MD, and David Lemak, MD. Yamarick went on to lead the emergency medicine department at Riverside Methodist Hospital.

Class of 1988

The class of 1988 included Kenneth Shildkrout, MD, Jonathan "Jon" Brooks, MD, Steve Eskin, MD, and Lee Lawrence, MD. Brooks completed medical school at the Medical College of Pennsylvania in 1985 and joined the Ohio State faculty post-residency. An early proponent of ultrasound, Brooks began to advocate for ultrasound and the purchase of a machine in 1988. In 1999 faculty meeting minutes he reported findings from a conference he attended that most machines would cost up to $30,000 and "there would be financial and political concerns" involved with its use by emergency physicians. The faculty consensus was to pursue more information regarding ultrasound in the ED.

Class of 1989

The class of 1989 included David F. Baehren, MD, Susan E. Churchill, MD, Jeffrey Lavanier, MD, and Linda Robinson, MD. At the end of her residency Robinson joined the faculty at Case Western Reserve in Cleveland but returned to Ohio State as a faculty member in 1990 and remained until 1992 when she moved to Miami to work in Jackson Memorial Hospital. Tragically she lost a battle to cancer and passed away in 2017. Following her death her family endowed a student scholarship in her name. Tributes from the faculty included the following:

> *I met Linda Robinson during my first year at Ohio State (1988-1989) as she was a senior resident and one of our two chief residents. She was one of the best clinicians I encountered as she managed multiple patients and multiple residents with ease. Her workups were more comprehensive than an internist but she was faster than any mere mortal emergency medicine physician. I would ask if she thought of this or if she ordered that and she would never just answer "no" and she could not be stumped. After a while I realized, I didn't have to ask her anything and could just watch in amazement. She was the perfect example of an ideal team player with excessive amounts of humility, hunger or drive and people smarts beyond her years.*
>
> *– Daniel M. Martin, MD, MBA (2017)*

Losing a role model, a colleague, and a friend is always difficult, but losing Linda is a loss for all of us in Emergency Medicine. I first met Linda when I was a medical student in Cleveland, and she was the first EM trained female physician I ever met. She was a strong leader without ever raising her voice and a trailblazer without ever intending to be. The first time I met her, I remember coming on a shift with her and she was telling me in detail about the subarachnoid hemorrhage she was seeing independently that she just intubated, placed an arterial line in, personally rolled over to CT, and started on pressure control, all in 15 minutes. She was breathless as she told the story and then in her usual Linda fashion turned to me and said "cool, huh?" I was hooked. She was the first physician I ever met who sparked the thought in me, "hey, maybe I can do this, and wouldn't THAT be cool?"

– Diane L Gorgas, MD (2017)

Class of 1990

The class of 1990 included Diana Johnson, MD, Genevieve "Genny" Messick, MD, Grace Nejman, DO, and Ronald Pirrallo, MD. Pirrallo went on to an academic career specializing in Emergency Medical Services. He eventually became the President of the National Association of EMS Physicians and Vice Chair of the Department of Emergency Medicine at the University of South Carolina School of Medicine.

Class of 1991

The class of 1998 included six residents, which was the largest in the history of the department to that date: Jeff Dreyer, MD; Kevin Bowman, MD; Margaret Hubbard, MD; David Lewis, MD; Charles "Charlie" Little, DO; and Keith Smith, MD. Little was the chief resident during the program restructuring. He joined the faculty following graduation and was an exceptional contributor to the research and educational missions.

Class of 1992

Michael "Mike" Dick, MD, joined the faculty immediately following residency and led the faculty group that began to staff Ohio State East in 1999. The trauma rotation at Baltimore Shock Trauma had been part of the residency since the program began but the program began to offer trauma experience at Grant hospital and additional experience at Ohio State.

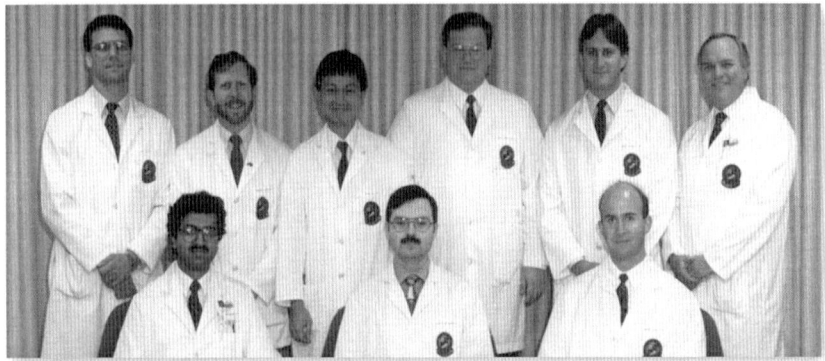

Figure 8: Residency class of 1992, back row, from left: Daniel M. Martin, MD (Program Director); Michael Dick, MD; Tuan A Luu, MD; Gary L. Swart, MD; Mark Darnell, MD; and Douglas A. Rund, MD (Department Chair). Front row: Prashanth Bhat, MD; David E. Davies, MD; and Robert W. Heck, MD.

Class of 1993

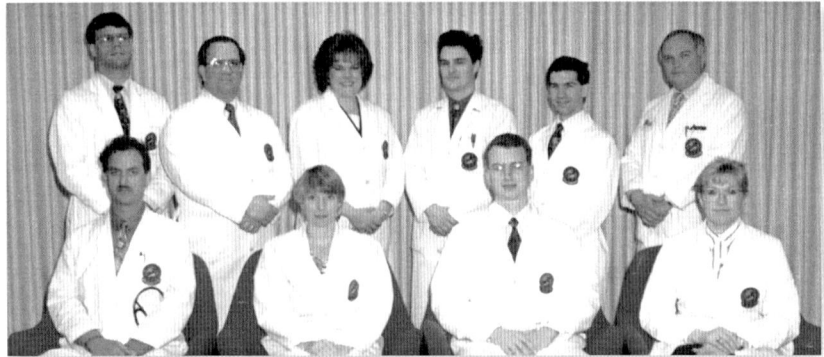

Figure 9: Residency class of 1993, back row, from left: Daniel Martin, MD (Program Director); Daniel Berndt, MD; Patricia Robitaille, MD; Blake Montana, MD; Marcel Casavant, MD; and Douglas Rund, MD (Department Chair). Front row: Roger Muller, MD; Carol Clinton, MD; Thomas Gavin, MD; and Rina Stein, DO.

Class of 1994

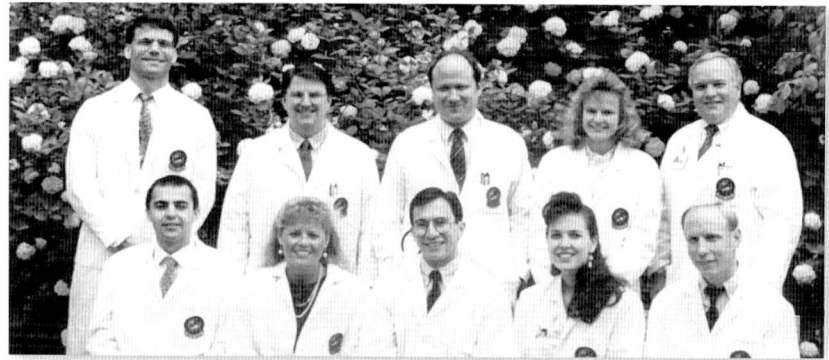

Figure 10: Residency class of 1994, back row, from left: Daniel Martin, MD (Program Director); Michael Vorbroker, MD; Bradford Cotton, MD; Mary Palte-Knapke, MD; and Douglas Rund, MD (Department Chair). Front row: Carlos Torres, MD; Letitia Overholt, MD; James Villereal, MD; Ann Stubbs, MD; and John Parker, MD.

Class of 1995

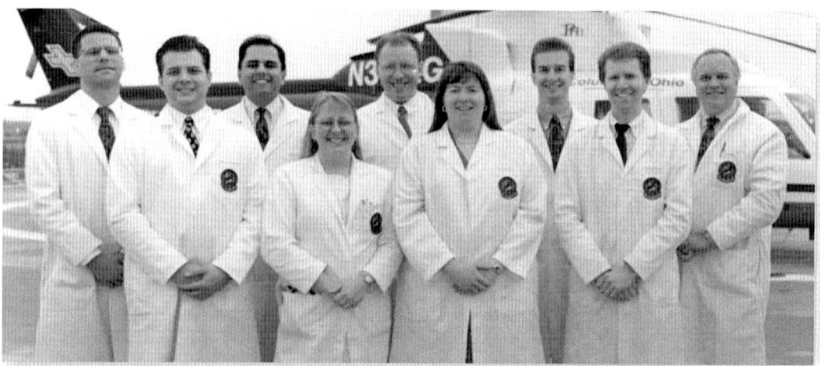

Figure 11: Residency class of 1995, back row, from left: Daniel Martin, MD (Program Director); David Reyes, MD; David Jones, MD; Alan Gora, MD; and Douglas Rund, MD (Department Chair). Front row: Michael Sotak, MD; Diane Gorgas, MD; Ann Haynes, MD; and Bruce Neely, MD.

Class of 1996

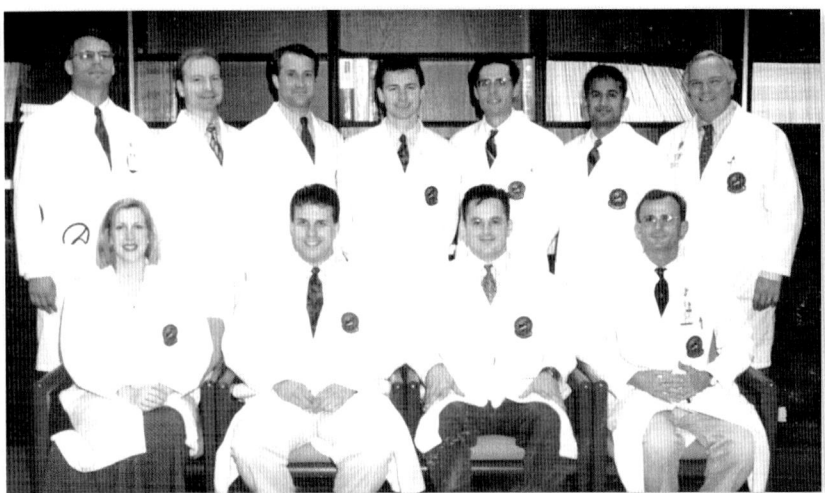

Figure 12: Residency class of 1996, back row, from left: Daniel Martin, MD (Program Director); Daniel Gorecki, MD; Michael Waite, MD; Phillip Bialecki, MD; Marcus Pesa, MD; Matthew Patel, MD; and Douglas Rund, MD (Department Chair). Front row: Leslie Browder, MD; Colin Kaide, MD; Richard Cavender, MD; and Stephen Dodds, MD.

Class of 1997

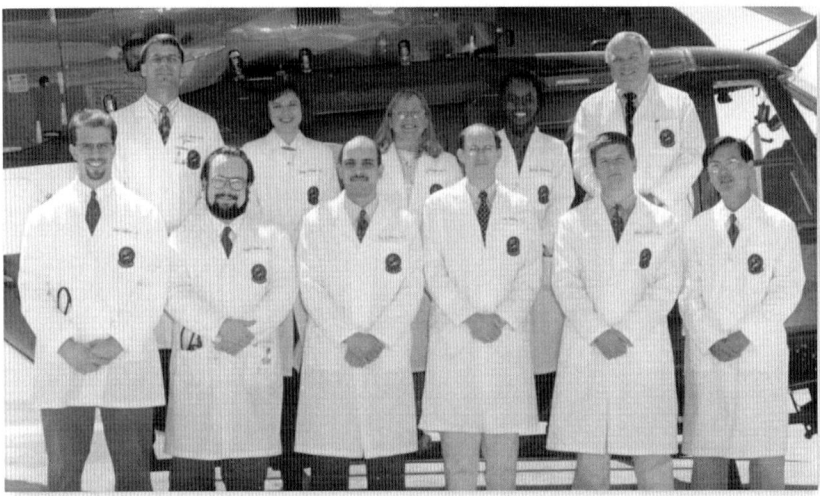

Figure 13: Residency class of 1997, back row, from left: Daniel Martin, MD (Program Director); Misty Arnold, MD; Diane Gorgas, MD; Michelle Flemmings, MD; and Douglas Rund, MD (Department Chair). Front row: Brian Seifferth, MD, Ralph Battles, MD, Emile El-Shammaa, MD, Eric Drobny, MD, Aaron Bender, MD, John Strayer, MD.

Class of 1998

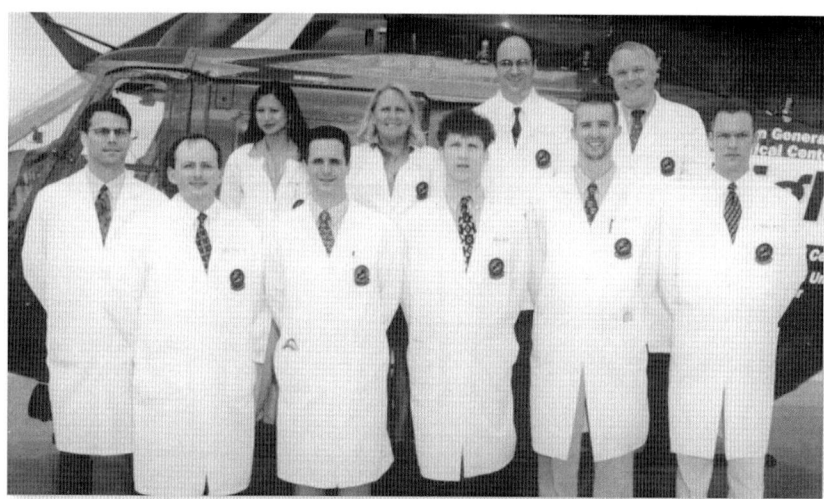

Figure 14: Residency class of 1998, back row, from left: Daniel Martin, MD (Program Director); Namchi Lee, MD; Diane Gorgas, MD; Steven Motarjeme, MD; Douglas Rund, MD (Department Chair). Front row: Timothy Reeder, MD; Gary Gechlik, MD; David Bahner, MD; Tadd Ferguson, MD; and Eric Stansby, MD.

Class of 1999

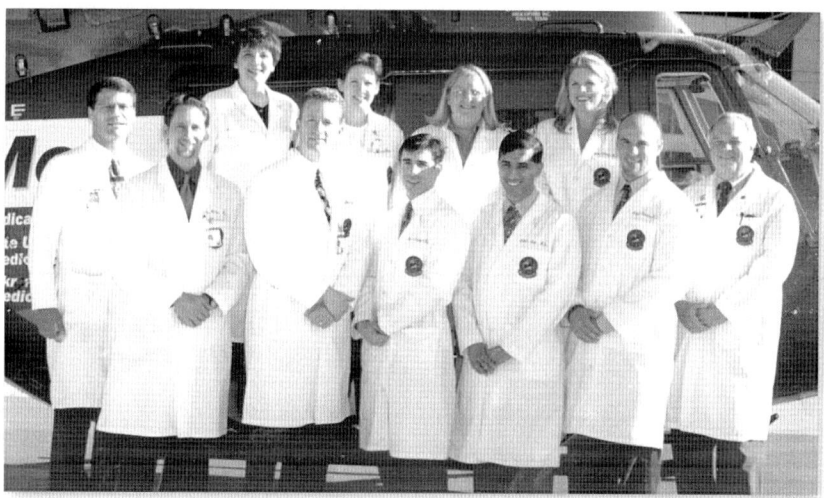

Figure 15: Residency class of 1999, back row, from left: Michelle Dayton, MD; Kimberly Moore, MD; Diane Gorgas, MD; and Colleen Casey, MD. Front row: Daniel Martin, MD (Program Director); Kenneth Michau, MD; Gregory Mosteller, MD; Marc Schnapper, MD; Manish Shah, MD; Wenzel Tirheimer, III, MD; and Douglas Rund, MD (Department Chair).

Class of 2000

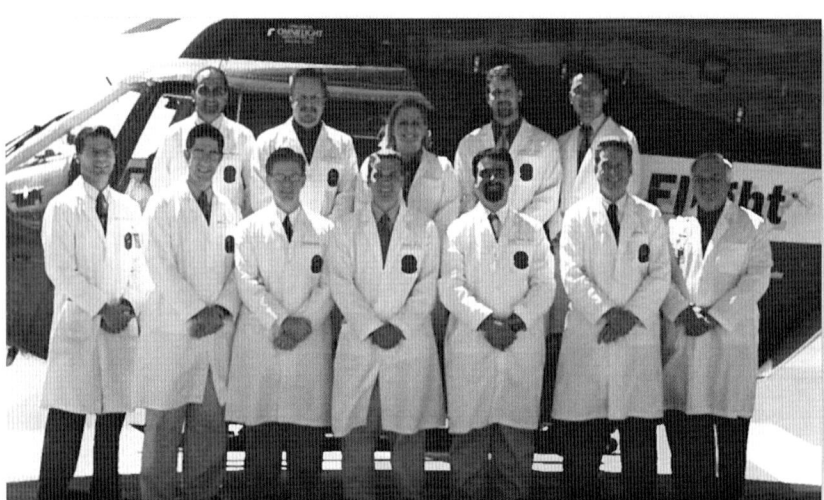

Figure 16: Residency class of 2000, back row, from left: Rizwan Pasha, MD; Joe Kohout, MD; Diane Gorgas, MD; Michael Ott, DO; and George Lew, MD, PhD. Front row: Daniel R. Martin, MD (Program Director); Matthew Kellar, MD; Frank Fraunfelter, MD; R. James Cretella, MD; Hamid Ehsani, MD; Paul Young, MD; and Douglas Rund, MD (Department Chair).

Class of 2001

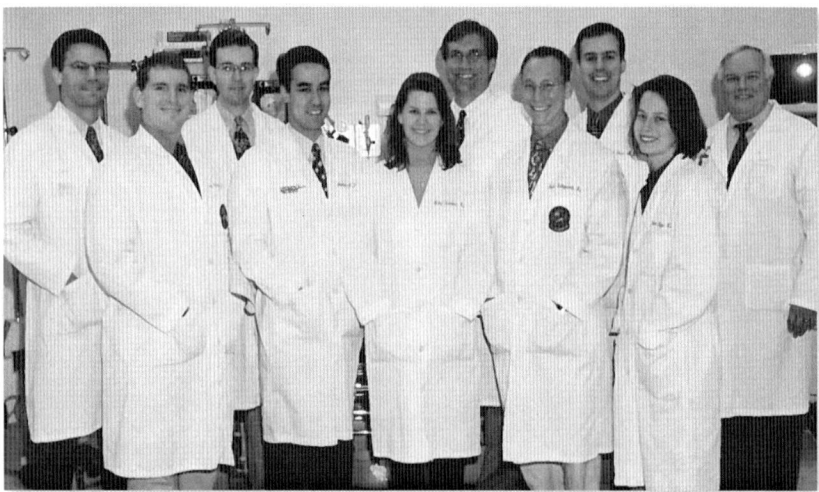

Figure 17: Residency class of 2001, back row, from left: Daniel Martin, MD (Program Director); David Schwegman, MD; Randall Knutson, MD; Steven Stack, MD; and Douglas Rund, MD (Department Chair). Front row: Brian Hiestand, MD; James Gerard, MD; Mary Osterlund, MD; Jason Hollingsworth, MD; and Catherine Glazer, MD.

Class of 2002

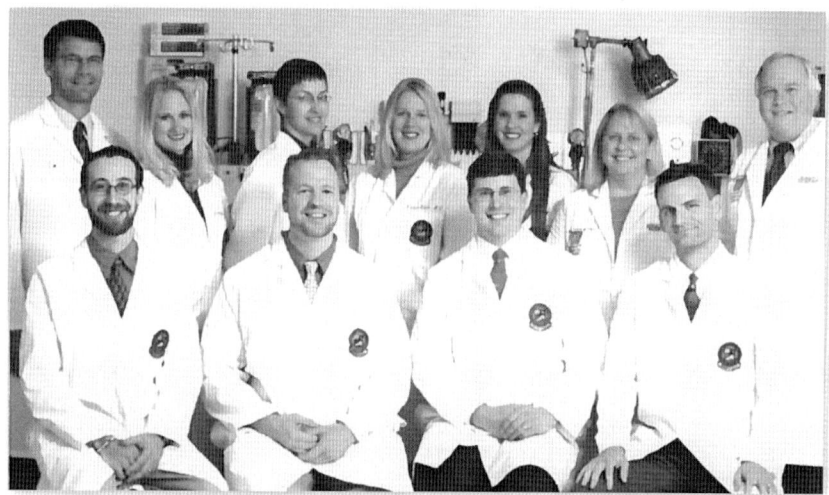

Figure 18: Residency class of 2002, back row, from left: Daniel R Martin, MD (Program Director); Brandy Helminiak, MD; Judy Brummer, MD; Melissa Fenner, MD; Allison Esenwine, MD; Diane Gorgas, MD; and Douglas Rund, MD (Department Chair). Front row: Brian Gelb, MD; David Dalton, MD; Matthew Lashutka, MD; and Christopher Schlanger, MD.

Class of 2003

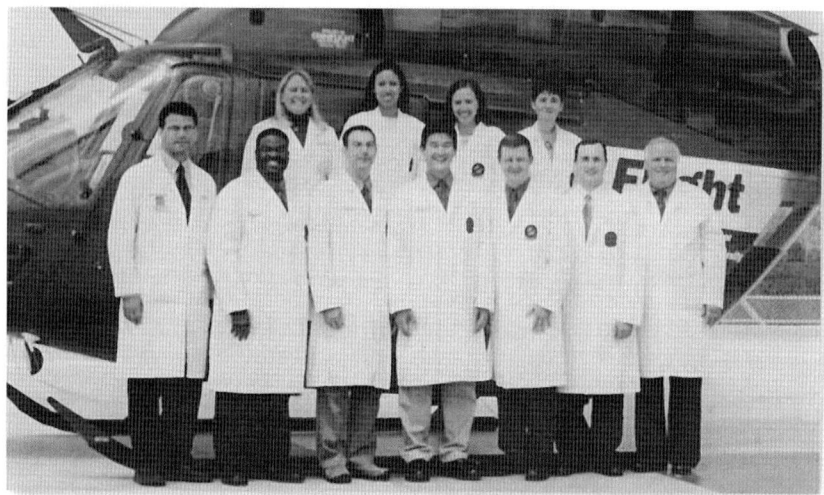

Figure 19: Residency class of 2003, back row, from left: Diane Gorgas, MD; Valerie Killian, MD; Kimberly Cordes, MD; and Dawn Prall, MD. Front row: Daniel Martin, MD (Program Director); Charles Washington, MD; Brett Forehand, MD, PhD; David Fujiwara, MD; Holt Murray, MD; Chad Miller, MD; and Douglas Rund, MD (Department Chair).

Class of 2004

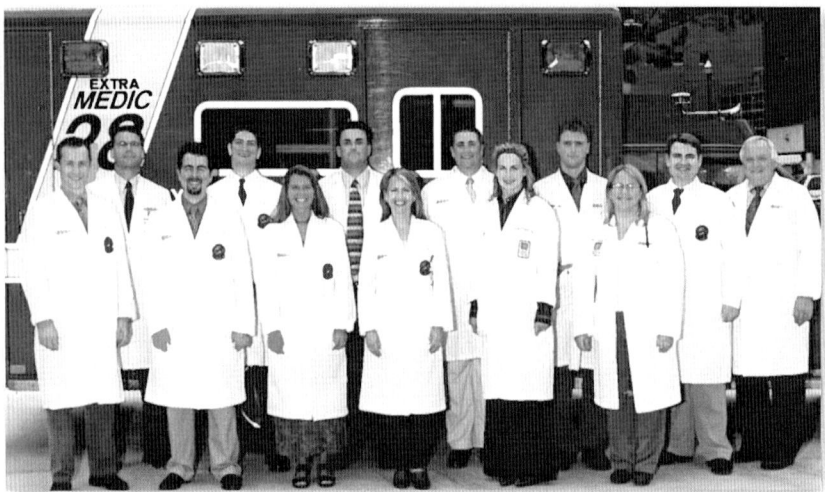

Figure 20: Resident class of 2004, back row, from left: Daniel R Martin, MD (Program Director); Robert Moskowitz, MD; Robert Paasche, MD; Marvin "Jake" Ott, MD; Fred Tzystuck, MD; Matthew Sanders, DO; and Douglas Rund, MD (Department Chair). Front row: Martin Schutte, MD; Richard Limperos, MD; Amy Ramey, MD; Cynthia Bowers-Lee, MD; Anna "Kate" Corbin, MD; and Diane Gorgas, MD.

Class of 2005

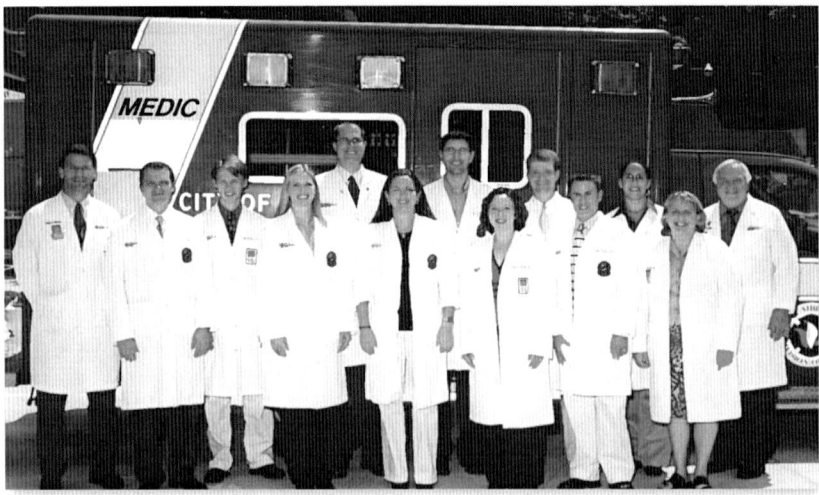

Figure 21: Resident class of 2005, back row, from left: Daniel R. Martin, MD (Program Director); Jeff Glinski, MD; Anthony "Koy" Lombardi, MD; Michael Argus, MD; Judson Garbarino, MD; Shoshone Richardson, MD; and Douglas Rund, MD (Department Chair). Front row: Timothy Corvino, MD, MBA; Katherine Mitzel, DO; Stefanie Huff, MD; Angela Minder Majino, MD, Chad Pritts, MD; and Diane Gorgas, MD.

Class of 2006

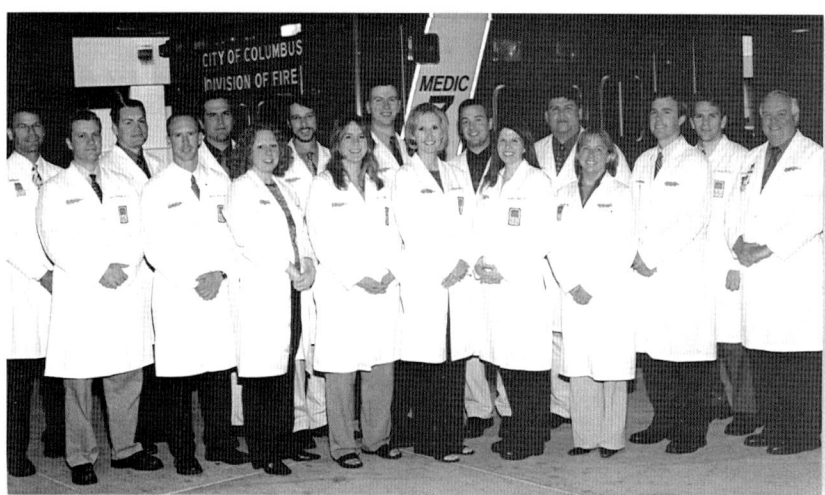

Figure 22: Resident class of 2006, back row, from left: Daniel R. Martin, MD (Program Director); Chad Nicholls, MD; Jonathan Stockdale, DO; Daniel Cheek, MD; Marc Wise, MD; Matt Kiefaber, MD; Scott Williams, MD; and Greg Hartt, MD. Front row: David Lancaster, MD; Scott Irvine, MD; Emily McNutt, MD; Sheri Knepel, MD; Erin Grimes, MD; Barbara Hapke, MD; Diane Gorgas, MD; Troy Madsen, MD; and Douglas Rund, MD (Department Chair).

Class of 2007

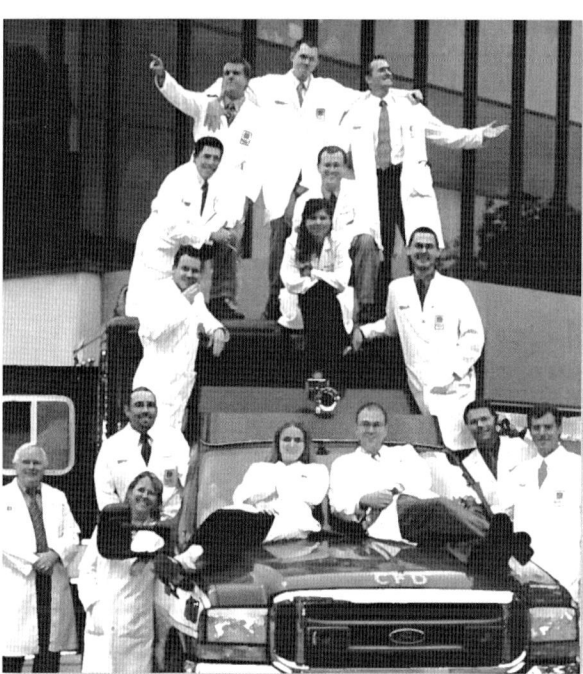

Figure 23: Resident class of 2007, top of ambulance, from left: Bryan MacWilliams, MD; William "Andy" Jenkins, MD; and Eric Kollai, MD. Sitting left to right: Brendan Sheridan, MD; Michael McCrea, MD; and Lesley Perez, MD. Standing near front of ambulance: Travis Ulmer, MD; and Nathan Angle, MD. Front of ambulance, left side: Douglas Rund, MD (Department Chair); Michael Borunda, MD; and Diane Gorgas, MD. Sitting on hood, left: Jamie Treseder, MD; and Jed Southwick, MD. (Right side): Daniel R. Martin, MD (Program Director); and Brian "Buck" Marshall, MD.

Class of 2008

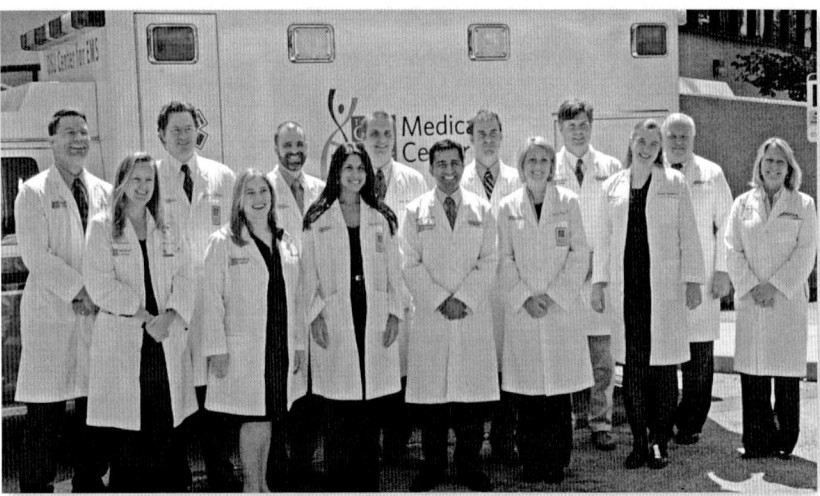

Figure 24: Resident class of 2008, back row, from left: Daniel R. Martin, MD (Program Director); Daniel Zelinski, MD, PhD; James Hirshberg, MD; Matthew White, MD; Daniel Marcus, MD; Mark Brauner, DO; and Douglas Rund, MD (Department Chair). Front row: Anne Ree Sumner Mitchell, MD; MPH, Jillian Schwaab, MD; Monique Mirshak, MD; Ashish Panchal, MD, PhD; Audry Slane, MD; Sarah Crockett, MD; and Diane Gorgas, MD.

Class of 2009

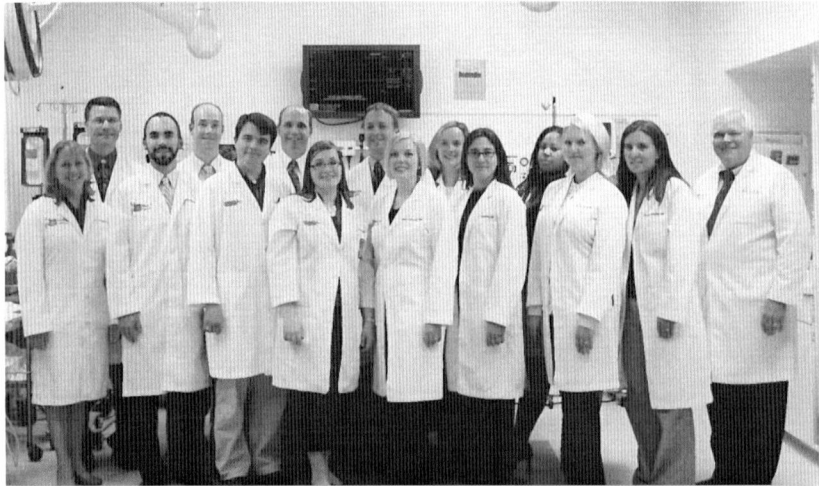

Figure 25: Resident class of 2009, back row, from left: Daniel Martin, MD (Program Director); Brock Franklin, MD; Jonathan Bowen, MD; John Ewing, MD; Erika Kube, MD; and Erica Brown, MD. Front row: Diane Gorgas, MD; Andrew Wagner, MD; Jason Reaves, MD; Christy Annis, MD; Sarah Orlousky, MD; Tracy Jalbuena, MD; Anna McCormick, MD; Evan Moore, MD; and Douglas Rund, MD (Department Chair).

Class of 2010

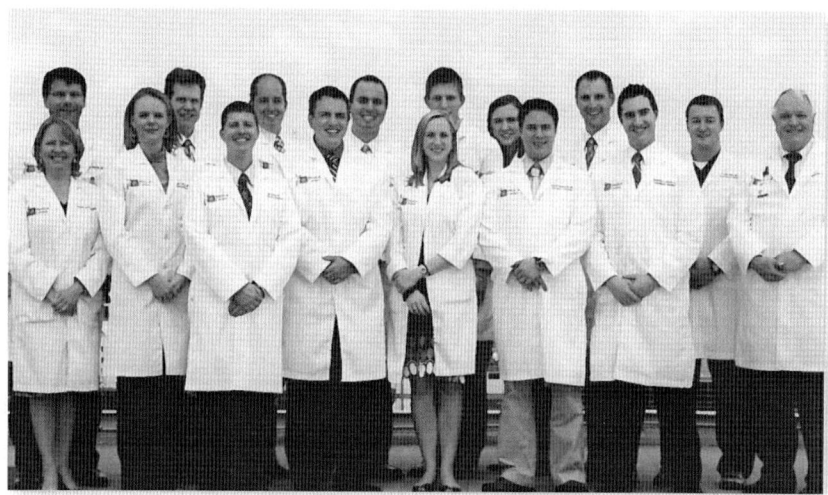

Figure 26: Resident class of 2010, back row, from left: Daniel R. Martin, MD; Andrew Bakke, MD; Kevin O'Rourke, MD; Nicholas Perchiniak, MD; Logan "Cole" Sondrup, MD; Melissa McConahy, MD; Daniel Bachmann, MD; and Mark Lanker, MD. Front row: Diane Gorgas, MD (Program Director) ; Ellen McDaniel, MD; Ryan King, MD; Matthew Roberts, MD; Anna Robinson, MD; Paul Robinson, MD; Timothy Comte, MD; and Douglas Rund, MD (Department Chair).

Class of 2011

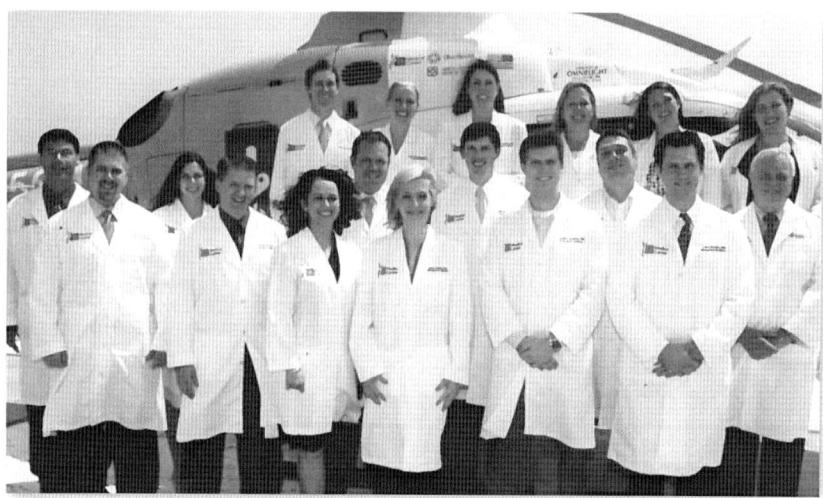

Figure 27: Resident class of 2011, back row, from left: Tyler Hoppes, MD; Amanda Aemisegger, MD; Carla Ralston, MD; Diane Gorgas, MD (Program Director); Creagh Boulger, MD; and Jillian Schwaab, MD. Middle row: Daniel Martin, MD; Hannah Hays, MD; Travis Eastin, MD; John Tanner, MD; Donald Norris III, MD; and Douglas Rund, MD (Department Chair). Front row: Timothy Brock, MD; Dallon Jones, MD; MPH, Laura Napier, MD; MBA, Lisa Colling, MD; Justin Adkins, MD; and Bradley Raetzke, MD.

Class of 2012

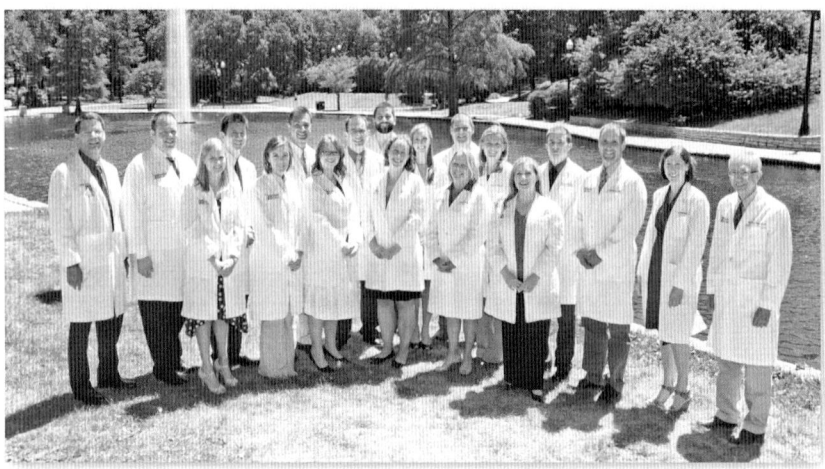

Figure 28: Resident class of 2012, back row, from left: Daniel Martin, MD; Travis Eastin, MD; James Chan, MD; Austin Wellock, MD; Stephen Rancour, MD; Michael O'Connell, MD; Rachel Smitek, MD; Chad Donley, MD; Karen Gustafson, MD; Andrew King, MD; Daniel Bachmann, MD; Sarah Greenberger, MD; and Mark Angelos, MD (Department Chair). Front row: Kristin Daugherty, MD; Kristina Mrowca, MD; Sara Sisbarro, MD; Jessica Miller, MD; Diane Gorgas, MD (Program Director); and Jillian Schwaab, MD.

Class of 2013

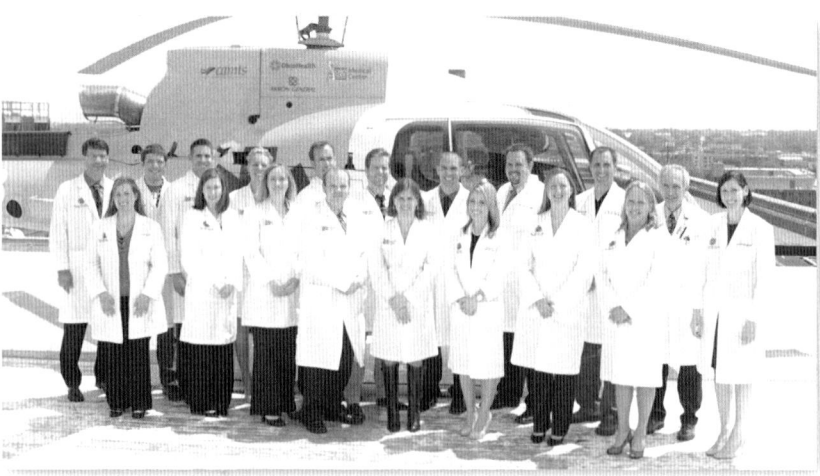

Figure 29: Resident class of 2013, back row, from left: Daniel Martin, MD; Andrew Retzinger, MD; Simas Laniauskas, MD; Anna Mandir Helms, MD; Brian Abbott, MD; Robert Cooper, MD, MPH; Eric Cortez, MD; Travis Eastin, MD; Daniel Bachmann, MD; Mark Angelos, MD (Department Chair); and Sarah Greenberger, MD. Front row: Jillian McGrath, MD; Cambria Baylor, MD; Ashley Patel, MD; Jonathan Stevens, MD; Hilary Yokley, MD; Lydia Sahlani, MD; Janice Jones, MD; and Diane Gorgas, MD (Program Director).

Class of 2014

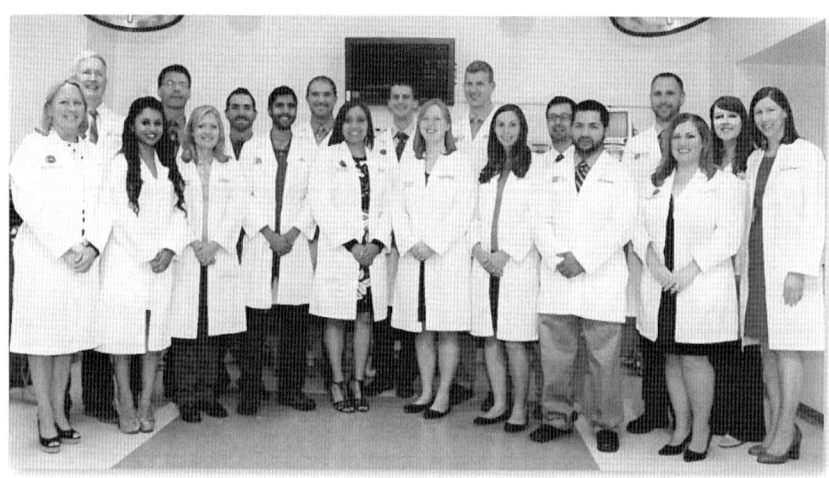

Figure 30: Resident class of 2014, back row, from left: Thomas Terndrup, MD (Department Chair); Daniel Martin, MD; Eric Cummins, MD; Kenneth Berg, MD; Benjamin Kartman, MD; Daniel Jeltes, MD; Maxwell Hill, MD; Daniel Bachmann, MD; Jennifer Hunnicutt, MD; and Sarah Greenberger, MD. Front row: Diane Gorgas, MD (Program Director); Meenal Sharkey, MD; Janice Shook, MD, MPH; Nilesh Patel, MD; Laura Espy-Bell, MD, MHA; Daralee Hughes, MD; Rebekah Richards, MD; Julian Macedo, MD; and Jillian McGrath, MD.

Class of 2015

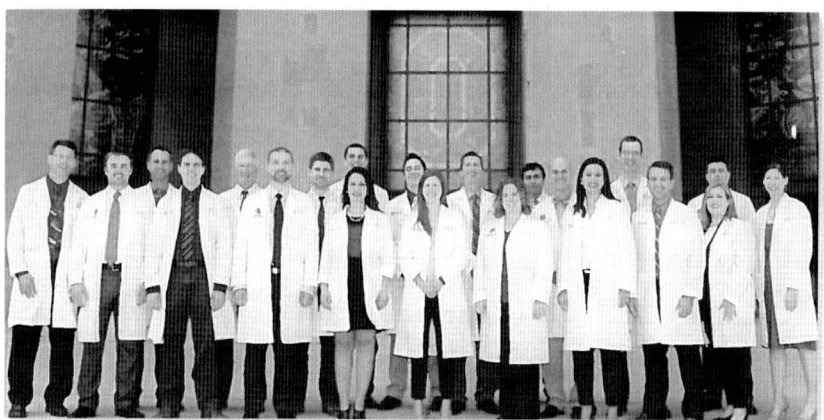

Figure 31: Resident class of 2015, back row, from left: Daniel Martin, MD; Daniel Bachmann, MD; Thomas Terndrup, MD (Department Chair); Ben Wallace, MD; Alex Fox, MD; Nicholas Libertin, MD; James Falk, MD; Sorabh Khandelwal, MD (Program Director); Andrew Gathof, MD; John Rosevear, MD; Andrew King, MD; and Sarah Greenberger, MD. Front row: Charles Burtis, MD; Michael Barrie, MD; David Notley, MD; Tamara Halaweh, MD; Leigh Giano, MD; Shari Robbins, MD; Alexandra Bush, MD; James "Matthew" Blickendorf, MD; and Jiliam McGrath, MD.

Class of 2016

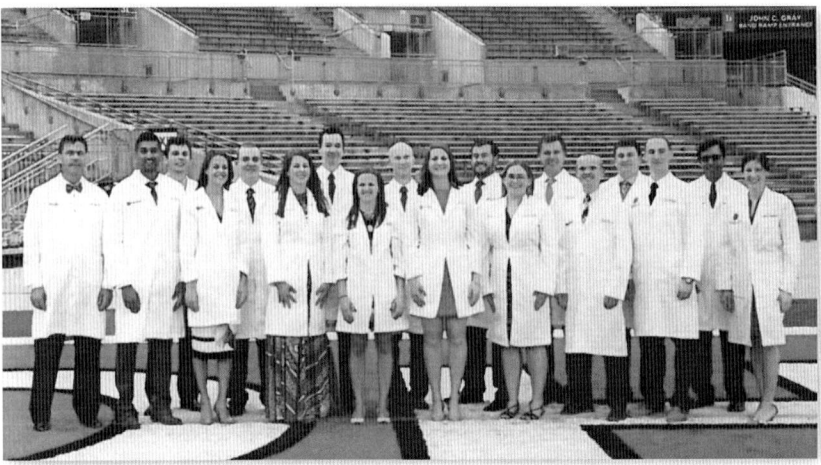

Figure 32: Resident class of 2016, back row, from left: Daniel Martin, MD; Douglas Romney, MD; Andrew Yocum, MD; Philip Kray, MD; Brett Ebeling, MD; Michael Roesch, MD; Andrew Krieger, MD; Andrew King, MD; Sorabh Khandelwal, MD (Program Director); and Sarah Greenberger, MD. Front row: Imran Shaikh, MD; Ashli Burns, MD; Ashley Heaney, MD; Lindsey Hogle, MD; Meghan Jones, MD; Kendal Herget, MD; Nathan Finnerty, MD; and David Calcara, MD.

Class of 2017

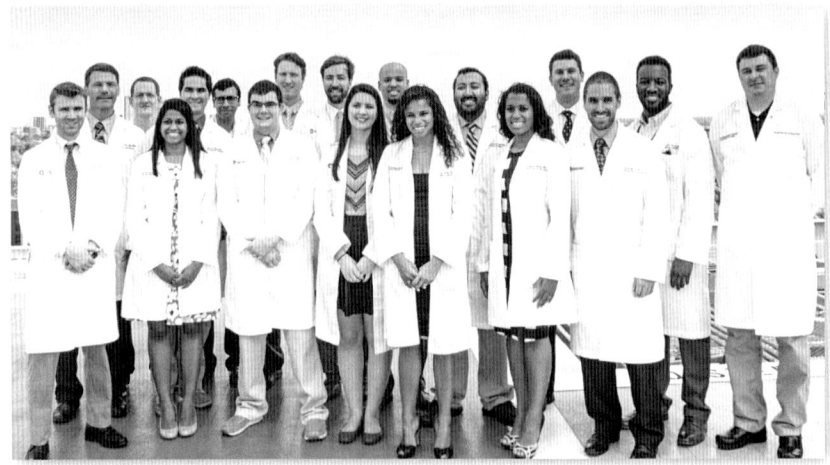

Figure 33: Resident class of 2017, back row, from left: Daniel Martin, MD; Geremiha Emerson, MD; George Ashby, MD; Sorabh Khandelwal, MD (Program Director); Eric Davis, MD; Samuel Dodson, MD; James Barton, MD; Christopher San Miguel, MD; Jason Bischof, MD; Jonathan Goss, MD, MPH; and Andrew King, MD. Front row: Michael Purcell, MD; Monica Mikkilineni, MD; Christopher Amick, MD; Joanna Le Parc, MD; Marlisa Mann, MD; Talitha Ashby, MD; and David Harris, MD.

Class of 2018

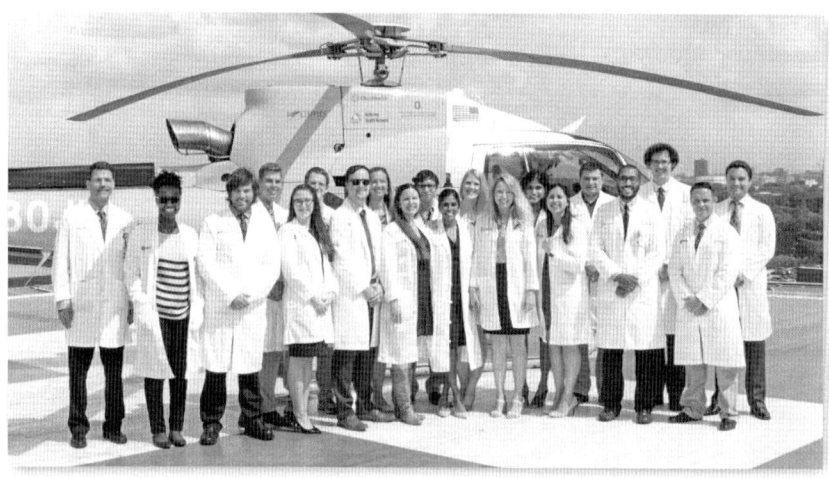

Figure 34: Resident class of 2018, back row, from left: Daniel Martin, MD; Austin Kosier, MD; Geremiha Emerson, MD; Alexis Hausfled, MD; Sorabh Khandelwal, MD (Program Director); Erin Wenzel, MD; Lalitha Nagaraj, MD;, Andrew King, MD; David Hartnett, MD; and Zachary Schirm, MD. Front row: Tatiana Thema, MD; Bradley End, MD; Margaret Krebs, MD; Chad Garthe, MD; Jennifer Cotton, MD; Sambita Basu, MD; Chloe Sidley, MD; Arwa Mesiwala, MD; Anand Patel, MD; and Daniel Adams, MD.

Class of 2019

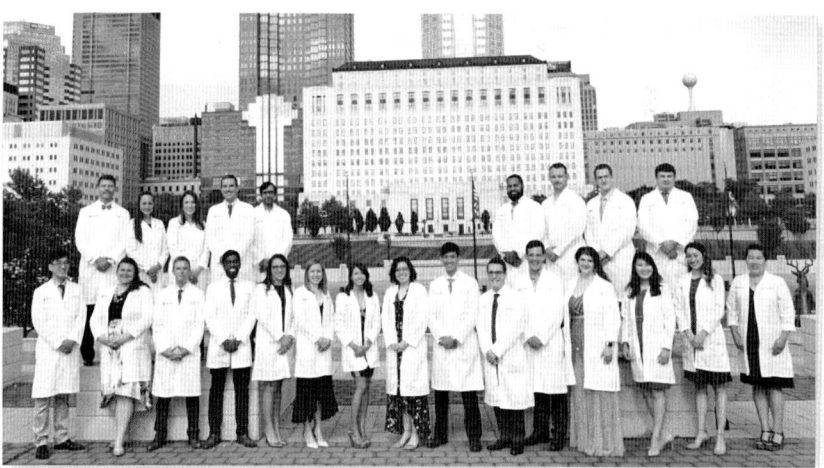

Figure 35: Resident class of 2019, back row, from left: Daniel Martin, MD; Lindsey Van Sambeek, MD; Caitlin Rublee, MD; MPH, Chad Mayer, MD; Sorabh Khandelwal, MD (Program Director); Justin Carroll, MD; Daniel Francescon, MD; Geremiha Emerson, MD; and Andrew King, MD. Front row: Christopher Lee, MD; Leslie Adrian, MD; Gregor Eisinger, MD; Kushal Nandam, MD; Krystin Miller, MD; Katherine Buck, MD; Emily Sanchez, MD; Carolyn Martinez, MD; Andrew Chou, MD; Joshua Faucher, MD; John Grantham, MD; Lisa Pursell, MD; Betty Yang, MD; Maya Hamilton, MD; and Simiao Li-Sauerwine, MD.

Class of 2020

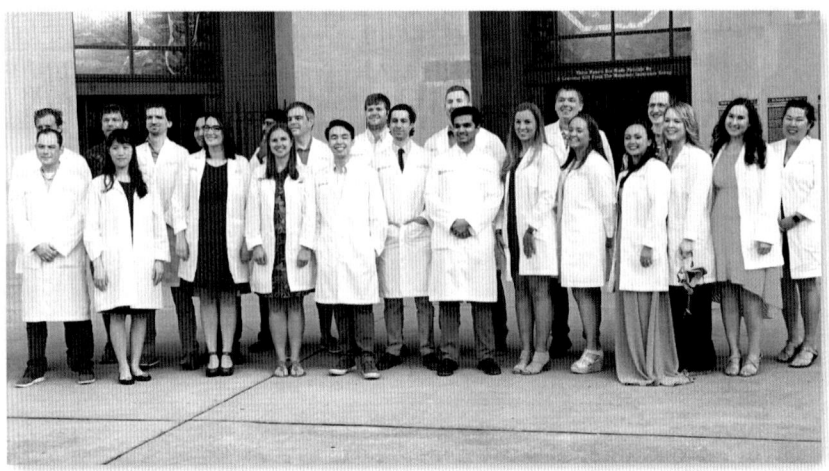

Figure 36: Resident class of 2020, back row, from left: Michael Howard, MD; Daniel Martin, MD; Travis Sharkey-Toppen, MD; PhD, Bryan Yeh, MD; Sorabh Khandelwal, MD (Program Director); Jeffrey Caterino, MD, MPH (Department Chair); Patrick Sylvester, MD; Ryan McGrath, MD; Matthew Schwab, MD; Geremiha Emerson, MD; and Simiao Li-Sauerwine, MD, MS. Front row: Matthew Huang, MD; Christine Luo, MD, PhD; Erica Ross, MD; Aubri Charnigo, MD; Alan Chu, MD; Paul Nicholson, MD; Milap Mehta, MD; Natalie Feretti, MD; Bridget Onders, MD; Michael Nassal, MD, PhD; Grace Rodriguez, MD; and Brooke Pabst, MD.

Class of 2021

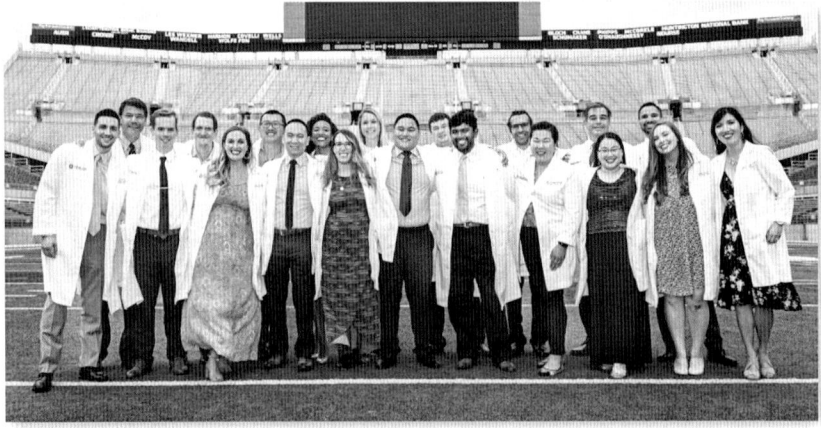

Figure 37: Resident class of 2021, back row, from left: Daniel Martin, MD; Geremiha Emerson, MD; Yuxuan "Tony" Qiu, MD; Kelli Robinson, MD; Jacqueline Furbacher, MD; Andrew King, MD; Sorabh Khandelwal, MD (Program Director); Jeffrey Caterino, MD, MPH (Department Chair); and Divyesh Mehta, MD. Front row: Paul DeJulio, MD; Eric Aaserude, MD; Lauren Moore, MD; Christopher Kao, MD; Kimberly Bambach, MD; Merrick Bautisa, MD; Rahul Rege, MD; Simiao Li-Sauerwine, MD, MS; Kelee Peyton, MD; Margaret Kirwin, MD; and Katherine Luu, MD.

Class of 2022

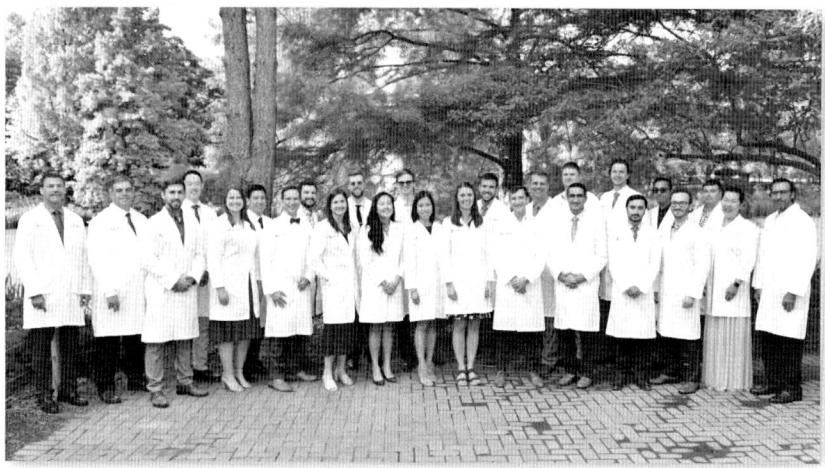

Figure 38: Resident class of 2022, back row, from left: Daniel Martin, MD; Jeffrey Caterino, MD (Department Chair); Peter Tsou, MD; James Fletcher, BM BCh; Timothy Hoffman, MD; Michael Scott Cardone, MD; Andrew Kendle, MD; Robert Bedenbaugh, MD; Michael Miles, MD; Michael Hollar, DO; Peter Rinne DO; Saket Kumar, MD; Andrew King, MD; Simiao Li-Sauerwine, MD; and Sorabh Khandelwal, MD (Program Director). Front row: Kevin Cofer, MD; Lauren Willoughby, MD; Thomas Powell, MD; Hannah Fox, MD; Serena Hua, MD; Jennifer Luong, MD; Dominique Dabija, MD; Madison Kommer, MD; Bobbak Tadayon, MD; Ashok Bhattarai, MD; and David Diaz, MD.

The Future

In 2023 the Department of Emergency Medicine's residency program had 406 residency alumni, and the program continued to offer 19 openings per year. This contrasts sharply with the program's beginning in 1981, when there was one second-year resident and four first-year residents. Despite its continued growth, the program has had only five program directors, which speaks to the high degree to which the program goals have been consistent in creating educational innovations, enhancing diversity and training academic emergency physicians.

More recently, a focused goal of promoting resident wellness has emerged, and an additional year of fellowship training following residency has become more popular as the specialty adds subspecialties and opportunities for practice beyond the emergency department.

One of the first programs in the country, the Emergency Medicine residency continues to attract the very highest quality individuals to continue their studies and become specialists in emergency medicine at The Ohio State University.

References

1. Khandelwal S. Interview with Sorabh Khandelwal by Douglas Rund. 2023: Columbus, Ohio.

2. Martin DM. Personal communication. 2023.

3. Lewis JW. Personal communication. 2022.

4. Smith MA. Interview with Mark Smith by Douglas Rund. 2022: Columbus, Ohio.

5. Birinyi F. Interview with Frank Birinyi by Douglas Rund. 2022: Columbus, Ohio.

Chapter 21

Subspecialties Indeed: Fellowships

David P. Bahner, MD
Douglas A. Rund, MD

From the beginning of the specialty, and certainly from the beginning of emergency medicine at Ohio State, there has been the strongest effort to create a department that shouted out: *"We are a specialty indeed."* In the earliest days this meant that the division had the goal of "looking like" the strongest departments among the most established specialties.

The largest departments at the time of the Division of Emergency Medicine's inception in 1978 were the Departments of Medicine and Surgery. Both had long histories of subspecialty fellowship training. In the beginning, moving toward proving specialty recognition required deliberate steps. Most critical were the establishment of an exceptional faculty, a research program, outstanding student courses, the residency program and a full and free-standing academic department.

Following the American Board of Emergency Medicine's (ABEM) creation in 1979, the specialty's first priority was to develop a certification examination, followed by achieving primary board status, which it did in 1989. Being a primary board would allow ABEM to offer subspecialty certifications. Pediatric Emergency Medicine was the first such subspecialty in 1991, followed soon after by Sports Medicine (March 1992) and Medical Toxicology (September 1992). One of the major advocates for sports medicine was Ohio State. Over the years subspecialty certificates were approved for the following: Undersea and Hyperbaric Medicine (2000), Hospice and Palliative Care (2006), Emergency Medical Services (2010), Internal Medicine Critical Care (2011), Anesthesiology

Critical Care (2013), Pain Medicine (2014), Neurocritical Care (2018), and Health Care Administration, Leadership and Management (2023) and Focused Practice Designation (FPD) in Advanced EM Ultrasonography (AEMUS) (2018).[1]

Ohio State and other institutions also recognized that other areas of specialization were possible. An extra year or two of focused development in a specific area could help launch one's career and provide an edge when looking for the best positions. Over time the department created fellowships in administration, emergency medical services (EMS), medical education, medical toxicology, hematologic and oncologic emergencies, research and ultrasound.

Administration

The fellowship in Emergency Medicine administration was started in 2007 by Gary Katz MD, MBA, and Mark Moseley, MD, MHA. Their vision: to create an educational program that combined real-life leadership experiences, longitudinal operations projects and formal executive leadership training. Using their own leadership experiences and previous degree training, they created a unique 24-month program for exceptional EM residency graduates.

Although Health Care Administration was not yet an accredited subspecialty of the American Board of Emergency Medicine, at the time of its inception in 2007, the program was unique in that it required the completion of an advanced management degree such as the Master of Health Administration (MHA) or a Master of Business Administration (MBA).

GARY KATZ, MD, MBA

Gary Katz, MD, MBA, received his master's degree in Business Administration from the Fisher College of Business and was an enthusiastic faculty member for the fellows in administration. An early proponent of free-standing emergency departments throughout the central Ohio area, he created detailed business plans to do so, and went on to become an effective leader of the specialty, particularly in the American College of Emergency Physicians.

MARK G. MOSELEY, MD, MHA, CPE, FACEP

Mark Moseley graduated in 2002 as Ohio State's very first combined five-year MD/MHA dual degree program offered through the College of Medicine and Public Health. He completed a residency in Emergency Medicine at Christiana Care Health System in Wilmington, Delaware, serving as Chief Resident in his final year of training. He then returned to his Ohio State alma mater in 2005, and began a journey of progressive leadership responsibility over the next 12 years. He and Katz shared a passion for formal education in business and health administration for emergency physicians seeking formal education that would lead to leadership positions in health care. He left Ohio State in 2017 to join the faculty at the University of South Florida in Tampa and became President of the newly combined University of South Florida (USF) and Tampa General Physicians practice corporation in 2022 (Figure 1). He is a full Professor in the Colleges of Medicine and Public Health at USF.

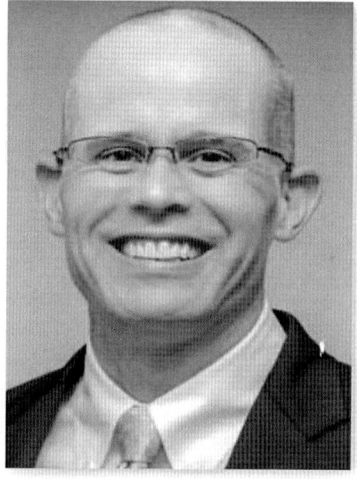

Figure 1: Mark G. Moseley, MD, MHA, was one of the founders of the administration fellowship at Ohio State. He left Ohio State in 2017 and became President of the combined USF Tampa General Physicians practice corporation in 2022.

Years later Moseley reflected on the beginning of the fellowship program:

> *It was a time of great challenges, but also of great opportunity at OSU. Due to the strength of our department's leadership (and particularly the investment by our Chair Dr. Rund), our department enjoyed exceptional strength and a national reputation in all three mission areas. This created a milieu that was conducive for innovation and program building. Dr. Katz and I thoroughly enjoyed working together, and the chance to create a program to equip the next generation of EM leaders was exciting and academically stimulating. We found ourselves tackling the significant operational and business challenges of our time, but wanted to also ensure we passed on those experiences to the physician leaders who came after us. The legacy of this program will be one of innovation and solving leadership challenges to better the lives of countless patients across the country.*[2]

ANDREW WAGNER, MD, MBA

The program's initial fellow was Andrew Wagner, MD, MBA (2009-2010), who obtained his executive Master of Business Administration degree (MBA) from Ohio State's Fisher College of Business. Wagner made significant contributions to operational and information technology (IT) advancements during his training. He also worked as an attending faculty member during his fellowship, which was the norm for non-accredited fellowship participants, and was instrumental in helping further define the program's leadership and project curriculum. Combining his entrepreneurial, IT, and leadership interest, Wagner became a national EM-IT thought leader in U.S. Acute Care, and became the Chief Clinical Officer for Dispatch Health in Colorado.

ROBERT D. COOPER, MD, MPH, MBA

Robert D. "Rob" Cooper, MD, MPH, MBA, graduated with his medical degree from Ohio State in 2010 (Figure 2) and completed the residency program in emergency medicine in 2013. He went on to complete the two-year fellowship in Emergency Medicine Administration in 2015 and received his MBA degree from the Fisher College of Business at that time. Cooper combined his passions for IT and population health, and currently serves as an Ohio State EM faculty member and Medical Director for the Ohio State University Health Plan. He was the program director of the administrative fellowship until 2022.

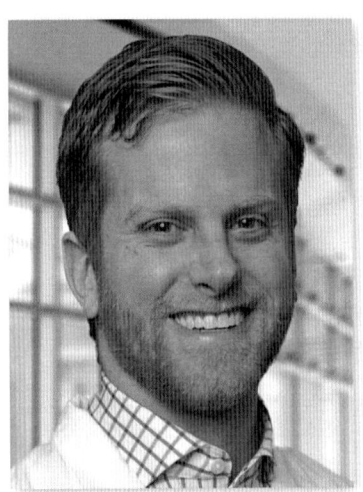

Figure 2: Robert D. Cooper, MD, MPH, MBA, graduated from the Administrative Fellowship in 2015 and became the Medical Director for the Ohio State University Health Plan.

Part of Cooper's responsibility for the health plan involves overseeing quality review, denials and appeals. He also serves on the Health Plan Quality Improvement Committee and is responsible for the credentialing and re-credentialing of providers.

In 2018 Columbus *Business First* newspaper named him one of the "40 under 40" awardees. A faculty advisor for the Columbus Free Clinic, Cooper was named the Ohio Free Clinic Physician of the Year in 2015.

PHILLIP A. DIXON, MD, MBA, MPH

Phillip A. Dixon, MD, MBA, MPH, was an administration fellow from 2017 to 2019 (Figure 3). He completed his undergraduate studies at Johns Hopkins University while playing four years of football. He completed medical school and his MPH degree at St. George's University School of Medicine in Grenada West Indies in 2013. He completed his residency in emergency medicine at the University of Mississippi Medical Center in 2017 and was Chief Resident during his third year.

During his residency, Dixon became interested in advocacy, physician leadership and administration. He was elected national secretary-treasurer for the Resident-Student Association of the American Academy of Emergency Physicians, and elected the resident representative for the Mississippi State Chapter of the American College of Emergency Physicians. He was also one of two chief residents among all specialties to co-chair the Chief Resident Committee and represented residents on multiple hospital administration committees.

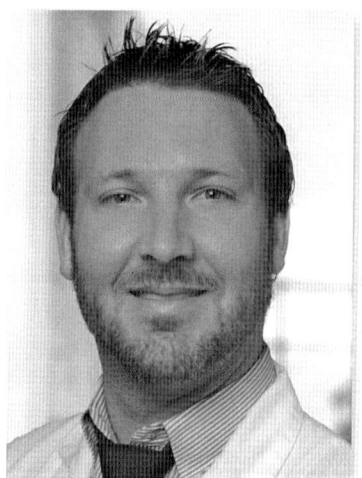

Currently an Associate Professor and the Assistant Medical Director for the Ohio State Emergency Department, Dixon developed the peer-to-peer program to connect physicians with medical directors of third-party payors to discuss patient coverages, medical conditions and patient payments. He also directs the physician advisor program, which trains physicians to address issues such as medical necessity, length of stay, and

Figure 3: Phillip A. Dixon, MD, MPH, MBA, was the third physician to become an administrative fellow in the department. His contributions included the establishment of programs focused on more effective patient care services operation.

issues with insurance carriers and others. The advisor acts as a liaison between hospital administration, clinical staff and support personnel to ensure compliance with regulatory issues and advise physicians on such issues as medical necessity. Dixon's professional interests include creating a more efficient and effective emergency department, as well as national and state health policy, advocacy and leadership and physician wellness.

MILAP MEHTA, MD, MBA

Milap Mehta, MD, MBA, completed his undergraduate education at Duke University and medical school at the University of North Carolina at Chapel Hill. He completed his residency in emergency medicine at Ohio State in 2020 and completed the administrative fellowship two years later, earning his MBA degree in 2022. He now works as an emergency medicine physician at Mid-Atlantic Emergency Medical Associates in Charlotte, North Carolina.

Emergency Medical Services

The Fellowship in Emergency Medical Services, accredited by the Accreditation Council for Graduate Medical Education (ACGME), began in 2013. The first Director of the program was Howard A. Werman, MD. Over time Ashish Panchal, MD, PhD, assumed leadership.

The purpose of the fellowship was to not only prepare emergency physicians to become EMS medical directors but to also foster skills that allowed them to be scholars and leaders in the field of prehospital care. The fellowship was structured to provide excellent clinical experience in the prehospital setting by teaching medical oversight and on-scene direction with the Columbus Division of Fire and the City of Worthington Division of Fire and EMS.

Columbus Fire, one of the largest metropolitan EMS agencies in the country, responds to 120,000 incidents per year. Fellows also work directly with MedFlight of Ohio, the largest aeromedical provider in the state and winner of many national awards for air medical services. Such experiences are supplemented by working with other affiliated fire departments and EMS agencies to form a well-rounded, urban and rural, EMS experience with ground, critical care and aeromedical transport.

Fellows have the opportunity to impact EMS culture and education though Ohio State's direct collaboration with the National Registry of EMTs, the national certifying organization for the United States with over 300,000 certified providers. Through this collaboration, the fellow gains an understanding of large database analysis, research methodology, scientific writing and reporting. This overall fellowship experience, combining a strong prehospital clinical background and abundant research opportunities, uniquely positions Ohio State to provide one of the best emergency medical services fellowships in the world.

ERIC J. CORTEZ, MD

The first Emergency Medical Services (EMS) fellow was Eric J. Cortez, MD, (Figure 4), who received his MD degree from the University of Toledo College of Medicine in 2010. Following graduation, he entered the residency in emergency medicine at Ohio State and completed the 3-year program in 2013. He started the fellowship in 2013 and finished in 2014. By that time, the American Board of Emergency Medicine had finally approved the subspecialty examination in EMS and gave the first examination in 2013. Cortez quickly became the Associate Medical Director for the Columbus Division of Fire. He went on to become the medical director for the OhioHealth Doctors Hospital emergency department and the EMS medical director for

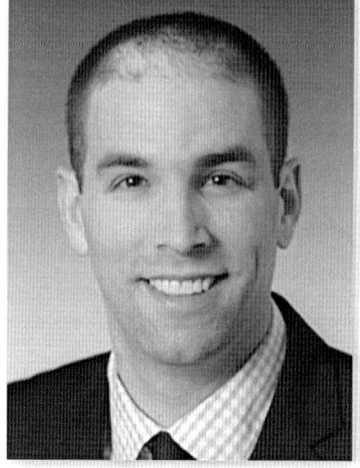

Figure 4: Eric J. Cortez, MD, completed his fellowship in Emergency Medical Services in 2015. An assistant director for the Columbus Division of Fire, he later became the EMS medical director for the entire OhioHealth System.

the entire OhioHealth System. He is associate program director for the EMS fellowship program at Doctors Hospital and also works closely with several EMS agencies in central Ohio.

Years later Cortez reflected on his training at Ohio State:

> *I am eternally grateful for the opportunity to train at OSU. I graduated residency and fellowship well prepared for a career in emergency medicine and EMS. I appreciate all of the knowledge, advice and wisdom from so many great faculty members.*[3]

WILLIAM A. "BILL" KREBS, DO

William A. Krebs, DO, completed the EMS fellowship from 2015 to 2016. He completed medical school at Ohio University Heritage College of Osteopathic Medicine in 2012 and completed his residency in emergency medicine in 2015 at Mercy St. Vincent Medical Center/Mercy Health Partners in Toledo. Krebs was always devoted to a career in air transport; after his fellowship he became the Medical Director of the Mercy Health Life Flight Network in Toledo. He is also Medical Director of the Northwest Ohio EMS Consortium, which provides medical direction for EMS agencies throughout northwest Ohio. The program director for the Mercy Health St. Vincent EMS fellowship, Krebs is also an active Life Flight physician (Figure 5).

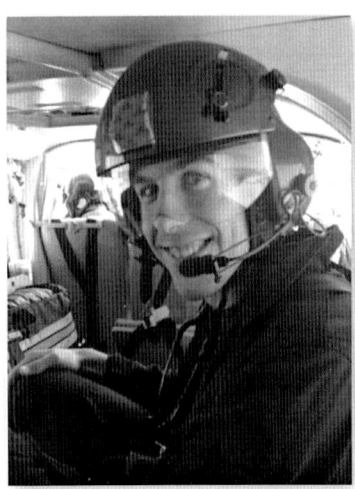

Figure 5: William A. "Bill" Krebs, DO, completed his EMS fellowship in 2016. His lifelong passion for air medical transport made him an ideal candidate for the medical directorship of the Mercy Health Life Flight Network in Toledo.

MATTHEW T. BALL, MD

Matthew T. Ball, MD, completed the Ohio State EMS fellowship in 2020. He received his MD degree from the University of Cincinnati in 2016 and completed his residency in emergency medicine at Henry Ford Hospital in 2019. After completing his fellowship, he returned to Henry Ford Hospital as an attending physician and Clinical Assistant Professor of Emergency Medicine at Wayne State University. He currently serves as faculty for the EMS Fellowship at Wayne State University and as the Deputy Medical Director of The Detroit East Medical Control Authority (DEMCA) and provides medical control for Henry Ford Health's mobile integrated health program. Years later he recalled the following about his experience:

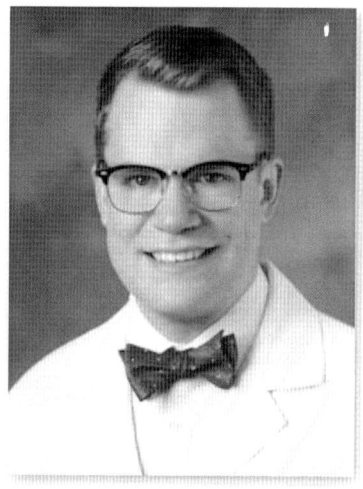

Figure 6: Matthew T. Ball, MD, completed his EMS fellowship in 2020.

> *The training that I received from The Ohio State University and the Columbus EMS community, including physicians and other allied health professionals, firefighters, EMS clinicians, students, and educators, was truly second to none. Above and beyond that, multiple brilliant, accomplished and extremely experienced EMS physicians, were so generous with their time and mentorship and that has had a profound effect on my development.*[4]

MICHAEL SETH KOZLOWSKI, DO

Michael Seth Kozlowski, DO, completed medical school at Lake Erie College of Osteopathic Medicine in Erie, Pennsylvania, and his residency in emergency medicine at the Grand Strand Medical Center in Myrtle Beach, South Carolina. Upon his completion of his EMS fellowship in EMS at Ohio State in 2021, he returned to the faculty at Grand Strand Medical Center.

TRAVIS P. SHARKEY, MD, PhD

Travis P. Sharkey, MD, PhD, grew up in a small town in Northeast Ohio. He moved to Columbus in 2003 to pursue an undergraduate degree in Computer Science and Engineering, including Electrical Engineering. While going on to pursue graduate school in Electrical Engineering, he was introduced to his PhD advisor, Subha V. Raman, MD, who was researching various roles for magnetic resonance imaging in understanding and identifying cardiovascular disease.

Months into graduate school, Sharkey found himself wanting to make a more direct impact on patient care by becoming a physician as well as an engineer. This would eventually lead him down the pathway to completing both a medical doctorate as well as a PhD through the NIH-supported Medical Scientist Training Program. His PhD largely focused on post-processing techniques to abstract accurate quantitative data from scarce data sources.

Although the natural pathway of his studies of the role of iron in atherosclerosis and cardiovascular MRI would have directed him toward a specialty in cardiology, he was enthralled by his experiences in the emergency department: Exploration into the curiosities of medicine mirrored that of engineering. To him one of the beauties of medicine was the opportunity to look at the still largely unknown human body, and try to understand the nuances of human behavior, physiology and disease processes that disrupt peoples' lives. Emergency Medicine especially requires a high level of diagnostic inquiry to stabilize, treat or even prevent such disruptions.

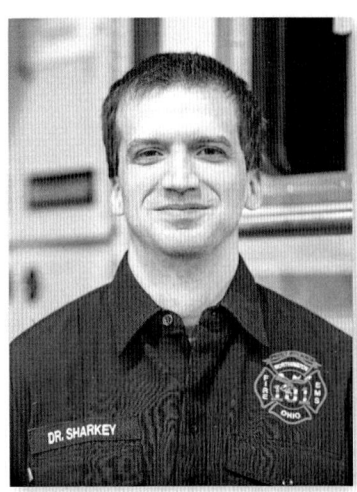

Figure 7: Travis P. Sharkey, MD, PhD, completed his medical education and fellowship in EMS at Ohio State. Post fellowship training in 2021, he quickly assumed medical direction of the City of Worthington Division of Fire and EMS, the Ohio State Center for EMS and the EMS fellowship program.

Sharkey matched at Ohio State's prestigious Emergency Medicine Residency Program in 2017. During his training, including a year as Chief

Resident ending during the COVID-19 pandemic, he was introduced to many arenas of research. Ultimately, however, his time with emergency medical services, working closely with Ashish Panchal, MD, and others in research, education and local medical direction, led him to an EMS fellowship and his new focus: strengthening prehospital care through evidence-based medicine, research and real-world educational experiences. He attributed this largely to the attitudes of EMS towards life-long learning and the challenge faced in the prehospital environment to provide life-preserving and life-saving care to often vulnerable populations.

Early on in fellowship, he was introduced to Douglas Rund, MD, pioneer of both emergency medicine and EMS in central Ohio as it exists today. Rund mentored him as Sharkey worked to develop new educational approaches to promote evidence-based practice in all aspects of prehospital care. He started this journey working with Rund at the City of Worthington Department of Fire and EMS where he is on track to assume Rund's role as medical director (Figure 7). He is similarly on track to become medical director of the Ohio State Center for EMS, an initiative started decades earlier by Rund to provide expert education, support and outreach to all central Ohio EMS agencies.

Not forgetting his roots in engineering, Sharkey also works closely with Henry Wang, MD, and Panchal in research about the use of emerging technologies in resuscitation and prehospital medicine. He often consults as a physician-engineer to support various technology-driven solutions for his colleagues in the Department of Emergency Medicine, seeking engineering solutions to clinical problems. He actively teaches and mentors graduate students in the College of Engineering in addition to his regular clinician duties and educational responsibilities within the department of emergency medicine.

Sharkey attributed his original interest in medicine to his wife Meenal Sharkey, MD, who finished the residency program in 2013 and continued to practice in Columbus. Sharkey credits her to introducing him to the "idea of practicing medicine and the joy specifically of practicing emergency medicine." She supported and encouraged him throughout his career in emergency medicine and EMS and he later credited her with his career successes.[5]

NICOLE T. McALLISTER, DO, MA

Nicole McAllister, DO, MA, completed medical school at the Arizona College of Osteopathic Medicine and her residency training at Nassau University Medical Center in New York. She was an EMT prior to medical school and remained interested in that field through her training (Figure 8). McCallister completed her fellowship in EMS at Ohio State, where she learned the fundamentals of prehospital medicine and stayed on as faculty to continue her work. She recently completed her training to be a physician with FEMA on the Ohio Task Force-1.

McAllister remembered this about her fellowship experience:

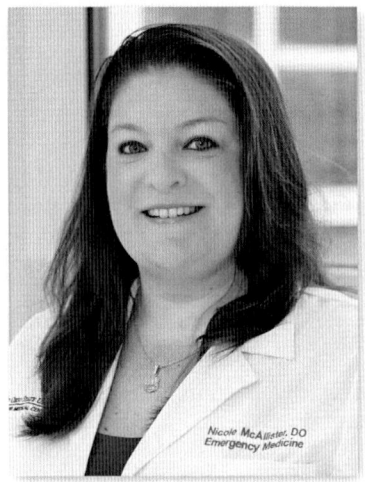

Figure 8: Nicole McAllister, DO, MA, completed the EMS fellowship in 2022, and continued on as a faculty member and medical director with the Center for EMS.

> *It was truly one of the best experiences in my career. I am so fortunate that I was afforded the opportunity to train with a program that was responsive and concerned about my education and allowed me to train with some of the best names in EMS. My experience with this program has completely shaped my career and impacted my future.*[6]

CHELSEA B. KADISH, MD, MS

Chelsea B. Kadish, MD, MS, began her EMS fellowship in 2022. She graduated from the University of California Berkeley with an undergraduate degree in molecular and cell biology in 2008 and received a master's degree in biomedical science in 2010 from the Mount Sinai School of Medicine Graduate School. She received her MD degree from Tulane in 2014 and completed a pediatric residency at New York University School of Medicine in 2017 (Figure 9). From 2017 to 2019 Kadish served as an attending physician in the Department of Emergency Medicine at the Langone Medical Center in New York, then completed a fellowship in pediatric emergency medicine at Nationwide Children's

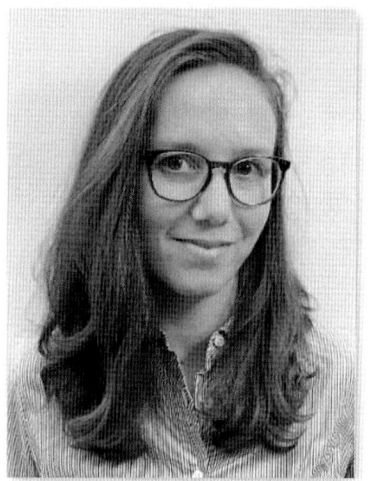

Hospital in Columbus in 2022.

Kadish brings exceptional skill and knowledge to the fellowship and the field of EMS for her essential skills in pediatrics and EMS.

Figure 9: Chelsea B. Kadish, MD, MS, became an EMS fellow in 2022. Her training and certification in pediatrics and pediatric emergency medicine contributed significantly to EMS in central Ohio.

Hematology and Oncology

MICHAEL G. PURCELL, MD

Michael G. Purcell, MD, completed the first fellowship in Hematologic and Oncologic Emergencies at the James Emergency Department from 2017 to 2018. During his fellowship, he studied acute presentation, diagnosis and management of hematologic and oncologic emergencies. During this time, he worked closely with the Division of Hematology, Division of Oncology, Division of Pain and Palliative Care, and the Division of Neuro Oncology to better understand emergent patient presentations for each of those specialties, improve patient management, foster interdepartmental cooperation, and improve the quality of care delivered to cancer patients in the emergency department.

Upon the completion of his fellowship, Purcell served as the Medical Director of the James Oncology Emergency Department. In 2018, he was approached by the Arthur G. James Cancer Hospital and Richard J. Solove Research Institute to serve as Medical Director of the novel James Immediate Care Clinic (ICC), which opened in March 2018.

Today, it continues to serve as an acute care site for established patients of The James who need immediate and acute level of care that cannot be provided in their clinics or at home. The service cares for patients who are too acute for routine outpatient care, but who may not need hospitalization or the full resources of an emergency department visit.

During his time as medical director of both sites, Purcell worked collaboratively with the Hematology and Oncology Divisions to institute pathways and guidelines that improved care, expedited workups and encouraged outpatient management of problems that had previously been addressed in the hospital. During his tenure as Medical Director of the ICC, there was a 4-fold growth in patient volume at that site. His pathways also helped to decrease boarding in the Emergency Department and unneeded admissions to the James Cancer Hospital. Furthermore, he oversaw an expansion of ICC hours and coverage, which led to fewer hospital admissions and emergency department utilization.

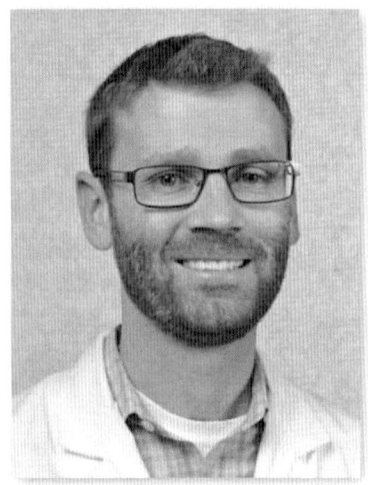

Figure 10: Michael G. Purcell, MD, completed the first fellowship in hematology and oncology in 2018. His training gives him unique qualifications to work with cancer patients and create important collaborative programs with the James Cancer Hospital.

In 2023, Purcell began to work closely with the Department of Radiology to improve throughput in CT imaging for emergency department patients. He has also worked to decrease oral contrast use in patients, decrease CT angiography of the brain and neck in non-stroke patients and improve the CT order-to-start turnaround time. These efforts have decreased turnaround time for imaging across the department. Purcell's current academic passions include hematologic and oncologic emergencies, palliative care in the Emergency Department, quality improvement and ED operations.

He graduated *cum laude* with a Bachelor of Science in Biochemistry from the University of Notre Dame in 2010 and received his medical degree from Emory University School of Medicine in 2014. He went on to complete a residency in emergency medicine at Ohio State where he served as Chief Resident during his final year of training (Figure 10).

Medical Education

The fellowship in medical education was started by Andrew King, MD, in 2017. The fellowship is a 1- or 2-year program intended to prepare EM graduates for academic careers as leaders and scholars in medical education. The fellowship provides training in educational methods and scholarship. Fellows engage in experiential learning through selected activities and work two clinical shifts per week in the emergency department. Two-year programs incorporate master's degree programs. Past fellows include the following individuals: Christopher San Miguel, MD (2017-2018); Krystin Miller, MD (2019-2020); Allison Beaulieu, MD (2020-2022); Kimberly Bambach, MD (2021-2022); and Andrew Kendle, MD (2022-2024).

CHRISTOPHER SAN MIGUEL, MD

Christopher San Miguel, MD, attended North Carolina State University as a Park Scholar and graduated with degrees in psychology, international studies and biological sciences. He received his medical degree from the University of North Carolina School of Medicine before coming to Ohio State for a residency in Emergency Medicine from 2014 to 2017, with a focus on procedural education and curriculum development. After residency he became the inaugural Medical Education fellow in the Department of Emergency Medicine (Figure 11).

Since completing the fellowship, he has served as a core educational faculty member within the department. In 2019, he became the clerkship director for the fourth-year medical student rotation in Emergency Medicine. In this role, he oversees 11 offerings of the course, which has over 200 students rotating at 9 different clinical sites annually. San Miguel also added a rural emergency medicine site in Lima, OH, updated the asynchronous lecture series, created new small group sessions focusing on evidence-based medicine and is developing differential diagnoses, procedural training, and updated student assessments.

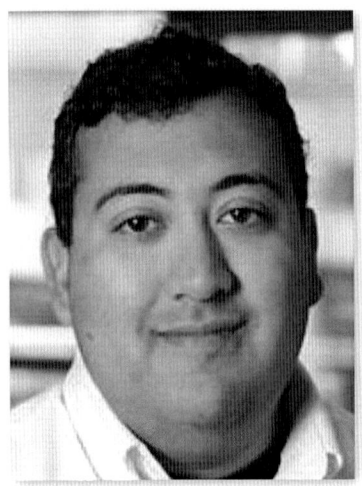

Figure 11: Christopher San Miguel, MD, was the first fellow in the Medical Education fellowship. The clerkship director for the fourth-year medical student rotation in Emergency Medicine, San Miguel has made important contributions to the curriculum and educational publications.

He also oversaw the implementation of a virtual reality-based simulation session to help students prepare to care for critically ill patients. Part of his role also involves overseeing the visiting student rotations in the department, including the creation of a new Emergency Medicine Ultrasound course.

In 2020, San Miguel and his colleague, Colin Kaide, MD, edited a book for Springer Publishing, *Case Studies in Emergency Medicine LEARNing Rounds*. This text has been downloaded over 75,000 times from the publisher's website and is the 2,034,257th best-selling book on Amazon.com. San Miguel has also contributed chapters to *CorePendium* (EM: RAP's online textbook) and *Rosen's Emergency Medicine: Concepts and Clinical Practice*. Since 2020, he has served as a Section Editor for the *Journal of Education and Teaching in Emergency Medicine*, and in 2021 he began serving as a Decision Editor for the Western Journal of Emergency Medicine's *Clinical Practice and Cases in Emergency Medicine*. Since graduating from residency, he has also given several regional and national lectures and workshops on various topics of EM core content and medical education.

KRYSTIN MILLER, MD

Krystin Miller, MD, completed all of her training at Ohio State, starting with a BS in Animal Sciences through the College of Food, Agricultural, and Environmental Sciences, followed by medical school and then residency in emergency medicine. During her residency she was involved in the medical education track and served as a Chief Resident. Following residency, she completed a medical education fellowship in 2020 while pursuing a masters in Biomedical Sciences Education degree at Ohio State. She was the second fellow to complete the program.

Miller took an interest in Graduate Medical Education during her fellowship, and that interest has continued to blossom in her first years as a faculty member. She currently serves as a faculty lead for Resident Didactic Programming, working closely with program leadership to bring innovative and engaging didactic sessions to the weekly emergency medicine conference sessions. She also has taken an interest in the education of off-service residents and fellows who rotate in the emergency department each month.

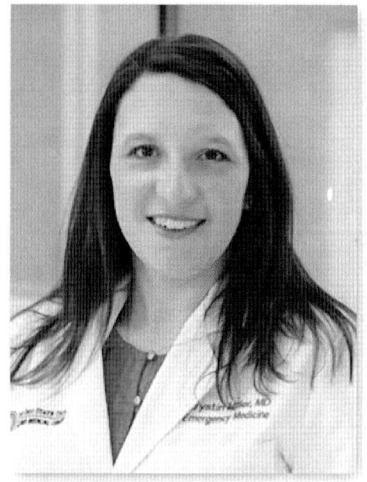

Figure 12: Krystin N. Miller, MD, completed the medical education fellowship in 2020. She joined the faculty and continued to make important contributions to the educational program including a special curriculum for residents outside emergency medicine who rotate in the department.

She was instrumental in developing a comprehensive rotator curriculum, including orientation, feedback and weekly didactic sessions for the off-service residents. Miller's passion for education has been recognized by the emergency medicine residents, as she was awarded the Educator of the Year in 2022 in just her second year as an attending (Figure 12).

KIMBERLY "KIM" BAMBACH, MD

Kimberly "Kim" Bambach, MD, is an Assistant Professor of Emergency Medicine and Assistant Director of the Kiehl Resident Wellness Endowment at Ohio State. She completed her undergraduate studies at Indiana University Bloomington with dual majors in Biology and Germanic Studies before attending medical school at Indiana University. She graduated residency at Ohio State in 2021, serving as Chief Resident in her final year and completed the medical education fellowship in 2022. Her academic interests include podcasting as an educational platform and she was a host of the Emergency Medicine Residents'

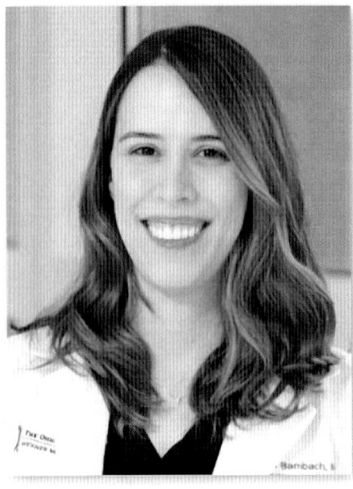

Association (EMRA) official podcast, EMRA*Cast, for two years.

Bambach is also a leader and founding member of the department's professional development program for women in Emergency Medicine, RAFFT (Resident and Faculty Female Tribe). She spearheaded extension of this successful program to undergraduate medical education, RAFFT PUPS (Providing UME Professional Support). She works alongside Simiao Li-Sauerwine, MD, as Assistant Director of the Kiehl Resident Wellness Endowment seeking promote wellbeing during residency (Figure 13).

Figure 13: Kimberly "Kim" Bambach, MD, completed the medical education fellowship in 2022. Her academic interests include podcasting as an educational platform and resident wellness.

ANDREW KENDLE, MD

Andrew Kendle, MD, completes his medical education fellowship in 2024. He grew up in Charlotte, North Carolina, prior to moving to Chapel Hill where he received his undergraduate degree in Chemistry and Biology (2014) at the University of North Carolina (UNC). He completed a year of cardiac surgical gene therapy research prior to obtaining his UNC medical degree (2019). He then went on to complete his emergency medicine residency at Ohio State (2022), during which he discovered a love of medical education thanks to his mentors, including Allison Beaulieu, Jennifer Yee and many others. With their assistance he has presented nationally at

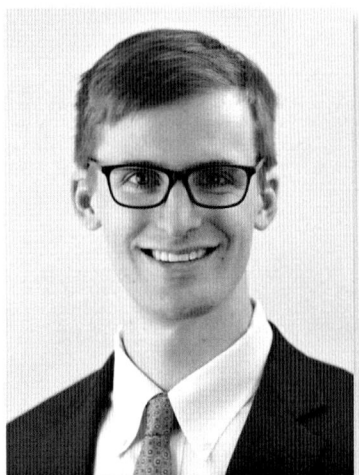

Figure 14: Andrew Kendle, MD, will complete his medical education fellowship in 2024. His interests include technological innovations and evidence-based teaching in emergency medicine.

CORD and SAEM and he hopes to bring his mixture of humor, photoshop/tech talents and passion for evidence-based medicine to more and more learners (Figure 14).

Medical Toxicology

The fellowship in medical toxicology started and stopped periodically over the years. A graduate of the second class of residents in 1984, Michael T. Kelley, MD, completed a toxicology fellowship at UC San Francisco, then returned to Ohio State as a faculty member and worked in both the University Hospital emergency department and the Central Ohio Poison Center with Phillip Walson, MD, who was a renowned and widely respected pediatrician and toxicologist. Walson headed the center and led a highly productive research program.

MARCEL J. CASAVANT, MD

Marcel J. Casavant, MD (Figure 15) completed his residency in emergency medicine at Ohio State in 1993 and began a 2-year fellowship in medical toxicology at the Columbus Children's Hospital (now Nationwide Children's) which was the home of the Poison Control Center. Casavant also studied under Walson.

Casavant graduated from Boston College in 1986 and the University of Massachusetts Medical School in 1990. Following his residency and fellowship, he served as an attending faculty member at Ohio State Main and East Hospitals and Nationwide Children's Hospital. In 2002 he became the Chief of the Division of Toxicology in the Department of Pediatrics. Years later

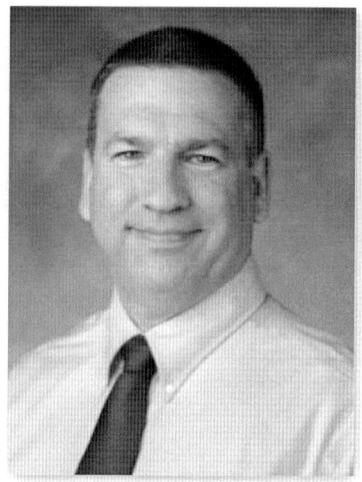

Figure 15: Marcel J. Casavant, MD, completed the Ohio State medical toxicology fellowship in 1995 and became the leader of the fellowship in medical toxicology and the Medical Director of the Central Ohio Poison Control Center until his retirement in 2023.

Casavant recalled that he was the last U.S. board certified physician to train in the Ohio State fellowship until 2011, when the fellowship began once again:

> *At your [Rund's] request we started an accredited tox fellowship in 2011. Several smart people wisely advised me NOT to take our first fellow until funding was locked up, but the residency was graduating Dr. Hannah Hays and we just couldn't pass on the opportunity to train her, so we opened the fellowship before funding was assured. Ohio State was willing to pay half of each fellow's salary, but there was no funding for the other half nor for faculty time and program expenses. We assigned Dr. Hays to work in the OSU ED part time to generate the other half of her salary.*[7]

HANNAH L. HAYS, MD

Hannah L. Hays, MD (Figure 16), was an outstanding resident in emergency medicine who completed the program in 2011, serving as Chief Resident in her final year. She became the first fellow in the re-incarnated toxicology fellowship, finishing in 2013. Hays came to Ohio State after graduating from the 6-year combined BS/MD program at Northeastern Ohio Medical University in 2008 (formerly Northeastern Ohio Universities College of Medicine-NEOUCOM). Following completion of her fellowship, she joined the attending faculty at OhioHealth Grady Memorial Hospital Emergency Department and subsequently served as the lead physician at Spero Health Columbus, an outpatient clinic that provides treatment for substance use disorders to underserved populations in Ohio.

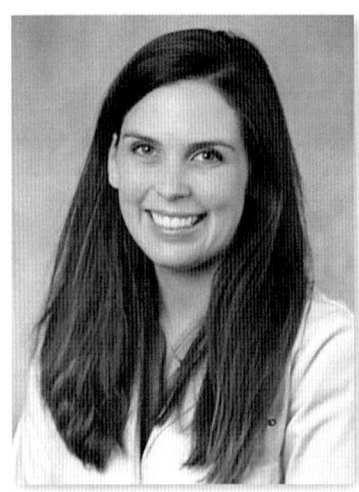

Figure 16: Hannah L. Hays, MD, completed her fellowship in toxicology in 2013. She became the Executive Medical Director of the Central Ohio Poison Center in 2023.

Following completion of her fellowship in 2013, Hays continued to work with the toxicology program, ultimately becoming medical director of the Central Ohio Poison Center and the division chief and section chief of toxicology at Nationwide Children's Hospital. She is currently an Assistant Professor of emergency medicine and pediatrics at The Ohio State University College of Medicine, where she serves as course director for the Toxicology Advanced Competency in Emergency Medicine. Her academic interests include addiction medicine, drug testing, laboratory detection of pediatric illicit drug exposures, and prevention of pediatric exploratory buprenorphine ingestions.

Years later, Hays remembered this about her medical toxicology fellowship:

> *I remember the time I spent on the toxicology rotation in residency. I had never encountered a topic as fascinating as toxicology felt to me then, and still does today. Making the decision to spend an additional two years in training was not easy, but I knew it was the right path. When I started fellowship, I could not believe how much time and energy the entire team was willing to pour into training me, especially Dr. Casavant, who spent long hours in the poison center, in clinic, and on the wards. I still look back with extreme gratitude to have been able to train at Ohio State.*[8]

Future Directions

Jason L. Russell, DO, completed the fellowship in 2014 and continues to staff the poison center on a part-time basis.

Glenn Burns, MD, completed the fellowship during the 2014-2015 time period. He published several studies with Casavant and became the President of the Medical Toxicology Fellows-in-Training Association from 2014 to 2015. He became a Colonel in the United States Air Force and a faculty member in the department of emergency medicine at Wright State University.

The toxicology program no longer operates a fellowship. Casavant related the history of the fellowship later in his career:

> *In 2012 Dr. Hays became a second-year fellow, and we later took on Dr. Devin Wiles (who brought military funding) and Dr. Jason Russell.*

In these years nationwide, there were almost as many tox fellowship applicants as there were accredited fellowship spots, with some programs fully funded and others, like ours, not fully funded so requiring fellows to work in the emergency department to earn their keep. Recruiting for us was more and more difficult. Dr. Russell continues to do part-time toxicology support of the poison center, but became first medical director of the emergency department at Memorial Hospital of Union County, and then CMO at that hospital. Dr. Wiles finished his tox fellowship and started working for the military as a toxicologist at the US Army Medical Research Institute of Chemical Defense. Dr. Burns was promoted to full Colonel in the USAF shortly after finishing his fellowship program, retired from his distinguished military career, and practices emergency medicine and medical education now in the Dayton area.[7]

Ultrasound

David Bahner, MD, envisioned an ultrasound fellowship during his residency and stayed on as faculty in emergency medicine to build the ultrasound program from the ground up, starting in the medical school and residency. Bahner had mentored faculty member and former Chief Resident Richard Limperos, MD, in the early 2000s to help him lead the ultrasound (US) program within the department.

Limperos was born and raised in Warren, Ohio (Figure 17). He graduated from Kent State University in 1997 with a Bachelor of Science degree and completed his medical degree at Northeast Ohio Medical University in 2001 and EM residency in 2004.

Some had called Limperos Bahner's first ultrasound fellow, but this was meant to imply that Limperos had been mentored by Bahner during his early years as a young faculty member. Limperos had never completed a formal ultrasound fellowship but used his faculty time to focus on teaching, and helping to run the many ultrasound activities, including residency scanning shifts, and interacting with clinical engineering to connect emergency department machines to the Picture Archiving and Communication System (PACS).

After completing his residency, Limperos became an Assistant Profes-

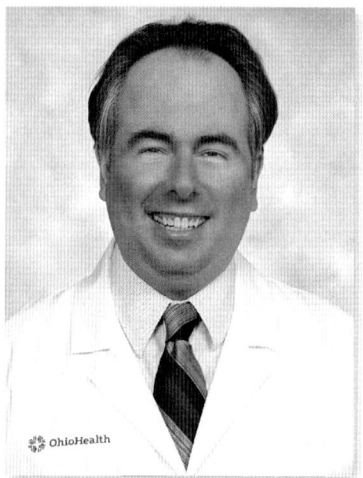

Figure 17: Richard Limperos, MD, completed his Emergency Medicine Residency at the Ohio State Wexner Medical Center in 2004 and served as Chief Resident. He soon distinguished himself in helping build the emerging ultrasound program. Later he completed the MBA curriculum at the University of Cincinnati Lindner College of Business in 2022.
Source: OhioHealth

sor of Emergency Medicine at Ohio State, continuing his mentorship under Bahner, and served as the first Assistant Ultrasound Director for the residency from 2005 to 2009. He was involved in developing and teaching the medical school ultrasound curriculum, including the Honors Ultrasound Course, and was awarded the Excellence in Teaching Award from the medical school in 2009 and awarded the residency's Outstanding Emergency Medicine Faculty Award in 2010. He was instrumental in implementing the billing process and image retention in PACS. He gave several national presentations on the novel wireless transmission of ultrasound images to PACS, which Ohio State pioneered with GE Ultrasound. Limperos also served as the Course Director for the nationally known Ohio ACEP Ultrasound Course from 2006 until 2018.

After leaving Ohio State, Limperos served as Ultrasound Director for Doctors Hospital Emergency Medicine Residency (Columbus, Ohio, 2009 to 2015), where he expanded ultrasound use in the emergency department and the intensive care unit.

As part of the emergency medicine contract group, EMP (now USACS), he served as the first National Ultrasound Director from 2012 to 2015, where he was implemented a companywide ultrasound education program and operations strategy. He served as faculty for the ACEP Ultrasound Management Course from 2013 to 2015, sharing his experience managing ultrasound for a large nationwide multihospital group. Ultimately, he became the Associate Medical Director for OhioHealth Urgent Care.

Bahner designed the framework for an ultrasound fellowship as an advanced extension of the graduate medical education opportunities he was providing the residency program each year. Under this model, the US fellow would become proficient in emergency ultrasound and the academic missions related to this burgeoning field. At the end of the fellowship, the physician would complete the Registered Diagnostic Medical Sonographer (RDMS) examination and thus certify their ultrasound skill and knowledge.

As emergency medicine progressed to offer a focused practice designation exam for advanced emergency ultrasonography in 2022, there was no longer a need for the RDMS certification. In the early 2000s, emergency medicine had strong representation on the hospital's credentials committee. Douglas Rund, MD, was committee chair until 2000 and Howard Werman, MD, was an influential member. Bahner navigated the credentials process to develop ultrasound privileges for faculty and worked to develop a novel curriculum for emergency ultrasound in developing the fellowship.

Codifying components from the emergency ultrasound guidelines published by ACEP in 2001 and updated in 2008, Bahner developed content, course material and ultrasound scanning shifts that became the foundation for a formalized ultrasound fellowship. In 2007 he applied for and received approval from the graduate medical education committee at Ohio State for a fellowship in emergency ultrasound. Bahner used his experiences in providing ultrasound education to residents but now he could go into greater depth and provide professional training over an entire year culminating in sitting for the RDMS examination.

Bahner's administrative lobbying efforts led to the establishment of the first successful EM ultrasound fellowship at Ohio State from 2009-2010. It existed outside a formal match process, so the fellow could work as an attending physician for a few shifts a week while completing the fellowship.

ERIKA C. KUBE, MD

After approval from the medical center to recruit an ultrasound fellow, Erika Kube, MD, interviewed and matched as the first Ohio State US fellow. An EMT from Colorado, Kube was recommended for a residency position by John Kendall, MD, an ultrasound expert from the University of Colorado, because of her ultrasound interest. She graduated from Rosalind Franklin University Medical School in 2006 and completed EM residency at Ohio State from 2006-2009.

Kube became an outstanding clinician. She was elected Chief Resident in her final year, was a leader in ultrasound during residency and completed the first US fellowship while the department had its offices in Cramblett Hall. Kube's fellowship year included ultrasound training of medical students and residents (Figure 18). She also proctored US events throughout the year. Kube's expertise expanded as the Quality Assurance (QA) system of review of PACS images was developed. The QA goal was to evaluate ED images, document the results and the bill payors for physician services.

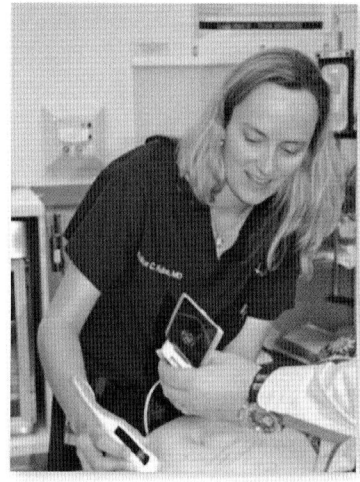

Figure 18: Erika Kube, MD, was the first ultrasound fellow in the Department of Emergency Medicine (2009-2010). Here she is shown performing one of what would become many ultrasound procedures throughout her career.

A stellar clinician and educator, Kube would later go on to work with the Ohio Chapter of the American College of Emergency Physicians and represent emergency medicine in the public policy arena. Kube continues practicing emergency medicine for Mid-Ohio Emergency Services, provides medical direction to many EMS services in central Ohio and writes a weekly column about emergency medicine in the *Columbus Dispatch* newspaper.

LYDIA M. SAHLANI, MD

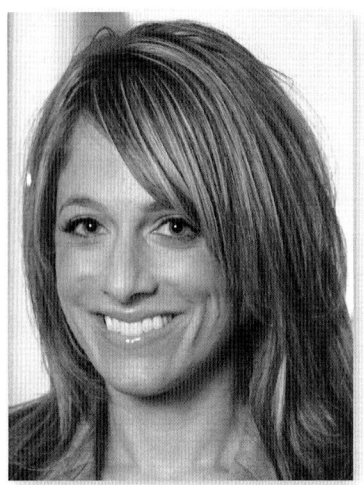

Figure 19: Lydia M. Sahlani, MD, completed her fellowship in ultrasound in 2014. She joined the faculty and became an exceptional teacher and resource for her students at all levels.

After Kube the fellowship was unfilled until 2013 when Lydia Sahlani, MD, enrolled in the program. Following her fellowship in 2014, Sahlani stayed on as a faculty member and continued as an enthusiastic teacher and an outstanding clinician. Having worked on procedural ultrasound efforts during her fellowship year, Sahlani presented her work at the American Institute of Ultrasound in Medicine (AIUM) annual conference (Figure 19).

AMAR VIRA, MD

Amar Vira, MD, completed his fellowship at Ohio State from 2014-2015. He was involved in research efforts looking at venous collapsibility and central venous pressures and co-authored articles about ultrasound guided procedures and transducer manipulation. Representing the Ohio State ultrasound program internationally at a conference in India at INDUS-EM Summit, Vira lectured about ultrasound in trauma, and presented studies on the correlation of inferior vena cava index to central venous pressure and other hemodynamic parameters during resuscitations. He also developed a passion for teaching bedside sonography to others and taught various courses around the country. Upon completion of his fellowship at Ohio State, Vira joined the faculty at the University of Texas and would eventually lead the ultrasound efforts at the University of Texas-Austin Dell Medical School (Figure 20).

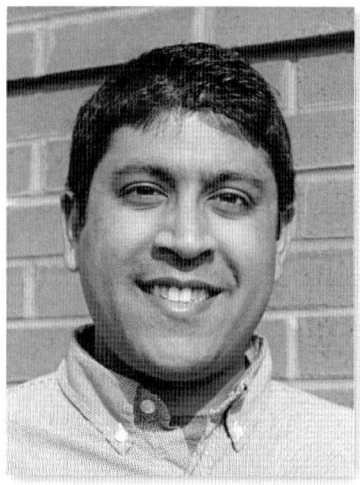

Figure 20: Amar Vira, MD, completed the ultrasound fellowship in 2015. A faculty member at the University of Texas, he travels the country to curate ultrasound courses and highlights the use of ultrasound in critical cases for a national publication. He was a part of the inaugural class awarded the Focused Practice Designation in Advanced Emergency Medicine Ultrasonography by the American Board of Emergency Medicine.

Vira continues to work in Austin, Texas, flipping the traditional teaching methods to match today's learners. He is a standing columnist for a national publication, highlighting the use of ultrasound in critical cases, and travels around the country to curate ultrasound courses. Although he earned his RDMS certification after fellowship, he was a part of the inaugural class to be awarded the Focused Practice Designation in Advanced Emergency Medicine Ultrasonography by the American Board of Emergency Medicine.

Bahner petitioned the ACGME committee at Ohio State—and received approval—for three emergency US fellowship spots for an increase in candidate applications, including several Ohio State medical students. The fellowship accepted three physicians in 2015-2016, including Ohio State College of Medicine alumni: Tyler Dschaak, MD, and Mike Prats, MD, and Sara Singhal, MD, who had trained in emergency medicine at the University of Kentucky. Prats would stay on as faculty in the department and became a founding member of the first Ultrasound Division within the Department of Emergency Medicine. After their fellowships, Dschaak and Singhal entered into community medicine and lead respective ultrasound programs.

MICHAEL I. PRATS, MD

An undergraduate of the University of Pittsburgh with dual majors in neuroscience and philosophy, and graduate of the Ohio State College of Medicine, Michael Prats, MD, first learned ultrasound in the Honors Ultrasound course that Bahner taught. He went on to complete his residency in emergency medicine at Drexel University, then returned to

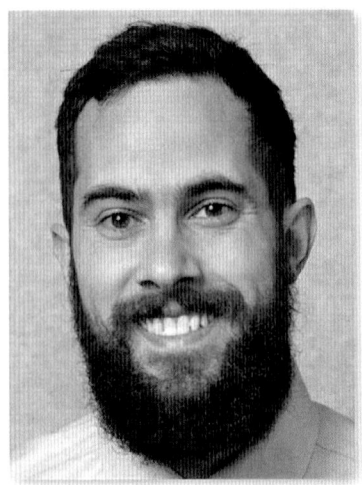

Figure 21: Michael Prats, MD, completed the ultrasound fellowship in 2016 and became an Associate Professor and Director of Ultrasound Research. He has established an international reputation for excellence in ultrasound teaching and research.

Ohio State for the emergency ultrasound fellowship, which he completed in 2016 (Figure 21). Post fellowship, Prats joined the Ohio State faculty and became the Director of Ultrasound Research in the Division of Ultrasound in the Department of Emergency Medicine.

During his fellowship, Prats co-founded and launched the Ultrasound GEL podcast, which reviews literature in point-of-care ultrasound. The podcast has an international audience in 200 countries and includes an educational blog edited by ultrasound experts worldwide. It has won multiple national awards and is one of the most accessed ultrasound podcasts. He has been an invited speaker and course instructor internationally. In addition, his experience in the realm of social media led him to found and chair the first Social Media Committee for the department in 2016. He also serves the medical center in the Institutional Point-of-Care Ultrasound Committee where he chairs the Policy Subcommittee. He has authored necessary policies regarding the use of hand-held ultrasounds and the documentation of ultrasound examinations.

Prats has been a strong advocate for expanding the role of ultrasound in the emergency department, helping to implement supplies and training for ultrasound-guided nerve blocks. He also worked with representatives in the Division of Cardiology and Cardiac Anesthesia in an effort to bring transesophageal echocardiography (TEE) to the emergency department. To this end, he co-authored an important publication regarding the use of resuscitative TEE in the *Journal of the American College of Cardiology*. In his role as Director of Ultrasound Research, he helped co-lead the first Ultrasound Research Interest Group for medical students. In addition, he has developed protocols and guidelines to encourage and assist the ultrasound research efforts

LAUREN D. BRANDITZ, MD

Bahner's final fellow was Lauren Branditz, MD, in 2016-2017. After that year Creagh Boulger, MD, officially took over as director of the fellowship. Branditz earned a Bachelor of Science degree in Biology and a medical degree at Ohio State and went on to complete a residency in Emergency Medicine at Christiana Care Health System in Delaware. She returned to Ohio State to complete an Emergency Ultrasound Fellowship, then stayed on as faculty.

Branditz became an Assistant Director in the Division of Ultrasound and is the course director for a 1-year longitudinal course titled, Advanced Topics in Emergency Medicine, which helps to prepare fourth-year medical students to apply for and enter Emergency Medicine residencies.

Due to her expertise, Branditz has been an invited speaker for other hospital systems and at conferences, and was recently elected Secretary of the Ultrasound in Medical Education group within the American Institute of Ultrasound in Medicine. After serving in this role for two years, she will continue on as Vice Chair, and then Chair (Figure 22).

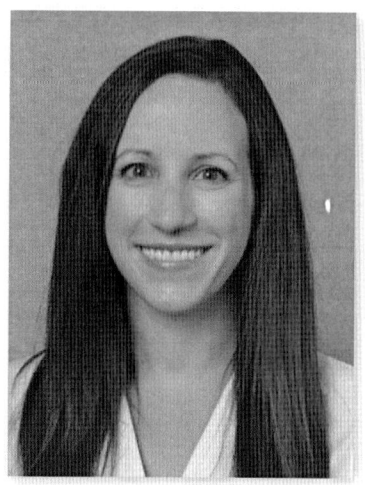

Figure 22: Lauren Branditz, MD, completed the ultrasound fellowship in 2017. She became an expert in ultrasound and medical student education.

In 2017 Creagh Boulger, MD, became the director of the fellowship. Under Boulger the program recruited Jess Everett, MD, and Irene Mynatt, DO. Carolyn Martinez, MD, completed the US fellowship in 2020, followed by Kim Fender, MD, and Hiten Patel, MD, in 2020-2021. Everett, Mynatt and Martinez would all join the Ohio

State Department of Emergency Medicine and the Ultrasound Division after their fellowships. Fender took a position leading the East Carolina Medical Center's Department of Emergency Medicine ultrasound program.

Hilary Davenport Stroud, DO, and primary care US fellow Natalie Nguyen, MD, completed ultrasound training from 2021- 2022 as the ultrasound fellowship successfully navigated the COVID pandemic and utilized videoconferencing.

CAROLYN MARTINEZ, MD

Carolyn Martinez is currently Assistant Fellowship Director and course director for the visiting medical student elective in the Division of Ultrasound. She completed her Bachelor of Science degree in Biochemistry at the University of California in San Diego and worked on biofuels in a small startup company prior to enrolling in the University of Kentucky College of Medicine. In medical school she started a student-run, ground-roots ultrasound program and became interested in medical education and point-of-care ultrasound.

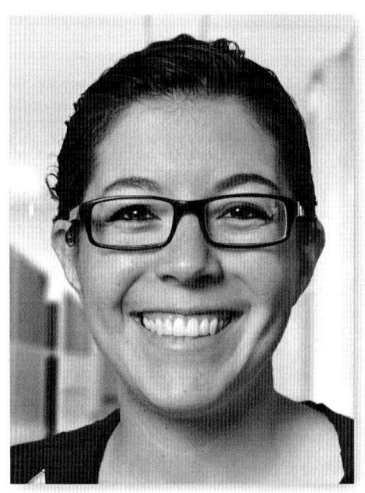

Figure 23: Carolyn Martinez, MD, is the Assistant Fellowship Director in the Division of Ultrasound at Ohio State.

She completed her emergency medicine residency at Ohio State in 2019 where she was Chief Resident. Her residency leadership team received the Chief Residents of the Year award from the Emergency Medicine Resident's Association. She stayed at Ohio State to complete the emergency ultrasound fellowship in 2020 before joining the faculty. During the fellowship she focused on education and was invited to teach hands-on sessions at multiple national conferences.

Currently, Martinez is active in the educational mission of the Ultrasound Division at all levels, including medical students, residents and fellows. She also has a strong interest in the administrative aspect of ultrasound, including quality assurance and is working to expand her involvement (Figure 23).

HILARY DAVENPORT STROUD, DO

Hilary Davenport Stroud, DO, grew up in Norwalk, Ohio, and graduated with her Bachelor of Science from the University of Mount Union in 2012. She completed medical school at Edward Via College of Osteopathic Medicine-Carolinas Campus in 2017, followed by a transitional year at Inspira Health in Vineland, New Jersey, in 2018. She started her emergency medicine residency at Hahnemann University Hospital/Drexel College of Medicine in Philadelphia where she was presented with the Ultrasonographer of the Year award in 2019. When Hahnemann University Hospital closed its doors the summer of 2019, she transferred to the University of Louisville to complete her residency.

In 2021-2022, Davenport Stroud completed the clinical ultrasound fellowship at Ohio State. During her fellowship she found her passion for teaching ultrasound and integrating ultrasound into the daily clinical lives of physicians. She has presented at American Institute of Ultrasound Medicine (AIUM) with her colleague Michael Prats, MD, on basic cardiac ultrasound. In 2022 she worked closely with the residents on their success at the Society for Academic Emergency Medicine's Sonogames, a resident ultrasound competition where the Ohio State residents placed 5th in the initial round and were awarded best costume and runner-up on most clever name.

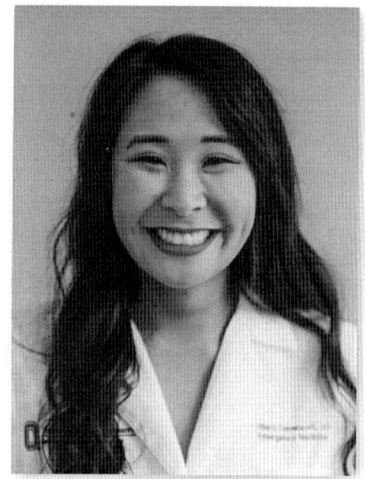

Figure 24: Hilary Davenport Stroud, DO, completed her ultrasound fellowship in 2022.

Davenport Stroud presents ultrasound cases monthly to the emergency medicine residents during their weekly conference and continues to have an interest in nerve blocks and the decreased use of opioids, geriatric emergency medicine and medical education. She is working on the inaugural longitudinal ultrasound curriculum, to be introduced in in 2023 (Figure 24).

Ultrasound and Primary Care

The fellowship was also offered to physicians in primary care. Hiten Patel, MD, graduated from the Ohio State family medicine residency program in 2020 (Figure 25). He became the inaugural primary care ultrasound fellow and, upon completion joined the family medicine faculty in 2021. He worked with the faculty in both emergency medicine and family medicine to institute ultrasound practice and education in outpatient family medicine. He developed an ultrasound curriculum for family medicine trainees. This led to a collaboration between departments to recruit and train a primary care ultrasound fellow each year. He has also worked with the Columbus Free Clinic and Latina Free Clinic to implement an ultrasound clinic during the free clinic. Hiten also sits on the Institutional Point-of-Care ultrasound (POCUS) committee and is the co-course director of the general POCUS provider course. Patel has taught ultrasound to medical students, EM/FM residents, and fellows.

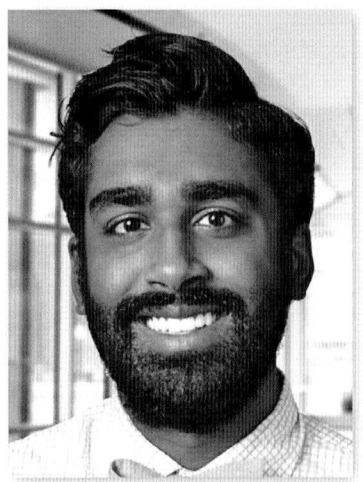

Figure 25: Hiten Patel, MD, was the first primary care ultrasound fellow in the department. He became an Assistant Professor in the Department of Family Medicine and is active in teaching ultrasound at Ohio State.

By 2022, an arrangement with Nationwide Children's brought a pediatric emergency medicine ultrasound fellowship to the Ohio State ultrasound program. Yamini Jadcherla, MD, filled this role as the first pediatric ultrasound fellow while Aaron Zabriskie, MD, was the 2022-2023 primary care ultrasound fellow and Rosalia Mahr, MD, was the emergency medicine ultrasound fellow. The ultrasound fellowship program continues to match motivated candidates and graduate trained ultrasound experts. Other activities in the early 2020s included a "learn from the leaders" conference hosted by Boulger where ultrasound experts from around the country connected with fellows to share their combined expertise and interact in small group sessions.

Future Directions

Over time the number of residents entering fellowships has increased from one to two per year, to approximately 50% of the residency graduating class.[9] The Department of Emergency Medicine's fellowships reflect the ever-present goal of continuing to being recognized as a respected academic discipline and to remove any possible doubts about being a specialty—"indeed".

References

1. American Board of Medical Specialties Board Certification Report 2021-2022.

2. Moseley MD. Personal communication. 2022.

3. Cortez EJ. Personal communication. 2022.

4. Ball MT. Personal communication. 2023.

5. Sharkey TP. Personal communication. 2023.

6. McAllister NT. Personal communication. 2023.

7. Casavant MJ. Personal communication. 2023.

8. Hays HL. Personal communication. 2023.

9. Khandelwal S. Personal communication. 2023.

Chapter 22

Leading the Way: Ultrasound

David P. Bahner, MD
Douglas A. Rund, MD

In 1794, Lazzaro Spallanzani, Bishop of Padua, was also a scientist. In one experiment he studied bats flying in total darkness. The bats flew breezily around his blackened study managing to avoid wires that he had hung from the ceiling. He knew that they were avoiding the obstacles because bells were attached to the ends of the wires. When the bats were blinded, they still flew confidently around the room. This ability was lost when their ears were blocked. As Gerhard Neuweiler wrote in his text *The Biology of Bats*:

> *The bats became irritated when Spallanzani placed brass tubes in their ear canals. When these tubes were closed, the bats hit the wires as they flew and rang the bells. As soon as the tubes were opened again these same bats regained their ability to fly in the darkness. Because they did not produce any sounds that were audible to Spallanzani as they flew through the darkness, he was not able to discover the secret of their orientation. Somewhat puzzled he ended his experiment in 1794 with the following entry in his journal "thus blinded bats are able to use their ears when they hunt insects…this discovery is incredible."*[1]

Spallanzani concluded that the bats navigated by sound rather than sight. After many such experiments he concluded that the "ear of the bat serves more efficiently (than the eye) for seeing or at least for measuring distances."[2] The matter remained a scientific mystery until 1938 when young Harvard students, Donald R. Griffin and Robert Galambos used a sonic detector to record directional ultrasound noises emitted by bats during flight.[2,3] Sounds were uttered through the mouth and nose and received by the ears. When the mouths of the bats were blocked, the bats could not avoid hitting obstacles. Many of the sounds were ultrasonic: unheard by the human ear because of their high frequency. The bats used the sound echo to determine the distance and location of potential obstacles, a phenomenon known as *echolocation*.

Ultrasound's Beginnings

Pioneering physicians recognized the potential for sound waves and echolocation to be used in medicine: A transmitter converted an electrical signal to sound waves and a receiver converted the sound wave into an electrical signal that could be read as an image on a screen. Though early diagnostic ultrasound devices were large, cumbersome, and complex, the technology offered a glimpse of a totally new imaging modality to innovative physicians. In 1942, Karl Dussik, a neurologist at the University of Vienna, attempted to locate brain tumors by measuring the ultrasonic beams through the head.[4,5] In obstetrics and gynecology, the great pioneer Professor Ian Donald of Glasgow recognized the possible uses of ultrasound in obstetrics.[6] Kane and colleagues outlined Donald's accomplishments in developing medical ultrasound in clinical practice:

> *Having gained initial experience in radar and sonar techniques while serving in the Royal Air Force during World War II, [Donald] was enthused in medical ultrasound on meeting John Wild while he was working at the Hammersmith in London. On becoming the Regius Professor of Midwifery of the University of Glasgow, Ian Donald and co-workers began a series of studies that would establish a role for medical ultrasound, overcoming initial clinical skepticism from his colleagues who believed that manual abdominal and pelvic examination provided sufficient diagnostic certainty. With the help of the engineering firm Kelvin Hughes Ltd, . . . Donald used a 'flaw detector' to differentiate cystic and solid abdominal masses—in one case altering a clinical diagnosis of terminal carcinoma to simple ovarian cyst—leading to the publication of their findings in* The Lancet *in 1958, a major milestone in medical history. With his colleagues, Donald first developed a two-dimensional scanner and then an automatic scanner in 1960, made the first ante-partum diagnosis of placenta previa using ultrasound, developed the method for measuring the biparietal diameter of the fetal head in 1962 and was the first to utilize the full bladder to allow*

the detection of very early pregnancy of about 6–7 weeks gestation in 1963. [2,7]

These early pioneers demonstrated that ultrasound could be used in the entire body to help answer common clinical questions. Ultrasound could help manage common complaints like knee or leg swelling. The first use of diagnostic ultrasound of the musculoskeletal system was reported in 1972 in a study to differentiate Baker's cysts from thrombophlebitis.[8]

Early Imaging at Ohio State

Ultrasound had a famous history at the Ohio State University Department of Radiology with Atis K. Freimanis, MD, a pioneer in B mode ultrasound development and imaging the abdomen and chest.[9] Freimanis completed his post-doctoral training in radiology at the Ohio State Department of Radiology in 1958. He became full professor in 1965 and published seminal works on abdominal ultrasound in 1969 and 1970. He left Ohio State in 1970 to become the inaugural chair in Toledo at the Medical College of Ohio Department of Radiology and Director of the Radiology Technology program. He returned to Ohio State as Chair of Radiology from 1976-1983 before moving on to the Department of Radiology at the Michigan State University Colleges of Human Medicine and Osteopathic Medicine. During Freimanis' tenure at Ohio State, ultrasound remained in the domain of radiology.

When the Ohio State University Division of Emergency Medicine was formed in 1978, imaging was a challenge for physicians. Computerized tomography (CT) of the head had just emerged, but was a scarce resource that had to be extensively discussed for its approved uses. Delores "Dee" Tschirner Goodwin, RT (R)(M), who came to Ohio State radiology in 1976, became for years the primary emergency radiology technician in the emergency department. She recalled those early days:

> *We had CT (called CAT scans then) but the first one had a huge separate room just for its computer. It was kept in the North Wing of the X-ray department. I remember the temp was kept at 68 degrees or so to keep the computer happy.*[10]

Plain X-ray studies were available for all parts of the human body, but the ability to detect pathology was limited due to the many boundaries of X-ray imaging at the time. Imaging was challenging before CT and ultrasound.

In the earliest days of the new specialty at Ohio State, ideal imaging alternatives for injured patients were not available in the emergency "room." In suspected abdominal bleeding plain X-rays were largely unhelpful unless there was intra-abdominal free air determined by supine and upright films. Victims of trauma with suspected abdominal injury were evaluated with diagnostic peritoneal lavage (DPL) to determine bleeding within the peritoneum. A small incision was made in the midline and a catheter was inserted into the abdomen and saline was introduced into the peritoneal cavity. At one time this was considered the "gold standard" for evaluating abdominal trauma. Detailed criteria were laid out for a positive result, including the number of red cells found in the effluent. There was always the possibility of injury from the procedure itself. The Focused Assessment with Sonography for Trauma (FAST) was years away and would eventually displace DPL

"Longing" to see inside the body

By Douglas Rund, MD

When I studied neurology at the National Hospital for Neurology and Neurosurgery, Queen Square, in London in 1970 as an elective in medical school, one of the ways to visualize the brain and spinal cord had been the pneumoencephalogram. The spinal fluid was partially drained by a lumbar puncture and air was injected into the subarachnoid space. The skull was then imaged with X-ray. The procedure resulted in incredibly intense headache and vomiting. I thought there had to be a better way to look at the brain.

When I first started practice in Columbus in 1976 and encountered a patient with head injury, the neurosurgeon on call would invariably ask about the pulse and blood pressure: If the heart rate was slow and the blood pressure high, there was a risk of intracranial swelling or bleeding (two parts of Cushing's triad).

Computerized tomography was not always available and plain X-rays of the skull were really no help. We were taught to look for a shift in a "calcified pineal gland" on a skull film which was rarely seen. The clinical examination sometimes determined the need for burr holes or craniotomy. We longed for a way to "see inside the body" to visualize pathology.

in the management of the unstable trauma patient.[11, 12, 13]

In evaluating the chest emergencies such as aortic dissection or thoracic trauma with plain X-ray, the clinicians had to hope for calcification in the vessel or nonspecific soft tissue enlargement to determine an abnormality on the plain film.

History of Ultrasound Nationally

In 1996, the field of ultrasound (US) in the United States was in a state of flux in emergency medicine (EM) for two main reasons: It was not yet incorporated into the EM residency, and traditional imaging specialists challenged the effort. Some specialists believed that emergency medicine either did not need ultrasound or that other clinicians were already adequately trained to deliver ultrasound care for those patients.

It is not that ultrasound technology wasn't in much use. In fact, from the 1950s through the 1970s, ultrasound technology grew exponentially around the world and in parts of the United States. From examining the kidney, bladder, and prostate in Japan (Watanabe),[14] pregnant patients in Scotland (Ian Donald)[15] or the eye in Australia (Gil Baum),[16, 17] to imaging the heart (Inge Edler),[18] ultrasound was taking shape as more sophisticated equipment gave innovators a platform to explore its use in the practice of medicine. Don Baker's group had advanced doppler ultrasound at the University of Washington,[19] while JJ Wild had discussions with Ian Donald in 1954 around using ultrasound more in obstetrics and gynecology. Many of these early ultrasound efforts paired innovative clinicians with engineers or technical experts to bridge into new territory as the technology improved.

In the United States, JJ Wild and John Reid's technical insights led to early B mode (brightness mode) grayscale imaging, M mode (motion mode) and the development of endoluminal transducers technology in the 1950s.[20] As more specialties started using ultrasound from around the world, its use would grow in radiology, cardiology, obstetrics/gynecology and within many other specialties as the technology improved and more physicians began to use it in medical care. As technology improved over time and machines became more affordable, the use of ultrasound in medicine grew. Notably, while ultrasound in medical education was common in Europe and Germany in the 1990s, it was not part of the medical education of every medical student, including in the United States.

A Specialty Indeed: Ultrasound at Ohio State Emergency Medicine

The possibility of real imaging that could look "inside the body" without harm to the patient or the tissues themselves presented a truly great opportunity for the burgeoning specialty of emergency medicine nationally and at Ohio State. Acquiring competence in using this novel form of imaging would reinforce the goal of demonstrating that emergency medicine was "a specialty indeed." If a new imaging technique could be mastered and studied by emergency physicians and used to diagnose patients with problems that were first seen in or unique to the emergency department, the specialty would advance substantially.

In the 1980s diagnostic ultrasound offered such a possibility. The work of Donald and others had shown its importance in obstetrics and gynecology, particularly in evaluating pregnant women with abdominal pain. A pelvic ultrasound could detect an empty uterus in a patient with a positive pregnancy test suggesting ectopic pregnancy. The obstetrics service seemed a natural ally in the procurement of a readily available ultrasound machine.

The topic of ultrasound continued to surface in the Ohio State emergency medicine faculty meetings and in December 1988 the faculty discussed purchase of an ultrasound machine. The topic arose sporadically over the next few years without conclusion. In 1991 resident Roger Muller, MD, presented a proposal to Rund summarizing the results of his study of the ultrasound literature. He outlined the essential nature of ultrasound in evaluating life threatening conditions: pericardial tamponade, electromechanical dissociation (is there heart wall motion?), symptomatic abdominal aortic aneurysm, ectopic pregnancy in patient with cardiovascular instability and documentation of intraabdominal fluid in trauma. He outlined other uses, including vascular access, aspiration of the bladder and foreign body location.

He recommended that the department purchase a Siemens model SI 200. The price was $40,500 with a lease option of $870 per month. Despite this persuasive review, no action was taken. In 1993 discussions were held with radiology and obstetrics-gynecology regarding an ultrasound machine but agreement could not be reached. It was not until early 1995 that the department's budget requests were prioritized with the first being an ultrasound machine and second, capnography. The hospital promised purchase of a machine but the problems with radiology continued and the purchase of a new ultrasound machine became "bogged down in committee."

The stalled attempts focused on several issues: Were the emergency physicians capable of performing and interpreting ultrasound studies? Were such studies more appropriately performed by the "experts' who devoted their careers and years of study to a given area of disease such as obstetrics or radiology? In reality, these issues were more about "turf"—ultimately, who would be billing and collecting for ultrasound procedures.

One of the early solutions to such problems for emergency medicine was to "work around" them by turning the conversation from practice provinces to education. In the earliest days of the Division of Emergency Medicine at Ohio State, faculty members were asked to participate in the development of educational materials for students and residents. The strategy relied on what should be common ground for university professors: education. David P. Bahner, MD, quickly learned the technique and broadened the acceptance of ultrasound through education.

DAVID P. BAHNER, MD, RDMS

When Bahner interviewed for an emergency medicine residency position at Ohio State in November 1994 (with James Hoekstra, MD, Douglas Rund, MD, and Dan Martin, MD), he did not have an answer for the question whether he wanted to go into academics or practice community medicine as he did not yet have the professional passion for his eventual career. Bahner knew he wanted to practice emergency medicine but had not yet set his eyes further on his future career in ultrasound, and at the time, no decision had been made about ultrasound.

Rund met with hospital leaders the following month, in December, to negotiate the future acquisition of the ACUSON 128XP ultrasound machine. There was still pushback despite the clear usefulness of the modality in obstetrics and trauma.

Beginning his residency in emergency medicine in 1995, Bahner continued his exploration of ultrasound throughout his training and on into the early part of his faculty career. Eventually and because of Rund's leadership, the ED finally received approval for an ultrasound machine, and Bahner used education as a way to initiate clinical practice discussions around its use. In theory, at least, education was a priority of all medical school faculty regardless of specialty. Over the next 2 decades of Bahner's career, he tried to find a variety of ways to integrate ultrasound into the undergraduate medical education curriculum. The eventual development of the Ultrasound Student Interest Group (USIG) was a key breakthrough made by empowering the medical students to get more involved and develop into future ultrasound leaders.

Bahner had felt the gaps in his own education in medical school with ultrasound and strived to create a better way. He used his academic career work to fill these gaps. Over time, this work helped promote and transform the use of ultrasound throughout the medical center from a tool from which images could only be acquired by a sonographer, vascular technologist, or echocardiographer and then read only by an imaging specialist to a Point of Care Ultrasound (POCUS) exam done in a variety of clinical settings. With POCUS any ultrasound-trained physician or provider caring for the patient at the point of care, usually the bedside, could perform a diagnostic ultrasound. This movement became known as POCUS, as covered in a 2011 *New England Journal of Medicine* article describing how almost all specialties use POCUS to care for patients.[21]

AMA HR 802-Scope of Practice and Credentialling—Dec 7, 1999

The early fight for "legitimacy" for using diagnostic ultrasound in the emergency department became contentious locally and nationally as traditional imaging specialists would clash with brash ED doctors who thought they could perform a focused ultrasound, save images, and generate a report, just like traditional imaging specialists in radiology and cardiology. This created animosity, as physicians of one specialty felt the other specialty was encroaching on their "turf." This sentiment and economic bullying motivated California ACEP members—led by Evelyn Cardenas, MD, who was Chair of National ACEP's Ultrasound Section, and in collaboration with urologists, presented a sentinel resolution at the Interim House of Delegates meeting in December, 1999 in San Diego. This resolution acknowledged the extensive application of ultrasound in medical practice and that its use was within the scope of practice of "appropriately trained physicians" (ie not limited to specific specialists). The resolution further stated that each specialty defines their own ultrasound scope of practice and that individual clinicians apply to local credentialing committees for ultrasound privileging.[22] This AMA Resolution 802 easily passed and became AMA policy. Among those voting for the resolution was Ohio State EM faculty member Richard Nelson, MD, who was a member of the Ohio delegation to the AMA House of Delegates.

AMA Resolution 802 was a game changer for the many emergency physicians who had been advocating for its expanded use and training in their field. The same night that 802 passed, Bahner was working with Steve Stack, MD, an EM resident at Ohio State and also an Ohio State medical school graduate. Stack had been politically active with the AMA since medical school and would eventually become AMA President, the first emergency physician to lead the AMA, in 2014. During their ED shift that night, Stack told Bahner about the AMA resolution on ultrasound that had just passed. The future of ultrasound in emergency medicine would never be the same.

Obtaining Advanced Ultrasound Certification

During his rotations at Riverside Methodist Hospital in the mid-1990s, Bahner met Jeff Bradley, RDMS. Bradley became an ultrasound mentor for Bahner, sharing many discussions about the field, new equipment, and techniques to improve image quality. Bradley told Bahner that if he wanted to acclimate into the ultrasound community, he needed to obtain his registered diagnostic medical sonography (RDMS) credential, a required credential for working in radiology and obstetrics ultrasound. Bahner pursued the RDMS certification, fulfilling the requirements to sit for the examination and began studying, using Hedrick's text on ultrasound physics[23] along with Rumack's two volume set on Diagnostic Ultrasound.[24] Bahner passed the RDMS certifying examination on January 26, 2000. Combined with his board certification in emergency medicine, this MD RDMS combination would establish him as a sonologist, a clinician who used and interpreted ultrasound for the care of patients.

At this time at the turn of the century, sonology was still an emerging field. Bahner and those like him would encounter roadblocks from a medical system not quite ready for what would become POCUS. The RDMS examination was a stopgap, based on radiology cases and ultrasound physics and was not specific to what Bahner saw on a daily basis in the ED. Now with an MD and an RDMS certification, Bahner networked with ultrasound experts from both the sonography side and the physician side as ultrasound's use expanded. These efforts paid off as Bahner participated in multiple conferences and met experts from around the world using ultrasound in unique ways for their patients. It was during these early years that Bahner conceptualized the idea for developing and expanding ultrasound education infrastructure at Ohio State.

Ultrasound Section of the Department of Emergency Medicine

After July 1998 when Bahner accepted a faculty position and agreed to lead the emergency ultrasound efforts, the hard work would begin. He became a focus for all things ultrasound in the Department of Emergency Medicine. While other faculty had ultrasound skills, few could take on the hours needed to teach ultrasound or help Bahner coordinate the various programs he was starting with medical students and residents. While writing a chapter for Hoekstra's book on cardiovascular emergencies, Bahner developed a novel ultrasound exam to assess the cause for hemorrhagic shock. What would develop into the Trinity protocol, this ultrasound approach to a patient in shock covered eight views of the torso that encompassed exams of the heart, aorta, and existing FAST scan.[25] He would later use this Trinity protocol to teach students how to use ultrasound to differentiate the cause of the patient in shock. Another early paper to address the quality of an ultrasound image, called the B QUIET assessment tool, focused on the elements of a "quality" ultrasound exam (e.g., depth and gain), elements that helped students and residents improve the quality of their saved ultrasound exams.[26]

As Bahner became more active at the national level presenting these papers and novel educational concepts and gained more expertise in the field, he became the de facto expert at the Ohio State Department of Emergency Medicine, and worked alongside colleagues in other departments and colleges, such as Allied Medicine, Engineering and Development, to promote ultrasound.

He also worked within the system to continue learning more about ultrasound and building experiences where others could learn and use ultrasound to help patients in the emergency department and medical center. A group of faculty members with ultrasound interest in the ED functioned as a section in the ED but had no formal governance until years later when the Division of Ultrasound medicine was formed. Bahner's early challenge during this period was to help EM faculty become trained with ultrasound, while at the same time train the residents and build a medical student experience toward a basic competency with ultrasound. No national models of these trainings existed, so Bahner and his team built each piece with novel curricula and innovative administrative solutions. All were important for the long-term growth of the ultrasound program.

Challenges remained. For one, faculty were some of the hardest to train and educate about ultrasound, which had not been a normal part of their own medical education in medical school or residency. Second, while the ultrasound machines used advanced technology, their sophistication meant they were not always intuitive to operate.

Bahner worked on simplifying the process of understanding ultrasound and developed steps to understand the physics behind ultrasound as a mechanical wave needing matter to travel through, and how that was different than electromagnetic waves like X-rays. He taught the fundamentals of echogenicity of ultrasound. Ultrasound beams passed through fluid without causing a reflection. On CT and X-ray, however fluid was white and reflected the beams of the X-ray. On ultrasound white indicated a high-density object such as bone or the calyceal portion of the kidney, or low density like air, which readily reflected echoes and appeared bright white (hyperechoic). Air on X-ray or CT was black while black on ultrasound was fluid(anechoic). These simple statements could cause much confusion and despite the utility and ubiquity of ultrasound, it remains "operator dependent" because these concepts need to be reinforced over time with spaced repetition and much practice.

These properties were confusing to novice ultrasound learners, however, and Bahner found methods to teach the basics of ultrasound. He began many of the presentations with the same principles of three colors of ultrasound (black, gray, white), four sides to the image and five probe motions to acquire B mode images. Brightness mode was the grayscale image that allowed reflections from tissues in the body to produce the high-resolution images that continued to improve as the technology advanced over the years. M mode was motion mode and was used to detect fetal heart rates and lung sliding and allowed the operator to take a slice of a B mode image and watch it move over time. The other two modes commonly used in ultrasound were color doppler that demonstrated the presence of blood flow and direction and pulsed wave doppler that quantified the velocity of flow and gave an audible output that could easily distinguish artery from vein.

These ultrasound basics were not always taught to students and residents across the country and Bahner's focus on solidifying the basic training served him well as he introduced new curricula for students, residents, and fellows eager to learn how ultrasound could help them in patient care. Bahner was determined to integrate ultrasound into the medical education infrastructure at Ohio State and tried to work with new succeeding iterations of leadership, including when the deans and leaders changed multiple times over the quarter of a century he was a faculty member. He himself would have to grow and change from a senior resident with interest, to a determined junior and then senior faculty member dedicated to integrate ultrasound into education, research and clinical care in the Department of Emergency Medicine.

At the graduate medical education (GME) level, an ultrasound rotation for emergency medicine residents began in 1999. The rotation was immensely popular. Fellows from the Surgical Intensive Care Unit (SICU) and residents from anesthesiology and internal medicine clamored for the opportunity to learn in the rotation. Several EM residents were outstanding during their rotations, including resident Creagh Boulger, MD. Her work ethic, professionalism and can-do attitude made her an exceptional faculty candidate. Bahner recruited Boulger to join as faculty in the department's ultrasound efforts—he knew her energy and technical savvy would be instrumental in building the program from where he had started it. Bahner and Boulger would later go on to launch a much-needed fellowship in ultrasound and worked to recruit ultrasound fellows and build the ultrasound program one graduate at a time.

CREAGH T. BOULGER, MD

Creagh T. Boulger, MD, began her academic career following EM residency at Ohio State (2008-2011) with a passion for education (Figure 1). She soon gravitated towards ultrasound as her academic niche. In her first year, her focus was primarily on medical student education, using the concept of gaming to build student knowledge. She began with the existing Ultrasound Olympics, which evolved into Ultrafest, a now immensely popular annual event at Ohio State and in the Midwest that attracts more than 200 students a year from surrounding states for a day of ultrasound education and games. Gamification eventually became a cornerstone of Boulger's career.

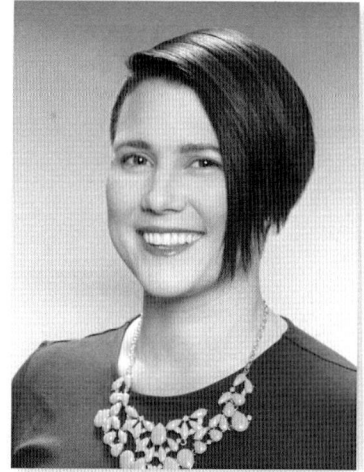

Figure 1: Creagh T. Boulger, MD, Professor of Emergency Medicine, was a graduate of the Ohio State emergency medicine residency program and rose to prominence in many areas of the specialty, including emergency medical services, trauma and ultrasound.

Boulger has been active at the national level with Sonogames through the Society of Academic Emergency Medicine (SAEM) and Sonoslam[27] at the American Institute of Ultrasound Medicine (AIUM). With interests in trauma, emergency medical services and sexual assault survivors, Boulger developed professional connections across the university and throughout the world. She lectured worldwide on gaming in education. In 2017 she was awarded Professor of the Year by the Ohio State University College of Medicine graduating fourth year class in honor of her passion for education.

As her career evolved, Boulger shifted some of her focus to ultrasound's administrative component, helping the division expand its fellowship offerings to family medicine and pediatrics in her tenure as fellowship director. She also became an inaugural member of the Emergency Ultrasound Fellowship Accreditation Council. In this role she became involved in the first cycle of national fellowship accreditation. While in her residency, Boulger not only mastered the technical skill of acquiring tough ultrasound images, she gave extra effort in the administrative quality assurance part of the rotation that Bahner initially built. Later as a new faculty member, she contributed immensely to the professionalization of the body of ultrasound knowledge at Ohio State. With the expansion of the original emergency medicine ultrasound fellowship to include other specialties in primary care and pediatrics, the fellowship grew under her leadership.

Boulger was promoted to full Professor in 2022. Characterized as the type of leader who would advance ultrasound education, training, and practice at Ohio State, Boulger essentially revolutionized the residency ultrasound training, the tracking and navigation of the milestones and the senior credentialing letters. As the program grew, Boulger used her technical savvy to make instructional videos and PowerPoints and to communicate digitally across many forums. Boulger's work with Carmen, the Ohio State learning management system, and Q Path, the ultrasound documentation middleware, distinguished her efforts into measurable outcomes. Her residency curricular efforts would be described in the literature for the resident track[28] and the advanced track, including the Ohio State residency curriculum she directed.

In addition to her fellowship lead and progress in updating the residency curriculum, Boulger became the second advisor for the Ultrasound Interest Group (USIG) and the sponsoring faculty for Ultrafest each year. An expert educator, Boulger easily connected with others and mentored many students. She was enthusiastic, knowledgeable, able to make sound decisions and able to identify and treat common conditions with a human touch. Her administrative leadership in EM was also recognized by hospital Medical Director Andrew Thomas, MD, who asked Boulger to lead the Interdisciplinary Point of Care Ultrasound Committee (I POCUS) with Scott Holliday, MD, the Associate Dean of Graduate Medical Education at Ohio State.

As the director leading I POCUS, Boulger's persistent advocacy for ultrasound quality led her to steward medical center systemwide credentialing for ultrasound, handheld device policies and a team-based approach to what had been contentious two decades previously. In retrospect, the Bahner and Boulger "one-two punch" was finally able to achieve what Bahner had envisioned early in his academic career. Focused ultrasound had become POCUS and was being taught and used throughout the medical center in a coordinated fashion to help patient care. In all components, Boulger was the brains and brawn behind I POCUS and its subsequent successes. Acquiring funding from the medical center and medical school were successes for Boulger even though the convoluted process took more than four years. The I POCUS framework was set for future collaboration, education and success for years to come.

The logistics of running the EM US program and administrating a professional program for training and revenue generation in the clinical setting were enormous. Bahner and Boulger became a team to lead these efforts but it became apparent early on that Boulger was a unique leader in her own right. She had built her national reputation with Sonogames at SAEM and her Sonoslam innovation at AIUM. Now with her leading I POCUS at Ohio State and expanding the US fellowship to other disciplines, she was promoting ultrasound to impact patient care far outside of the emergency department.

The Medical Student Ultrasound Interest Group

Ultrasound was known to be operator dependent, meaning it was an important challenge for the learner to learn and scan with aplomb and acumen. It was difficult, however, because the many knobs and components could confuse the uninitiated, and the techniques could be quite daunting for the residency graduate who would likely join a practice group where expertise in ultrasound was expected. It was up to the new clinician to catch up and take the necessary time and attention to learn and practice.

Bahner knew that if he was going to solve this gap in ultrasound education, he would need to come up with a long-term plan and focus on mentorship. This meant starting with basic programs beginning year one in medical school and develop advanced ultrasound opportunities for the most motivated of students and residents. Eventually both students and residents were brought together on ultrasound projects, many of which became publications focused on ultrasound education, innovations, curricula and clinical cases.

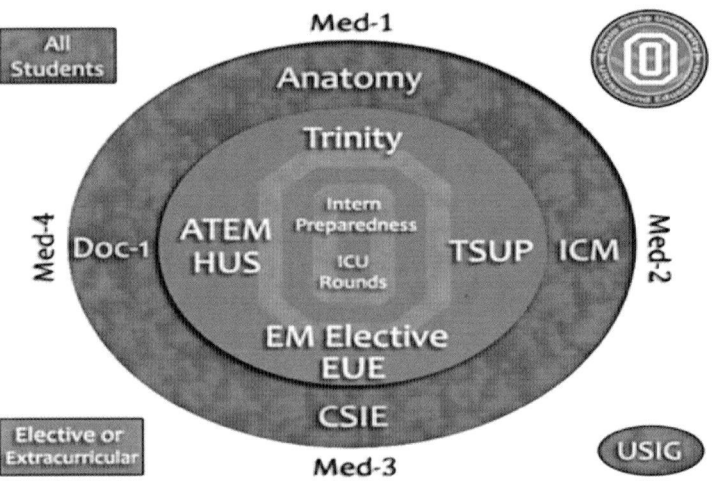

Figure 2: This schematic illustrates the medical student courses per year open for all students and those in the center that are elective or extracurricular for the more motivated students. This 2000-2010 framework existed before USIG modified the extracurricular ultrasound offerings to allow all students to participate regardless of year of training into basic, intermediate and advanced ultrasound training.

Medical students had many ways to get involved with ultrasound outside of the curriculum and these paths became more sophisticated each year. In 2006, the Ultrasound Sound Interest Group (USIG) was formed, with medical students serving as formal group leaders and members of the executive committee to also serve later. This group was responsible for parts of the extracurricular sessions to develop core competencies in ultrasound. The extracurricular ultrasound offerings were initially offered to each class each year, but did not allow students to catch up if they did not get involved in the first year.

As the program progressed, student leaders decided to collate the educational offerings into groups of graded learning from basic to advanced. These courses became known as basic ultrasound (BUS), intermediate ultrasound (IUS) and advanced ultrasound (AUS). Curricula were developed with saved lectures, protocols, guides and materials on the website, www.osuultrasound.com. When the new programs opened to the entire student body, the third-year student who was not ready to participate in Years 1 or 2, could easily find US education through USIG and BUS (Figure 2).

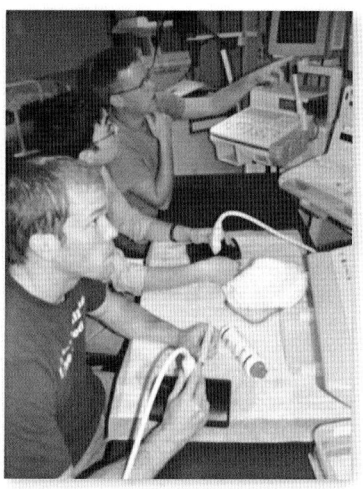

Figure 3: Medical students practice vascular access in the Clinical Skills Education and Assessment Center in the basement of Prior Hall.

Bahner's goal was to work with medical students and provide them with opportunities so they could participate in the excitement surrounding point of care ultrasound. He created them systematically, providing curricular and extracurricular options for every year of medical school, helping multiple students participate in the various programs as they progressed from year to year. For the most motivated of students during their fourth year, Bahner developed an honors ultrasound program and published this novel curriculum in *Academic Medicine* (Figure 3).[29] Many of these students went on to become leaders after medical school, noting that the ultrasound experiences helped shape their careers.

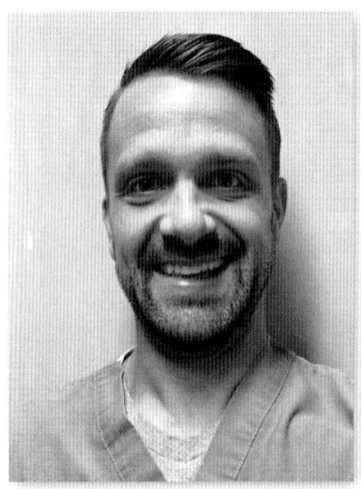

Figure 4: As a medical student, Matthew Blickendorf, MD, was one of many who helped contribute to the Ohio State ultrasound culture through his continued participation, innovation, and leadership. He served as Chief Resident in Emergency Medicine and received the Clinical Excellence Award and the Top Pediatric Resident Award at graduation in 2015.

One medical student, Matt Blickendorf, was attracted to the ultrasound program as a way to gain early access to patient care and hands-on clinical teaching (Figure 4). Blickendorf served as a trained simulated ultrasound patient (TSUP) as a second-year student and continued to learn ultrasound through his clinical years. While an honors ultrasound student, Blickendorf worked with Bahner to develop a formal curriculum for TSUPs and published this work in the *Journal of Ultrasound in Medicine* in 2014.[30] Perhaps his greatest contribution to the Division of US at Ohio State was his work in codifying the terms of probe motions for efficient bedside teaching and learner feedback.[31] AIUM invited Blickendorf to present this work in 2014; it was published in 2016. Throughout residency he regularly served as instructor of POCUS for medical students and fellow residents in the ED and ICU.

Another key figure in the US program at Ohio State was Eric Adkins, MD, who completed his residency in Emergency Medicine and Internal Medicine at Christiana Hospital in Delaware, where he worked with renowned national leaders in the field. Adkins entered the pulmonary and critical care fellowship at Ohio State and then joined the faculty in both Emergency Medicine and Internal Medicine. Adkins worked with Bahner to develop a curriculum for the pulmonary fellows including a checkout exam at the end of the Pulmonary and Critical Care fellowship.

Adkins and Bahner worked together on ICU rounds where fellows could scan with Bahner and Adkins on interesting ICU patients. Adkins would change the culture of US in the MICU and worked with trauma surgeon Stan Stawicki, MD, in the Surgical Intensive Care Unit (SICU) on ultrasound research in the critically ill. Bahner, Boulger and Adkins went on to author a number of clinical ultrasound papers with Stawicki and their surgical colleagues to continue promoting ultrasound use in the critically ill to assess volume status.[32, 33] Adkins became the Medical Director of the emergency department and a respected intensive care physician. Later he also became one of the experts in information technology within the institution and ultimately the Vice Chair for Clinical Affairs in the Department of Emergency Medicine.

Sonographers were not available at all hours for focused exams in the ICUs similar to the emergency department. Bedside ultrasonography still had to be mastered by the physicians caring for the patient at the time it was needed. After a series of discussions with medical center leadership, Bahner finally began receiving financial support for his ultrasound teaching in critical care unit of the hospital including the ICUs.

Division of Ultrasound in the Department of Emergency Medicine

In May 2017 the combined diverse funding sources—from the College of Medicine, Graduate Medical Education, billing for the professional services of fellows working in the emergency department, and other funds—set the foundation for a solvent enterprise within the Department of Emergency Medicine: The Division of Ultrasound Medicine. The Ultrasound Division was the first division within the Department of Emergency Medicine. Since then, advanced emergency ultrasonography has become an official ABEM board certification. With the successful launch in March 2022 of the certifying exam for a Focused Practice Designation (FPD) in Advanced Emergency Medicine Ultrasonography (AEMUS), the pathway for advanced ultrasound certification in emergency medicine now exists.

Within emergency medicine, ultrasound has become a subspecialty indeed. The growth of the emergency medicine practitioner and the development of the ultrasonologist or POCUS practitioner has been the academic aim since the beginning of the Ohio State EM ultrasound program. Currently, Ohio State medical students can learn and practice ultrasound in all three parts of the Lead. Serve. and Inspire. (LSI) curriculum, as well as participate in an advanced ultrasound competency. Ultrasound is prominent at the graduate medical education level during intern orientation in addition to ED ultrasound rotations during the three-year residency. After residency, an ultrasound fellowship is ideal for those residency graduates with an academic career goal. Staying on as faculty and having a practice in emergency ultrasound increases expertise. Now with board certification, the end point of a career dedicated to EM and ultrasound is feasible.

Emergency physicians require the ability to take care of the sickest patients in time sensitive windows for optimal care on a daily basis. Ultrasound helps in that effort in many ways, such as visualizing the heart and assessing its function or using US to guide a needle, start a line, insert a catheter, drain a fluid collection, as well as determine hydronephrosis, pneumothorax, the presence of an intrauterine pregnancy and a number of pertinent EM procedures.[34, 35] In emergency care, this can apply to a number of disease processes that can cause traumatic, cardiopulmonary, or multiorgan collapse.

Funding for the new Ultrasound Division included institutional support for a fellowship director, professional fees from clinical exams, institutional support for training house staff throughout the hospital, and agreement with other departments to provide ultrasound instruction to faculty and residents. To bill and receive professional fees, a detailed quality assurance program had to be in place. Scans had to be properly performed and recorded. Timely documentation from residents and faculty were needed and oversight was required by the division faculty team. These processes take considerable time to oversee and physicians need to be reminded constantly to complete their charts. While the technical efficiency has improved with middleware software, refining the process of billing and collection remains a priority.

The effective practice of emergency medicine now requires competency in ultrasound. All the faculty are now credentialed according to the 2016 ACEP ultrasound guidelines. All residents participate in a graduate medical education (GME) ultrasound curriculum to fulfill requirements to generate a certifying letter at graduation according to individual ultrasound skill and competency.

In 2023 the Ultrasound Division hired a new coordinator and entered the year with much momentum. The ultrasound fellowship has two

EM ultrasound fellows and a primary care ultrasound fellow who started in 2023. The division faculty continue to make a presence in the medical school, medical center and in the practice of medicine at Ohio State.

As Bahner's vision of an integrated ultrasound education ecosystem at Ohio State became a reality with Boulger's implementation of an Institutional Point of Care Ultrasound program (I POCUS), the stage is set for even greater growth. Now learners from students, residents, fellows and faculty have institutional resources, equipment, websites, simulators and courses available to learn and practice ultrasound. Striving to impact patient care with novel uses of ultrasound, Bahner, Boulger and their team in the ultrasound community at Ohio State continue to promote ultrasound education for the ultimate goal of improved, evidenced-based patient care.

References

1. Neuweiler G. *The Biology of Bats*. Oxford University Press; 2000:140.

2. Kane D, et al. A brief history of musculoskeletal ultrasound: 'from bats and ships to babies and hips.' *Rheumatology*. July 2004;43(7):931-933.

3. Griffin D, Galambos R. The sensory basis of obstacle avoidance by flying bats. *J Exp Zool A Ecol Integr Physio*. April 1941;86(3):481–505.

4. Dussik KT. On the possibility of using ultrasound waves as a diagnostic aid. *Neurol Psychiat*. 1942;174:153-68. (In German).

5. Shampo M, Kyle R. Karl Theodore Dussik—pioneer in ultrasound. *Mayo Clinic Proceedings*. December 1, 1995; 70(12):1136.

6. Donald I, MacVicar J, Brown TG. Investigations of abdominal masses by pulsed ultrasound. *The Lancet*. 1958;271:1188–1195.

7. Kurjak A. Ultrasound scanning-Prof Ian Donald (1910-1987). *Eur J. Obstet Gynecol Reprod Biol.* 2000;90:187-9.

8. McDonald KG, Leopold GR. Ultrasound B-scanning in the differentiation of Baker's cyst and thrombophlebitis. *Br J Radiol.* 1972;45:729-32.

9. Chase SP, Freimanis AK. Abdominal echography. *Ohio State Med J.* 1971; Oct;67(10):901-6.

10. Goodwin D. Personal communication. 2023.

11. Mateer J, et al. Model curriculum for physician training in emergency ultrasonography. *Ann Emerg Med.* 1994;23:95-102.

12. Jarawenko DG, et al. Ultrasonography in the initial evaluation and follow up of blunt abdominal trauma. https://surgjournal.com. 1985.

13. Gruessner R, Mentges B, Duber CH, Ruckert K, Rothmund M. Sonography versus peritoneal lavage in blunt abdominal trauma. *J Trauma.* 1989; 29: 242-244.

14. Watanabe H. History of ultrasound in nephrourology. *Ultrasound Med Biol.* April 2001;27(4):447-53. doi: 10.1016/s0301-5629(00)00352-5.

15. Erjavic, N. Ian Donald (1910–1987). *Embryo Project Encyclopedia* (2018-01-30). ISSN: 1940-5030 http://embryo.asu.edu/handle/10776/13050.

16. Goldberg B. Gilbert Baum, MD, 1922–2002: A pioneer in ultrasound. *J. Med. Ultrasound.* First published June 1, 2003;22(6). https://doi.org/10.7863/jum.2003.22.6.660

17. Baum G, Greenwood I. A critique of time-amplitude ultrasonography. *Arch Ophthalmol.* March 1961;65(3):353-365. doi:10.1001/archopht.1961.01840020355007

18. Edler I, Lindström K. The history of echocardiography. *Ultrasound Med Biol.* 2004;30:1565-644.

19. Baker DW. Pulsed ultrasonic blood flow sensing. *IEEE Trans Sonics Ultrasonics.* 1969;17:170.

20. Wild JJ, Reid JM. Diagnostic use of ultrasound. *Br J Phys Med*. Nov 1956;19(11):248-57.

21. Moore CL, Copel JA. Point-of-care ultrasonography. *N Engl J Med*. 2011; Feb 24;364(8):749-57. doi: 10.1056/NEJMra0909487.

22. American Medical Association HR 802. December 7, 1999. Privileging for Ultrasound Imaging H-230.960

23. Hedrick, Hykes, Starchman. *Ultrasound Physics and Instrumentation*. 1st ed. Mosby;1995.

24. Rumack, Wilson, Charboneau. *Diagnostic Ultrasound*. 2nd ed. Mosby; 1998: Vol 1, 2.

25. Bahner DP. Trinity: A hypotensive ultrasound protocol. *J Diagn Med Sonogr*. 2002 July;18(4).

26. Bahner DP, Adkins EJ, Nagel R, Way D, Werman HA, Royall NA. Brightness mode quality ultrasound imaging examination technique (B-QUIET): quantifying quality in ultrasound imaging. *J Ultrasound Med*. 2011 Dec;30(12):1649-55. doi: 10.7863/jum.2011.30.12.1649.

27. Boulger C, Liu RB, De Portu G, Theyyunni N, Lewis M, Lewiss RE, Soucy ZP, Dinh VA, Chiem A, Singhal S, Di Salvo D, Pellerito JS, Bahner D. A National Point-of-Care Ultrasound Competition for Medical Students. *J Ultrasound Med*. 2019 Jan;38(1):253-258. doi: 10.1002/jum.14670.

28. Boulger C, Adams DZ, Hughes D, Bahner DP, King A. Longitudinal ultrasound education track curriculum implemented within an emergency medicine residency program. *J Ultrasound Med*. 2017 Jun;36(6):1245-1250. doi: 10.7863/ultra.16.08005.

29. Bahner DP, Royall NA. Advanced ultrasound training for fourth-year medical students: a novel training program at The Ohio State University College of Medicine. *Acad Med*. 2013 Feb;88(2):206-13. doi: 10.1097/ACM.0b013e31827c562d.

30. Blickendorf JM, Adkins EJ, Boulger C, Bahner DP. Trained simulated ultrasound patients: medical students as models, learners, and teachers. *J Ultrasound Med.* 2014 Jan;33(1):35-8. doi: 10.7863/ultra.33.1.35.

31. Bahner DP, Blickendorf JM, Bockbrader M, Adkins E, Vira A, Boulger C, Panchal AR. Language of transducer manipulation: codifying terms for effective teaching. *J Ultrasound Med.* 2016 Jan;35(1):183-8. doi: 10.7863/ultra.15.02036.

32. Kent A, Bahner DP, Boulger CT, Eiferman DS, Adkins EJ, Evans DC, Springer AN, Balakrishnan JM, Valiaveedan S, Galwankar S, Njoku C, Lindsey DE, Yeager S, Roelant GJ, Stawicki SPA. Sonographic evaluation of intravascular volume status in the surgical intensive care unit: a prospective comparison of subclavian vein and inferior vena cava collapsibility index. *J Surg Res.* 2013 Sep;184(1):561-6. doi: 10.1016/j.jss.2013.05.040.

33. Stawicki SPA, Adkins EJ, Eiferman DS, Evans DC, Ali NA, Njoku C, Lindsey DE, Cook CH, Balakrishnan JM, Valiaveedan S, Galwankar SC, Boulger CT, Springer AN, Bahner DP. Prospective evaluation of intravascular volume status in critically ill patients: does inferior vena cava collapsibility correlate with central venous pressure? *J Trauma Acute Care Surg.* 2014 Apr;76(4):956-63; discussion 963-4. doi: 10.1097/TA.0000000000000152.

34. Mateer JR, Plummer D, Heller M, Olson D, Jehle D, Overton D, Gussow L. Model curriculum for physician training in emergency ultrasonography. *Ann Emerg Med.* 1994 Jan;23(1): 95-102. doi: 10.1016/s0196-0644(94)70014-1.

35. Mateer JR, Jehle. Ultrasonography in emergency medicine. *Acad Emerg Med.* 1994 Mar-Apr;1(2):149-52. doi: 10.1111/j.1 2712. 1994.tb02746.x

Chapter 23
Diversity, Equity and Inclusion

Diane L. Gorgas, MD

"The greater the diversity, the greater the perfection."
— Thomas Berry, Catholic priest*

The Department of Emergency Medicine at The Ohio State University has had an ever-advancing commitment to diversity, equity and inclusion. Historically, this pledge was demonstrated in an openness to consider applications and interest from diverse faculty and residents, but as this chapter shows, it has now morphed into active efforts to increase diversity in all aspects of the department.

Gender Diversity

"None of us can know what we are capable of until we are tested."
— Elizabeth Blackwell, MD, first woman medical school graduate, 1849

The "Firsts"

In 1849, Elizabeth Blackwell became the first woman to graduate from medical school in the United States.[1] Blackwell was a fierce advocate for indigent women and children, and often facing resistance from male physicians who barred her from practicing at their institutions.

Women have made great strides in medicine since then, yet the "firsts" among women in medicine are still fairly recent. The first woman resident in the Emergency Medicine residency training program at Ohio State was Cheryl Lee, MD, in 1986. When Lee began her training, there were no women in the program. It was not until she completed her training that more women had joined the residency. Now, still practicing emergency medicine, Lee recalled her time at Ohio State:

> *I was the only woman in the program for one year...until Teresa Bridges [1987] joined a year later. When I was a senior, we participated in the interviews, and I remember interviewing my successors, Susan Churchill [1989] and Linda Robinson [1989]. I am not sure Doug (Dr. Rund) knew what to do with us, particularly on outside rotations like toxicology where there were dress codes. We didn't wear ties, and skirts and heels were impractical. Can you imagine trying to work in heels? It was torture. I think that because the Chair's (Dr. Martin Keller's) wife Geraldine was an academic, she had our backs.[2]*

The first woman faculty member in the department was Linda Robinson, MD. Robinson's faculty career started at Case Western Reserve University but she shortly returned to Columbus and became a pioneer in Emergency Medicine (EM), a specialty where few women were trained and even fewer went on to become academic faculty. Tragically she lost a battle to cancer and passed away in 2017. Today, a scholarship in her name honoring her leadership is awarded each year to a graduating medical student who matches in EM at Ohio State.

Another Ohio State Department of Emergency Medicine first was Diane L. Gorgas, MD, the first woman faculty member to be promoted within the department, both as associate and subsequently the first woman at a full professor rank. Gorgas also is the first female program Director of the residency in Emergency Medicine at Ohio State. Creagh Boulger, MD, was the first woman fellowship director (Ultrasound) and Lauren Southerland, MD, was the first woman awarded a National Institutes of Health grant in the department.

Southerland was also the first clinical researcher in the department. Breaking into a male-dominated specialty with an even greater proportion of male researchers speaks to her groundbreaking career in the research realm. Her leadership allowed the Ohio State Main ED to gain "Level 1 Geriatric Emergency Department Accreditation" (GEDA).

Women have held clinical leadership roles at the Ohio State Main and East campuses throughout the more recent eras in the department's history, including Lauren Southerland, MD, Director of the Observation Unit; Maegan Reynolds, MD, Director of Emergency Oncology at Ohio State Main; and Sondra "Soni" Shellman, MD, Associate Medical Director at Ohio State East.

Ohio State East has been a particularly strong community of accomplished women emergency physicians. Shellman has spoken of the success of women working at the Ohio State East clinical site:

> *When I consider the women on faculty at OSU East, I think that we were at times in our career with even young children or perhaps a young marriage. And we were allowed to do that, encouraged to do that. East was a site that was and remains flexible. Once the demands of home or personal life lightened, you took on a project or two, mostly to help the cause of a department that had helped you—a department you believed in because it believed in you. I think that's a philosophy that I learned from Mike [Dick, medical director of the ED] and try to employ as much as possible.*[3]

"*The first rule of the Dunning-Kruger club is you don't know you're a member of the Dunning-Kruger club. People miss that.*"[4]

— *David Dunning, PhD, American social psychologist and professor of psychology, University of Michigan*

The Dunning-Kruger effect, as first published by David Dunning and Justin Kruger in 1999, is a theory that there is a cognitive bias whereby people with limited knowledge or competence in a given intellectual or social domain greatly overestimate their own knowledge or competence in that domain relative to objective criteria or to the performance of their peers or of people in general.[4] The meta-cognition of social inequities for women in the department was unrecognized and parity was assumed, but as the number and productivity of women in the department grew, the potential for inequities caught the attention of leadership.

As such potentials surfaced, under the leadership of Douglas Rund,

MD, a Parity and Equity Committee was convened. The goal of the committee was to: 1) identify metrics that could demonstrate parity and equity between women and men physicians in the department; 2) create an action plan to achieve parity in these areas, if any inequities were discovered; and 3) develop interventions to reach the goal of parity. Metrics from the committee showed disparities in the rate of advancement and likelihood of women moving into leadership in the department, and delays in promotion of women faculty.

Very few efforts at achieving parity of an under-representative group in medicine are successful without a majority member group champion. For the Parity and Equity committee, those men were Nicholas Kman, MD, Howard Werman, MD, and Daniel Bachmann, MD. Their commitment to the cause of elevating women faculty to an equal level as men was critical in the metrics the department now demonstrates today (see page 556, on "The Department Today"). Regarding their work as allies, Kman recalled his thinking at the time:

> *I learned quickly that if people in our group weren't happy, the organization was not healthy. I realized that I could best function in the role of an ally as I learned more about becoming an advocate in this space.*[5]

Werman discussed his motivation for being part of the early leadership in saying this:

> *I got involved because the history of the department, including its early policies, were developed by a leadership that was male dominated and not racially diverse. As we became more gender diverse, it was important to hear and support the perspectives of our younger female colleagues who were becoming a greater percentage of our faculty.*[6]

Bachmann recalled: "I think the pay and promotion advances that have occurred to bring opportunities more into alignment across gender/race are the greatest success."[7]

Their efforts not only advocated for formal recognition of advancement and leadership, but also a "down-in-the-trenches" day in and day out accounting for language, attitudes and culture that supported parity for women. Both the men and women faculty were encouraged to "lean in" to the discussions in meetings, the clinical environment, and teaching sessions when sexist language or attitudes was used to call out these instances in the moment and suggest non-sexist alternatives.[8]

The departmental efforts and action plan would not have been nearly as successful without a champion outside of the department as well. Quinn Capers IV, MD, an interventional cardiologist who was Associate Dean for Admissions at the Ohio State College of Medicine and Vice Dean for Faculty Affairs, served as that advocate and catalyst. Along with The Women's Place at Ohio State, he led gender divided groups in the department through Implicit Bias Training, and raised the cultural awareness of the perspectives and voices of both sets of colleagues in the department. Focused mentorship programs followed along with efforts to increase gender diversity in search practices for new faculty. These efforts, along with the progressive leadership of both Mark Angelos, MD, and Jeffrey Caterino, MD, resulted in closing the gender gap by moving women into more supervisory and leadership positions as opposed to "assistant" positions.

Ethnic Diversity

*"If not us, then who?
If not now, then when?"*

— John Lewis, American politician, civil rights activist and
U.S. Representative for Georgia's 5th congressional district, 1987-2020

The population of the city of Columbus and Franklin County as a whole is one of the most ethnically diverse areas in the nation. Census data show that Central Ohio has more foreign-born residents than any other region in the state, and the population continues to grow. Around 150,000 residents of Franklin County (11% of the population) were born outside the United States, the highest total of any Ohio county. In Columbus, the number exceeds 13%. Refugee populations in the city include those from Somalia, Nepal, The Democratic of Congo and Bhutan.

The emergency departments at Ohio State Main and East see a diverse population. In the last academic year, the Department of Emergency Medicine at the main campus saw over 25% Black patients whereas Ohio State East's percentage was more than 65%. Four to ten percent of the Ohio State ED patients identify as Latina/Latino annually. If our goal as physicians is to be able to deliver culturally competent and synesthetic care, striving to reflect the ethnic complexity of our population must be our goal as caregivers.

The Ohio State College of Medicine's commitment to ethnic diversity reaches back long before racial disparities and social injustices came to the forefront of the nation's consciousness with the murder of George Floyd in 2020. The College has been on the front lines of increasing diversity in its faculty and training programs, and has deliberately moved the needle by increasing the number of ethnically diverse students in the pipeline. Specific programs and deliberate measures have been developed, including "MD Camp," a program offered to low-income high school students to foster an interest in medicine.

The College also received the 2021 Insight into Diversity Health Professions Higher Education Excellence in Diversity (HEED) Award, and holds the distinction of being the 14th most racially integrated medical school in the United States, including among Historically Black Colleges and Universities. Annually, the College recruits incoming classes with at least 25% representation of under-represented ethnic populations in medicine

The Department of Emergency Medicine was similarly an early adopter of diversity values and initiatives. Gorgas received the university's Shining Star award in 2014 for her efforts at recruiting the most diverse EM residency training class in the history of Ohio State graduate medical education and nationally among EM. She was also the keynote speaker at the Society of Academic Emergency Medicine's Academy of Diversity and Inclusion in Emergency Medicine conference, discussing her success and strategy for increasing diversity in the program. Since then, the Associate Dean of Graduate Medical Education, Scott Holiday, MD, developed a second look program for ethnically under-represented minoritized groups in medicine (URMs) and Lesbian, Gay, Bisexual, Transgender and Queer (LGBTQ) students with an interest in Ohio State as a residency training location. The program comprised a funded return to the medical center for a more in-depth look at the training programs.

The department applied the same philosophy in moving towards an ethnically and racially representative faculty with respect to finding champions, within our department and from without. An invitation to speak at the residency program's grand rounds was extended to Sheryl Heron, MD, MPH, Associate Dean for Community Engagement, Equity & Inclusion and Vice Chair of Faculty Equity, Engagement and Empowerment in Emergency Medicine at Emory University. At Ohio State, Heron spoke of her own experience:

> *My origins are I was the first black woman at Emory University College of Medicine. My parents came to the United States the year Martin Luther King was assassinated, but I didn't start my career thinking I wanted to be a DEI expert. It was hard to ignore that when I came in when there were no people who looked like me. The Black woman, the Jamaican – it all helps me serve many of the people who look like me in the ED.*[9]

Heron challenged the audience, the leadership and the faculty in examining the role of diversity in our setting. How committed were we? What concrete steps were we taking to address the issue? Did minoritized applicants to any rank or position feel that we as a department were "truly invested in you and your potential"?

In addition, Capers and Leon McDougle, MD, MPH, Chief Diversity Officer for the Ohio State Medical Center and Associate Dean for Diversity and Inclusion for the College of Medicine, were invaluable resources to the department in understanding perspective on the need for diversity and helping to break down the barriers while intentionally seeking diversity for trainees and faculty.

The pendulum moving towards a more diverse faculty had begun its swing. The intentional building of a culture accepting and valuing diverse candidates began. This was not an effort at implementing "tokenism", but rather a concerted movement to recruit faculty who could better mirror our patients and increase cultural competency of all faculty. Skills and abilities remained the center focus for choosing faculty and searching for these diverse candidates who represented excellence in the practice of Emergency Medicine and also brought a perspective of diversity had to be well-devised and intentional.

The Dean of the College of Medicine, Carol Bradford, MD, recommended that all departments create a Vice Chair position for Diversity, Equity and Inclusion (DEI). Caterino, as chair, went above and beyond College of Medicine practices and completed a national search for a leader in DEI to serve as Vice Chair. The search was a significant educational experience for the department as we considered the highest quality and most advanced leaders in emergency medicine DEI nationally. The department welcomed Henry Young, MD, from the University of Florida as the new Vice Chair in 2022 (Figure 1). Young spoke about the Ohio State commitment to DEI efforts and his motivation:

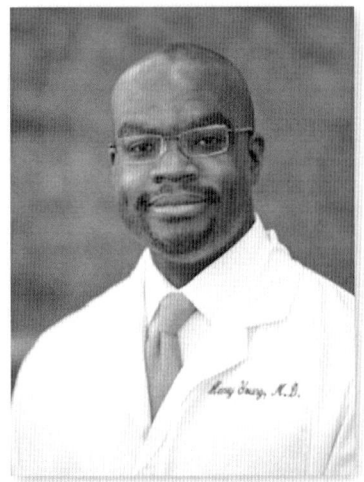

Figure 1: Henry Young, MD, became Vice Chair of Diversity, Equity and Inclusion in the Department of Emergency Medicine in 2022.

> *I took the job at OSU because the department and institution were already well established in the field of diversity long before 2020, and nationally recognized for what they were doing—that combined with Columbus being such a diverse city – 12.5% are foreign born and 15% speak English as a 2nd language. I love seeing beautiful cultures and ethnicities mix here. I find there is still room to innovate in the area of DEI, and that this innovation is supported from the top down. I have always been very interested in mentorship and I am finding my path moving more and more toward marginalized groups. COVID was a motivator for me since I lost a lot of loved ones and friends who were young, and I realized time was short. I had the opportunity to do something meaningful to make a better future for the nation and for my children. Creating diverse workspaces and giving people a voice, especially for people who don't usually have a voice, makes us stronger.*[10]

Young was an outstanding addition to the department faculty. In his own words he recalled his career:

> *I became enamored with science from his parents. My mother was a special education teacher and my father a family medicine physician in rural Georgia. Both were very active in serving their community. Following*

my father's footsteps, I attended medical school at the Medical College of Georgia and completed emergency medicine residency at the University of Florida where I served as Chief Resident in my final year. After residency, I completed an NIH NIDA T32 Post-Doctoral Research Fellowship at the University of Florida Substance Abuse Training Center in Public Health. As Vice Chair of Diversity, Equity and Inclusion in the Department of Emergency Medicine, my passions include diversity, health care equity and community engagement. I believe that with meaningful community engagement I can use my position to advocate more effectively for the community that I serve and promote equitable health care for all.[8]

Other early champions and pioneers in diversity in Emergency Medicine include Jennah Morgan, MD, who joined the faculty in 2021 from King's County, New York, where she completed training in both emergency medicine and internal medicine (Figure 2). She spoke of her choice to practice emergency medicine "We're in a unique position to help vulnerable people. Illness makes people honest. When you're sick, you're sick and illness makes everyone the same."[11]

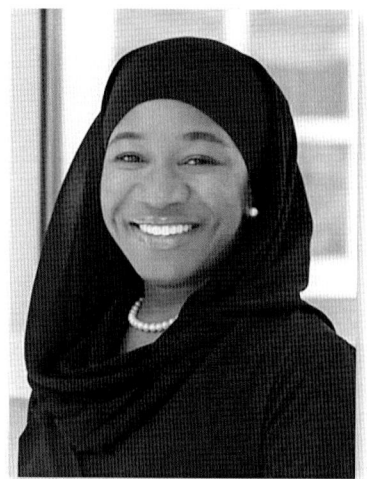

Figure 2: Jennah A. Morgan, MD, Assistant Professor of Emergency Medicine and Internal Medicine works as both an emergency physician and a hospitalist at Ohio State.

Being an avid reader of socially focused nonfiction, Morgan goes on to say, "So much of the history of this country is tied to systemic racism and as we work as a society to undo it, EM is a unique position to do that."[11]

The Department Today

"Our intention creates our reality."

— Wayne Dyer, American self-help author and motivational speaker

Nationally, 27% of all academic emergency physicians are women, despite medical school graduation ratios of women to men being roughly 50/50.[12] In contrast, the Ohio State Department of Emergency Medicine has seen significant progress in closing gender disparities and is significantly exceeding the national average with over 40% women faculty and fellows. Advancement of women has accelerated in the department, with more women than men being promoted within the last two promotion and tenure cycles, to both associate professor and full professor.

Women in the department have also taken on significant national leadership roles including these individuals:

- **Creagh Boulger, MD**: American Institute of Ultrasound in Medicine (AIUM) national conference chair, Emergency Ultrasound Fellowship Accreditation Council (EUFAC) chair

- **Katie Buck, MD**: Academy of Geriatric Emergency Medicine, Society of Academic Emergency Medicine (SAEM), Executive Board, Geriatric Emergency Department Accreditation (GEDA) Board of Governors

- **Diane Gorgas, MD**: American Board of Emergency Medicine (ABEM) Board of Directors and President-elect, Accreditation Council for Graduate Medical Education (ACGME) Review Committee, Emergency Medicine

- **Simiao Li-Sauerwine, MD**: Chief Academic Officer of Research Lab and Incubator, Academic Life in Emergency Medicine (ALIEM)

- **Cynthia Leung, MD, PhD**: Director of Advanced Topics in Emergency Medicine student course

- **Lauren Southerland, MD**: President, Academy of Geriatric Emergency Medicine, Society of Academic Emergency Medicine (SAEM), Chair, American College of Emergency Physicians (ACEP) Geriatric Emergency Medicine Section

- **Jennifer Mitzman, MD**: National speaker, FeminEM Idea Exchange to discuss and discover the challenges and unique opportunities of women in emergency medicine (Figure 3)

Clinical leadership has been significantly impacted by women in the department. Southerland, who is Director of the Clinical Decision Unit and Observation Medicine, leads the Geriatric Accreditation of the Emergency Department. Shellman continues to lead at OSU East, where projects led by women include work in sepsis, ultrasound and prevention and tracking of sexually transmitted infections. Emily Kauffman, DO, has been a vocal advocate for improved treatment of patients with Opioid Use Disorder (OUD) and has been well-funded in initiating programs for Medication Assisted Treatment of OUD throughout central Ohio and her work with the grant "Helping to End Addiction Long-term (HEAL) Initiative" through the National Institutes of Health.

Maegan Reynolds, MD, an Assistant Professor of Emergency Medicine and Pediatrics, completed an Emergency Medicine residency at Denver Health and a Pediatric Emergency Medicine fellowship at Nationwide Children's Hospital (NCH) prior to joining the faculty at Ohio State in 2016 (Figure 4). Reynolds continues to split her clinical time between the university

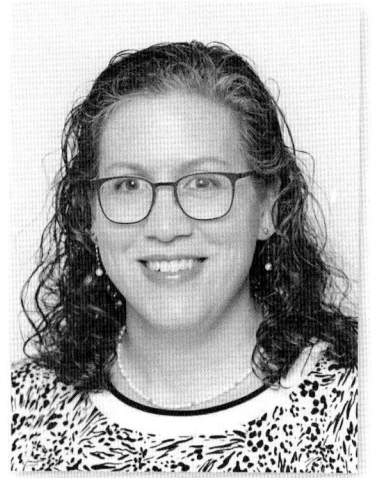

Figure 3: Jennifer Mitzman, MD, Assistant Professor of Emergency Medicine, leads national discussions regarding discovery of the challenges and unique opportunities of women in emergency medicine.

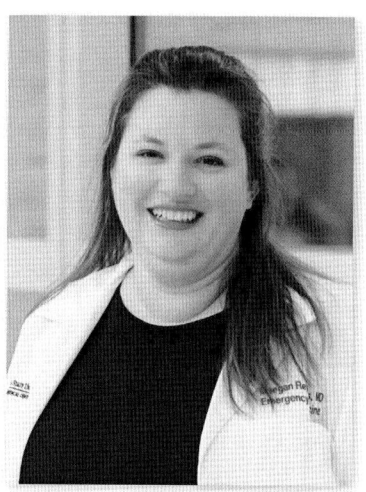

Figure 4: Maegan Reynolds, MD, Assistant Professor of Emergency Medicine and Pediatrics, is the Ohio State lead physician for the Oncology Pod and Quality Improvement in the department.

and NCH. Reynolds was the Director for the NCH Emergency Department resident rotation for several years prior to transitioning to the Director of Quality Improvement Education for the Ohio State Emergency Medicine Residency. Reynolds also serves as the department's lead physician for the Oncology Pod and lead physician for Quality Improvement. Reynolds completed her Lean Six Sigma Black Belt Training through The Ohio State University Fisher School of Business and has ongoing research interests that include quality improvement initiatives and education with a current focus on sepsis care, oncology care pathways, pediatric emergency medicine education, and the management of febrile infants.

Ashley Larrimore, MD, serves as co-medical director of MedFlight, central Ohio's largest and well-respected aero-medical and ground patient transport system (see Chapter 15-Air Medical Transport), along with ground crew EMS work by Brooke Moungey, MD.

Women researchers in the department are now at parity in volume to our men researchers, and have established themselves with a significant national presence (Southerland, Buck, Nassal) with Rebekah Richards, MD, spanning the distance between research and education in providing Evidence-Based Medicine education and spearheading best practices for the Emergency Department through Clinical Guidelines.

Irene Mynatt, DO (Figure 5), and Jennah Morgan, MD, have been instrumental in developing community outreach programs and working to deliver socially just and equitable care at both Ohio State Main and East. Mynatt attended medical school at Midwestern University at the Arizona College of Osteopathic Medicine campus and completed her residency in Emergency Medicine at Hahnemann Hospital. After practicing for a year in the community in Austin, Texas, she returned to Ohio State to complete a fellowship in Ultrasound. She serves as an Assistant Professor of Emergency Medicine, continues to teach ultrasound and is heavily involved in community outreach with the Diversity, Equity and Inclusion Committee.

The education arena is populated with women at both the undergraduate and graduate medical education level, with Lauren Branditz, MD, Jillian McGrath, MD, Kimberly Bambach, MD, and Krystin Miller, MD, all providing educational leadership and mentorship. Jennifer Yee, DO, created and leads a robust simulation curriculum and Simiao Li-Sauerwine, MD, serves as Assistant Program Director for the EM residency. A group of women educators has created the RAFFT (Resident and Faculty/Fellow Tribe) in EM, a collaborative mentorship and education program for women residents and students, which has been spotlighted nationally.[13]

DEI initiatives have manifested in the clinical setting as well as the search practices for diverse candidates. Robert Cooper, MD, Irene Mynatt, DO, and Farhad Aziz, MD, have spearheaded these efforts in the department. As a faculty leader of the cause of health care equity and social justice in health care, Cooper notes: "The emergency room is the front door to the hospital. More than any other department we interface with the community and see community members at their best and worst. If we really want to impact our patients' health, we have to impact their communities. The health of these communities relies on Diversity, Equity and Inclusion. We all have to be advocates for our patients to ensure they have equal access to food, health care, voting rights, education, and dignity."[14]

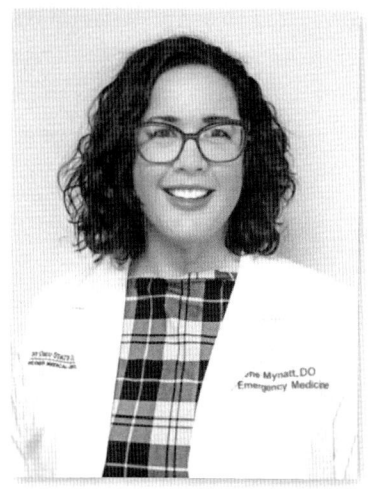

Figure 5: Irene Mynatt, DO, Assistant Professor, is developing a community outreach program and working to deliver socially just and equitable care at both Ohio State Main and East.

Mynatt adds: "One of the reasons I went into emergency medicine was because we see everyone at every time. My work with the DEIC has given me so much. Through my monthly outreach events with a local church, I have gotten to know the surrounding community first hand."[15]

Specific initiatives developed in response to the focus on health equities include: 1) creating a Social Determinants of Health screening tool used in all Ohio State emergency facilities to identify vulnerable patients and barriers to care; 2) incorporating into resident education team work with social workers and being exposed to a designated curriculum focused on Social Determinants of Health; 3) establishing community outreach programs to integrate OSU EM into the community at large; 5) developing policies and changing culture in interacting with the discriminatory patient, allowing residents, students, and fellow faculty to know they are protected against micro and macro aggression; and 6) empowering and educating patients about their rights and responsibilities to vote in local and national elections to have a voice in their community through a voter registration campaign.

As the department prepares for the challenges and opportunities of the decades to come, diversity will remain a central driver of providing excellence in emergency care.

References

1. https://en.wikipedia.org/wiki/Elizabeth_Blackwell
2. Lee C. Personal communication. 2022: Columbus, Ohio.
3. Shellman S. Personal communication. 2022: Columbus, Ohio.
4. Dunning D, Johnson K, Ehrlinger, J, Kruger J (1 June 2003). Why people fail to recognize their own incompetence. *Curr Dir Psychol Sci* 12(3): 83–87. doi:10.1111/1467-8721.01235.
5. Kman N. Personal communication. 2022: Columbus, Ohio.
6. Werman HA. Personal communication. 2022: Columbus, Ohio.
7. Bachmann D. Personal communication. 2022: Columbus, Ohio.
8. Sandberg S: *Lean In: Women, work and the will to lead*. New York: Knopf, 2013.
9. Heron S. Personal communication. 2022: Columbus, Ohio.
10. Young H. Personal communication. 2022: Columbus, Ohio.
11. Morgan J. Personal communication. 2022: Columbus, Ohio.
12. Oh L, Linden JA, Zeidan A, Salhi B, Lema PC, Pierce AE, Greene AL, Werner SL, Heron SL, Lall MD, Finnell JT, Franks N, Battaglioli NJ, Haber J, Sampson C, Fisher J, Pillow MT, Doshi AA, Lo B.

Overcoming barriers to promotion for women and underrepresented in medicine faculty in academic emergency medicine. *J Am Coll Emerg Physicians*. 2021 Dec 21;2(6):e12552. doi: 10.1002/emp2.12552. PMID: 34984414; PMCID: PMC8692182.

13. Agrawal P, Madsen TE, Lall M, Zeidan A. Gender Disparities in Academic Emergency Medicine: Strategies for the recruitment, retention, and promotion of women. *AEM Educ Train*. 2019:Dec 12;4(Suppl 1):S67-S74. doi: 10.1002/aet2.10414. PMID: 32072109; PMCID: PMC7011407.

14. Cooper R. Personal communication. 2022: Columbus, Ohio.

15. Mynatt IA. Personal communication. 2022: Columbus, Ohio.

Recommended reading: Wilkerson, Isabel. *The Warmth of Other Suns: The Epic Story of America's Great Migration*. New York: Random House, 2010.

* A cultural historian and student of the earth's evolution, Berry called himself a "geologian."

Chapter 24

Growth of the Department's Research Mission – from Infancy to National Prominence (1991-2021)

Mark G. Angelos, MD

Laboratory Research (1991-2013)

In 1991, Charles G. "Chuck" Brown, MD, successfully recruited Mark G. Angelos, MD, a new research faculty member, to the Department. At the time of his recruitment, Angelos was a faculty member in the Department of Emergency Medicine at Wright State University, where he was actively developing his own laboratory-based research program focused on cardiac arrest reperfusion. Prior to his appointment at Wright State, Angelos had completed a critical care fellowship at the University of Pittsburgh, where he spent one year in the laboratory of Peter Safar, MD, one of the pioneers of cardiopulmonary resuscitation. Under Safar's guidance, Angelos developed an interest in resuscitation techniques to treat cardiac arrest, in particular, reperfusion with extra corporeal cardiopulmonary bypass.

Three factors played prominently in Angelos' recruitment. First, moving to Ohio State allowed Angelos to work with Brown, one of the early pioneers and leaders in the fledging field of cardiac arrest research. Second, the Department of Emergency Medicine was itself a new academic department established in 1990. The department had excellent young faculty, excellent leadership and great growth potential. Third, research was viewed as an important mission area within the department and within the Ohio State University College of Medicine. Faculty were strongly encouraged to engage in research and support was provided through faculty tenure track support and research seed funding.

At that time, all departments within the College of Medicine were required to have a majority (at least 51%) of their faculty on the tenure track. To attain promotion and tenure, a faculty member on the tenure track could only be successful by developing a research skill and demonstrating success in obtaining external funding and publishing the results in high quality academic journals. Successful research was also vital to the success of the specialty of emergency medicine. Leading academic centers were still skeptical that emergency medicine was indeed a specialty as discussed earlier.

From fall of 1991 until Brown's departure from Ohio State in 1995, Brown and Angelos worked together in the laboratory along with the department's research fellow, Charles "Charlie" Little, DO, whom Brown recruited. Little had completed his Emergency Medicine residency at Ohio State and then a two-year research fellowship from (1990 to 1992), which focused on large animal models of cardiac arrest resuscitation. Post fellowship, Little accepted a full-time faculty position in the department and continued his work in the laboratory for the next six years before moving to a faculty position at the University of Colorado in 1998.

The 1990s were a fruitful time of laboratory collaboration, with three young faculty members, all from a very young department, presenting at national meetings, publishing papers and training research fellows. The most prestigious peer-reviewed publication from this era was Brown's first author paper in *The New England Journal of Medicine* in 1992. Brown and his colleagues reported their findings in a multi-center trial of high-dose epinephrine in pre-hospital cardiac arrest patients.[1] This was one of the first multi-centered research studies conducted by emergency physicians.

In these early years, there was very little grant funding available for emergency medicine. Much of the early research in emergency medicine was being done with small internal grants or departmental funds derived from clinical practice and directed toward research. The number of academic Emergency Medicine departments in the country was also relatively small. In 1991, there were 23 academic emergency medicine departments in U.S. medical schools representing only 18% of LCME accredited schools.[2] The department at Ohio State was the 16th in the country. Departments of Emergency Medicine also had essentially no representation at the National Institutes of Health (NIH), either as funded investigators or study section members.

Some research funding, however, was available in the Ohio State College of Medicine in the form of seed grants that were awarded on a competitive basis. Such funding opportunities included the Ohio State University Seed Grant Program, the Davis Scholarship Funds and the Bremer Foundation. Brown, Angelos and Little were all successful in obtaining these small one-year grants, which, together with some department funds, were the principal funding sources in the laboratory's early years.

However, with time, the laboratory successfully obtained its first, external national, multi-year grant funding. In 1993, Angelos as Principal Investigator (PI) was awarded a three-year (1993-1996) national American Heart Association (AHA) grant, "In vivo Metabolism During Perfused Ventricular Fibrillation," for $119,680. Angelos subsequently successfully obtained other grants from the Emergency Medicine Foundation (EMF), the AHA and the Society of Academic Emergency Medicine (SAEM).

In 1997, the department was awarded a three-year EMF Center of Excellence grant for which Angelos was the PI. This $250,000 grant supported the research, "Studies in Myocardial Metabolism During Ischemia and Reperfusion." The Center of Excellence award was the largest and most competitive grant offered in Emergency Medicine, awarded to only one center a year. These and other grants provided continuous external funding for the laboratory over the next 20 years.

The EMF was established in 1972 as a non-profit organization by visionary leaders of the American College of Emergency Physicians (ACEP) who recognized that emergency medicine had created new knowledge about challenging problems in the field. In the early years, however, only small amounts of money were raised and there was a sense that funds were used to support the needs of the large practice groups that seemed to dominate ACEP. Among others, John Wiegenstein, MD, ACEP's founder, was troubled by so little funding for research and so much paid for fund administration. Ohio State was among the institutions that pushed for higher research funding. The Center of Excellence grant program was an example of true, substantial funding for emergency medicine scientists.

Laboratory Focus: cardiac arrest resuscitation and cardiac reperfusion injury (1993-2013)

During the years between 1993 and 2013 the lab's research focus remained on reperfusion injury of the ischemic myocardium with particular attention to reperfusion free radical formation, oxygen delivery and mitochondrial function. For two decades, Alan Blumberg was a key part of the laboratory managing supplies, equipment, budgets and also working as an excellent technician (Figure 1).

Blumberg joined the university in 1989 working as a research assistant in the Department of Anesthesiology investigating the outcomes of hypoxia at different times in the swine model. In 1993 he joined the Department of Emergency Medicine working with Brown and Angelos and medical students interested in emergency medicine research. Years later Blumberg remembered this early research:

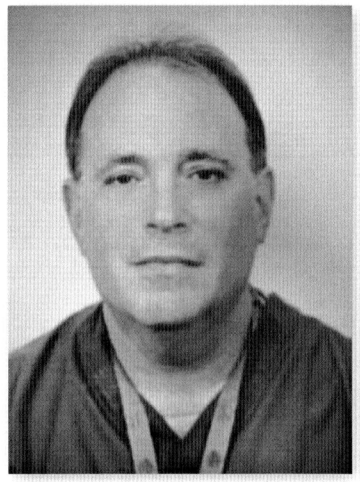

Figure 1: Alan Blumberg managed the laboratory experiments for many Ohio State investigators, particularly those studying issues related to cardiac resuscitation.

> We had excellent fellows and students working with us. One of the students, Holt Murray, encouraged us to switch our animal model to the Langendorff perfused rat heart model which he had learned prior to enrolling in medical school. He showed us how to accomplish this. It allowed us to do 16 experiments per day as opposed to one per day which we had been doing. This really increased our research productivity.[3]

Over time Blumberg transitioned to a more administrative role in the department handling department relocations and renovations, information technology support and new staff onboarding. He had many administrative talents and managed tasks unassigned to other staff members.

A number of peer-reviewed research papers resulted from this work with multiple publications in *Critical Care Medicine, Annuals of Emer-*

gency Medicine, Resuscitation, Academic Emergency Medicine, Journal of Molecular Cellular Cardiology and *American Journal of Physiology – Circulation Physiology*. Each year, faculty working in the laboratory were presenting their research at national research meetings. The most frequent meetings were the annual meetings of the Society of Academic Emergency Medicine (SAEM), the American Heart Association (AHA) and later the Resuscitation Science Symposium (ReSS).

Angelos was invited to present the laboratory's work at the AHA, as visiting professorships and multiple times at the Wolf Creek Conference for Cardiopulmonary Resuscitation Research, established in the late 1970s to bring together a core group of researchers interested in different aspects of cardiac arrest resuscitation.

Research Trainees in the Department

After the departure of Charles Brown in 1995 and Charles Little in 1998, Angelos continued the laboratory research program, working with fellows and later on, graduate students. Part of the maturation of the research program involved mentoring trainees in the laboratory. Such individuals brought manpower, new ideas and collaborations. As the fellowship director, Angelos mentored seven EM research fellows in the laboratory over an 18-year period (1993-2011). Each of these fellows made valuable contributions to the research program, resulting in many peer-reviewed publications (Table 1).

Table 1. Research fellow mentees of Mark Angelos, MD (1993-2011)

Years	Name	Institution
1993-1994	Kevin Ward, MD,	University of Pittsburgh
1995-1997	Carlos Torres, MD,	Ohio State University
1997-1998	Michael Waite, MD,	Ohio State University
1998-2002	Paul Klawitter, MD,	SUNY Upstate Medical University
2002-2004	Jason Stoner, MD,	Henry Ford Hospital
2002-2004	Carlos Torres, MD,	Ohio State University
2009-2011	Daniel Zelinski, MD, PhD	Ohio State University

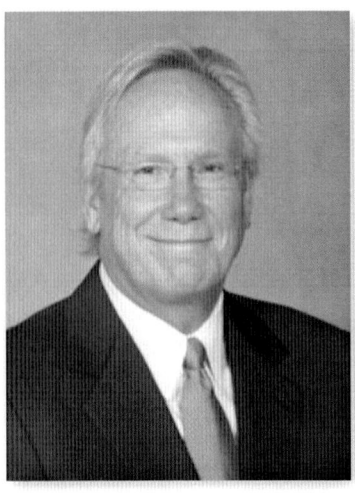

Figure 2: Thomas Clanton, PhD, was an important collaborator for emergency medicine researchers. He worked closely with investigators studying the effects of myocardial ischemia.

A critical component for the success of the research fellowship program was the ability to obtain external grant support for the fellows, which afforded them significant clinical release time in order to devote quality time to perform research. During this time period, Angelos was successful in obtaining six, one-to-two-year grants from the EMF and SAEM to support such fellows. Thomas "Tom" Clanton, PhD, was an important partner in the department's research efforts (Figure 2).

Initially educated in the field of respiratory therapy following college in the early 1970s, Clanton pursued research and received his PhD from the University of Nebraska in 1980. He accepted a position as Director of the Pulmonary Diagnostic Laboratory at Ohio State and held that position from 1982 to 1997. He eventually became Professor of Internal Medicine until his transition to Emeritus status in 2007. Clanton established a research laboratory investigating respiratory physiology and free radical biology and was successful in assisting faculty members in pulmonary medicine and emergency medicine during his career.

Angelos (PI) and Clanton obtained the first NIH grant for the laboratory in the form of a 3-year, NIH F32 training grant (2000-2003) to support Paul Klawitter during his PhD work. Another important key to the success of the fellowship was linking the fellowship with a master's program offered through the College of Medicine.

In addition to the Emergency Research fellows, Angelos mentored other trainees in the laboratory, including graduate students, a post-doctoral fellow and a research scientist, all of whom brought new skills and interests to the laboratory based on their prior training. They also facilitated broader collaborations with other laboratories and investigators. Being a clinical department, Emergency Medicine also drew a number of medical student and MD mentees to pursue the master's degree program through the College of Medicine, with Angelos serving as their advisor. The first Doctor of Philosophy (PhD) candidate was Paul Klawitter, MD (Figure 3), who came to Ohio State in 1998 having finished an Emergency Medicine residency at The State University of New York (SUNY) Upstate Medical University in Syracuse, New York. He worked on his PhD in Angelos' and Clanton's labs for four years. Clanton served as Klawitter's PhD advisor, which further strengthened the collaboration between the two labs. Klawitter was awarded his PhD in 2002.

Years later Klawitter reflected upon his years at Ohio State:

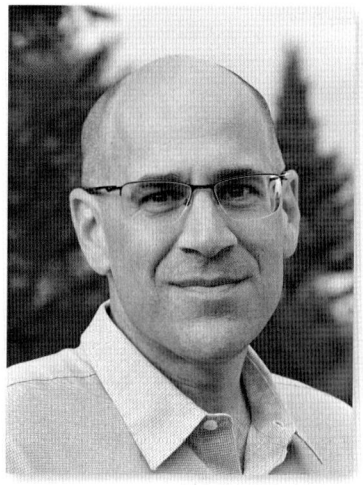

As an undergraduate I was a physics major at Clarkston University in upstate New York and considered going to graduate school for physics or medical school. I ended up going to medical school at SUNY upstate in Syracuse and then did an emergency medicine residency at SUNY upstate but always kind of missed doing research. I ended up applying to the fellowship at Ohio State because I decided I really wanted to give back and didn't want to just do clinical medicine. I joined the fellowship and became a graduate student. I worked with my PhD advisor, Tom Clanton, who had an appointment in biophysics as well as pulmonary and critical care. He and Mark Angelos guided my research efforts. We did a lot of work studying energetics or control of metabolism and energetics in cardiac and skeletal muscles that were under stress. We were studying the heart in a cardiac ischemia model and skeletal muscle: it was a fatigue model. We studied the role of free radicals and reactive oxygen in controlling energy availability in those muscles and the injury that occurs when reperfusion occurs. The whole thing took a little more than four years.

Figure 3: Paul Klawitter, MD, PhD, was the first emergency physicians to earn his PhD in the Department of Emergency Medicine. He was mentored by Clanton and Angelos.

About halfway through I wrote a grant application to the NIH and got a small NIH grant, and which I think at the time was the first NIH grant the emergency department at Ohio State had received. This was a fun thing and something I was proud of. The lab and the research opportunities were phenomenal and Ohio State in general had a ton of resources, Mark had a lot of support from the department, which was nice and which was not always true for other places, so I really appreciated then and appreciate it more now.

I think I might have been the very first Ohio State doctor to work a shift at Ohio State East back when we were first taking over, I think I ended up working a night shift there. The day guy didn't show up, and no one else in our department was credentialled to work there. I ended up having to stay most of the next day after working the night shift. I'm laughing about it now...

[When I decided to leave Ohio State] I was too afraid to go to your [Rund's] office because I thought "Doug is going to try to convince me to stay and it is going to be really, really hard to say no." [4]

Three additional researchers working in the Angelos lab would later earn their PhD degree. In 2006, Angelos received a graduate faculty appointment in the Ohio State Biophysics Graduate Program, which allowed him to advise PhD candidates. Beginning in 2006, Angelos began advising two PhD students who were in his lab: Ting-Yuan (Steve) Yeh, MD, and Sverre Aune. Yeh received his PhD in 2010, Aune in 2012. Later, Carlos Torres, MD, an emergency physician who had earned his master's degree in Angelos' lab, returned for his PhD in 2010. His advisor was Paul Janssen, PhD, and Angelos served on his PhD committee. Torres was awarded his PhD in 2014, the fourth individual in the department to do so.

Laboratory Focus: post-ischemic myocardial regeneration (2013-present)

In 2013, Angelos recruited Mahmood Khan, PhD, into the laboratory as a research scientist (Figure 4). In 2015 Khan was appointed Assistant Professor on the tenure track in the Department of Emergency Medicine; he was promoted to Associate Professor in 2017 and awarded tenure in 2020. With the appointment of Angelos as Department Chair in 2015, Khan assumed day-to-day supervision and the position of laboratory director.

Table 2. Graduate students and faculty members mentored by Mark G. Angelos, MD

Graduate School Mentees of Mark Angelos, MD (1995-2012)

1995-1997: Carlos Torres, MD – Master's Program Advisor

2010-2014: Carlos Torres, MD – PhD committee member, PhD Advisor: Paul Janssen; Dissertation title: "On the role of heart rate variability and pyruvate on cardiac contractility"

1998-2002: Paul Klawitter, MD-PhD committee member, PhD Advisor Tom Clanton, PhD; Dissertation title: "The Role of Antioxidants in Cardiac and Skeletal Muscle During Conditions of Energy Deficit"

2001-2004: Brian S. Palmer, PhD – Post-Doctoral Fellow Advisor

2002-2004: Jason Stoner, MD – Master's Program Committee

2006-2007: Ryan Butke, MS II – Graduate Student Advisor

2008-2009: Cameron Hypes, MD, MPH - Master's Program Advisor

2006-2010: Ting-Yuan Yeh, MD, PhD – PhD Advisor; Dissertation title: "The Role of Oxygen in Cardiopulmonary Resuscitation and Post-Resuscitation Period – a Mitochontrial Perspective"

2006-2012: Sverre Aune, - PhD Advisor, Dissertation title: "The Role of Reactive Oxygen Species in Post-Ischemic Low Flow in the Myocardium"

Research Faculty Mentored by Mark Angelos, MD

2012-2018: Chun-An (Andy) Chen, PhD, Assistant Professor, Department of Emergency Medicine (tenure track)

2013-2020: Mahmood Khan, PhD, M. Pharm, Associate Professor (tenured), Department of Emergency Medicine

---

After joining the department in 2013, Khan introduced his myocardial stem cell work to the laboratory. The laboratory research focus began to shift to post-ischemic myocardial regeneration with an emphasis on stem cell therapy. A collaboration led to the development of a bioengineered nanofiber cardiac patch to promote angiogenesis in the post ischemic heart. New collaborative relationships were formed with investigators both at Ohio State and other institutions. As this was a relatively new area for the laboratory, Khan and Angelos worked to develop preliminary data in support of new grants, targeting the NIH. The initial research project R01 applications to the NIH were not funded. However, in 2016 the laboratory and collaborators obtained their

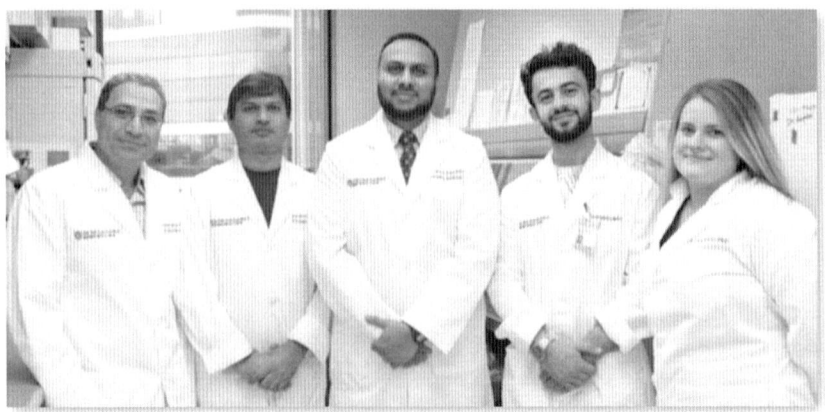

Figure 4: Mahmood Khan, PhD, (center) and laboratory associates worked closely with Mark Angelos, MD, in the area of post-ischemic myocardial regeneration with an emphasis on stem cell therapy.

first NIH R01 grant ($2.8 million) in this area, with Khan as the principal investigator, for the five-year study entitled "Biomimetic Cardiac Patch Capable of Rapid Angiogenesis."

After Angelos' retirement in 2020, Khan continued to have success growing and expanding the laboratory research program. In 2021, he received his second five-year NIH R01 grant ($5.1 million) with

Table 3. Research Mentees of Mahmood Khan, PhD

2014: Serena Hua – Medical student, Ohio State

2015: Dall Christopher – Medical student, Ohio State

2016-present: Julie Dougherty, PhD – Post-Doctoral associate

2016: Muhamad Mergaye – Research volunteer, Undergraduate, Ohio State

2016: Lindsey Van Sambeek, MD – Research intern, Clinical instructor, Ohio State

2017-present: Naresh Kumar – Post-Doctoral researcher

2017-present: Jordon Prox – Graduate student

2017-present: Noor Momin – Undergraduate student

2017-present: Nil Patel – Undergraduate student

2018-2019: Bryan Gardiner – Undergraduate student, University of Cincinnati

2018-present: Zahra Naseer – Undergraduate student,

2019-present: Nooruddin Sahal – Undergraduate student

2019-present: Sridhar Fanghyi – Graduate Student

2019-2021: Ali Akhtar – Research assistant

multiple principal investigators (MPI) entitled, "Molecular Identity and Role of BK Channels in Exosomes." As of spring 2022, Khan had five R01 grants (three as PI and two as MPI) under review at the National Institutes of Health (NIH). In addition, Khan and the lab have additional funding from the AHA and the Shriners Hospital for Children.

An effective mentor with trainees in the laboratory, Kahn mentored multiple students, residents and post-doctoral in the laboratory over eight years, from 2013 to 2021.

In 2019, Angelos recruited another young outstanding basic science investigator to the Department: Venkata Srikanth Garikipati, PhD, from Temple University, who also came with AHA funding (Figure 5). In collaboration with the College, a startup package was created to support him in developing his research program to study the role of a novel class of RNAs (circular RNAs) in cardiovascular disease. In 2023 he received a $2.8 million R01 grant from the NIH to study the role of small RNAs in ischemic tissue repair.

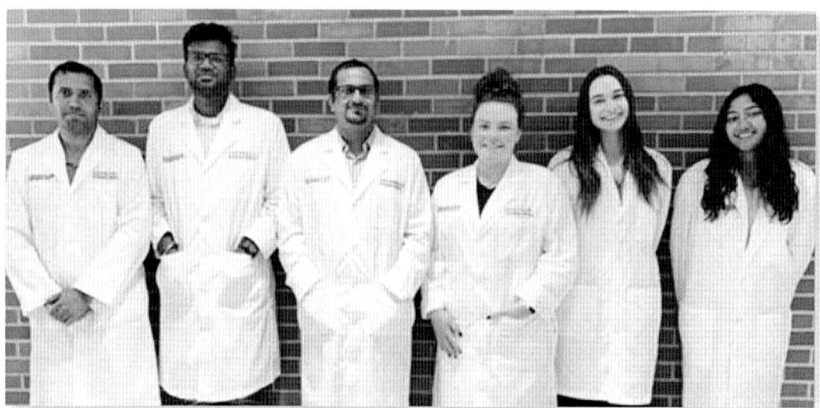

Figure 5: Venkata Srikanth Garikipati, PhD, (third from left) and his laboratory staff. He developed a research program to study the role of a novel class of RNAs (circular RNAs) in cardiovascular disease.

2021 Khan Research Laboratory Focus

The Khan laboratory continued to focus on establishing the role of stem cells and/or evaluating cell-free products such as extracellular vesicles in cardiac repair for acute myocardial infarction (AMI). The lab studied the role of intramyocardial delivery of stem cells or biomimetic nanofiber cardiac scaffolds to repair the damaged heart and other important projects.

Also, work progressed on the reprogramming of stem cells (human induced pluripotent stem cells) into cardiac and endothelial lineage to repair and regenerate the failing heart muscle. Another interesting new research focus area was to evaluate the role of non-coding RNAs (both small and long) in the myocardial infarction mouse model. The next step is to translate the findings from the small animal AMI model into a pre-clinical large-animal AMI model, which could be utilized for clinical translation in the future.

Clinical Research in the Departments

In the early years after the Department of Emergency Medicine was established, its research efforts were primarily focused in the laboratory. However, it was Howard A. "Howie" Werman, MD, who was one of the first faculty members to engage in clinical research and one of the first Ohio State emergency medicine residents. Werman stayed on as a resuscitation research fellow, then joined the faculty immediately following his residency to work with Charles Brown in the laboratory. Also one of the earliest faculty members (1984), Werman began to focus on aeromedical transport and took on leadership positions with SKYMED and later MedFlight. In such roles he began to write and conduct research studies regarding important issues in aeromedical medicine. Much of this work was unfunded, but the resulting publications have been impactful in the field. He remained very active in the end of his career.

As the department continued to grow, interest in clinical research began to grow. Growth was accelerated with the recruitment of Jeffrey "Jeff" Caterino, MD, in 2004. Douglas Rund, MD, recruited Caterino to Ohio State after he completed an emergency medicine-internal medicine (EM/IM) residency at Allegheny General Hospital in Pittsburgh. In Caterino's early years in the department he developed his own clinical research interests. While Angelos provided general research mentorship, it was important for Caterino to find research mentors who more closely fit with his clinical research interests. He did this successfully and the new mentorship enabled him to obtain a five-year (2010-2015) National Institutes of Aging/National Institutes of Health (NIA/NIH) mentored Patient-Oriented Research Career Development Award K23 grant award entitled "Expanding Antimicrobial Stewardship for Long Term Facility Patients: Implementation in Novel Clinical Settings using Information Technology."

Caterino's grant was the first K award in the department's history, and also enabled him to complete a Master of Public Health (MPH) degree. He turned this K award into an R01 one year after finishing his K award with a $2.8 million five-year (2016-2021) R01 grant from NIA/NIH entitled, "Urine Antimicrobial Proteins in Older Adults; Aging, Infection, and Innate Immunity." This grant was the first R01 in the department, an important research milestone. As Caterino progressed along his research path, he mentored other clinical EM faculty, fellows and students. Caterino's mentees who were faculty members are listed in Table 4.

Table 4. Faculty Mentees of Jeffrey Caterino, MD (2013-2018)

2013: Lauren Southerland, MD Faculty, Department of Emergency Medicine
  Mentoring role: Research mentor
2016: Ashish Panchal, MD, PhD Faculty, Department of Emergency Medicine
  Mentoring role: Research mentor
2018: Xia Ning, PhD Faculty, Department of Biomedical Informatics
  Mentoring role: Research mentor
2018: Jason Bischof, MD Faculty, Department of Emergency Medicine

> **Table 5. EM Research Fellow and Master's Degree Mentees of Jeffrey Caterino, MD (2012-2019)**
>
> 2012: Jessica Wall, MD, MPH; MPH student, Ohio State College of Medicine, MPH culminating project research advisor
>
> 2012: Amy Raubenolt, MD, MPH; MPH student, OSU College of Medicine, MPH culminating project research advisor
>
> 2015: Rebekah Richards, MD Research Fellow, Department of Emergency Medicine, Fellowship director
>
> 2016- 2017: Carmen Cantemir, PhD Fellow, Ohio State Department of Biomedical Informatics, Fellowship research advisor
>
> 2019-2020: Katherine Hunold Buck, MD Research Fellow, Department of Emergency Medicine, Research mentor
>
> 2020: Michelle Nassal, MD, PhD, Research Fellow, Department of Emergency Medicine, Research mentor

Growth of Clinical Research in the Department

With Caterino's influence, other faculty with clinical research interests joined the department. Lauren Southerland, MD, was an early key recruit in support of the clinical research mission (Figure 6). Southerland came to Ohio State in 2013 after completing a geriatrics fellowship at Beaumont Hospital in Michigan. She worked with Caterino on some preliminary geriatric research as applied to patients presenting to the Emergency Department. She also managed a number of industry-sponsored clinical studies in the department. In 2019, she received a K23 NIH grant from the National Institute on Aging with Caterino as her mentor. In 2020 she was named Director of Clinical Research in the department.

LAUREN SOUTHERLAND, MD, AND THE OHIO STATE GERIATRIC EMERGENCY DEPARTMENT AND GERIATRIC RESEARCH PROGRAM

Southerland completed her emergency medicine residency at Duke University, followed by her fellowship in Michigan. She joined as Ohio State faculty with the purpose of training under Caterino as a clinical researcher with an accompanying goal: Making the Ohio State Emergency Department more aging friendly.

Southerland gathered a multidisciplinary group of case managers, physical therapists, nurses and nurse practitioners to design protocols to better care for older adults. She took over the management of the ED Observation Unit (EDOU) in 2015, creating the first Geriatric Observation Unit in the United States. Under Southerland as the Director of Geriatric Emergency Care, the unit nurses received special training in caring for older adults and screening for delirium, fall risk, and home needs after their ED encounter. The unit also had special equipment, such as walkers and canes, to help older adults stay mobile

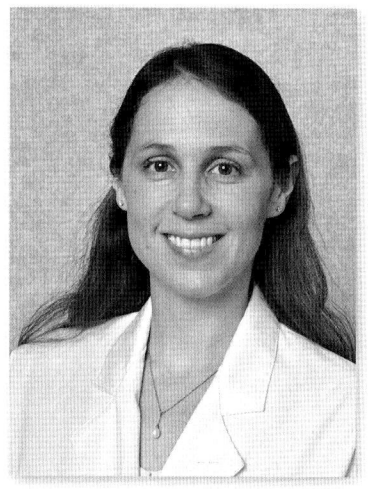

Figure 6: Lauren Southerland, MD, established the geriatrics care unit in the emergency department and achieved national recognition for her work in geriatric research.

Ohio State also gained its first geriatric consult service in 2015 with the hiring of Tanya Gure, MD, a geriatrician from the University of Michigan. The geriatric consult team would see older adults in the EDOU who had cognitive issues, multiple comorbidities and concern for polypharmacy, or were not thriving well. This allowed the providers to obtain quick, holistic evaluations for complex medical patients that didn't have an "acute" problem that required hospital admission. The patients could be placed in EDOU and see geriatrics, physical therapy and case managers, all with an average length of stay of 15 hours.

When the American College of Emergency Physicians decided to develop an accreditation process for Geriatric EDs, Ohio State was asked to be one of the trial sites. Southerland and her team worked to put together quality improvement protocols for 20 different geriatric measures and increase their equipment options for delirium, sensory impairment and fall risk.

In 2018 Ohio State was accredited as the first Level 1 Geriatric ED in the Midwest. Since then, the program has been a model for other institutions, including the Cleveland Clinic, Massachusetts General Hospital and the Kaiser Permanente System. In 2019 Southerland was awarded an NIH K23 training grant to research how to implement geriatric screening tools into the ED. Katie Hunold Buck, MD, took over as Director of Geriatric Emergency Care and Geriatric Emergency Department medical director.

Buck was an Ohio State EM resident from 2016-2019 and her prowess included obtaining an EMF grant to study pneumonia on older adults during her residency and while becoming Chief Resident. She stayed on as a research fellow, obtaining a coveted NIH Grant for Early Medical/Surgical Specialists' Transition to Aging Research (GEMSSTAR) grant during her fellowship. This grant allowed her to obtain MPH training and continue her research evaluating biomarkers for pneumonia infection in older adults.

The Geriatric ED at Ohio State was pioneering due to its use of the observation unit to allow for collaboration and consultation, but also for the research underpinning the program. Southerland, Caterino and Buck published many articles on the care of older adults in regards to infections, trauma and fall evaluations, transitions of care, hospice, the needs of oncology patients and implementation/process improvement. Later Southerland recalled this about her accomplishments:

> *OSU's investment in Geriatrics began with the recruitment of Jeffrey Caterino. His research interest in diagnosing infections in older adults was awarded with a NIH Beeson grant in 2010. The Beeson was a prestigious training grant that provides five years of protected time for training and research. During that time, he published numerous papers and was involved in national Geriatric Emergency Medicine groups. This gave Ohio State's Geriatric ED a national reputation for evidence-based care. This would also not have been possible without the support of Dr. Mark Angelos, who provided protected time and resources to build the clinical and research teams in Geriatric Emergency Medicine.*

In 2013 Tom Terndrup, MD, was recruited from Penn State University by Ohio State Dean Charles Lockwood, MD, to serve as Chair of the Department of Emergency Medicine. He remained in this position until 2015. He brought with him two-year (2012-2015) grant funding consisting of a Research Dissemination and Implementation (R18) NIH Grant titled, "Improving Patient Safety through Simulation Research." While at Ohio State he successfully became co-PI for the Ohio Consortium Clinical Center for the National Heart, Lung and Blood Institute (NHLBI) Prevention and Early Treatment of Acute Lung Injury (PETAL). The grant ran from 2014 to 2021; the total amount awarded was $1.45 million over seven years. The clinical research mission continued to grow with the addition of new young faculty with previous research experience and training.

In 2013, Ashish "Ash" Panchal, MD, PhD, was recruited back to the department by Angelos. Panchal had earned a research PhD from Case Western Reserve University prior to medical school and had done his EM residency at Ohio State before taking a faculty position at the University of Arizona. His research efforts focused on improving pre-hospital cardiac arrest and airway management as well as defining the risks faced by EMS professionals while providing high quality care. In 2016, Panchal was named the Research Director for the National Registry of Emergency Medical Technicians, a national organization for all EMTs with its headquarters based in Columbus, Ohio.

In 2019, Katie Buck, MD, finished her EM residency at Ohio State and worked as a clinical research fellow for one year (Figure 7). In 2020, Buck joined the department as a faculty member and was the recipient of an NIH small research grant (R03) award to study improving pneumonia diagnosis in older adults with Caterino as her mentor. This was a GEMSSTAR award, which provides Grants for Early Medical/Surgical Specialists Transition to Aging Research.

KATHERINE "KATIE" HUNOLD BUCK, MD

Katherine "Katie" Hunold Buck, MD. completed her Bachelor of Science in Public Health in 2012 at The University of North Carolina at Chapel Hill, with a major in biostatistics and minors in mathematics and chemistry and earned her MD from the University of Virginia in 2016. She and her husband came to Ohio State in June of 2016 for emergency medicine and internal medicine residencies, respectively. She was selected as one of the Chief Residents for the program along with Carolyn Martinez, MD, Krystin Miller, MD, and Caitlin Rublee,

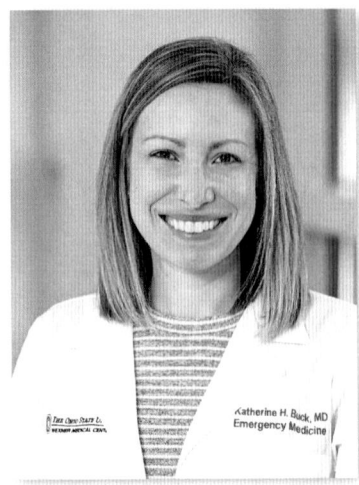

Figure 7: Katie Hunold Buck, MD, joined the faculty in 2020 after completing her research fellowship in the department. Her special interests are research about the clinical problems associated with aging and clinical care.

MD, MPH. After completing her emergency medicine residency in 2019, she completed a one-year research fellowship at Ohio State. She joined the faculty as an Assistant Professor in July 2020.

Buck's academic interests focused on clinical geriatric emergency medicine research with a focus on improving diagnostic accuracy. Her research in clinical geriatric emergency medicine began as an undergraduate student and she was awarded a Summer Undergraduate Research Fellowship and selected as a Medical Student Training in Aging Research (MSTAR) scholar as a medical student to pursue these interests. As a resident, Buck obtained her first research funding under the mentorship of Caterino: The Emergency Medicine Residents' Association/Emergency Medicine Foundation Resident Research grant. The results from this formed preliminary data for her successful National Institute on Aging (NIA) R03 GEMSSTAR grant that was successfully funded and completed enrollment in March 2022. Buck is a Co-Investigator, with Caterino, on an R01 with the Department of Bioinformatics. Dr. Buck also received a NIA K76 Paul B. Beeson Emerging Leaders Career Development Award in Aging.

Buck is an emerging national leader in both geriatric emergency medicine research and clinical care. She took over as the Director of Geriatric Emergency Care from Southerland in 2019 and oversees Ohio State's Level 1 Geriatric ED. This facility is regarded as a national leader and serves as an example for other EDs around the country.

Buck has been recognized with local and national awards for her research and has served on SAEM's Academy of Geriatric Emergency Medicine Executive Board as a medical student, resident and now faculty member. Most recently, she was elected to serve on the Board of Governors for ACEP's Geriatric Emergency Department Accreditation.

JASON BISHOF, MD

In 2018, Jason Bishof, MD, was recruited as a clinical investigator from the University of North Carolina where he had completed a research fellowship (Figure 8). Bishof received his MD degree from the University of North Carolina School of Medicine in 2014. He completed his residency in emergency medicine at Ohio State in 2017 and the research fellowship in 2018. Bishof was extremely productive in authoring and publishing clinical studies, particularly in the area of cancer and emergency medicine.

As the clinical research and investigators in the department grew, efforts were made to prioritize resources for infrastructure support. This plan included recruiting research personnel beginning with a research nurse, Michael Hill, RN, in 2009. Under Caterino's and Hill's direction, a group of students were recruited and trained to identify and enroll ED patients in the various clinical research studies. ED coverage by the research staff and these students then grew to nearly 24 hours a day, seven days a week, which greatly allowed multiple clinical research protocols to be managed simultaneously. As the number of clinical studies continued to grow, so did the funding to support the clinical research infrastructure. Thanks to grant funds, primarily from industry sponsored projects supplemented by the department, additional research personnel were hired. In 2017 Jennifer Frey, PhD, was hired as the clinical research and grants manager working directly with Caterino and other faculty investigators.

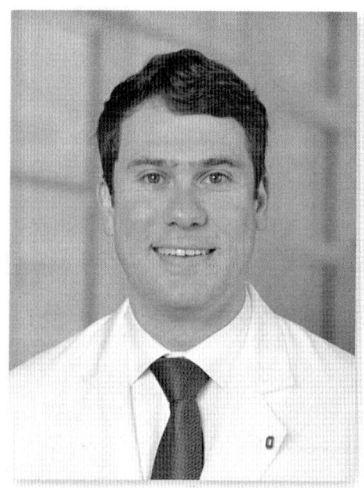

Figure 8: In 2018 Jason Bischof, MD, joined the faculty. He completed his residency in emergency medicine at Ohio State in 2017 and his research fellowship at the University of North Carolina in 2018. He later joined the Ohio State faculty to begin his research, under the direction of Jeffrey Caterino, MD.

Emily Kauffman, DO, received a $950,000 grant from Franklin County and the Centers for Disease Control and Prevention (CDC) to improve care for opioid dependent patients. Kauffman began her studies regarding opioids at her primary clinical site, Ohio State East Hospital.

With a more mature research infrastructure—i.e., a critical mass of clinical research faculty and department support for research projects—the department clinical research mission now included a much wider swath of the faculty. Most of those faculty members, although not primary researchers themselves, participated in research relative to their primary focus. Clinical track faculty, with the support of the department's research infrastructure, participated in various clinical research studies and at times led the projects.

Education track faculty developed a much stronger academic foundation through education research. As a group, they have been prolific in publishing education research, even to the point of making the Department of Emergency Medicine the top department in terms of the number of educational research publications at the Ohio State College of Medicine. The relatively new Division of Ultrasound also benefited: researchers developed a body of published work around teaching new learners about bedside ultrasound techniques.

As a larger proportion of faculty participated in such research-related activities, a greater number of residents and medical students became involved as well. One result was a greater diversity of presentations at each Spring Research Day. This cumulative involvement of faculty and trainees further added to the breadth and impact of the Department's research mission.

Annual Spring Research Day

In support of both the laboratory and clinical research groups in the department, the first Spring Research Day was instituted in 2005. As part of the now annual event, a nationally prominent Emergency Medicine researcher is invited to provide a keynote address, after which members of the department—faculty, fellows, residents, students and research staff—present their research with short oral presentations followed by questions from the audience. In 2017 with the generosity of Matt Lashutka, MD, a former chief resident in Emergency Medicine at Ohio State and his wife Melinda, an endowed lectureship was established in conjunction with Spring Research Day. The Lashutka endowed lectureship allowed the department to bring nationally acclaimed researchers into the department to interact with trainees and faculty as part of the annual Spring Research Day. Tom Aufderheide, MD, from Medical College of Wisconsin presented the first Lashutka lecture at the 2017 Spring Research Day.

Endowed Research Chair

In 2018 Angelos established The Ohio State University Emergency Medicine Endowed Research Chair utilizing funds from the OSU Emergency Medicine LLC, and with departmental and College of Medicine support. The vision of the research chair is to support recruitment of an established nationally prominent researcher with a track record of external funding, including NIH funding. This effort was a major step to support and grow a renowned research program. A faculty member, Henry Wang, MD, MS, MPH, was soon recruited to be a centerpiece for growing the clinical research program, which then provided opportunities for research fellow training, mentorship for other faculty members and senior leadership for the department research mission. This was the second endowed chair established in the department and the first one devoted to research.

Department Research Mission Rises to National Prominence

In the 30 years since the Ohio State Department of Emergency Medicine was established in 1990, the department's research mission developed, matured and attained national prominence within the specialty of Emergency Medicine even as the specialty itself, particularly academic Emergency Medicine, has experienced extensive growth: In 2023 there were academic departments in nearly all medical schools in the country in contrast to the 20 academic departments reported in 1990.

The early vision of Douglas Rund, MD, Charles Brown, MD, and Mark Angelos, MD, to build research within a newly formed department was so successfully carried forward that the department's research mission reputation continues to garner national prominence, as noted by the

Blue Ridge Institute for Medical Research's annual report, which ranks U.S. medical schools' NIH funding (Figure 9). In addition, several investigators, including Angelos, Caterino and Khan regularly serve on NIH and AHA study sections. They review established research training programs, including research fellowships, graduate student programs, post-doctoral and research scientist programs. Their activities show the number of research publications each year and national meeting research presentations.

In 2017, the Blue Ridge Institute ranked the Ohio State Department of Emergency Medicine #10 nationally in NIH funding among other EM departments nationwide. That same year, the Department of Emergency Medicine was the highest ranked department in the Ohio State College of Medicine for NIH funding within specialty, another indicator of how much the department's research output grew dramatically since the department's creation.

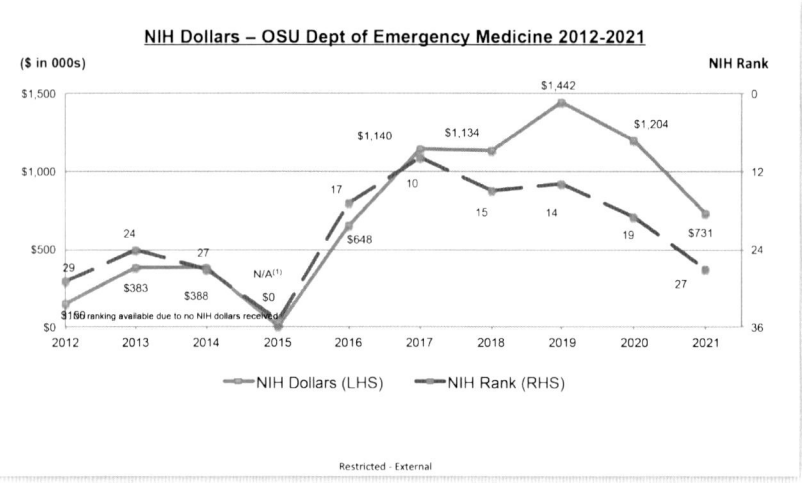

Figure 9: Grant Support and Blue Ridge Institute NIH Rankings* Ohio State Department of Emergency Medicine, 2012-2021

*Reference: The Blue Ridge Institute for Medical Research
<http://www.brimr.org/NIH_Awards/NIH_Awards.htm>

References

1. Brown C. A comparison of standard-dose and high-dose epinephrine in cardiac arrest outside the hospital. The multicenter high-dose epinephrine study group *N. Engl J Med*. 1992 Oct 8;327(15):1051-5.

2. Gallagher E, Henneman P, Schropp M. SAEM Task Force (Bivins H): Changing status of academic emergency medicine. *Academic Emergency Medicine*. 1997; 4:746-751.

3. Blumberg A. Interview with Alan Blumberg by Douglas Rund. 2022: Columbus, Ohio.

4. Klawitter PF. Interview with Paul Klawitter, MD by Douglas Rund. 2022: Columbus, Ohio.

Chapter 25
Leadership: Advancing the Specialty

Douglas A. Rund, MD
Richard N. Nelson, MD

Ohio State faculty, residents and administrators have held important leadership positions in national organizations and academic departments over the years. Their contributions to the specialty have been consequential and helped Emergency Medicine (EM) create and solidify its identity as a true specialty in the house of medicine.

Academy of Administrators in Academic Emergency Medicine (AAAEM)

GREGORY M. ARCHUAL, MBA

Gregory M. "Greg" Archual, MBA, Chief Operating Officer and Administrator of the Department of Emergency Medicine, was elected President of the Academy of Administrators in Academic Emergency Medicine (AAAEM) in 2018. He is currently co-chair of the AAAEM Benchmark Committee. During his years as president, he established associate and emeritus membership categories, and two separate committees addressing education and wellness. He also resurrected the Insight AAAEM member newsletter, the first editions since 2013.

He updated the strategic plan and implemented a member assistance program to provide financial assistance to AAAEM members who are unable to attend annual educational meetings because of their institutions' financial constraints.

Association of Academic Chairs in Emergency Medicine (AACEM)

DOUGLAS A. RUND, MD

When the Association of Academic Chairs in Emergency Medicine (AACEM) was formed in 1989 there were 12 academic departments of emergency medicine nationwide. The chairs of those departments had the foresight to realize that an organization of department leaders could be invaluable.

First, new ideas and developments could be shared and presented in a small enough circle that real discussion could develop and even the smallest concerns and opinions could be shared among an empathetic group. Second, the networking of leaders turned out to be essential for effective functioning as a department chair. Academic faculty promotion required external evaluation. Since all chairs were full professors, each was called upon many times a year to help in the faculty promotion process in universities, which was invaluable. Third, the group could help with advocacy and represent a unified voice from the academic side.

Among the leaders of this group of 12 were two chairmen from Ohio: Glenn Hamilton, MD, of Wright State University in Dayton and Richard Levy, MD, of the University of Cincinnati. Their departments had been established in 1980 and 1984 respectively. In 1989 three additional academic departments were added and the new chairs were invited to membership. At this point Ohio State was slowly moving in the process of establishing an academic department.

Douglas Rund, MD, Division Director, met in person with Hamilton and Levy to advocate that division directors should also be able to join. The answer was a polite "no" with a postscript: When Ohio State *did establish* an academic department there would be a great celebratory event—a "big party." In 1990 the Ohio State Department of Emergency Medicine was the 16th established in the country and Rund was finally invited to join the AACEM. The association held a banquet at Le Lion d'Or in Washington, DC.

Rund became the third AACEM President in 1992. The organization's

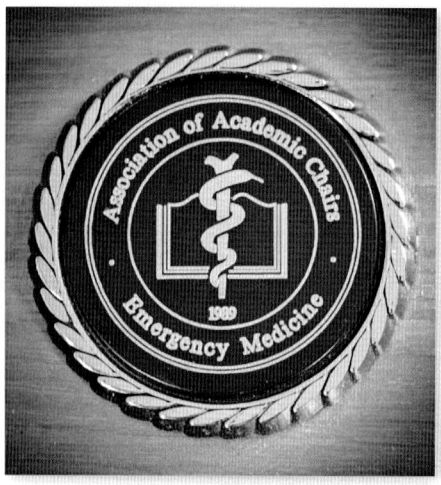 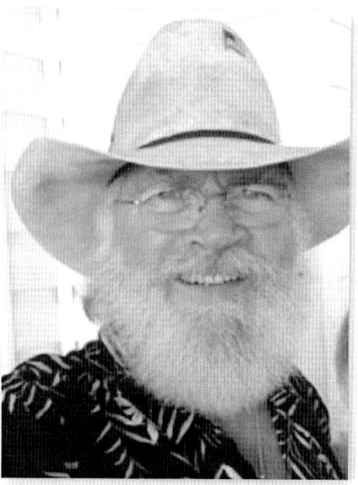

Figure 1: The original logo of the Association of Academic Chairs in Emergency Medicine (Figure 1) was designed by Ohio State medical illustrator and artist Robert "Cowboy Bob" Hummel (Figure 2) in 1992.

Figure 2: Robert Hummel, Ohio State designer of the AACEM logo.

logo was designed by Ohio State medical illustrator and artist Robert L. "Cowboy Bob" Hummel (Figures 1 and 2). The logo shows the Staff of Aesculapius atop an open book and the 1989 founding date. Hummel was also known by "Cowboy Bob," signifying his guitar playing role in the Columbus band Rainbow Canyon, which was enormously popular at that time.

American Board of Emergency Medicine (ABEM)

DOUGLAS A. RUND, MD

The American Board of Emergency Medicine (ABEM) was finally approved by the American Board of Medical Specialties (ABMS) in 1979 as a "conjoint board," which meant that seven other boards had to be represented on the ABEM board. The first examination was given in 1980; Rund passed and became one of the new examiners. In 1988 he was elected to the ABEM board of directors and in 1995 became President.

One of Rund's goals as president was to make an examination and resulting certification in critical care available to diplomates. Still fearful of the new specialty, other specialty boards such as medicine and surgery were at first opposed to any possible inroad into hospital practice. There was a vague assertion circulating that a previous leader of emergency medicine had promised that emergency physicians would never practice in the inpatient environment, rather only prehospital or in the emergency department. This was supposedly part of a bargain to gain support from other specialties to establish the specialty board in emergency medicine. No known document or source of such a promise was ever found, but in 1995 the powerful existing boards' resistance to allowing critical care certification for emergency physicians was palpable.

A possible breakthrough occurred at an ABMS meeting. Leaders of the ABEM had finally convinced leaders of the American Board of Anesthesiology (ABA) that, following an ABA fellowship in critical care, emergency medicine graduates were qualified to take a critical care examination and practice in a critical care unit. The proposal with ABA was to go forward on a Friday. On Wednesday, during a reception, Rund was approached by the leadership of the American Board of Internal Medicine (ABIM). Their proposal was that ABEM withdraw its application to take the anesthesiology critical care examination and instead take the internal medicine critical care fellowships and sit for the ABIM examination to attain certification in critical care. The ABIM rationale was that both boards were highly motivated by high quality certifications. One of the individuals posited that emergency medicine and internal medicine were "blood brothers," joined by their mutual commitment to quality medical practice. They also stated that if ABEM did not withdraw the proposal, ABIM and allies would vote against the proposed certification with anesthesiology and, moreover, the offer of the ABIM pathway would be withdrawn forever.

The ABEM leadership hastily reconvened. The final decision: ABEM had to proceed on the assurance that the internal medicine proposal would be approved, and the proposal to attain certification through anesthesiology was withdrawn. In the end the proposal was approved by the critical care subcommittee and executive committee of ABIM but rejected by the entire ABIM board later that year. It was felt that emergency physicians were too aggressive and would soon take over all the intensive care units. It would take the efforts of subsequent Ohio State ABEM President Richard N. Nelson, MD, to finally attain a pathway to certification in critical care for ABEM diplomates.

RICHARD "RICK" N. NELSON, MD

Nelson joined the Ohio State faculty in 1981, passed the ABEM examination in 1982 and, at the urging of Rund, became an oral examiner for the certification examination. He was later asked to participate as an oral examiner for the recertification examination in 1990, which was then required of ABEM diplomates every 10 years. Most diplomates took the written recertification examination; however, there was also an oral exam option. The oral recertification exam was different than the oral certification exam in that it was based on actual emergency department cases submitted in advance by the examinees themselves. Very few diplomates choose this option. The low demand and the extensive time commitment for its examiners ultimately led to its early demise. Nelson fondly recalled the experience of administering the oral recertification exam to EM legend Peter Rosen, MD, who, of course, passed easily.

In 1987 Nelson was invited to be an ABEM item writer, in essence, to create questions for the written exams, including Certification, Recertification, and In-training. The first two exams were later renamed Qualifying and ConCert. For the next 14 years Nelson wrote questions for all three primary ABEM exams, becoming the most prolific item writer in ABEM history. He later also became a writer for ABEM's oral examination.

In 2004, Nelson was elected to the ABEM board of directors and served nine years. In 2008 he was asked to chair both the Test Development Committee and the newly created Initial Certification Task Force (ICTF), which was charged with updating and upgrading the ABEM exams for the first time since their establishment 30 years prior. This task force led to the establishment of the eOral exams in 2013, which added computer screens and real-time imagery to the oral exam. The task force also upgraded the written exam, which by then was being administered electronically through local Pearson-Vue testing centers rather than in-person at large proctored testing sites in Chicago and Dallas.

In 2011 Nelson was elected ABEM President. During his term, he focused on the ICTF and test development. Another important part of his presidential year involved successfully negotiating with internal medicine to allow emergency medicine diplomates who had completed fellowships in critical care medicine to take the examination in critical care offered by ABIM, a proposal strongly opposed by internal medicine during Rund's efforts 16 years earlier. On November 14, 2012, 25 ABEM diplomates took the ABIM critical care medicine exam. All 25 passed, thus easily validating this decision. The success and momentum of ABEM's negotiating team, which was composed of Nelson, ABEM executive director Earl Reisdorff, MD, and board members Debra Perina, MD, Mark Steele, MD, Francis Counselman, MD, and John Morehead, MD, also paved the way for complementary critical care pathways in Anesthesiology and Surgery.

After his ABEM board term ended in 2013, Nelson continued to be active in the organization. He served as both a writer and team leader examiner for the oral exams. He was also the first examiner to be named "Consultant Team Leader," a designation that included serving as mentor and consultant to both new and experienced oral examiners. He also encouraged and nominated other emergency physicians, both at Ohio State and across the country, to volunteer for ABEM as writers and examiners. One of his nominees, Diane Gorgas, MD, not only would become an examiner, but would also go on to become President-elect of ABEM, the third emergency physician from Ohio State to be elected to this office.

DIANE L. GORGAS, MD

Gorgas began serving as a volunteer for ABEM in 1995 as an oral examiner. She was chosen to become a Team Leader, Senior Case Reviewer and the chair of the Modified Singles Advisory Panel prior to being elected to the Board of Directors.

She continued the Ohio State tradition for ABEM leadership and was elected to the board in 2018 and served as an item writer, case developer and case administrator. She was elected Secretary-Treasurer of the Board in 2022 and President-elect in 2023. She is the Chair of the crucial Test Administration Committee and Chair of the Becoming Certified Initiative (BCI) and its task force to reimagine and design the future of initial certification in Emergency Medicine.

Gorgas is the current chair of the Test Administration and Finance Committees. Much of her focus within the Board has been with her appointment as BCI chair. The last revisions of the initial certification process were chaired by Nelson in 2014 and resulted in the pivot from paper oral exam cases to an electronic format, which was delivered in person (the Oral Certification Exam, or OCE).

When Gorgas was appointed BCI Chair, the growing pressures on the capacity of the current system to examine a seemingly ever-expanding number of residency graduates met head-on with the COVID pandemic. This perfect storm necessitated a total shift of not only practical aspects of delivering an oral examination, but also the philosophical questions of what initial certification was to assess beyond that demonstrated by passing a multiple-choice question written exam. Gorgas led studies to show the validity of the post-COVID system of delivering the OCE in a virtual format via teleconferencing. The now Virtual Oral Certification Exam (VOCE) was successfully administered in 2021, holding true to ABEM's promise of seating all the residents sidelined by cancelled exams in 2020.

ABEM supported a subsequent study by Gorgas showing the correlation and distinct purposes between the OCE and the written Qualifying Exam (QE). The correlation emphasized that the VOCE measured knowledge and abilities as compared with the QE's assessment of "just" a resident's medical knowledge. However, key components of competency remained largely unmeasured in the testing rubric (QE + VOCE). As the BCI leads, ABEM and Gorgas convened a national initial certification summit with all major EM organizations leaders in conjunction with the ACGME, ABMS, the newly formed ABEM Becoming Certified Task Force (BCTF) and ABEM's Stakeholder Advisory group (SAG).

The BCTF and SAG's summit and independent work pointed toward a new direction for the VOCE, focusing on patient and family interaction skills, procedural mastery, trouble-shooting and complex higher-order decision making. The new initial certification system planned for rollout over the next three years will be revolutionary in the ABMS world and will assure the public, ABEM diplomates and residents in Emergency Medicine that their physicians and colleagues will have the capacity to deliver clinical care to the highest standards.

Gorgas was elected to the Board's executive track in 2021. She was selected as the group's treasurer in 2022 and will be president of the ABEM Board in 2024. No other Emergency Medicine practice site, academic or community, can boast three ABEM presidents within its ranks like Ohio State can.

JILLIAN McGRATH, MD

Jillian McGrath, MD, is continuing the ABEM leadership tradition. She was appointed to ABEM's LLSA (Lifelong Learning and Self-Assessment) CME committee and in 2015 became an oral board examiner. She was among the first examiners to be trained in the newly created Structured Interview portion of the exam.

The American College of Emergency Physicians (ACEP)

MARK L. DeBARD, MD

Mark DeBard, MD, was elected to two terms on the National American College of Emergency Physicians (ACEP) Board of Directors from 1992 to 1998 and as Speaker of the ACEP Council from 2003 to 2005. He received ACEP's highest honor, the John G. Wiegenstein Award, in 2013. DeBard's research and expertise included his leadership in describing, identifying and listing the dangers of the Excited Delirium Syndrome, which the ACEP Council and Board subsequently endorsed as a medical diagnosis in 2009. He also convinced national ACEP to establish a task force to establish national standards for the examination of sexual assault patients. He served as President of Ohio ACEP in 1990-1991.

GARY R. KATZ, MD

Gary Katz, MD was Speaker of the ACEP Council from 2019 through 2021. He developed and set up the first virtual council meeting and followed up with a hybrid meeting during the COVID-19 pandemic. This allowed the council to complete college business when other organizations were outright cancelling their meetings. During his time at Ohio State, he also served as President of Ohio ACEP from 2009 to 2011 and was Chair of the AMA Young Physician section from 2007 to 2008. Katz also serves as Lt. Colonel with Ohio Air National Guard and in 2023 was selected to receive the prestigious ACEP Council Meritorious Service Award.

HENRY E. WANG, MD, MS, MPH

In 2019 Henry E. Wang, MD, MS, MPH, Professor of Emergency Medicine, became the Founding Editor-in-Chief of the new emergency medicine journal, *Journal of the American College of Emergency Physicians Open (JACEP Open)*. The new online journal, published by the American College of Emergency Physicians (ACEP), offers a user-friendly route to early publication for scientific papers and reviews. The publication is subscription free and available to all readers internationally. The first edition was published in July 2019. Early editions in 2020 featured the first articles in emergency medicine journals addressing the COVID-19 pandemic.

Wang recalled the journal's inception:

> *In late 2018, ACEP decided to start a second medical journal to expand publication opportunities for the entire emergency medicine world. Part of this was realizing that* Annals of Emergency Medicine *was receiving a high number of submissions and turning away many high quality papers worthy of publication.*
>
> *While starting a second journal was logical and strategic, many were apprehensive. The plan was for JACEP Open to use an open access model, charging authors publication fees for accepted papers. However, we had to fight the predatory reputation of online journals and the fear of creating a second-rate product. There was also fear that a second ACEP journal*

would diminish the perceived quality of all of ACEP's publications.

I had my work cut out for me. I had to jump into a new role, quickly design a new journal, recruit a board of 40 editors and design processes for all aspects of manuscript submission, review and publication. For jump-start content, we reached out and personally invited dozens of prominent authors to contribute works to the new journal. We had to ensure a highest quality product and leverage social media to spread the word. We settled on the title Journal of the American College Emergency Physicians Open *(JACEP Open), drawing upon the original name of* Annals of Emergency Medicine *and pairing it with a bold and flashy cover.*

The journal smashed all expectations in the first year. We planned for 200-300 manuscript submissions; we received about 750 in that first year. Article downloads totaled 750,000. Knowing that we had designed a speedy production timeline as the pandemic broke out, we immediately sought to become the first emergency medicine journal to publish on COVID-19. We recruited authors to write COVID-19 papers, giving them 1-2 weeks to write the work, 3 days for peer review, and on-line publication one week later. Our first three years have been highly successful. Today, JACEP Open *is widely recognized as a major force in the emergency medicine publication world.*[1]

Academy of Emergency Ultrasound (AEUS)

CREAGH BOULGER, MD

Creagh Boulger, MD, was the President of the Academy of Emergency Ultrasound from 2018 to 2019. During her presidency the organization refreshed the peer review process for the narrated lecture series to increase access for junior faculty and fellows and created a question bank based on the lectures that numerous residencies and medical schools utilized during the pandemic and continue to use. Some of the efforts lost some momentum with the pandemic, but the program has grown since.

Academy of Geriatric Emergency Medicine (AGEM)

JEFFREY M. CATERINO, MD, MPH

Jeffrey M. Caterino, MD, MPH, was President of the Academy of Geriatric Emergency Medicine (AGEM) from 2012 to 2013. A highly successful National Institutes of Health-funded investigator, he conducted important studies in conditions affecting the elderly, including urinary tract infection and sepsis. Caterino was the second chair of the Academy. A major focus of his time was fostering the creation of the first guideline statements for geriatric emergency medicine, which was a collaboration among the Society for Academic Emergency Medicine (SAEM), ACEP, Emergency Nurses Association, and the American Geriatrics Society. These guidelines were ultimately released in 2014. Another focus was fostering the next generation of EM physicians with interest in geriatrics. Caterino introduced the concept of resident and medical student representation on the executive committee of the Academy. The Academy also organized its first annual meeting dinner, which continues each year at the annual meeting. The steps helped facilitate the pipeline of young emergency physicians into geriatrics and expand its scope within the specialty. In 2022 he received the AGEM's academic career achievement award. In 2023, he received the Academy's Gerson-Sanders award, which recognizes individuals who have made significant contributions to improving care for older adults in emergency medicine and is considered the Academy's highest award.

LAUREN T. SOUTHERLAND, MD

Lauren Southerland, MD, served as President of the AGEM for the 2017-2018 year; she served on the board of the academy from 2014 to 2019. Under her leadership the Academy improved outreach and education and initiated a junior board member program with a medical student and resident/fellow position. The organization also started a scholarship for medical students, residents and fellows to present a case or a research interest at the SAEM annual business meeting.

Southerland has also been active in ACEP and on the board of the

ACEP Geriatric Emergency Medicine Section (GEMS) from 2018 to 2024. She later recalled her leadership years:

> *I was Chair from 2020 to 2022, some rather tumultuous years. We focused on giving our members access to colleagues and shared tips and tricks for dealing with staffing crises, boarding crises and the increased difficulties of the pandemic. We developed a virtual pre-conference that provided 4 hours of geriatric-focused CME. This was important as 4 hours of geriatric CME a year is necessary to being a Geriatric ED Medical Director. I also instituted the highly popular GEMS "Boxing Match," where junior faculty and trainees get a chance to debate topics in clinical care such as stopping anticoagulants after a fall in someone with stroke risk factors. Our section received the 2021 ACEP Service to Section Award, given for best Section Leader and Section accomplishments. This was the first time GEMS received this award.*[2]

KATHERINE H. "KATIE" BUCK, MD

Katherine "Katie" Hunold Buck, MD, is President-Elect of AGEM in 2023-2024. Previously she served as student member, resident member and member at large.

American Institute of Ultrasound in Medicine (AIUM)

DAVID P. BAHNER MD

David P. Bahner, MD, served on the AIUM Board of Governors and as the third vice president of the organization and currently is an ex officio member of the board as an AIUM delegate to the AMA House of Delegates, which represents all 50 states and all major medical specialty societies. He helped to pioneer and was the first leader of the AIUM medical education section (community of practice).

LAUREN BRANDITZ, MD

Lauren Branditz, MD, is continuing as a leader in AIUM, serving as Secretary in the Ultrasound in Medical Education Community. She will ascend to become Chair in 2026-2028.

The American Medical Association (AMA)

STEVEN J. STACK, MD, MBA

In 2015, at age 43, Steven J. "Steve" Stack, MD, MBA became the youngest President of the American Medical Association (AMA) since 1854 and was also the first emergency physician to be elected to the position. He was a graduate of the Ohio State College of Medicine and completed his Emergency Medicine residency at Ohio State in 2001. In 2020 he became Commissioner of the Kentucky Department for Public Health and in 2022 he was elected President-Elect of the Association of State and Territorial Health Officials, headquartered in Washington, DC.

Clerkship Directors in Emergency Medicine (CDEM)

SORABH KHANDELWAL, MD

Sorabh Khandelwal, MD, served as President of the Clerkship Directors in Emergency Medicine (CDEM) in 2013. He served on the first executive board of the group from the time of its founding. The group is now an Academy of the Society of Academic Emergency Medicine. He was part of a group that developed an EM Clerkship Primer, educational sessions, and a track at the Council of Residency Directors (CORD), educational sessions at SAEM, acceptance into the Alliance for Clinical Education (ACE), SAEM Tests, CDEM self-study modules, and assisted the National Board of Medical Examiners (NBME) to create the EM Advanced Clinical Examination.

During Khandelwal's leadership years, CDEM grew to become the national voice of medical student educators. He has also served on the Advisory Council for the NBME and on many committees for the

USMLE, including the Management Committee and the Step 3 Computer-Based Case Simulations Committee.

NICHOLAS "NICK" E. KMAN, MD

Nicholas E. Kman, MD, served as CDEM President from 2014 to 2015. The organization is now an Academy of the Society of Academic Emergency Medicine, although the scholarly presentations happen during the CORD meeting. One of the greatest accomplishments during Kman's term was the establishment of the CDEM/CORD *Western Journal of Emergency Medicine Education Supplement.* Manuscripts accepted for publication were part of the October 2015 supplement. The leadership under Kman accepted manuscripts in original research, brief research reports and brief educational innovations for the online version of the journal.

The CDEM/CORD *WestJEM* Special Issue in Educational Research & Practice still publishes educational scholarship that supports emergency medicine clinical educators in their mission to promote and provide a culture of education for medical students, residents, fellows and faculty. The clerkship directors also produced a short video to teach medical students how to make streamlined presentations to their supervisors in the emergency department. This was a joint collaboration between CDEM and EMRA to produce a professional grade instructional video for medical students on how to present patients in the emergency department. Kman sought to create a high quality and engaging video that reflects modern learning styles. The video can be seen here: https://www.emra.org/students/advising-resources/patient-presentations/.

In 2015 Kman and his colleagues began work to establish a CDEM-sponsored End of Shift Feedback Card. A two-day national consensus conference was held in March 2016 in the CDEM track at the CORD Academic Assembly in Nashville. The goal of the conference was to standardize assessment practices and to create a national clinical assessment tool for use in EM clerkships across the country. Conference leaders synthesized the literature, articulated major themes and questions pertinent to clinical assessment of students in EM, clarified the issues, and outlined the consensus-building process prior to consensus-building activities. The National Clinical Assessment Tool for Medical Students in the Emergency Department (NCAT-EM) was born from this effort.[3]

Comprehensive Oncologic Emergencies Research Network (CONCERN)

JEFFREY M. CATERINO, MD, MPH

Jeffrey M. Caterino, MD, MPH, was co-chair of the CONCERN network from its inception in 2015 through 2022. The network was formed as part of a National Cancer Institute-supported initiative to increase research on patients with cancer in the emergency department. The network included representatives from both emergency medicine and oncology at over 50 academic institutions. Caterino led the first multicenter observational study to characterize presentation, emergency department treatment and disposition of patients with cancer presenting to the ED.

National Association of Emergency Medical Services Physicians (NAEMSP)

RONALD G. PIRRALLO, MD

Ronald Pirrallo, MD, MHSA, completed the residency program in 1990 and became the President of the National Association of Emergency Medical Services Physicians (NAEMSP) in 2011. He is currently Vice Chair of the Department of Emergency Medicine at The University of South Carolina School of Medicine.

Years later Pirrallo recalled the accomplishments of his presidency:

> *Emergency Medical Services became an ABEM Subspecialty during my NAEMSP Presidency. It was the culmination of decades of publishing the unique science and critical care provided by many EMS physicians. One of the most rewarding moments of my term on the board was welcoming the first group of physicians who passed their certification examinations and proudly claimed their well-earned acknowledgement of their expertise.*[4]

Society of Academic Emergency Medicine (SAEM)

DANIEL M. MARTIN, MD, MBA

Daniel M. Martin, MD, MBA served as chair of the SAEM Medical Education Research Interest Group from 2006 to 2016.

Other Leaders

Eric Drobny, MD, residency class of 1997, was elected President of the Ohio State Medical Association (OSMA) in 2023. He had been an active member serving on the Focused Task Force on State Legislation and on the OSMA Council, where he chaired the Audit and Appropriations Committee. He was named OSMA Advocate of the Year in 2019 for his work on the Ohio Surprise Billing Law. He also served on the boards of the Ohio ACEP and the Columbus Medical Association. He joined the Mt. Carmel Emergency Services Incorporated (ESI) group after residency and serves as their Chief Financial Officer.

Timothy Reeder, MD, MPH, residency class of 1998 and Chief Resident, graduated from the Ohio State University College of Medicine in 1995. He went on to earn his Master of Public Health degree at the University of North Carolina. He served as medical director of the ED at Pitt County (NC) Memorial Hospital/Vidant Medical Center from 1999 to 2018 and was Chief of Staff in 2009. He was elected President of the North Carolina Medical Society in 2019 and subsequently was elected to the North Carolina House of Representatives, starting his term in 2023.

Academic Department Chairs

CHADWICK D. MILLER, MD, MS

Chadwick D. Miller, MD, MS, a clinician-scientist, completed emergency medicine residency training at Ohio State in 2003 and served as a Chief Resident in his final year. In 2016 he was appointed Chair of the

Department of Emergency Medicine at Wake Forest School of Medicine. He also became a leader of the Emergency Medicine Service Line at Atrium Health across the Southeast Region of Advocate Health. The clinical mission spans more than 1 million patient encounters annually across three states.

Miller's research addresses cardiovascular emergencies and critical illness. He co-directs the Critical Illness, Injury, and Recovery Research Center (CIIRRC), and the Southeastern Clinical Center for the NIH funded PETAL Network. He also collaborates on a portfolio of investigations testing new methods to evaluate patients with chest pain presenting to the Emergency Department. At Atrium Health Wake Forest, Miller also leads the Clinical Operations Committee of the Wake Forest University Group Practice and the Operational Excellence Committee. He received his Master of Science degree with a major in Clinical and Population Translational Sciences at Wake Forest University in 2009. He was selected and has served as a member in the North Carolina Institute of Medicine since 2018.

JAMES W. HOEKSTRA, MD

James W. Hoekstra, MD, became chair of the Department of Emergency Medicine at Wake Forest University in 2003 and served in that capacity until 2015. Previously he was Professor of Emergency Medicine at Ohio State.

ROBERT W. NEUMAR, MD, PHD

Robert Neumar, MD, PhD, was a Sarnoff Medical School Research Fellow under Charles "Chuck" Brown, MD, at Ohio State from 1988 to 1989. He became the Chairman of the Department of Emergency Medicine at the University of Michigan in 2012. He is a renowned researcher focused on molecular mechanisms of post-cardiac arrest brain injury, therapeutic strategies to improve neurologic outcomes after cardiac arrest and extracorporeal cardiopulmonary resuscitation for refractory cardiac arrest.

He is also co-Chair of the International Liaison Committee on Resuscitation and a member of the National Academy of Medicine. Years later he recalled that his experience at Ohio State "basically launched my career to this day where I continue to continue to do research focused on cardiac arrest and resuscitation, both in animal models and humans."[5]

MANISH N. SHAH, MD, MPH

Manish Shah, MD, MPH, completed his residency in emergency medicine at Ohio State in 1999. He was Chief Resident in his final year. He was appointed Professor and Chair of the BerbeeWalsh Department of Emergency Medicine at the University of Wisconsin in 2022. He is a national leader in prehospital and geriatric emergency medicine research with over $150 million in grants and contracts as principal or co-investigator and over 175 publications. His work has helped establish the fields of geriatric emergency medicine and community paramedicine. He is passionate about developing the next generation of emergency care researchers and research leaders.

Years later he recalled his experience:

> *I wanted to come to OSU because I wanted the incredible clinical training to give me that solid foundation before I moved on to a research fellowship. I will never forget the neurosurgery and ICU rotations (or lose the scars from those months), my first shift in the ED as a new intern, or being expected to run the ED as an R3. Those experiences gave me the essential clinical, organizational and leadership skills that I have used every day in my career as an ED physician, EMS physician, researcher and now department chair. I wanted to complete a research fellowship after residency and I must credit Dr. Rund for getting me to the right fellowship. I was interested in the Robert Wood Johnson Clinical Scholars Program and happened to mention it to him. He had been involved in the program [since its beginning as one of the first clinical scholars] and strongly encouraged me to apply as it would be the best research training option for an emergency physician. And he was correct.*[6]

References

1. Wang HE. Interview with Henry Wang by Douglas Rund. 2023: Columbus, Ohio.

2. Southerland LT. Personal communication. 2023.

3. westjem.com/articles/the-national-clinical-assessment-tool-for-medical-students-in-the-emergency-department-ncat-em.html

4. Pirrallo RG. Personal communication. 2023.

5. Neumar RW. Interview with Robert Neumar by Douglas Rund. 2022: Columbus, Ohio.

6. Shah MN. Personal communication. 2023.

Chapter 26

Recollections

Douglas A. Rund, MD
Richard N. Nelson, MD
David P. Bahner, MD
Jeffrey M. Caterino, MD, MPH

In 2021 the editors asked faculty and residents, current and former, for their recollections about their experiences in the department. The reason for the request was to collect "eyewitness accounts," and add more texture to the narrative. The book is a representation of the continual evolution of academic emergency medicine and some of the stories that have made up the Ohio State experience. We have recorded a number of the responses here. The editors are so very grateful for these contributions.

CAROL CLINTON, MD (RESIDENCY CLASS OF 1993)

After completing medical school and her residency in emergency medicine at Ohio State in 1993 and practicing emergency medicine for 15 years, Carol Clinton, MD, was ready for a new approach to the healing arts (Figure 1). In 2004, at the dawn of the aesthetics industry, she launched a new type of service in Columbus. She created *Timeless Skin Solutions*, a practice that provided a new patient experience whereby they could maximize their skin health and appearance.

Clinton sold Timeless Skin Solutions in 2020. An educator at heart, she always found great joy in sharing her knowledge with medical practitioners, her co-workers and potential newcomers in this type of venture. One of the hallmarks of her practice was the multi-year educational curriculum (based on her residency model) she designed for her employees. "The University," as she called it, gave rise to a generation of elite aesthetics practitioners.

Years after her residency she recalled the following:

> First, as a medical student rotating through the department, the hands-on teaching and one-to-one mentorship for students was second to none of any other department I rotated through. The attendings, Dan Martin, Howie Werman, Charles Brown, Rob Griffith, and Jim Hoekstra are a few that come to mind. There were enough females who had rotated through the department and Genevieve Messick, I believe, was a chief resident that year. Tales of Grace Nejman and Linda Robinson were legendary and very encouraging to a female medical student looking for a career path.

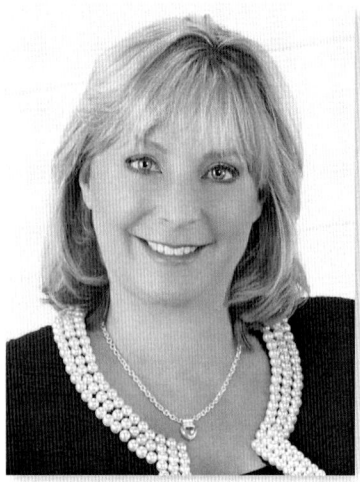

Figure 1: Carol Clinton, MD, completed her residency in emergency medicine at Ohio State in 1993. In 2004 she launched a new kind of practice in aesthetic medicine, Timeless Skin Solutions, in Dublin, Ohio.

> Listening to Doug Rund and his plans to take what he created as a Division out of the Preventive Medicine Department at the College of Medicine and bring the life to a Department of Emergency Medicine was a big factor in my choice of Residency Programs in Emergency Medicine. He had a vision for where the profession needed to go and this was an instrumental time in that development.

> As residency began, the staff of residents began to increase and the coverage of multiple hospitals ED around the city gave great exposure to intense pediatric cases, community practice and the academic setting at Ohio State. Enough trauma was being generated in our city and the removal of the rotation in Baltimore occurred. There was also enough knowledge in the department so teaching was outstanding as well. Of course, the "old fellas" felt like we had it easy not travelling to Shock Trauma and all that entailed. Chuck Brown's deep academic research in resuscitation, with Charlie Little spending a good bit of time in his lab, gave exposure to that

aspect of Emergency Medicine. While the Department was launched in 1990, my intern year, it was also highlighted by a wonderful party at the home of Dr. Rund! I am surprised I ever became Chief Resident after that as it was a night filled with libations and celebrations and my key memory besides being very happy for the forward movement of this profession, was Rund telling me to "not peak too early" as there was more to come!

Throughout my time at Ohio State in the residency program, more research was accomplished, the department and faculty increased, and the teaching and opportunities for the residents were second to none. When I left at the end of my Chief year— I had been the first female resident to have a child during my tenure— and complicated with hyperemesis, great support from the faculty and staff to help me end on time. I am sure we all learned through that process! Linda Robinson had returned to faculty by the time I left and she was a great mentor to all and a friend to me and we had great times together over the years even with her relocation to Florida. A fellow originally from Pittsburgh during my third year wrote an outstanding letter to our graduating class encouraging us to continue to learn, strive and grow and remember our heritage.

The influence of [Rund's] vision, and the entire faculty being on board and supporting [Rund] thoroughly was not lost on me. As I traversed my years in Emergency Medicine, when an opportunity to look into a new emerging area of medicine, I was not afraid to try. As one patient told me after I started my private practice in Aesthetic Medicine, "I know you will know what to do, no matter what happens!".

When I was diagnosed and hospitalized at The James for ovarian cancer in 2005, many of the faculty from the Emergency Medicine Department came to visit me and encourage me. Many had also become my colleagues in my community practice, prior to my departure from Emergency Medicine. It was a great privilege to learn from this esteemed group and I always felt 100% comfortable with a graduate of our program at my side or me referring the transfer of a patient to one of them.[1]

Sadly, Carol Clinton lost her long and determined battle with cancer and gracefully passed away surrounded by her family on June 24, 2023. She contributed much to the department over the years including the establishment of the Alumni Society. In her honor, her family established The Dr. Carol Lee Clinton Emergency Medicine Career Accelerator Endowed Fund to support early to mid-career faculty members with as many resources as possible. (https://www.dispatch.com/obituaries/pwoo0515023)

JAMES W "JIM" HOEKSTRA, MD

James W. Hoekstra, MD, graduated from the University of Michigan Medical School in 1984 and completed his Emergency Medicine residency at the University of Cincinnati (Figure 2). He joined the emergency medicine faculty at Ohio State in 1988. Following 14 years on faculty of The Ohio State University College of Medicine (see Chapter 8), he was recruited to the position of Professor and Chair of the Wake Forest Department of Emergency Medicine.

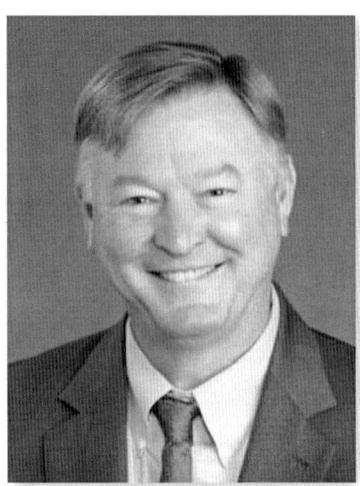

In that capacity he built a network of more than a dozen Wake Forest Baptist-managed emergency departments across North Carolina. Instrumental in the integration of Cornerstone Healthcare with Wake Forest Baptist Health, he was named Vice President for Business Development in 2015 and Senior Vice President and Associate Dean, Clinical and Academic Network Development in 2017. His work reflected a deep commitment to creating strong community, academic and provider relationships that advance Wake Forest Baptist's mission to improve health. In 2018 he was named President of High Point Medical Center, a 350-bed hospital system that joined Wake Forest Baptist Health that year.

Figure 2: James W. Hoekstra, MD, FACEP, now President of the Wake Forest Baptist Health High Point Medical Center, was one of the early leaders in Ohio State emergency medicine.

Years later he recalled his days at Ohio State:

> *I transitioned from basic science research in resuscitation to clinical research in emergency cardiology. We were studying the use of CKMB and eventually troponin as potential serum markers for acute myocardial in-*

farction. The Ohio State ED became a clinical site for several clinical trials on serum markers, short stay protocols, and novel ECGs in the diagnosis of MI and unstable angina. We set up a research lab in the ED and even hired clinical coordinators to enroll patients in clinical trials.

I remember once we were doing a bedside serum marker trial on patients with chest pain, utilizing a rapid CKMB test that required just a minute or two to run. As per our usual routine, in my copious free time, I was running tests on consented chest pain patients in the ED while I was doing my hyperbaric oxygen shifts down the hall. One patient that I was working with got anxious and decided to leave the ED against medical advice while we were still analyzing his blood. I ran the test and found out it was positive. I remember chasing him out into the parking lot and convincing him to come back to the ED because he was having an MI. Whew!!

Working clinically in the ED at Ohio State was a joy. We had such a collegial environment when we worked. There are a few situations that stand out in my memory: I was working a day shift in the ED. There was an explosion at a local factory or warehouse. We had a handful of victims in the ED with burns. I was asked to come outside to do an interview with a local TV station about the incident. I was on camera, describing the patient injuries to the TV reporter when Diane Gorgas, who was watching it all on TV at home, decided it would be a good idea to call me on my pocket phone in the middle of the interview. I'm reaching in my pocket to silence the phone on live TV. Good stuff!

We were working a day shift when someone brought in a family member of a high official who was suffering from sinus congestion. As would be predictable, the patient was placed in the trauma room, and the Chiefs of Medicine, ENT and Pulmonary Medicine were there. We emergency physicians, of course, were there as "standby" (if anyone had logistic concerns). It was decided that the patient had a sinus infection. At which point the division chief of pulmonary quietly asked me "what antibiotics are you using now to treat sinusitis?" I rest my case.

Working in the ED was often the highest form of theatre. The relationships between residents and faculty from non-EM services was often touch and go. I remember one cardiac surgeon ripping me because his post-transplant patient had died of sepsis and we had not used maximal doses of beta agonists to resuscitate him. He asked me, "does anyone use Isuprel anymore?" If only he knew how wrong he was. Some of these folks needed to take a walk in our shoes.

Doug Rund was our chairman and Rick Nelson was our medical director throughout my tenure at OSU. Howie Werman ran Air Care, and Dan Martin was the Residency Director. Most importantly Chris Dailey ran the office, and so much more! The department was extremely stable. We never had financial trouble. We never had turmoil or upheaval. We grew the research and educational programs, and grew our clinical programs. In short, we were a very successful and stable department. I have a few memories of the group that deserve mention:

Doug Rund was the epitome of a quiet leader. He led through departmental performance and through relationships. He had friends in every department and in the dean's office. He was the chair that did not make waves, and was always even keeled. As such, he was often placed in leadership positions in the practice group and in the medical school. Leading through relationships is a lesson for us all.

Rick Nelson was the medical director. His quiet demeanor and wry sense of humor were well known to all of us. Whenever he would come up to you and motion you over quietly, with his finger, you knew you had screwed up, and were in trouble. But he was always on your side.

We had corporate meetings once a quarter where all the department faculty who were corporate partners would get together to go over financials. Corporate partner status was always a moving target, up for debate. Doug was the Chair of the corporation's board of directors. Rick was President and did the financials. Our business administrator would talk billing and coding, etc. The meetings were always fun, and always in the Hunan Lion Chinese restaurant private dining room. It was Chuck Brown's first choice, and we all loved the dumplings and Tsing Tao beer. We didn't know anything about how to run a group, or how to read a balance sheet, but we muddled through and did just fine. We all learned a lot too, and have a lot of great memories.[2]

DIANE L. GORGAS, MD

Diane L. Gorgas, MD, was a leader in the residency program from the beginning of her tenure as a faculty member. One of her roles was to advise residents and beginning faculty members about their careers. She recalled the following regarding David Bahner, who eventually became one of the most eminent authorities on emergency ultrasound:

> *I do recall telling Dave Bahner in 1997 that "Maybe you should think about something besides ultrasound to choose as a focal point for your career. I think this modality has limited applications and may be just a flash in the pan.".*
>
> *(Don't take any stock tips from me!)*[3]

BRUCE K. NEELY, MD
(RESIDENCY CLASS OF 1995)

Bruce Neely, MD, was a resident from 1992-1995 and Chief Resident during his senior year (Figure 3). Years later he recalled some of his experiences:

> *Our class started out with 8, but as I recall one member was asked to repeat the first year and subsequently changed to a different specialty, and one member was asked to repeat the second year and was subsequently released from the training program, which left us with 6 graduates for the 1995 residency class. The member of the class who repeated the second year had issues taking direction from the attendings and as I recall after one particularly heated discussion with Dr. Dick, he looked towards his waist and asked me, "are they still there?". That was a pretty good indicator to me that the resident in question was not long for the program.*

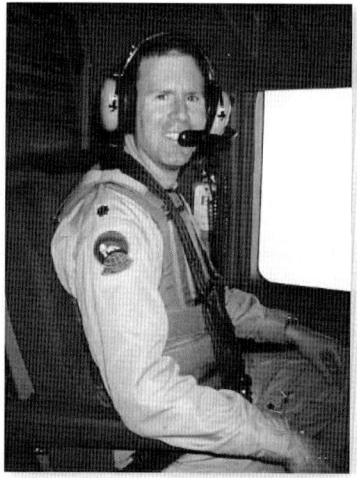

Figure 3: Bruce Neely, MD, graduated from the residency program in 1995. He went on to practice emergency medicine in the state of Washington following his residency.

Two other particularly memorable events in the OSU ED occurred during my 3rd year. It was a very busy day and as the senior resident on duty and working on the surgery side of the old ED, I was responsible for treating patients with trauma as well as supervising the junior residents on that side. The surgery side also included E4, which was the psychiatric seclusion room. After taking care of a patient with trauma I walked by the unit secretary desk and looked up at the CCTV monitor and there was a patient in E4 who was pacing around the room. I got a brief report from the junior (Dr. Emile El-Shammaa as I recall).

About that time there was another trauma. After finishing that trauma activation, I again walked by the back desk and the patient in E4 was now naked and "marking his territory" by urinating on the walls. A third trauma came in about that time. After that trauma, the patient in the seclusion room had figured out how to rearrange the foam rubber furniture in the room to barricade the door (the door opened into the room... bad design choice). Security was trying to pry the door open with a broom handle which broke and the patient grabbed the broken pointy end and was now also armed with a sharp stick. I think a fourth trauma came in about that time.

When that was done, I remember standing in the hall outside the trauma room with Dr. Rund, looking down the hall towards the room. On the floor in front of the room there was a firefighter, in full gear, kneeling down starting a chainsaw. He got the saw started and yelled down the hall to have someone look at the monitor and make sure the patient didn't get near the saw as he proceeded to turn the blade horizontal to the door and began cutting it, effectively making a Dutch door. Unfortunately, when you turn a chainsaw on its side like that the exhaust blows straight up, and there was a smoke detector right outside the room, which of course, caused fire alarms to go off all over the hospital. This caused numerous calls to the ED about "where's the fire," which were answered with "it's ok, it's just the fire department with a chain saw."

After the door was cut the patient was dragged out of the room, placed in restraints on a gurney, had a covering placed over his naked backside and was taken directly to the psychiatric facility. I remember Dr. Rund commenting afterwards, "Why did they cut the door? He would have gotten hungry at some point and would have asked to come out." Still makes me smile and laugh nearly 30 years later.

The second memorable event involved Dr. Rick Nelson. Dr. Nelson was always very serious and dour and many of the residents thought he had no sense of humor. I am here to tell you he had a fantastic sense of humor and impeccable comedic timing. At that time the overhead page for a fire was "Paging Captain Thermo" and then a floor number or unit. One day the one-inch water line that fed the X-ray processor broke. This caused a large stream of water to pour from the room and out across the hall towards the trauma room. Dr. Nelson and I walked around the corner at about the same time and saw this flood of water. Without a pause, and in a very deadpan voice, Dr. Nelson commented, "I see we have a Captain Noah," and just went on about what he was doing. The perfect comment, with perfect timing and perfect delivery. Dr. Nelson was a complete and total gem! [4]

DAVID R. JONES, MD (RESIDENCY CLASS OF 1995)

David R. Jones, MD, completed the residency in emergency medicine in 1995 (Figure 4). He was the first resident to complete an ultrasound elective and helped recruit ultrasound pioneer David Bahner, MD, to the residency program. In the past he served as Chief of Emergency Medicine at Doctors Hospital in Columbus. He continued his commitment to the department by participating in weekly conferences and the oral board simulated examinations for residents. He has also worked in sports medicine as a team physician, The Arnold Classic, various running events, and OHSAA State Wrestling Championships. He has practiced emergency medicine in many states. Years later he recalled some of his residency experiences:

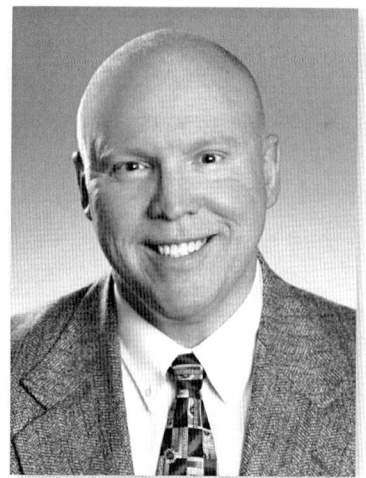

Figure 4: David R. Jones, MD, graduated from the emergency medicine residency program in 1995 and continued his affiliation with the residency program, participating in residency conferences and the oral board simulations.

One memorable encounter 15 minutes prior to the end of a busy second year shift I attempted to "grease the runway" for the oncoming resident. I went to see the next patient, who was in the seclusion room. I introduced myself to the patient and asked him why he presented to the emergency department. He was a tall, husky male who was wearing a leather jacket and worn boots and he resembled a bar bouncer of the late 1980s. He informed me that he was depressed and suicidal. I asked him if he had a plan. He informed me that he planned to kill himself with a machete.

Surprised by his response, I asked him if he had access to a machete. He said, "Sure," and continued to reach toward his right boot: he pulled out a 2-foot-long machete. In my calmest voice, I asked him if I could get him a sandwich and something to drink. He said, "Sure." I asked if he would give me his machete to make sure he was safe. I got the patient a drink and sandwich, and then signed the patient out to a fellow resident. It was the only time I passed on a machete at change of shift. I attempted to make my best Bryan Adams reference, and said it "Cuts Like a Knife" but it is machete.

I am constantly entertained and amazed by our patient encounters. I have actually looked for cameras to see if I was being "punked!" Sometimes patient interactions are unbelievable. I remember a gentleman asking me, "Is it serious Doc?" He presented with draining right thigh MRSA abscess with over 20 centimeters of cellulitis, fever and inguinal lymphadenopathy. I had initiated IV antibiotics and arranged admission. I informed patient that it was serious enough where we are admitting him to the hospital as he had the potential for limb or life-threatening infection. The patient replied, "I knew when I had my dog lick it for a week and it didn't get better, I had to come in." And to this day, he isn't wrong.

I have experienced burn out, been bitten, threatened and punched by patients. But over 99% of my patient interactions have been extremely positive. I still practice Emergency Medicine full time. If I go more than a week without working a clinical shift, I miss the human interactions with the patients and their families, and the staff, and all the people at the hospital.

I think of the Ohio State Emergency Medicine residency program as a close fraternity, and I have learned so much from each one of you. Thanks for teaching an old dog some new tricks, and for that I will forever be grateful. I'm not sure you realize how much of an impact each of you have had on my life. I still remember my Chief Residents: Alan Gora and Bruce Neely.

I have had moments to keep up with Al, but I wish I could catch up with Bruce and all the other members of our extended work family. A special thanks to Creagh Boulger, who has been extremely kind, inclusive and understanding as she shares her ultrasound knowledge.[5]

BRENDAN P. SHERIDAN, MD (RESIDENCY CLASS OF 2007)

Brendan Sheridan, MD, completed his residency in emergency medicine in 2007. He recalled a story from his residency he entitled: "Addressing your Residency Director or When to Wash your Mouth out with Soap"

The story begins with the OSU EM co-ed basketball team in a heated game against some co-ed undergraduates on one of the middle courts at the recreation center. Our team was not very formidable, but had a fun time getting exercise in between shifts. Our team was mostly composed of attendings, residents and undergraduate research assistants. Our team's tallest player was Dr. Dan Martin, our resident co-director at the time. The rest of the team was about as tall as I at a diminutive 5 feet 9 inches, which explains why one may not have heard of our team ever before.

Despite my height disadvantage I could jump and so was asked to do the tip-offs against opponents at least half a foot taller. I tried to take it upon myself to help with rebounding as well. In this game I leaped to get a rebound and had it grasped securely between my hands only to realize that I had grabbed this over the back of an opponent who was half a foot taller. He locked onto both the ball and my right hand. As gravity pulled me to earth, I was stuck with my extended right arm over his shoulder with my feet dangling 6 inches above the court. The other player then tried to jerk both the ball and my hand away, dislocating my shoulder in the process. I heard the clunking pop of my shoulder, the other player's astonishing gasp, and the referee's insulting whistle (she called me for an over the back foul). I was left kneeling and wincing in pain; I could neither feel nor move my hand as it dangled motionless.

Fortunately, if you are going to dislocate a joint it is best to do it when you are surrounded by group of OSU EM physicians! Dr. Martin expeditiously ran over and examined me diagnosing the obvious deformity. He then compassionately asked if I wanted him to reduce it then and there. With-

out hesitation I nodded yes as I could neither speak through my grunting nor did I want to wait at least another hour until I got registered, signed consent, was X-rayed, and had to wait for a respiratory therapist to come do a conscious sedation to get it reduced. I took a deep breath and concentrated on trying to slow down my breathing and relaxing what was left of my shoulder that I could control.

Dr. Martin then began his attempt of reducing my shoulder on the court by direct traction off to my right side. After a few painful unsuccessful attempts, he inquisitively asked, "is it in?" Meanwhile at least two of the other team's players were nearly passed out, all the players on all four courts were silent, and the referees stood by speechlessly as the other residents tried to explain to them that we were doctors and knew what we were doing. With all of this, my shoulder refused to move and the searing pain was increasing with every tug. Getting frustrated with the lack of Dr. Martin's progress I felt a pep talk was in order and so I turned to him and shouted through tears of pain:

"MARTIN, YOU [disrespectful expletives], PULL HARDER!"

He seemed to have heard the message and went fully Hippocratic. He grabbed my arm, placed his foot below my armpit, and fell to the floor eventually pulling the shoulder into successful alignment. And now, after what I had yelled at the top of my lungs, even all the residents were also standing speechlessly on the sidelines. Dr. Martin's daughter Jackie was also on our team and had a priceless look of disbelief seeing both a live reduction without anesthesia but also seeing her father be spoken to in such a fashion.

I am truly apologetic to the Martin family for this, but beyond this am enormously grateful. After this, both he and Travis Ulmer escorted me to the ED for x-rays and the very next morning Dr. Martin had personally gotten me an appointment with Grant Jones at the orthopedic center where I was enrolled in an immobilization study (they still call me every 5 years) and I was successfully rehabilitated without recurrence. OSU is a special place where I learned an enormous amount, some of which was medicine. More importantly I learned how to treat people especially those in the OSU family. Dr. Martin remains an inspirational model for how to be an EM physician, mentor and person and I am honored to have had a chance to be part of this unique Buckeye family.[6]

DELORES "DEE" TSCHIRNER GOODWIN, RT, (R)(M)

Delores "Dee" Tschirner Goodwin, RT, (R)(M) was an outstanding radiologic technologist who was devoted to the emergency department and never failed to help in any way she could. Years later she recalled some of her experiences in the emergency department:

I have some great memories. Great experiences!

I was standing in the hallway with Jack Sells (ED paramedic and original crew member of the Heartmobile—great guy). We were talking about how our morning was going and someone got out of a car in front of the ER and yelled that they needed help. Jack and I went out and found this woman in the back seat crying, "My baby's out." Yep, we could see the shape of a large softball between her legs. Poor thing was stuck! Jack and I got her into a wheelchair and then to a cart that sat in the hall. I think I must have said something like, "Honey, you gotta lift your bottom so I can get these pants down." She lifted and I started to help her remove her sweatpants and as I pulled, baby appeared. Jack and I just looked at each other and said, "baby!"

Within a few seconds and help from more staff, she was on her way to Labor and Delivery. I loved that I was in the right place at the right time. X-ray techs don't get to deliver babies![7]

JAMES CHAN, MD, PHD
(RESIDENCY CLASS OF 2012)

James Chan, MD, PhD (Figure 5) was the first President of the Ohio State Emergency Medicine Alumni Society established by Mark Angelos, MD, during his time as chair. The Interim Dean of the College of Medicine, Christopher Ellison, MD, strongly advised that it be named for a founding faculty member. The only other residency alumni group at that time

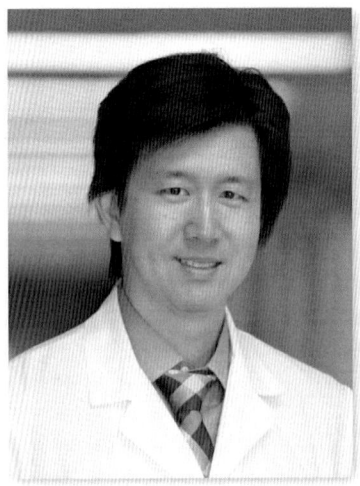

Figure 5: James Chan, MD, PhD, was the inaugural President of the Douglas A. Rund Emergency Medicine Alumni Society. Under his leadership the Society was established and soon earned "Scarlet" status, which is the highest level attainable by an Alumni Association.

was the Zollinger Surgery Residency Alumni Society and so the emergency medicine society was named the Douglas A. Rund Emergency Medicine Alumni Society. Chan was outstanding as president and devoted the time and energy necessary to make the endeavor successful. He also provided the organization and connection with Ohio State that was needed at the time. A few years later Chan recalled the following about the founding of the society:

It should be noted that while student alumni groups are widely prevalent it is uncommon to have a university-sponsored resident alumni group. In the spring of 2016, David Bahner, Greg Archual, Sam Kiehl and I had dinner one fine evening at Akai Hana restaurant to discuss the formation of [the alumni society]. Little did I know that, over sushi and sake, I was being recruited to become the founding president and chief recruiter of the inaugural board of directors. We were able to successfully assemble a wide swath of graduates from our program to serve as inaugural board members. Greg Archual took charge to set up a meeting with the OSU Alumni Association (OSUAA) to get the ball rolling. By late summer of 2016, a working group, including parliamentarian Mike McCrea, got together to draft the constitution. The first official board meeting of the Emergency Medicine Alumni Society took place on January 5, 2017.

The inaugural Board of Governors included the following people: Mark Angelos, MD, Chairman; James Chan, MD (2012) President; Michael McCrea, MD (2007) President-Elect; Hannah Hays, MD (2011) Secretary; Carol Clinton, MD (1993) Treasurer; Frank Birinyi, MD (1986); Bradford Cotton, MD (1994); Andrew Gathof, MD (2015); Tamara Halaweh, MD (2015); Brian Hiestand, MD (2001); Monica Mikkilineni, MD (2017); Richard Nelson, MD (COM 1978); Matthew Roberts, MD (2010); Douglas

Rund, MD, Founder; Travis Ulmer, MD (2007); and Michael Waite, MD (1996).

The mission of the Society is to connect and enrich the relationships between former graduates and OSU's Department of Emergency Medicine. Moreover, we want to be a resource to current residents as well as to promote emergency medicine as a specialty. MJ Fortney and David Way became tireless allies in coordinating meetings as well as creating quarterly newsletters, respectively. The Douglas Rund Emergency Medicine Alumni Society successfully achieved scarlet status within the first year of existence, by simply following the guidelines set forth by the OSU Alumni Association. In the 2017 calendar year, we held numerous events, including serving as medical volunteers at the Arnold Expo in Columbus, networking dinner at ACEP Las Vegas, Buckeye football tailgate, Columbus Zoo family picnic, and Clippers baseball family outing. In 2018, virtual mentorship was another community building endeavor that was introduced by the Alumni Society to connect current EM residents with former graduates.

References

1. Clinton CL. Personal communication. 2022: Columbus, Ohio.
2. Hoekstra JW. Personal communication. 2022: Columbus, Ohio.
3. Gorgas DL. Personal communication. 2022: Columbus, Ohio.
4. Neely BK. Personal communication. 2022: Columbus, Ohio.
5. Jones DR. Personal communication. 2023: Columbus, Ohio.
6. Sheridan BP. Personal communication. 2022: Columbus, Ohio.
7. Goodwin DT. Personal communication. 2023: Columbus, Ohio
8. Chan J. Personal communication. 2023: Columbus, Ohio.

Chapter 27
Biographies

Douglas A. Rund, MD
Richard N. Nelson, MD

This chapter focuses on four people who have served the department for 40 years or more: Christine A Dailey, Douglas A. Rund, MD, Howard A. Werman, MD, and Richard N. Nelson, MD. These individuals created a common vision in the earliest days of the department and never wavered in their dedication and perseverance. Their biographies are presented here in recognition of their service to The Ohio State University Department of Emergency Medicine, the College of Medicine, and the specialty of emergency medicine.

The Early Years

In 1973 a young cardiothoracic surgeon, Thomas E. Williams, Jr., MD, was appointed director of the emergency room. In that era, it was the norm in many academic centers for a practicing surgeon to be appointed director. It was a very part-time position for a busy surgeon early in his career. The search for a full-time director began in 1975. The search was unsuccessful for several years. By 1976 Williams could no longer manage both his busy practice and the emergency room. Another surgeon was appointed: William E. Evans, MD. Evans was a popular and successful vascular surgeon. He was only able to meet with the head nurse "once a week."[1] Both he and Williams were eager to find an emergency physician replacement— and someone dedicated to building the specialty of emergency medicine.

Despite Evans' limited time commitment, the hospital decided to provide a secretary, Carleen Burwell (Figure 1). She had begun her Ohio

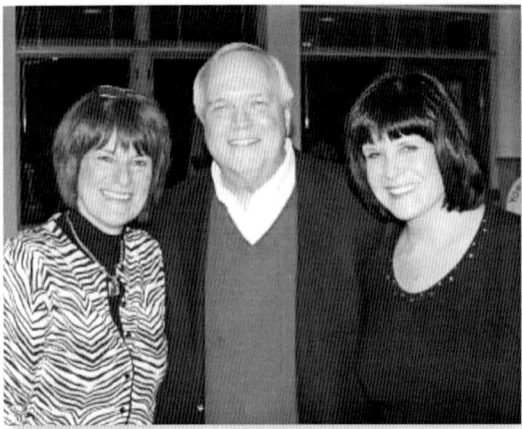

Figure 1: Carleen Burwell Mueller, Douglas Rund, MD, and Chris Dailey Shoemaker at the celebration of Rund's retirement in 2012.

State employment in the hospital billing office in 1973. She later remembered that, with Evans, she was sequestered in a small space in the Department of Surgery and had very little to do. In 1977, Burwell transitioned from surgery to assist the newly hired Chief of Emergency Services, Douglas Rund, MD.

Years later Burwell recalled those early days:

> *I worked with you from mid-1977 to December of 1979. [For a few months] we were part of the Department of Family Medicine. We met in a very small office in the clinic building. [Eventually] office space was assigned on the second floor of the clinic building. I was there during the opening of the new facility. In today's lingo I was the Administrative Assistant.*[2]

Burwell and Rund found recruiting difficult but managed to hire a few faculty members to staff the emergency room and supervise the residents. When Burwell left Columbus in 1979, she recruited Chris Dailey to replace her. Burwell and Dailey had both worked together in the business office years earlier.

CHRISTINE A. "CHRIS" DAILEY

The oldest of six children, Christine A. "Chris" Dailey grew up in Columbus (Figure 2). She began working at Ohio State in 1971 in several departments before joining emergency medicine, including the hospital billing department and the Department of Surgery. In December 1979 Dailey joined the new Division of Emergency Medicine as a secretary to the Director. At the time she was the only administrative person in a department, which had four full-time emergency physicians. Dailey expertly performed all secretarial and managerial tasks. In an era before the introduction of word processors, she created all these documents—correspondence, agreements between departments, research papers, grant applications, textbooks, and work schedules—on a typewriter. She typed the entire manuscripts of the *Triage and Essentials of Emergency Medicine* textbooks on a typewriter in an era when edits were made with liquid white-out or the text had to be completely retyped. Edits involved literally cutting and pasting pieces of paper onto a new sheet of paper and retyping by hand.

She managed the student education program, provided the student orientation, created the didactic schedule, typed the 35mm slides used in the lectures and arranged the student schedules at all the Columbus hospitals. She also coordinated the schedules for the rotating residents in the departments of Medicine and Surgery before the official launch of the residency in emergency medicine.

When the practice plan dispute was finally resolved in 1979, Dailey managed the business side of both the division and the newly created physician partnership. She created and kept the written records of the finances, managed the checkbook, paid all invoices, and sent refunds to patients when needed. She kept the written records of the partnership and all faculty meetings. She recorded all meeting minutes and worked with the accountants to manage the payroll.

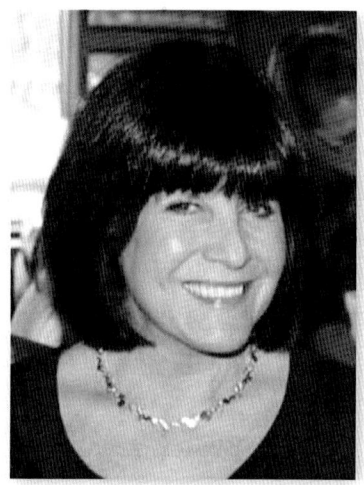

Figure 2: Christine A. "Chris" Dailey Shoemaker began her administrative responsibilities in the Department of Emergency Medicine in 1979.

She also prepared the initial application for the new emergency medicine residency program. When the program started in 1981, Dailey served as the residency coordinator for the first few years until the program grew and a full-time coordinator could be recruited.

While never really receiving all the accolades she deserved, she was recognized as the College of Medicine Employee of the Month in the early 1990s and the Administrative Staff of the Year Award for both 2015 and 2020. In 2015 she was recognized with the prestigious Gail Johannes Award, which recognizes excellent service by employees with a minimum of 25 years at Ohio State.

Over the years Daily's responsibilities increased and her job titles changed to office associate and then administrative associate. In 2023 she continues to work with the department doing the enormously challenging task of creating attending physician and advanced practice providers' work schedules. In 2023 she creates monthly schedules for 129 providers covering 43 shifts per day at five sites.

DOUGLAS A. RUND, MD

Douglas A. Rund, MD, grew up in Clintonville, a suburb just north of the university district in Columbus (Figure 3). As a child he was fascinated by the house call visits of the family doctor when he was ill with common childhood illnesses of the time, including measles. The doctor's office was in the doctors home two blocks away on High Street. Rund dreamed about someday opening a general practice where he could practice in a nice office and make house calls.

Rund and his friends would occasionally walk or take the bus to the Ohio State campus, usually to visit the Ohio Archeological and Historical Museum located in Sullivant Hall (1913) on High Street. In an era of popular horror films, they were invariably frightened by the dimly-lit Egyptian mummy exhibit on the second floor. When his parents bought their home, they wanted to be close to the High Street bus line so he could take the bus to Ohio State, where, it was assumed, he would attend college. The family's means were modest. They didn't own an automobile. He graduated from North High School, where he was active in speech and debate. He was elected President of the Senior Class and attended the American Legion's Buckeye Boys State program, where he was elected Lieutenant Governor, and the Legion's Boys Nation, an educational program in how the federal government works, in Washington, DC. His Boy's Nation group was disappointed that they could not meet with President Kennedy in 1962.

Rund attended Yale University where he majored in history and com-

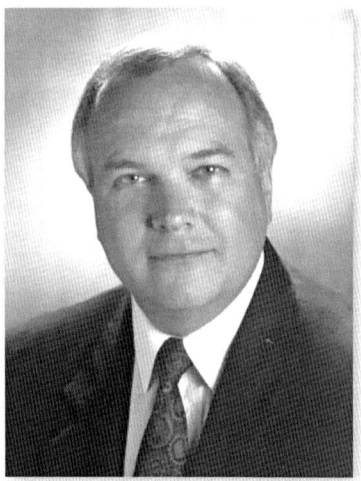

Figure 3: Douglas A. Rund, MD, served as Chief of Emergency Medicine at Ohio State from 1978 to 2011. Pictured here is his photo as President of the American Board of Emergency Medicine in 1995.

pleted the premedical curriculum. He was elected Speaker of the Yale Political Union in his sophomore year. He briefly considered a career in law and politics but on reflection had little name recognition and no financial resources whatsoever. He soon moved back to his lifelong dream of becoming a physician. He left student politics in his junior year to concentrate on the sciences. Years later, as Chair of the Department of Emergency Medicine at Ohio State, and interim Chair of two other departments, President of two national emergency medicine organizations and long-standing President of Ohio State University Physicians, he utilized some of the skills he had learned in student politics: Create and communicate a clear and compelling vision that others can support, recruit and promote the best people, and listen carefully to all constituents so that their views can be carefully considered.

During his senior year at Yale, he was accepted by the Stanford School of Medicine. At that time, Stanford had a three-year preclinical curriculum prior to the clinical experience. The intent was to encourage students to engage in scientific research with the faculty. Eager to begin seeing patients as soon as possible, Rund met with Halstead Holman, MD, an immunologist who was the Chairman of the Department of Medicine. Holman was a scientist and a visionary who was willing to explore the effect of an early clinical experience on subsequent learning of the basic sciences. Both he and Rund wanted to see if the existing four-year curriculum represented the most efficient way to educate future physicians.

Holman assigned the Chief Resident in Medicine to teach Rund about physical diagnosis. In the summer following Rund's first year, he began the medical clerkship, which was normally reserved for fourth-year students. Rund remembers that his "learning curve shot up dramatically." Finally able to wear the white coat and take care of patients, he was highly motivated to learn as much as possible about medicine. The clerkship, he felt, made learning the rest of the basic sciences easy; he could study them with the perspective of one who had been working on the wards. Realizing the importance of the preclinical curriculum and their ultimate importance to patient care, Rund completed the remainder of the basic science curriculum in one year, graduating in 1971 as a member of Stanford's Alpha Omega Alpha, the medical honorary society.

He joined the residency program in Internal Medicine at the University of California at San Francisco (UCSF) and quickly realized that his favorite rotations were in the emergency room, where first-year medical interns were supervised by a second-year resident who retired to sleep at night, leaving the interns in charge. Rund had a significantly more organized experience at the San Francisco General Emergency Room, which had a larger patient population and handled virtually all major trauma cases from around the city. Rund recalled that, for many trauma victims, his sole responsibility was to perform a "cut down" on the greater saphenous vein at the ankle, which involved making a surgical incision, identifying and mobilizing the vein, and inserting a large catheter for fluid or blood transfusion. At the time, the thinking was that this was a definitive way to get a catheter into the bloodstream and that the procedure was far away enough from the head of the bed that the rest of the resuscitation could proceed unhindered.

Despite Rund's interest, emergency medicine as a career was relatively unheard of at the major academic institutions. He initially considered a "general practice" in a remote location where a wide variety of services could be provided. Looking for a broader range of skills, he joined the residency program in general surgery at Stanford following his intern year at the University of California.

But the second-year surgical residency following a first year of internal medicine was a challenge. Surgical skills had to be learned quickly and a whole new body of knowledge acquired for each new rotation: neurosurgery, orthopedics, general surgery, and cardiovascular surgery. The residents were completely in charge at the affiliated county hospital. During his very first night on call, a patient presented with a knife embedded in his skull. The patient was still talking incoherently. Rund called his supervising resident, who was moonlighting in another hospital. The resident was irritated and admonished Rund to "shave the head and take him to the operating room. I will meet you there."

Despite the enjoyment of the operating room, he realized that the emergency room really provided the greatest satisfaction. It was the part of medicine for which he was searching. He began to realize that if emergency medicine was to be his career, he needed additional training. He consulted with Holman, his medical mentor, who was just then creating the Clinical Scholars Program at Stanford, which was sponsored by the Robert Wood Johnson Foundation. In July 1974, Rund became one of the first clinical scholars in the nation and began work on research to streamline medical education, including early clinical experiences, the use of "programmed patients" and student-taught courses in physical diagnosis. He and Holman were also exploring the idea of a patient-owned, patient centered clinical practice and together they formed the Mid-Peninsula Health Service affiliated with Stanford in Palo Alto. Rund became the Medical Director in 1976.

In his early years as a clinical scholar, Rund also began creating his own residency experience in emergency medicine. He completed two months of residency in obstetrics-gynecology at a private hospital with many deliveries and surgeries, and no other residents competing for procedures. He also completed a month of anesthesiology at Stanford. In addition, his clinical experience in emergency medicine was accumulating in hospitals throughout the Bay Area. He was creating the physician schedule at San Mateo County hospital and physicians in practice were applying for shifts to earn extra income at the rate of $15.00 per hour. Although not recognized officially as "emergency medicine," the experience of creating one's own residency was like that of Bruce Janiak, MD, the first official emergency official medicine resident in 1970, at the University of Cincinnati.

Rund's self-styled post MD training lasted five years. He completed the Clinical Scholar Fellowship in 1976 and joined the faculty at Stanford, his main responsibility being the expansion of the Mid-Peninsula Health Service. Family illness arose in Ohio, however, and he took a 90-day leave of absence to return to Columbus to be with his mother, who was seriously ill with cancer. In order to earn money in the interim, he began working for Emergency Medical Associates, mainly in the emergency room, at Grant Hospital. The group had been founded by T. William Evans, DDS, MD, in 1969 as the first emergency medicine practice in Columbus. Rund soon realized that the need to help with the illness (and meeting his future wife, Sue) would require him to relocate back to Columbus where he was to find a great new opportunity.

In 1976 Rund also joined the Ohio State Department of Family Medicine. Early in 1977 he met with Manuel Tzagournis, MD, the Medical Director of University Hospital. Unknown to Rund, Evans had recommended him to Tzagournis as a good fit for someone to become Director of Emergency Services. Tzagournis offered Rund the position and he accepted on the spot without hesitation. Tzagournis cautiously seemed to agree with Rund's vision that the future direction must include starting a residency program and establishing an academic department at Ohio State.

Rund became the Chair of Emergency Medicine when the department was established in 1990 and served in that capacity until 2011. He became Professor Emeritus upon his retirement in 2012. He and his wife, Sue, live in Worthington and enjoy time spent with their three daughters and three grandsons.

HOWARD A. "HOWIE" WERMAN, MD

Howard A. "Howie" Werman, MD (Figure 4), was born in Glen Cove, New York, in 1955. His parents, Paul and Marilyn, moved to Long Island in 1952 when the area was underdeveloped and was mostly potato and corn farms. His parents met when they were undergraduates at New York University. Paul had graduated from Brooklyn Law School but was actually more interested in real estate development and the opportunities seemed ideal for that pursuit in the early 1950's.

While Paul had grown up in Brooklyn, Marilyn was originally from Akron. Ohio. Both of her parents had extended family in the Akron area. Her father, Joseph Sholiton, graduated the Ohio State University in 1926 with a degree in Pharmacy. Ironically, Howie was a fan of the Ohio State University Buckeyes for as long as he could remember.

The family moved to Syosset, New York, in 1957 into a typical neighborhood that was springing up in the area as the Long Island suburbs were being heavily developed. Werman attended Robbins Lane Elementary

School, Harry B. Thompson Middle School, and Syosset High School. He was an above average student who only began to take his school work seriously in the 10th grade. Students at Syosset High School were generally high-achievers and like most parents in that environment, success was measured by pursuit of a professional degree. He had a neighbor who was a volunteer at Meadowbrook Hospital (now Nassau County Medical Center) and she invited him to volunteer on Saturdays in the Emergency Department. It was there that he got his first exposure to the medical profession during the years 1971-1973 although admittedly, as a high school volunteer the exposure was modest at best. It was also during this time that Werman befriended a classmate at Syosset, Gwen Zanar, who would become his life partner.

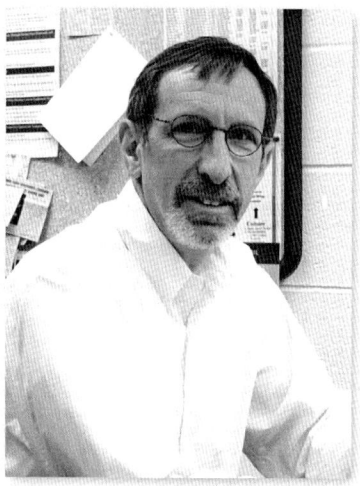

Figure 4: Howard A. Werman, MD, was a member of the first full class of emergency medicine residents at Ohio State. He graduated from the residency program in 1984 and immediately joined the faculty and conducted research in cardiac arrest. He rose to the rank of full Professor and became an international expert in emergency medical services and air medical transport.

Werman graduated Syosset High School in 1973 with a respectable place in his class. He fell in love with Duke University during a campus visit in his senior year and chose to sit out a semester and enter Duke as a 'January freshman.' What would have been his fall semester in 1973 was spent packing furniture for shipment in a factory in Queens. It was a challenging time for him, receiving phone calls and letters from high school friends describing their exciting college-life experiences while he remained behind working. But it also reinforced within him the desire to take every advantage of his opportunities once he arrived on campus.

He worked extremely hard as a college student pursuing a major in mathematics but, also continued to explore a career in medicine, volunteering at Nassau County Medical Center when he was back home, as well as Memorial Hospital in Chapel Hill. He also conducted summer research, looking at the impact of alcohol use on mitochondrial function in rats to further define the underlying causes of fetal alcohol syndrome.

He was accepted to the State University of New York at Buffalo to attend medical school. As he entered his clinical years, he enjoyed many of the medical specialties but could not settle on one specific specialty that he could envision as a lifetime career. During several of those rotations, he would be called upon to evaluate patients in the Emergency Department which at that time was staffed by surgical and medical residents.

He remembered very vividly an incident which was discussed during his rotation in the surgical intensive care unit (ICU). One of the patients was a young man who had fallen off the hood of a moving car while horsing around with friends. The patient presented to the Emergency Department quite lucid but began to decline neurologically as he was being evaluated. After a significant amount of time had elapsed, it was finally recognized that the patient had an epidural hematoma; however, surgical intervention had been delayed too long and his neurologic prognosis was poor. It is clear today that any emergency medicine resident would recognize this story of an epidural hematoma. Werman realized that the resident staffing model that he was witnessing did not provide adequate training and was not up to the standards that he was hearing about in other parts of the country, particularly the Midwest.

Werman arranged an away rotation at Akron City Hospital during November 1980 and lived with his grandparents. He enjoyed his time at Akron City Hospital, observing how emergency medicine residents trained under attending physicians. He witnessed the breadth and depth of emergency medicine practice and the broad knowledge that was required. He was impressed with the knowledge of those he encountered, including William Roush, MD, John Weigand, MD, and Michael Mackan, MD. Roush and Mackan not only demonstrated an interest in emergency medicine practice in the Emergency Department, but were also interested in the practice of paramedics *on the street*. Thus, a budding interest was born.

Werman had clearly become committed to the specialty and he interviewed for positions in Akron. When he learned of a new program opening in Columbus jointly sponsored by Ohio State University Hospital and Riverside Methodist Hospital, he called for and was granted an interview there, meeting with Rund, Samuel Kiehl, MD, and Nancy Trhlik, MD, during his visit.

It is important to describe the Emergency Department offices at that time. The academic division consisted of two offices within the emergency department itself. There was an outer and an inner door. The outer office belonged to Chris Dailey who at that time was the department's only administrator. She was the residency administrator, bookkeeper, scheduler, faculty and resident administrative supporter and any other duties that were required to run the Department. The inner office was Rund's office.

Impressed with the proposed program, Werman returned to Akron, where senior resident Richard Nelson, MD, had expressed an interest in joining the faculty of the Columbus program. As fate would have it, Werman matched at Ohio State and started his residency on the morning of July 1, 1981. In the first room he found David Roberts, MD, who was one of the early faculty members initially trained in Internal Medicine and Cardiology performing a difficult nasal intubation on a young female who was lethargic after an apparent drug overdose – there was bleeding. Werman immediately began reconsidering his residency choice. Fortunately, he decided to persist.

The early residency days were challenging, as other medical specialties did not seem to understand or respect emergency medicine. In one instance, Robert Behrendt, MD, Werman's residency classmate, was seen vigorously pushing a cart onto the elevator with a medical resident just as strenuously pushing back insisting on a longer work-up even though the ED bed was desperately needed for a new critical patient. With only four residents each year, the idea of graded responsibility was difficult to institute. On the other hand, the residents were fortunate to have great role models, including the first residency-trained faculty member, Richard Nelson, MD, who challenged the residents to have a strong depth and breadth of knowledge and excellent clinical skills so that they would be able to prove true worth on the services on which they rotated.

In the early 1980s, two new faculty were added: Thomas Bullock, MD, and Charles "Chuck" Brown, MD. Brown was recruited to develop a research program and he ultimately recruited Werman to become the program's first research fellow in 1984 and a member of the faculty.

In reflecting on his long career in academic Emergency Medicine, Werman remained grateful to so many faculty for contributing to his successful career in Emergency Medicine. However, three individuals truly stand out in terms of his career development. The first was Rund, who demonstrated a commitment of service to the Department, the Medical Center, and the College of Medicine. He made it clear that as a young specialty, the faculty would have to say 'yes' to any opportunities that presented themselves.

Rund was also chair of the Corporate Credentials Committee, a position which he bequeathed to Werman, who went on to serve in that capacity for 10 years and as a committee member for over 30 years. Werman also published many scholarly publications authoring, at Rund's request, a chapter on laryngotracheitis with Robert Schaefermeyer, MD, in Rund's book, *Emergency Medicine Annual 1983*.

Nelson provided Werman significant mentorship as well, possessing a tremendous clinical knowledge base and an adept skill set. Nelson, who served as medical director for the Westerville Division of Fire and EMS, took Werman on as an 'assistant' medical director' and fostered his love and interest in prehospital medicine. This eventually led Werman to serve in many emergency medicine roles over the years, including Medical Director for SKYMED and MedFlight, Chair of the Board of Directors of the National Registry of EMTs, ACEP and Ohio ACEP EMS Committees, the State EMS Board and Trauma Subcommittee and liaison representative to NREMT from the National Association of EMS Physicians.

Werman also credits Brown for teaching him how to conduct basic science research and encouraging him to participate in national presentations and publications. After dabbling in scientific writing during his residency, Werman was shocked to see how an initial draft of a manuscript could be 'corrected' by Brown, leaving the pages riddled with red ink. From these experiences he learned the importance of scientific exploration and publication. Additionally, Brown networked with colleagues involved in the publication of *Annals of Emergency Medicine*, for which Werman continues to serve as a Senior Reviewer, and the *American Journal of Emergency Medicine*, on whose editorial board Werman has served for many years.

Werman recognizes some of the great nurses who helped him in the early days to become a better clinician. He notes that he may have learned more from nurses like Patty Finerty, Pam McKinley, Barb Beck, Kim Lascola, Helena Collier, and Polly Hansplant than he did from the faculty. Sally Betz and Lynette Halstead taught Werman not only the basics of emergency medicine, but shared their ICU experience as well. He fondly remembers the weekend night crew of Judy Rykowski, Randi Carnahan, and Glen Lundgren (of blessed memory).

Werman retired from his EMS activities in July 2020 but continues to work many shifts in the emergency department and urgent care centers. He and his wife, Gwen, live in Bexley and enjoy their family, including 4 children and 10 grandchildren.

RICHARD N. NELSON, MD

Richard "Rick" Nelson, MD (Figure 5) was born in Akron, Ohio, in 1953. His parents, Milton and Sarah, were both musicians. Milton was a superb trumpet player and music educator performing with the Akron Symphony and ultimately became the Director of Instrumental Music for the Akron Public Schools. He was a WWII veteran and Bronze Star winner, serving in an anti-tank battalion that was among the first units to liberate Dachau concentration camp in April, 1945. Sarah was also a trumpet player and was one of the first, if not the first, female trumpet major at Dana School of Music, now part of Youngstown State University. She also played viola with the Akron Symphony as well as her own string quartet. She continued to play trumpet in community bands well into her eighties, and taught her three children, Marcia, Richard, and Linda, how to play trumpet.

The family lived in a middle-class neighborhood on West Hill, later moving to the suburbs where Rick began tenth grade at Norton High School. There he was quite active in band, debate, and science clubs. He was also active in a healthcare-oriented Explorer post at Barberton Citizens Hospital. He also was quite serious with trumpet playing, occupying first chair his junior year and first chair/soloist his senior year. He also performed with various local ensembles, including Akron Youth Symphony and various brass groups and summer band at the University of Akron. By the time he finished high school, he was torn between a career in music versus one in medicine. Ironically, both his musician

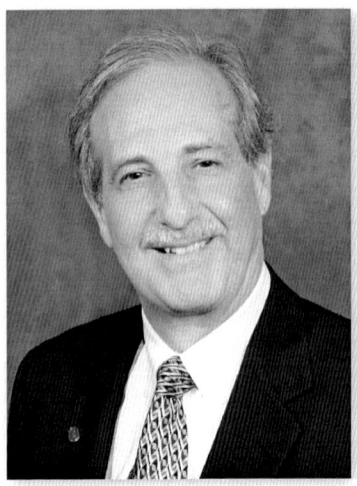

Figure 5: Richard N. Nelson, MD, Professor, Department of Emergency Medicine as President of the American Board of Emergency Medicine in 2011.

parents encouraged him to go the pre-med route.

He began college at the University of Akron, a predominantly commuter state college, in the summer of 1971 with both music and academic scholarships. He did well academically while also remaining active in marching and symphonic bands as well as brass choir. He also worked part time as a custodian with some friends at a local Ford dealership and earned some money doing various gigs on trumpet.

One of his favorite memories from college was his involvement in a hoax he and a friend perpetrated on the University of Akron student newspaper, *The Buchtelite*. Over a two-month period in 1974 the two students, neither of whom worked for the newspaper, submitted sports articles about the university's table tennis team of which they were captains. By the time the newspaper discovered that no such team existed, the story of the hoax was picked up by the wire services and received widespread coverage across the country.[3]

Nelson graduated in December, 1974, and the day after graduation received his letter of acceptance to the Ohio State University College of Medicine, which he entered in July 1975. At the time, The Ohio State University College of Medicine was a three-year program which students attended year-round. The equivalent of the basic science first year in a traditional four-year curriculum was the most challenging, being completed in just five and a half months. Classes and labs went all day on weekdays with evenings and weekends reserved for studying.

An opportunity available to first year students interested Nelson if only because it was grounded in medical reality: a ride-along program with Columbus Division of Fire medic units. The program, developed by the College of Medicine in cooperation with the Columbus Division of Fire, had students spend the evening and night in the firehouse, joining the crew whenever there was a call. The students' function was primarily observing; however, they would typically help carry equipment, which served a useful purpose in helping the students get through the police barricades on some of the sketchier runs. The paramedics took Nelson under their wing, teaching him a great deal and demonstrating the value of a well-designed and run prehospital care system. Nelson says experience provided valuable insight into prehospital care, and helped break up the tedium of the first-year curriculum.

One of his later core clinical rotations was General Surgery, which he opted to do at Akron City Hospital in June 1977. He would often spend his nights on-call in the emergency department, where the residents would gladly give up procedures such as laceration repairs and abscess drainages to the student from Ohio State. He participated in code blues, performed CPR, and was invited to perform endotracheal intubations after the fact in cases in which resuscitation efforts were unsuccessful. It was during these codes that he met his future wife, Susan Pickenpaugh who worked the night shifts as an EKG tech while majoring in Speech and Hearing. They of course began seeing each other and the relationship eventually became permanent.

After Akron, Nelson continued his rotations at Ohio State. One of his most memorable rotations was Neurosurgery, which he began on July 1, 1977, immediately after the Akron rotation. One reason the rotation was so memorable was that, effective June 30th, the entire neurosurgery residency class had quit and either left the field or transferred to other programs, leaving Nelson as the lone student and Stephen Hill the lone first year neurosurgery resident to run the busy service. Nelson had the opportunity to first-assist on many surgical procedures, one of his most memorable experiences being on a traumatic head bleed case with Joseph Goodman, MD, a junior neurosurgery faculty member.

The patient was a young man who had fallen and had brief loss of consciousness followed by a short period of lucidity, followed again by unconsciousness. Goodman, of course, immediately recognized this was likely an epidural hematoma that required immediate decompression with burr holes. Because CT scans were not yet available, all medical decisions had to be made clinically. The patient had a unilateral dilated pupil on the left, which correlated to both the likely side of the bleed and the impending burr holes. Using a hand drill worthy of Home Depot, he drilled the first hole and was rewarded with a large gush of blood. He then allowed Nelson to drill the second and third holes. This was a seminal educational experience for the future emergency physician.

In 1977 Nelson chose to pursue a career in emergency medicine even though emergency medicine (EM) was not yet a boarded specialty and many of the early pioneers and many then entering the field were specialists in internal medicine. Not surprisingly, very few of the College of Medicine's class of 1978 included EM on their match lists, though many of his classmates would later switch to an emergency medicine career during or after their residencies in traditional specialties. One thing that convinced him to pursue an EM residency was his experience at Akron City, including an EM elective there in the fall of 1977. Nelson remembers noticing that the EM attendings who had trained in traditional specialties, knew about emergencies within their specialties, however only those who had completed EM residencies demonstrated a mastery of virtually all conditions presenting to the ED. On Match Day Nelson got his first choice, Akron City Hospital.

Residency began in July, 1978 with a rotation in the ED. It was a busy summer month with many medical and surgical patients to manage under the watchful eyes of senior residents and attendings. One patient he remembers vividly and who helped solidify his decision on choice of specialty, was a middle-aged man who presented with chief complaint of leg cramps after spending a good part of the day mowing his lawn. Nelson initially thought this was a silly complaint to seek care in the emergency department; and indeed, the patient's vital signs and general appearance were benign. Nelson did notice a spotty rash on both legs, which the patient thought was related to contact with grass and weeds.

He presented the case to John Weigand, MD, an EM trained attending who did his residency across town at Akron General, a rival hospital. Dr. Weigand was an attending who epitomized the well-trained emergency physician, one who could diagnose and manage whatever came through the door. Weigand examined the patient and suggested the patient required a more extensive work up than what Nelson initially proposed. Weigand suggested obtaining lateral lumbar x-rays to include the soft tissue anterior to the lumbar spine.

Those who trained in the 1970s would immediately recognize what he was looking for: an abdominal aortic aneurysm, and in Weigand's determination, one that contained an intraluminal thrombus that was showering his lower extremities with small emboli, thus explaining the rash. Today, this would be easily diagnosed with CT angiogram or ultrasound of the abdomen, however, in those days neither study existed. The only way to make the definitive diagnosis was by contrast angiography, which was not an easy test to obtain, especially on a weekend, and generally required hospital admission. The lateral lumbar film did indeed show calcification of the aorta with characteristic aneurysmal bulge, the so-called egg shell sign (present in 50% of aneurysms). Weigand then had to convince the vascular surgeon and the radiologist to come in from home and admit and manage the patient, which both did reluctantly. Of course, Weigand's diagnosis, including the intramural thrombus, was totally accurate and the patient went to the operating room and ultimately did well. The lesson Nelson learned was that life-threatening conditions can be present in well-looking patients with seemingly trivial presentations, and they require an expert diagnostician like Weigand to figure it out. Nelson decided then that he wanted to be such an expert diagnostician.

Near the end of his residency, Nelson learned that his alma mater, Ohio State, was starting up an EM residency program in July 1981. He had always been interested in resident education and had presented well-received lectures on emergency related topics to his fellow residents in conferences. He called the Ohio State emergency department to inquire about a job. Division Director Rund spoke with him, confirming they were looking to recruit faculty for their new residency program. Nelson's background was so impressive that he was offered a position soon after his interviews, ultimately becoming the first emergency medicine residency graduate hired into the Division.

On arrival, Nelson set to work preparing the teaching program for the new emergency medicine residents largely based on his curriculum in Akron. Nelson eventually became active with the Ohio American College of Emergency Physicians (ACEP), serving as the first state medical director of a new pre-hospital trauma program called Basic Trauma Life Support (later called International Trauma Life Support). He also served on the program's national board of directors and editorial board. Other activities he pursued during the 1980s included participating in 1983 as an oral examiner for the American Board of Emergency Medicine (ABEM), then in 1987 as an item writer, writing questions for ABEM's written certification exam.

By the late 1980s Nelson had transitioned from Associate Residency Director to Medical Director of the emergency department. He became President of Emergency Care Associates, Inc, the department's practice plan, and among other things, negotiated better group rates for liability insurance and established a group pension and profit-sharing plan. In 1993 he became Medical Director of Hyperbaric Medicine at the Ohio State Medical Center and was instrumental in establishing a hyperbaric medicine unit in the emergency department, one of the few programs in Ohio that provided 24/7 emergency hyperbaric services.

Nelson also became active in organized medicine and before the decade was out had served as President of both Ohio ACEP and the Columbus Medical Association, during which he helped establish Central Ohio Trauma Systems and served on its executive committee for many years. He was also elected to the American Medical Association House of Delegates as an Ohio representative. In addition, he was active in political and legislative efforts and was the lead physician behind Ohio H.B. 361, passed in 1998, which established the prudent layperson standard for defining an emergency medical condition in Ohio. By then, Nelson had become Vice Chair of the department. Other leadership roles included ABEM board member in 2004 where he ultimately became ABEM President in 2011-2012.

In 2013 Nelson stepped down as Vice Chair of Clinical Affairs after almost 25 years, transitioning to directing the new AfterHours Care Clinics. Nelson officially retired at the end of 2014, and then was hired back as Professor Emeritus, working clinically in the AfterHours and Advanced Immediate Care clinics, and providing administrative support to the medical center as one of several Emergency Department Physician Advisors (EDPA), physicians who help determine inpatient versus observation status for patients admitted to the hospital.

In 2015 he was honored as the first recipient of the newly established Richard N. Nelson Distinguished Alumni Award, given annually to a graduate of the College of Medicine or EM residency/fellowship programs who distinguish themselves through significant contributions to the specialty of Emergency Medicine. At the time of this book's printing, Nelson continues in his Advanced Immediate Care (later called Advanced Urgent Care) and EDPA roles, and also has been active in helping to establish the Douglas A. Rund EM Alumni Association as well as the College of Medicine Emeritus Professor Society and Medical Heritage Center.

Nelson has rekindled his interest in music. During the 1980s he developed an interest in Irish music and the guitar. Although, according to Ancestry.com, he has zero percent Celtic heredity. He now performs and records with different Irish musicians throughout the country. He and his wife, Sue, live in Westerville and enjoy visits and vacations with their three daughters and grandchildren.

References

1. Evans WE. Interview with William E. Evans, MD by Douglas Rund. 1977: Columbus, Ohio.

2. Burwell Mueller C. Personal communication. 2023.

3. Price, Mark J: Local history: Fake pingpong team pulls off hoax at University of Akron in the 1970s. *Akron Beacon Journal*, April 9, 2012. (https://www.beaconjournal.com/story/lifestyle/2012/04/09/local-history-fake-pingpong-team/10606400007/)

Chapter 28

The Future and the Ohio State Department of Emergency Medicine

Jeffrey M. Caterino, MD, MPH

The preceding chapters have told the story of emergency medicine at Ohio State during its first 45 years as an academic structure. The foundational work done by the pioneers and those who followed set the stage for the department to continue to grow as a world-class entity. Even though the specialty itself is undergoing stress in the post COVID-19 years, the strong foundations of the department ensure that emergency medicine at Ohio State will be among the leaders in the nation as the specialty evolves in the coming years.

Health care systems throughout the country are overwhelmed. Increasing patient numbers and insufficient staffing have caused a growing crisis. Emergency departments, the entry point for the sickest patients, are the front lines and are facing unpredictable surges in demand. Inpatient units are also inundated. The result is that patients destined for hospitalization are kept in the emergency department for indefinite periods, sometimes days. The phenomenon, known as inpatient boarding, creates distressing challenges.

Emergency medicine has had to develop innovative care pathways and models out of necessity. Leaders have been challenged to apply such innovations both within the emergency department and the institution. The COVID-19 pandemic taught nimbleness and innovation and brought both to the culture of the department. As a result, the current generation of leaders can rapidly adapt to challenges and adopt new initiatives to meet them. This chapter includes a brief review of what the future might look like for various mission areas.

Clinical Operations

The emergency department footprint will not be increasing in the next decade as it has in previous years. As a result, all care providers will have to make the most effective use possible of available space and resources. This is a challenge that academic emergency departments throughout the country will also face. At Ohio State new strategies have been deployed. Much of the effort has been led by Mark Conroy, MD, Director of Emergency Services (Figure 1). Conroy works collaboratively with the Director of Nursing and the Business Operations Manager to oversee the University Hospital ED, the Observation Unit, the Center for EMS and the Hyperbaric Unit. Conroy played an essential role in creating the emergency procedures during the COVID-19 pandemic.

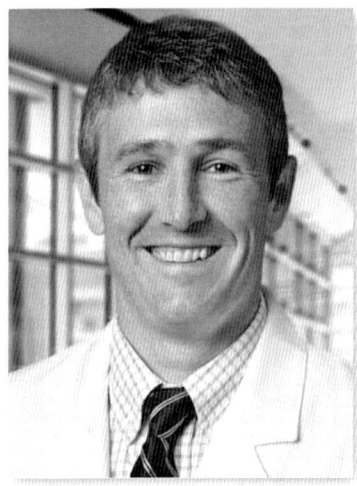

Figure 1: Mark J. Conroy, MD, Director of Emergency Services in the Ohio State Department of Emergency Medicine, played a critical role in creating COVID-19 emergency procedures during the pandemic.

Strategies developed by the leadership are based upon sound principles of management and operational improvement. One example is the redesign of the front-end processes to efficiently move patients through the department. Appropriate patients are now seen by a physician and care team before reaching an ED bed, with many able to be dispositioned as a result of this initial evaluation. Such improvements also include well-defined effective search processes to rapidly find available beds. The next steps include closely working with consultants and other departments to ensure optimal collaborations and jointly developed patient care strategies. Thanks to the front-end redesign and other process improvements, Conroy's operations leadership team has already been successful in decreasing ED boarding and eliminating the chance that patients would not first be seen by a physician and care team before directed to an ED bed. A particular challenge will be to ensure that all these innovations are provided both in the University Main and East emergency departments.

In fall of 2023, the advanced *immediate* care centers will be renamed advanced *urgent* care centers. This will put them clearly in the lineup of patient options within the health care system. The first of the centers—in New Albany and Dublin—have been tremendously successful. As of spring 2023, the two centers combined are already seeing over 40,000 patient visits per year. These facilities will continue to offer the services of Ohio State emergency physicians, but to a much larger community than possible through the current two urban emergency departments. They are tremendous assets both for the entire Ohio State health system and the emergency department. Additional capacity will also be available with the expansion of Martha Morehouse hours as well as the addition of a new urgent care facility in Powell. Current plans call for the addition of more centers at the end of the decade.

While patients seeking care at these outpatient centers typically have less acute conditions than might have been treated previously in the larger hospital, the level of care provided in the centers is high and patients with more serious conditions can be managed expertly—at least in the early stages. The physicians are emergency physicians, and advanced testing and imaging are available. Most patients can be managed completely on site without the need for hospital transfer. The expansion of these advanced urgent care/advanced immediate care centers enables the faculty to increase the clinical services provided to the entire central Ohio community.

The leadership team is excellent and their expertise will allow the department to continue to succeed. Gregory M. "Greg" Archual, MBA, Chief Operating Officer and Administrator of the Department of Emergency Medicine, manages financial, regulatory, and institutional issues, and is a nationally recognized leader in emergency department administration. Likewise, the department benefits from the services of finance manager Elizabeth Savage, who is indispensable given the ever-increasing complexity of the department's business. Mary-Jayne Fortney, who has years of experience in handling administrative issues as Administrative Coordinator to the Chair, has a long history of excellence, including working closely with former Deans and Vice Presidents.

Education

A number of new leaders are emerging in the education space. For the emergency medicine/internal medicine residency program, Jennah Morgan, MD, and Greg Eisinger, MD, are new assistant program directors. Emergency medicine categorical residents Krystin Miller, MD, and Jennifer Yee, DO, join assistant program directors Geremiha G. Emerson, MD, and Simiao Li-Sauerwine, MD. The residency programs already draw from a national group of outstanding candidates. Many are from top medical schools.

In the 2023 match, the specialty of emergency medicine faced substantial challenges nationwide. The pandemic reduced patient volumes in emergency departments, and the continued boarding and operational challenges after the pandemic ebbed discouraged many students from pursuing the specialty. This fallout led to a significant decrease in medical school graduates' applications to emergency medicine residency programs. The phenomenon was compounded by the release of a questionable workforce study indicating concerns over the availability of jobs following emergency medicine residency training.[1]

Despite the study findings, however, all signs indicate that emergency medicine physicians will continue to be in demand for the foreseeable future.[2]

In addition, operational improvements implemented in many emergency medicine departments nationwide, and certainly at Ohio State, have had an increasingly positive effect. As emergency medicine emerges from the pandemic, the faculty anticipates that applicant numbers will again rise to fill the positions available. In fact, the 2023 resident match at Ohio State was successful with all positions filled with excellent candidates.

Program leaders and faculty at Ohio State have addressed any concerns head on with ever new and evolving ideas and teaching modalities. For example, the residency program has now implemented coaching programs, flipped classroom didactics, mastery procedural curricula and residency tracks in a variety of disciplines. Program leaders and faculty have also focused on ensuring that the residents who train here are of the highest quality and have the best experience possible. In fact, Ohio State emergency medicine faculty members are national leaders in resident wellness and innovative curriculum development.

Our education faculty also continues to be one of the leading departments in the College of Medicine in education scholarship output. Several education faculty members have presented their research and innovations at national meetings such as the Society for American Emergency Medicine, Council of Residency Directors in Emergency Medicine and the American College of Emergency Physicians. In 2023, Kelsey Jordan, PhD, joined David Way, MEd, Senior Medical Education Research Scientist, to help with our education and ultrasound scholarship and resident projects.

The relationship with medical students is also increasingly important and the undergraduate medical education group will remain heavily involved in the College of Medicine curriculum. The leaders in this space include Nick Kman, MD, Chris San Miguel, MD, Cynthia Leung, MD, Ben Ostro, MD, Matt Malone, MD, and Henry Young, MD, among others. This group also emphasizes mentoring and student engagement as critical efforts to ensure the pipeline for the future of emergency medicine.

Finally, the department will continue to recruit and train physicians through its fellowship programs. Some fellowship graduates will, of course, stay on as faculty, but all, including those who move on to other institutions, are destined become leaders within their area of expertise. A new social emergency medicine fellowship will be recruiting for 2024 and will join the other currently active fellowships. Training excellent fellows is critical for the continued advancement of the department's reputation and sows the seeds with future leaders in the specialty.

Diversity, Equity and Inclusion

Departmental diversity, equity and inclusion (DEI) efforts continue to expand with active collaboration between faculty and residents and under the leadership of Henry Young, MD, Vice Chair of DEI for the Department of Emergency Medicine and Assistant Dean of Diversity and Inclusion for Learners at the Ohio State Wexner Medical Center. DEI efforts will touch on all aspects of the mission, including clinical operations, community outreach, education and research. A key goal in the next several years is to ensure that emergency medicine faculty members collaborate effectively with those of other College of Medicine departments and the institution.

These efforts will create the greatest faculty impact particularly in community outreach and improved clinical operations. The plan is to continue our early wins in areas such as support of local churches, health fairs, vaccination efforts and other community outreach. One goal is to continue providing services in Ohio State East Hospital's after-hours clinic adjacent to the ED which provides, at present, the only urgent care option for the residents of the near east side of Columbus.

In regard to education, faculty and trainees alike are increasingly involved in efforts to ensure a diverse and equitable training experience. Likewise, efforts in research encompass areas of particular concern to underrepresented communities such as access to care and provision of early intervention services. Most important, in all recruitment efforts for faculty, ATPs, residents and fellows, the department will continue to follow diversity principles as established by all components of the College of Medicine.

Division of Ultrasound

The Division of Ultrasound is already internationally recognized for its excellence and innovation. In addition to its ongoing programs, the next decade will see Department of Emergency Medicine ultrasonography faculty training not just solely for emergency medicine physicians, but also for physicians in departments across the institution and even those outside Ohio State. The goal is to bring point-of-care ultrasound (POCUS) to the bedside regardless of the department or prior training of the treating physician. The POCUS effort has begun with the acceptance of faculty from other departments into the ultrasound fellowship training program, which expands the Department of Emergency Medicine's excellence-in-training model across the entire Ohio State health sciences. The strong research program will also continue.

Novel areas of point-of-care ultrasound are being investigated such as transesophageal echocardiogram in cardiac arrest. These efforts will allow point-of-care ultrasound to take the next step in its development.

The future of the US Division will be bright. Key faculty such as David Bahner, MD, helped establish an ultrasound ecosystem and he continues work to expand the ultrasound education infrastructure he has been building since the 20th century. Now, the next generation of leaders can thrive and personalize their ultrasound career path. Creagh Boulger, MD, leads I POCUS, Institutional Point of Care Ultrasound, a medical center wide committee addressing credentialing, policy and educational needs surrounding point of care ultrasound. Her mentorship and fostering of ultrasound fellows like Lauren Branditz, MD, Carolyn Martinez, MD, Hilary Stroud, DO, Irene Mynatt, DO, and Jessica Everett, MD, have led them to join the Ultrasound Division and lead educational and administrative initiatives. Mynatt leads outreach programs like MD Camp, which brings high school students from underserved communities to campus. As faculty, they teach ultrasound to high school students, administer a plan for an undergraduate course in ultrasound, and implement the 4 Year advanced competency that starts in 2023. The Division is a leader in ultrasound education for all ages.

The Ultrasound Division aims to be the best program in the world and thus the monetization of each service line becomes important. Generating research dollars and continuing to publish innovative ultrasound techniques and teaching tips as well as clinical impact of ultrasound programs will help the US Division grow. Mike Prats, MD, leads the US Division research efforts and his Ultrasound G.E.L. podcast, citing evidence from the literature, is broadcast to over 100 countries.

The educational footprint in the medical school and medical center can also help foster the next generation of ultrasound leaders with proper support. The continued miniaturization of ultrasound equipment, improved image resolution and augmented technical features makes ultrasound technology even more impactful in medical care.

As more specialties, specialists and generalist providers become interested in learning ultrasound, the lessons learned from the EM US journey are applicable to help shepherd more nascent programs in other specialties. Boulger's leadership with I POCUS helps to bring a

POCUS priority, medical center wide, to education, credentialing, and best practice with ultrasound. As the Ultrasound Division continues to share knowledge and experience with others, its reputation and impact within the medical center and beyond will continue to grow.

Clinical Research

The Department of Emergency Medicine research program has undergone unprecedented growth over the last five years, transforming from a program featuring the work of one or two individuals to a large team with diverse expertise.

The department now has nine NIH-funded investigators at all career stages, a number that eclipses all but a few departments of emergency medicine in the nation. Several internationally recognized investigators joined the department in 2021-2022, bringing unparalleled breadth and depth to the department's areas of scientific expertise. Adding to existing programs in geriatrics, oncology and implementation science are new teams immersed in prehospital care, resuscitation, substance use disorders and public health.

Led by Henry Wang, MD, MS, MPH, Ashish Panchal, MD, PhD, and Michelle Nassal, MD, PhD, the prehospital and resuscitation science group is focused on prehospital care and novel approaches to resuscitation from cardiac arrest. Wang joined the department in 2021 as the new Vice Chair for Research, bringing his vast experience with prehospital, resuscitation and acute care research. His current efforts entail innovative approaches to clinical trial design and implementation. He is poised to receive an NIH UG3/U24 grant of over $10 million to conduct a multicenter clinical trial of pediatric prehospital airway resuscitation. Nassal's program includes using noninvasive biomarkers to guide resuscitation of out-of-hospital cardiac arrest and she will receive her first NIH K grant in Fall of 2023. Panchal's STOP-COVID project, a team collaborative involving multiple Ohio State clinical and basic sciences departments, is tracking first responders and health care workers to identify not just the biological mechanisms of COVID-19 immunity and recovery, but also the linkages to health stressors and beliefs.

Led by Michael S. Lyons, MD, Brittany Punches, RN, PhD, and Emily Kauffman, DO, MPH, the public health and substance use disorders group demonstrates the vital opportunities in the ED for public health screening and intervention. Kauffman previously created clinical programs of ED-based treatments for opiate use orders. Lyons and Punches (formally affiliated with the College of Nursing) arrived at Ohio State in the spring of 2022, bringing their vast experience with ED-based public health intervention programs. This team is also highlighting the important opportunities intersecting research and clinical care.

Also joining the clinical research program is world renowned toxicologist Edward Boyer, MD, PhD. Boyer's work explores how to utilize advanced technologies at the intersection of substance abuse, HIV and human behavior. Boyer is also one of the few emergency physicians nationally funded by a prestigious NIH K24 mid-career mentoring award; in this capacity, Boyer has trained dozens of young scientists. Boyer's skills will set the stage for Ohio State to become a major training ground for EM scientists internationally.

Division of Basic and Translational Sciences

In 2023, the department established a new Division of Basic and Translational Sciences with Mahmood Khan, PhD, as the division director. This is a recognition of the bright future seen for basic and translational sciences within the department. The division initially consists of two NIH-funded investigators, Khan and Venkata Garikipati, PhD. Over the next decade, the plan is to support continued aggressive growth of this division. In collaboration with the Dorothy M. Davis Heart Lung Research Institute, Ohio State will be making an investment in regenerative medicine. Regenerative medicine uses a variety of techniques to repair tissue or organs that have been damaged by heart disease, aging, trauma or other processes. This is a new frontier in medical therapy. The goal is to bridge the gap between basic scientists and clinicians within the department and to enhance collaboration between investigators in various departments in the Ohio State College of Medicine and investment in the processes and techniques of regenerative medicine. With the combined efforts, the department is positioned to lead in the development of new therapies and establish itself as a national leader in the field.

Philanthropy

Alumni and faculty have been extremely generous in supporting the department through philanthropy. The most recent endowment is the Dr. Carol Lee Clinton Emergency Medicine Career Accelerator Endowed Fund, named in her honor.

A graduate of the Emergency Medicine residency program in 1993, Clinton lost her 18-year battle with ovarian cancer in June 2023. In her last hours she expressed that it was her desire to support early- to mid-career faculty with as many resources as possible with a focus on supporting underrepresented folks in the medicine space. She was especially passionate about this endeavor. This fund is going to impact the futures of numerous physicians in perpetuity, and she expressed hope that the fund would grow with future contributions from alumni and friends of the department.

Great Expectations

This book—telling the story of emergency medicine at Ohio State—has been a labor of love and a gesture of respect and admiration for those who have spent all or parts of their career in making the Ohio State Department of Emergency Medicine one of the most successful in the country. In 45 short years, the department has gone from justifying its existence to demonstrating national leadership in clinical care, research and education. The specialty of emergency medicine will continue to remain strong and continue to serve as the safety net for our health care system.

Over the coming decades, the Department of Emergency Medicine will continue both to provide care to the people of central Ohio and to lead the way in developing and deploying new clinical innovations to improve care for people across the country and the world. The education team will continue to impact the education of every single medical student who comes through the College of Medicine. They will also continue to generate both excellent emergency medicine physicians and leaders for the specialty and health care in general in the years to come.

The research team will continue pushing the envelope in both the basic and clinical sciences, developing new theories therapies, new operational processes and new interventions to help the most ill and the most vulnerable in our population.

It is with profound gratitude that we thank those who have made and will continue to make the Ohio State Department of Emergency Medicine truly great.

References

1. Marco CA, Courtney DM, Ling LJ, Salsberg E, Reisdorff EJ, Gallahue FE, Suter RE, Muelleman R, Chappell B, Evans DD, Vafaie N, Richwine C. The emergency medicine physician workforce: projections for 2030. *Ann Emerg Med.* 2021; Dec;78(6):726-737. doi: 10.1016/j.annemergmed.2021.05.029. Epub 2021 Aug 2.

2. Gettel CJ, Courtney DM, Janke AT, Rothenberg C, Mills, AM, Sun W, Venkatesh AK. The 2013 to 2019 emergency medicine workforce: clinician entry and attrition across the U.S. geography. *Ann Emerg Med.* 2022; Sep;80(3):260-271. doi: 10.1016/j.annemergmed.2022.04.031. Epub 2022 Jun 16.

Selected List of Figures

Chapter 1
1-2	T. William Evans, DDS, MD, FACS	8
1-3	Samuel J. Kiehl, MD	11
1-4	Thomas Williams, MD, PhD	15
1-5	Peter Rosen, MD	18
1-6	Douglas A. Rund, MD	21

Chapter 2
2-2	E. Christopher Ellison, MD	30
2-4	David E. Roberts, MD	35

Chapter 3
3-1	Manuel Tzagournis, MD	43
3-2	Martin D. Keller, MD, PhD	44
3-4	Nancy Thrlik, MD	48
3-5	Tom Sutton, MD, Richard Cline, MD, and John Gaeuman, MD	49

Chapter 4
4-2	Richard N. Nelson, MD	64
4-3	Kendel Kidwell, MD	69
4-4	Robert Behrendt, MD	70
4-5	Michael Kelley, MD, Howard A. Werman, MD, and Robert Behrendt, MD	71

Chapter 5
5-1	Emergency Medicine Faculty Mid 1980s: Werman, Brown, Roberts, Bullock, Rund and Nelson	84
5-9	Geraldine Keller, PhD and Martin D. Keller, MD, PhD	95

Chapter 6
6-1	Charles G. Brown, MD	104
6-3	Robert Hamlin, DVM, PhD	108
6-4	Robert Neumar, MD, PhD, Charles G. Brown, MD, and Kevin Ward, MD	114

Chapter 7
7-6	Thomas R. Bullock, MD	126
7-7	James W. Hoekstra, MD	131
7-8	Daniel R. Martin, MD, MBA	132
7-9	Emergency Medicine Faculty 1990s	133
7-10	David G. Cornwell, PhD	135

Chapter 8
8-1	Mark G. Angelos, MD	142
8-2	Charles M. Little, DO	144
8-4	Robert Griffith, MD	147
8-5	Robert Guthrie, MD	150
8-6	Diane L. Gorgas, MD	153
8-7	Michael Waite, MD	156
8-8	Emile El-Shammaa, MD	157
8-9	Leo Richard Boggs Jr., MD	158
8-10	David P. Bahner, MD	160
8-11	Sorabh Khandelwal, MD	161
8-12	Thomas J. Gavin, MD	165
8-13	Craig B. Key, MD	166
8-14	Colin G. Kaide, MD	167
8-15	Stephanie Cook, DO	170
8-16	Grant Morrow, MD	174

Chapter 9
9-3	Christine A. "Chris" Dailey	187
9-6	James Coleman	201
9-7	Richard J. Sobieray, MHA	204
9-8	Kelly J. Scheiderer, RHIA, MHA	205

Chapter 10
10-1	Brian C. Hiestand, MD, MPH	211
10-2	Carlos A. Torres, MD, PhD	212
10-3	Jeffrey M. Caterino, MD, MPH	215
10-4	Michael R. Sayre, MD	216
10-5	Michael R. Dick, MD	221
10-6	Nicholas E. Kman, MD	224
10-7	Aaron W. Bernard, MD	226
10-8	Donald L. Norris, MD	229
10-10	Jillian McGrath, MD	230
10-11	Ayesha Khan, MD	231
10-12	Mark G. Moseley, MD	237
10-13	Gary Katz, MD, MBA	239
10-14	Eric J. Adkins, MD	241
10-15	Daniel J. Bachmann, MD	242
10-16	Emergency Medicine Faculty: 25 Anniversary, 2003	244
10-17	Douglas A. Rund, MD: portrait, 2012	245

Chapter 11
11-1	Thomas E. Terndrup, MD	247
11-2	Andrew M. King, MD, MEd	249
11-3	Luca R. Delatore, MD	253
11-4	Ashish R. Panchal, MD, PhD	257

SELECTED LIST OF FIGURES

Chapter 12
12-1	Mark G. Angelos, MD	263
12-2	Gregory Archual, MBA	264
12-3	Samuel J. Kiehl, MD Endowment recognition event, 2021	273
12-4	Matthew Lashutka, MD	274
12-5	Linda A. Robinson, MD	275

Chapter 13
13-1	Jeffrey M. Caterino, MD, MPH	281
13-3	Henry E. Wang, MD, MS, MPH	295
13-4	Edward W. Boyer, MD, PhD	296

Chapter 14
14-9	David P. Keseg, MD	310
14-10	Ronald G. Pirrallo, MD	313
14-13	Brooke M. Moungey, MD	316

Chapter 15
15-5	Ashley Larrimore, MD	329

Chapter 17
17-6	Richard Nelson, MD, Sara O'Neilly, RN, Marla (Unterzuber) Milstead, RN, and Kathleen "Kate" Bullock, RN	356
17-9	Julie Mitchell, RN, Glen Lundgren, RN, Dee Tschirner Goodwin, RT	366
17-10	Paulina "Polly" Hansplant, RN, and MedFlight crew	368

Chapter 18
18-3	Michael R. Dick, MD	408
18-4	Ann M. Haynes, MD	410
18-5	Kurt Neltner, MD	411
18-6	Sondra "Soni" Shellman, MD	412
18-7	Mark L. DeBard, MD	414
18-8	Melissa Fenner, MD	416
18-9	Brandy (Helminiak) Zimmer, MD	417
18-11	Daralee R. Hughes, MD	420
18-12	Emily B. Kauffman, DO, MPH	421
18-13	Andrew Gathof, MD	423

Chapter 19
19-3	Sharon Pfeil	440
19-4	David Way, MEd	441
19-7	Jennifer Yee, DO	447

Chapter 20
20-5	Geremiha G. Emerson, MD	462
20-6	Simiao Li-Sauerwine, MD	463

Chapter 21
21-2	Robert D. Cooper, MD, MPH, MBA	492
21-3	Phillip A. Dixon, MD, MPH, MBA	493
21-4	Eric J. Cortez, MD	495
21-5	William A. "Bill" Krebs, DO	496
21-6	Matthew T. Ball, MD	497
21-7	Travis P. Sharkey, MD, PhD	498
21-8	Nicole T. McAllister, DO, MA	500
21-9	Chelsea Kadish, MD, MS	501
21-10	Michael G. Purcell, MD	502
21-11	Christopher San Miguel, MD	504
21-12	Krystin N. Miller, MD	505
21-13	Kimberly Bambach, MD	506
21-14	Andrew Kendle, MD	506
21-15	Marcel J. Casavant, MD	507
21-16	Hannah L. Hays, MD	508
21-17	Richard Limperos, MD	511
21-18	Erika C. Kube, MD	513
21-19	Lydia M. Sahlani, ND	514
21-20	Amar Vira, MD	515
21-21	Michael Prats, MD	516
21-22	Lauren Branditz, MD	517
21-23	Carolyn Martinez, MD	518
21-24	Hilary Davenport Stroud, DO	519
21-25	Hiten Patel, MD	520

Chapter 22
22-1	Creagh T. Boulger, MD	535

Chapter 23
23-1	Henry Young, MD	554
23-2	Jennah A. Morgan, MD	555
23-3	Jennifer Mitzman, MD	557
23-4	Maegan Reynolds, MD	557
23-5	Irene Mynatt, DO	559

Chapter 24
24-1	Alan Blumberg	566
24-2	Thomas Clanton, PhD	568
24-3	Paul Klawitter, MD, PhD	569
24-4	Khan Lab	572
24-5	Garikipati Lab	573
24-6	Lauren Southerland, MD	577

24-7	Katherine "Katie" Hunold Buck, MD	580
24-8	Jason Bishof, MD	581

Chapter 26

26-1	Carol L. Clinton, MD	608
26-3	Bruce K. Neely, MD	613
26-4	David R. Jones, MD	615
26-5	James Chan, MD, PhD	620

Chapter 28

28-1	Mark J. Conroy, MD	644